PHARMACOLOGICAL TREATMENT OF ALZHEIMER'S DISEASE

PHARMACOLOGICAL TREATMENT OF ALZHEIMER'S DISEASE

MOLECULAR AND NEUROBIOLOGICAL FOUNDATIONS

Edited by

Jorge D. Brioni and Michael W. Decker

Abbott Laboratories
Abbott Park, Illinois

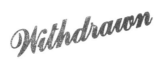

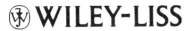

ⓌWILEY-LISS

A JOHN WILEY & SONS, INC., PUBLICATION

New York • Chichester • Brisbane • Toronto • Singapore • Weinheim

Address All Inquiries to the Publisher
Wiley-Liss, Inc., 605 Third Avenue, New York, NY 10158-0012

Copyright © 1997 Wiley-Liss, Inc.

Printed in the United States of America

While the authors, editors, and publisher believe that drug selection and dosage and the specifications and usage of equipment and devices, as set forth in this, are in accord with current recommendations and practice at the time of publication, they accept no legal responsibility for any errors or omissions, and make no warranty, express or implied, with respect to material contained herein. In view of ongoing research, equipment modifications, changes in governmental regulations and the constant flow of information relating to drug therapy, drug reactions and the use of equipment and devices, the reader is urged to review and evaluate the information provided in the package insert or instructions for each drug, piece of equipment or device for, among other things, any changes in the instructions or indications of dosage or usage and for added warnings and precautions.

Library of Congress Cataloging-in-Publication Data

Pharmacological treatment of Alzheimer's disease : molecular and
  neurobiological foundations / Jorge D. Brioni, Michael W. Decker, editors.
        p.   cm.
     Includes index.
     ISBN 0-471-16758-4 (cloth : alk. paper)
     1. Alzheimer's disease—Chemotherapy.   2. Alzheimer's disease—
  Molecular aspects.   3. Cognition—Physiological aspects.
   I. Brioni, Jorge D., 1956–   . II Decker, Michael W., 1951–
     [DNLM: 1. Alzheimer's Disease—drug therapy.   2. Alzheimer's
  Disease—genetics.   3. Cognition—physiology.   WT 155 P536 1997]
RC523.P44   1997
616.8′ 31061—dc20
DNLM/DLC
for Library of Congress   96-30137
                                                                           CIP

The text of this book is printed on acid-free paper.

10   9   8   7   6   5   4   3   2   1

CONTENTS

▬▬▬ PREFACE

During the past several years, we have witnessed enormous growth in scientific information regarding Alzheimer's disease (AD). To this point, however, little of this information has been translated into effective treatments. In this volume, we have assembled chapters focused on potential treatments for this devastating disease, attempting to bring together basic science and industrial perspectives. In so doing, we hope to foster improved communication and understanding between the several areas of science at academic, clinical, and industrial levels and ultimately enhance our ability to find a treatment for patients suffering from AD.

Alzheimer's disease must be studied on multiple levels. A multidisciplinary approach will be the key to success. This is a critical point, and this book takes this tack, as only with a multidisciplinary understanding of AD will we be successful. Genetics, molecular and cellular biology, and biochemistry provide insights into potential causes of and treatments for AD. Basic science aimed at unraveling the neurobiological mechanisms of cognitive function will help in understanding how AD might disrupt cognitive function and, more importantly, what treatments might be helpful in ameliorating the cognitive deficits produced by this disease. The therapeutic approaches suggested by these basic science findings will yield new treatments only after extensive drug discovery and development efforts that are likely to take place within an industrial framework. Thus, diverse approaches will be required to find treatments for this uniquely human disease.

In the present book we have gathered contributions from specialists in each of these fields to cover specific topics of critical importance and have organized them into three parts: Neurobiology of Cognition, Molecular Aspects of Alzheimer's Disease, and Alzheimer's Drug Discovery and Development.

Given the prominence of the effects of AD on cognition, we have devoted a section of this book to basic research on the neurobiology of cognitive function. This section surveys relevant information on the way the brain encodes and stores information. Much of the work reviewed in this section has been conducted with rodents and nonhuman primates, but its relevance to understanding cognitive deficits in AD is made clear by the parallels between human and animal studies drawn by Kesner and Ragozzino in Chapter 1. Neurochemical systems important in modulating rodent memory are discussed extensively in Chapter 2 by Guzowski and McGaugh. An understanding of this content will be important in developing symptomatic treatments for the cognitive deficits associated with AD, and further consideration of this topic from the perspective of nonhuman primate studies and their potential relevance to work in humans is found in Chapter 3 by Arnsten and van Dyck. The cholinergic hypothesis, which has been central in attempts to understand and treat AD in the last 20 years, is the topic of two chapters in this section. Chapters 4 by Baxter and Gallagher and Chapter 5 by Sarter and Bruno make the case that the idea that cholinergic dysfunction underlies the memory deficits in AD is no longer tenable. Instead, they propose that cholinergic dysfunction in AD produces marked deficits in attentional processes. Finally, this section concludes with Chapter 6 by Salmon, surveying the neuropsychological findings in Alzheimer's patients. This information, when combined with our knowledge of brain structures involved in cognitive processes, provides hypotheses regarding the relative importance of pathological changes observed in AD for producing cognitive deficits. Identification of the types of memory deficits present in AD patients (declarative, procedural, attentional, etc.) is also important in validating animal models of AD, which goes back to a major theme of Chapter 1.

The topic of brain pathology observed in AD and the relevance of these changes for producing cognitive deficits is the focus of Chapter 7 by Solodkin and Van Hoesen, which provides a transition between the behavioral studies of the first section and the mechanisms of AD explored in the second section. This section emphasizes investigations of possible etiological factors. To begin this analysis, in Chapter 8 Grewal and Finch discuss a major etiological question: is Alzheimer's just an acceleration of normal aging or is it a separate condition? The answer to this question will have important public health and treatment implications. In Chapter 9 by Clark and Goate, the genetics of AD are reviewed. Genetic studies can reveal the location of mutations associated with the disease, and molecular biology can be used to identify the candidate mechanisms involved in producing the disease. The potential role of the classical histopathological features of the disease, neurofibrillary tangles and senile plaques, are discussed in separate chapters. In Chapter 10 Clark, Trojanowski, and Lee review evidence that neurofibrillary tangles are an important causal factor in AD and reflect on some implications for treatment. Interestingly, no animal models overexpressing tangles have been reported yet. In Chapter 11 Mattson, Bruce, Mark, and Blanc provide an extensive review of potential mechanisms of the toxicity of β-amyloid, the primary component of senile plaques. The recent discovery that the apolipoprotein E genotype may be a risk factor for AD is the topic of Chapter 12 by Falduto and LaDu. The authors describe the relationship between apolipoprotein E and AD and discuss potential mechanisms involved. In Chapter 13 Borchelt, Martin, Hsiao, Gearhart, Lamb, Sisodia, and Price review novel animal models of AD, particularly animal models based on recent findings in the molecular biology of the disease. Transgenic models are being developed exclusively in mice for practical reasons, but we will need to develop transgenic models in rats or other higher mammals in the near future.

The lack of good animal models for AD has hampered efforts both to understand disease processes and to test potential treatments. Conversely, the lack of effective treatments precludes the pharmacological validation of the animal models under consideration. By analogy to other central nervous system (CNS) disorders such as epilepsy or anxiety, we are at a stage equivalent to the prebarbiturate or prebenzodiazepine era with respect to AD. Thus, we should not be hypercritical of the small advances or limited efficacy of present treatments. As was true for other CNS disorders, even incremental progress in therapeutics will likely accelerate future advances.

The need for animal models to test potential therapeutics provides transition from basic science approaches to AD to treatments, the topic of the last section of the book. In this last section, a variety of issues important in developing treatments are discussed. Chapter 14 by Whitehouse opens the section with a discussion of AD as a public health concern and regulatory issues related to developing a drug for treating AD. Improved ability to diagnose AD and to develop surrogate markers for the disease are clearly important in conducting clinical trials, and these issues are the subject of Chapter 15 by Seubert, Galasko, and Boss on biochemical markers. Clinical trials for AD are complex, and proper design is critical for providing appropriate information on compounds in clinical development. Cutler and Sramek tackle this important issue in Chapter 16 on clinical trials and assessment.

The final seven chapters of this section deal with specific treatments. Since cholinergic-based treatments have been prominent in efforts to develop therapeutics for AD, this approach is the topic of three separate chapters. Gracon and Berghoff (Chapter 17) describe the clinical results with tacrine, a cholinesterase inhibitor that was the first compound approved in the United States for the treatment of AD. Jaen and Schwarz (Chapter 18) review the development of muscarinic cholinergic agonists for AD, and our chapter (Chapter 19) describes efforts to develop compounds acting as nicotinic cholinergic receptors. Pelleymounter and Williams (Chapter 20) provide information on neurotrophins and discuss the therapeutic potential of this approach. The next two chapters are devoted to classes of compounds approved for other therapeutic targets but that may also be useful in treating AD. Rogers (Chapter 21) focuses on issues related to the role of neuroinflammation in AD and the therapeutic potential of anti-inflammatory agents. Simpkins, Green, and Gridley (Chapter 22) discuss the possible therapeutic role of estrogens and suggest some potential mechanisms underlying these apparent beneficial effects. Finally, this section concludes with Chapter 23 by Williams and Arneric that provides an overview and an update on the status of a variety of treatment approaches currently under development in industry.

We are indebted to our colleagues who agreed to participate in this endeavor and allowed us to cover so many areas of importance in understanding AD. We are deeply grateful to Dr. James McGaugh and Dr. Michela Gallagher for all the lessons learned from them, to Dr. Michael Williams for guidance in the development of our original book proposal, and to Dr. Williams and to Dr. Stephen Arneric for their support. We would also like to acknowledge the help of the staff at Wiley for their excellent editorial work.

This book is dedicated to our wives, Elsa Daprati-Brioni and Elisa Trombetta Decker, as they have shared with us this long journey from graduate school, years full of dreams and sacrifice, doubts and accomplishments, in essence and in retrospect, a gratifying adventure.

JORGE D. BRIONI
MICHAEL W. DECKER

■■■■■■■ CONTRIBUTORS

Stephen P. Arneric, Neuroscience Discovery, Pharmaceutical Products Division, Abbott Laboratories, Abbott Park, Illinois 60064-3500

Amy F. T. Arnsten, Section of Neurobiology, Yale Medical School, New Haven, Connecticut 06510-8001

Mark G. Baxter, Curriculum in Neurobiology, University of North Carolina, Chapel Hill, North Carolina 27599

William G. Berghoff, Parke-Davis Pharmaceutical Research, Division of Warner-Lambert Company, Ann Arbor, Michigan 48105

Emmanuelle M. Blanc, Sanders-Brown Research Center on Aging and Department of Anatomy & Neurobiology, University of Kentucky, Lexington, Kentucky 40536

David R. Borchelt, Departments of Pathology and Neuropathology Laboratory, The Johns Hopkins University School of Medicine, Baltimore, Maryland 21205

Michael A. Boss, Athena Diagnostics, Inc., Four Biotech Park, 377 Plantation Street, Worcester, Massachusetts 01605

Jorge D. Brioni, Neuroscience Discovery, Abbott Laboratories, Abbott Park, Illinois 60064-3500

Annadora J. Bruce, Sanders-Brown Research Center on Aging and Department of Anatomy & Neurobiology, University of Kentucky, Lexington, Kentucky 40536

John P. Bruno, Department of Psychology and Neuroscience Program, Ohio State University, Columbus, Ohio 43210

Christopher M. Clark, Department of Neurology, School of Medicine, University of Pennsylvania, Philadelphia, Pennsylvania 19104

Robert F. Clark, Department of Psychiatry, Washington University School of Medicine, St. Louis, Missouri 63110

Neal R. Cutler, California Clinical Trials, Beverly Hills, California 90211

Michael W. Decker, Neuroscience Discovery, Abbott Laboratories, Abbott Park, Illinois 60064-3500

Michael T. Falduto, Immunoscience Discovery, Pharmaceutical Products Division, Abbott Laboratories, Abbott Park, Illinois 60064

Caleb E. Finch, Department of Neurology, School of Medicine, and Division of Neurogerontology, Andrus Gerontology Center, University of Southern California, Los Angeles, California 90089-0191

Katsutoshi Furukawa, Sanders-Brown Research Center on Aging and Department of Anatomy & Neurobiology, University of Kentucky, 40536

Douglas Galasko, Department of Neurosciences, University of California at San Diego and Veteran's Affairs Medical Center, San Diego, California 92161

Michela Gallagher, Department of Psychology, University of North Carolina, Chapel Hill, North Carolina 27599

John D. Gearhart, Departments of Obstetrics & Gynecology and the Division of Reproductive & Developmental Biology, The Johns Hopkins University School of Medicine, Baltimore, Maryland 21205

Alison M. Goate, Department of Psychiatry, Washington University School of Medicine, St. Louis, Missouri 63110

Stephen I. Gracon, Parke-Davis Pharmaceutical Research, Division of Warner-Lambert Company, Ann Arbor, Michigan 48105

Pattie S. Green, Department of Pharmacodynamics and the Center for the Neurobiology of Aging, University of Florida, Gainesville, Florida 32610

Raji P. Grewal, Department of Neurology, School of Medicine, and Division of Neurogerontology, Andrus Gerontology Center, University of Southern California, Los Angeles, California 90089-0191

Kelly E. Gridley, Department of Pharmacodynamics and the Center for the Neurobiology of Aging, University of Florida, Gainesville, Florida 32610

John F. Guzowski, Center for the Neurobiology of Learning and Memory, University of California, Irvine, California 92717-3800

Anne Marie Himmelheber, Department of Psychology and Neuroscience Program, Ohio State University, Columbus, Ohio 43210

Karen K. Hsiao, Department of Neurology, University of Minnesota Medical School, Minneapolis, Minnesota 55455

Juan C. Jaen, Parke-Davis Pharmaceutical Research, Division of Warner-Lambert Company, Ann Arbor, Michigan 48105

Raymond P. Kesner, Department of Psychology, University of Utah, Salt Lake City, Utah 84112

Mary Jo LaDu, Department of Pathology, University of Chicago, Chicago, Illinois 60637

Bruce T. Lamb, Departments of Obstetrics & Gynecology and the Division of Reproductive & Developmental Biology, The Johns Hopkins University School of Medicine, Baltimore, Maryland 21205

Virginia M.-Y. Lee, Department of Pathology and Laboratory Medicine, School of Medicine, University of Pennsylvania, Philadelphia, Pennsylvania 19104

Robert J. Mark, Sanders-Brown Research Center on Aging and Department of Anatomy & Neurobiology, University of Kentucky, Lexington, Kentucky 40536

Lee J. Martin, Departments of Pathology and Neuroscience and the Neuropathology Laboratory, The Johns Hopkins University School of Medicine, Baltimore, Maryland 21205

Mark P. Mattson, Sanders-Brown Research Center on Aging and Department of Anatomy & Neurobiology, University of Kentucky, Lexington, Kentucky 40536

James L. McGaugh, Departments of Psychology and Pharmacology, University of California, Irvine, California 92717-3800

Mary Ann Pelleymounter, Department of Neurobiology, Amgen Inc., 1840 DeHavilland Drive, Thousand Oaks, California 91320

Donald L. Price, Departments of Pathology, Neuroscience, Neurology, and the Neuropathology Laboratory, The Johns Hopkins University School of Medicine, Baltimore, Maryland 21205

Michael E. Ragozzino, Department of Psychology, University of Utah, Salt Lake City, Utah 84112

Joseph Rogers, Sun Health Research Institute, 10515 West Santa Fe Drive, Sun City, Arizona 85372

David P. Salmon, Department of Neurosciences, School of Medicine, University of California, San Diego, La Jolla, California 92093-0948

Martin Sarter, Department of Psychology and Neuroscience Program, Ohio State University, Columbus, Ohio 43210

Roy D. Schwarz, Parke-Davis Pharmaceutical Research, Division of Warner-Lambert Company, Ann Arbor, Michigan 48105

Peter Seubert, Athena Neurosciences, Inc., 800 Gateway Boulevard, South San Francisco, California 94080

James W. Simpkins, Department of Pharmacodynamics and the Center for the Neurobiology of Aging, University of Florida, Gainesville, Florida 32610

Sangram S. Sisodia, Departments of Pathology, Neuroscience, and the Neuropathology Laboratory, The Johns Hopkins University School of Medicine, Baltimore, Maryland 21205

Ana Solodkin, Departments of Anatomy and Neurology, University of Iowa, Iowa City, Iowa 52242

John J. Sramek, California Clinical Trials, Beverly Hills, California 90211

John Q. Trojanowski, Department of Pathology and Laboratory Medicine, School of Medicine, University of Pennsylvania, Philadelphia, Pennsylvania 19104

Christopher H. van Dyck, Department of Psychiatry, Yale Medical School, New Haven, Connecticut 06510-8001

Gary W. Van Hoesen, Departments of Anatomy and Neurology, University of Iowa, Iowa City, Iowa 52242

Peter J. Whitehouse, University Hospitals of Cleveland, Case Western Reserve University, Cleveland, Ohio 44120

Lawrence R. Williams, Department of Neurobiology, Amgen Inc., 1840 Dehavilland Drive, Thousand Oaks, California 91320

Michael Williams, Neuroscience Discovery, Pharmaceutical Products Division, Abbott Laboratories, Abbott Park, Illinois 60064-3500

PHARMACOLOGICAL TREATMENT OF ALZHEIMER'S DISEASE

PART I

NEUROBIOLOGY OF COGNITION

CHAPTER 1

Structure and Dynamics of Multiple Memory Systems in Alzheimer's Disease

RAYMOND P. KESNER and MICHAEL E. RAGOZZINO

Department of Psychology, University of Utah, Salt Lake City, Utah 84112

INTRODUCTION

Given that one of the cardinal features of dementia of the Alzheimer's type (DAT) is a severe memory loss accompanied by the presence of high density of senile plaques and neurofibrillary tangles in a large number of neocortical and limbic brain structures, it is imperative to develop a neurobiological model of memory to provide a theoretical framework within which one can assess potential memory dysfunctions and their neural substrates in both animals and humans. Currently, the most established models of memory can be characterized as dual memory models with an emphasis on the hippocampus for one component of the model and a composite of other brain structures as the other component. For example, Squire (1994) has proposed that memory can be divided into a hippocampal-dependent declarative memory, which provides for conscious recollection of facts and events, and a nonhippocampal-dependent nondeclarative memory, which provides for memory without conscious access for skills, habits, priming, simple classical conditioning, and nonassociative learning. Others have used different terms to reflect the same type of distinction, including a hippocampal-dependent explicit memory versus a nonhippocampal-dependent implicit memory (Schacter, 1987), and a hippocampal-dependent declarative memory based on the representation of relationships among stimuli versus a nonhippocampal-dependent procedural memory based on the representation of a single stimulus or configuration of stimuli (Cohen and Eichenbaum, 1993). A different dual memory system (Olton, 1983) proposes

Pharmacological Treatment of Alzheimer's Disease: Molecular and Neurobiological Foundations,
Edited by Brioni and Decker
ISBN 0-471-16758-4 © 1997 Wiley-Liss, Inc.

that memory can be divided into a hippocampal-dependent working memory defined as memory for the specific, personal, and temporal context of a situation and a nonhippocampal-dependent reference memory defined as memory for rules and procedures (general knowledge) of specific situations. Different terms have been used to reflect the same distinction, including episodic versus semantic memory (Tulving, 1983).

However, memory is more complex and involves many neural systems in addition to the hippocampus. To remedy this situation, Kesner and DiMattia (1987) proposed a neurobiology of multiple attributes or forms of memory model. Based on extensive research aimed at testing the attribute model, the model has been refined and updated. In this chapter we will first present an updated version of the attribute model; then we will clarify how the assumptions of the model have utility in describing the neural bases of mnemonic dysfunction in various stages of DAT. Finally, we will analyze and evaluate one extant animal model of DAT within the context of the attribute model.

NEUROBIOLOGY OF AN ATTRIBUTE MODEL

In this comprehensive model, it is assumed that any specific memory is organized into a data-based memory system and a knowledge-based memory system. The data-based memory system is biased in providing for temporary representations of incoming data concerning the present, with an emphasis upon facts, data, and events that are usually personal or egocentric and that occur within specific external and internal contexts. The emphasis is upon bottom–up processing. During initial learning great emphasis is placed on the data-based memory system, which will continue to be of importance even after initial learning in situations where unique or novel trial information needs to be remembered. The data-based memory system is composed of different independently operating forms or attributes of memory. Even though there could be many attributes, the most important attributes include *space, time, response, sensory-perception,* and *affect.* In humans a *language* attribute is also added.

A spatial attribute within this framework involves memory representations of places or relationships between places, which are usually independent of the subjects's own body schema. It is exemplified by the ability to encode and remember spatial maps and to localize stimuli in external space. Memory representations of the spatial attribute can be further subdivided into specific spatial features including allocentric spatial distance, egocentric spatial distance, allocentric direction, egocentric direction, and spatial location.

A temporal attribute within this framework involves memory representations of the duration of a stimulus, the succession or temporal order of temporally separated events or stimuli, and from a time perspective the memory representation of the past.

A response attribute within this framework involves memory representations based on feedback from motor responses (often based on kinesthetic and vestibular cues) that occur in specific situations as well as memory representations of stimulus–response associations.

A sensory-perceptual attribute within this framework involves memory representations of a set of sensory stimuli that are organized in the form of cues as part of a specific experience. Each sensory modality (olfaction, auditory, vision, somatosensory, and taste) has its own memory representations and can be considered to be part of the sensory-perceptual attribute component of memory.

An affect attribute within this framework involves memory representations of reward value, positive or negative emotional experiences, and the associations between stimuli and rewards.

A language attribute within this framework involves memory representations of phonological, lexical, and morphological information.

The organization of these attributes within the data-based memory system can take many forms and are probably organized hierarchically and in parallel. Some interactions between attributes are important and can aid in identifying specific neural regions that might subserve a critical interaction. For example, the interaction between spatial and temporal attributes can provide for the external context of a situation, which is important in defining when and where critical events occurred. The interaction between sensory-perceptual attributes and the spatial attribute can provide for the memory representation of a spatial cognitive map.

Within the data-based memory system there are operational characteristics associated with each attribute, which include a number of processes: (a) selective attention, selective filtering, or attenuation of interference associated with temporary memory representations of new information; (b) short-term memory of working memory of new information; (c) consolidation or elaborative rehearsal of new information; and (d) retrieval of new information based on flexibility and action.

Based on a series of experiments, it can be shown that within the data-based memory system different neural structures and circuits mediate different forms or attributes of memory. The most extensive data set is based on the use of paradigms that measure the short-term or working-memory process, such as matching or nonmatching to sample, delayed conditional discrimination, or continuous recognition memory of single or lists of items.

Spatial Attribute

With respect to spatial attribute information, it can be shown that with the use of the above-mentioned paradigms to measure short-term memory for spatial information there are severe impairments for rats, monkeys, and humans with right hippocampal damage or bilateral hippocampal damage (Kesner, 1990; Olton, 1983, 1986; Parkinson et al., 1988; Smith and Milner, 1981; Chiba et al., submitted; Hopkins et al., 1995a).

With respect to specific spatial features, such as allocentric spatial distance, egocentric spatial distance, and spatial location, it has been shown in both rats and humans with bilateral hippocampal damage that there are severe deficits in short-term memory of these spatial features (Long and Kesner, 1994, in press;

Kesner and Hopkins, unpublished). These data are consistent with the recording of place cells (cells that increase their firing rate when an animal is located in a specific place) within the hippocampus of rats and monkeys (Kubie and Ranck, 1983; McNaughton et al., 1983; O'Keefe, 1983; O'Keefe and Speakman, 1987; Rolls et al., 1989). Short-term memory for the spatial direction feature has not yet been investigated, but based on recording data indicating that head direction cells (cells that increase their firing rate as a function of the animal's head direction in the horizontal plane, independent of the animal's behavior, location, or trunk position) are not found in the hippocampus, it is possible that the hippocampus does not represent spatial head direction information. The hippocampus is not the only neural region that mediates short-term memory for spatial information. Using a continuous spatial short-term recognition task, it has been shown that lesions of the dorsal lateral thalamus, pre- and parasubiculum, medial entorhinal cortex, and pre- and infralimbic cortex produce profound deficits similar to what has been described for hippocampal lesions, suggesting that other neural regions contribute to the spatial attribute within the data-based memory system (Kesner, unpublished). It should be noted that place cells have also been recorded from medial entorhinal cortex (Quirk et al., 1992) and parasubiculum (Taube, 1995) and that head direction cells have been recorded from the lateral dorsal nucleus of the thalamus (Mizumori and Williams, 1993). Thus, the hippocampus represents within short-term memory some if not all the spatial features associated with the spatial attribute.

The hippocampus also plays a role in the acquisition or learning of new spatial information requiring the consolidation of spatial attributes. This is readily observable in the acquisition of spatial navigation tasks in a water maze, dry-land version of the water maze, and inhibitory avoidance tasks requiring an association of a painful stimulus with a specific spatial location, in that rats with hippocampal lesions are markedly impaired in these tasks (O'Keefe and Nadel, 1978; Morris et al., 1982; Kesner et al., 1991). Whether the hippocampus promotes the transfer of spatial information to the knowledge-based system or whether the hippocampus promotes the consolidation of information already processed in the knowledge-based system still needs to be resolved.

Based on ample evidence that almost all sensory information is processed by hippocampal neurons, perhaps to provide for sensory markers for space, and that the hippocampus mediates spatial information, it is likely that one of the main process functions of the hippocampus is to encode the spatial order of events. This would ensure that new highly processed sensory information is organized within the hippocampus and enhances the possibility of remembering and temporarily storing one place as separate from another place (spatial order). It is assumed that this is accomplished via selective attention or selective filtering of event information in order to reduce spatial interference. This process is akin to the idea that the hippocampus is involved in representation differentiation (Myers et al., 1995) and indirectly in the utilization of relationships (Cohen and Eichenbaum, 1993).

To assess this function rats are trained in a *spatial* order task. In this task rats are required to remember a spatial location dependent on the distance between the study phase object and an object used as a foil. More specifically, during the study phase an object that covers a baited food well was randomly positioned in one of six possible spatial locations on a cheese board. Rats exited a start box and displaced the object in order to receive a food award and were then returned to the start box. In the ensuing test phase rats were allowed to choose between two objects that were identical to the study phase object. One object was baited and positioned in the previous study phase location (correct choice), the other (foil) was unbaited and placed in a different location (incorrect choice). Five distances (min. = 15 cm, max. = 105 cm) were randomly used to separate the foil from the correct object. Following the establishment of a criterion of 75% correct averaged across all separation distances, rats were given either large (dorsal and ventral) hippocampal or cortical control lesions dorsal to the dorsal hippocampus. Following recovery from surgery the rats were retested. The results indicated that whereas control rats matched their presurgery performance for all spatial distances, hippocampal-lesioned rats displayed impairments for short (15–37.5 cm) and medium (60 cm) spatial separations, but performed as well as controls when the spatial separation was long (82.5–105 cm). It can be shown that the ability to remember the long distances was not based on an egocentric response strategy, because if the study phase was presented on one side of the cheese board and the test originated on the opposite side, the hippocampal-lesioned rats still performed the long distances without difficulty. It is clear that in this task it is necessary to separate one spatial location from another spatial location. Hippocampal-lesioned rats cannot separate these spatial locations very well, so that they can perform the task only when the spatial locations are far apart. It is important to note that these same hippocampal-lesioned rats have no difficulty in discriminating even the shortest distances, implying that the difficulty in separating places is based on the memory requirement of the task. Similar deficits have been observed for new geographical information in patients with hippocampal damage due to an hypoxic episode (Hopkins and Kesner, 1993).

Does spatial interference play a role in the acquisition (consolidation) of a variety of hippocampal-dependent tasks? A few examples will suffice. Because rats are started in different locations in the standard water maze task, there is a great potential for spatial interference. Thus, the observation that hippocampal-lesioned rats are impaired in learning and subsequent consolidation of important spatial information in this task could be due to enhanced spatial interference. Support for this idea comes from the observation of Eichenbaum et al. (1990) who demonstrated that when fimbria-fornix-lesioned rats are trained on the water maze task from only a single starting position (less spatial interference), there are hardly any learning deficits, whereas training from many different starting points resulted in learning difficulties. In a somewhat similar study it was shown that total hippocampal-lesioned rats learned or consolidated rather readily that only one spatial location was correct on an eight-arm maze (Hunt et al., 1994). In a different study, McDonald and White (1995) used a place preference procedure in an eight-arm maze. In this procedure food is placed at the end of one arm and no food is placed at the end of another arm. In a subsequent preference test normal rats prefer the arm that contained the food. In this study fornix-lesioned rats acquired the place preference task as quickly as controls if the arm locations were opposite each other; but the fornix-lesioned rats were markedly impaired if the locations were adjacent to each other. Clearly, it is likely that there would be greater spatial interference when the spatial locations are adjacent to each other rather than far apart. Thus, spatial interference can play a role in the acquisition of new spatial information.

If short-term memory and consolidation processes associated with mnemonic processing of spatial information are both subserved by the hippocampus, is it possible to dissociate the two? The answer to the question is positive. It has been shown that phencyclidine [an N-methyl-*d*-aspartate (NMDA) antagonist] injections into the dentate gyrus of the hippocampus at dose levels to block electrical stimulation of the medial entorhinal cortex-induced long-term potentiation (LTP) disrupts consolidation of new learning in a dry-land version of the water maze, but the same dose of phencyclidine has only a mild effect on a short-term memory task for spatial location information in an eight-arm maze (Kesner and Dakis, 1995). In contrast, naloxone (an opiate antagonist) injections into the dentate gyrus of the hippocampus at dose levels to block electrical stimulation of the lateral entorhinal cortex-induced LTP disrupts completely performance within the short-term memory task, but has no effect on consolidation of new learning in the dry-land version of the water maze spatial navigation task (Dakis et al., 1992). These results suggest that short-term memory and consolidation processes can operate independent of each other and that perhaps each process is mediated by a different form of LTP.

Temporal Attribute

With respect to temporal attribute information, it can be shown that with the use of the above-mentioned paradigms to measure short-term memory there are severe impairments for duration information for rats and humans with bilateral hippocampal damage (Jackson-Smith et al., 1994; Hopkins and Kesner, 1994), suggesting that the hippocampus plays an important role in short-term memory representation of duration of exposure of a stimulus as an important feature of temporal attribute information.

Based on ample evidence that almost all sensory information is processed by hippocampal neurons, perhaps to provide for sensory markers for time as well as space, and that the hippocampus mediates temporal information, it is likely that one of the main process functions of the hippocampus is to encode the temporal order of events. This would ensure that new highly processed sensory information is organized within the hippocampus and enhances the possibility of remembering and temporarily storing one event as separate from another event in time.

In the *temporal* order task, rats are required to remember an event (e.g., spatial location, visual object) dependent on the temporal order of occurrence of events. More specifically, on an eight-arm maze during the study phase of each trial, rats were allowed to visit each of eight arms once in an order that is randomly selected for that trial. The test phase required the rats to choose which of two arms occurred earlier in the sequence of arms visited during the study phase. The arms selected as test arms varied according to temporal lag or distance (0–6) or the number of arms that occurred between the two test arms in the study phase. After the rats reached a criterion of 75% or better performance on all the distances but zero, the rats received large (dorsal and ventral), small (dorsal) hippocampus, cortical control lesions dorsal to the dorsal hippocampus or medial prefrontal cortex (anterior cingulate and medial precentral cortex) lesions. Following recovery from surgery, the rats were retested. The results are shown in Figure 1 and indicate that for both pre- and postsurgery tests, the control rats performed at chance at a temporal distance of zero, but their performance was excellent for the remaining temporal distances. In contrast, on postsurgery tests dorsal hippocampal lesions disrupted performance for temporal distances of 0 and 2 but did not affect performance for the longest temporal distances of 4 and 6. Furthermore, on postsurgery tests large (dorsal plus ventral) hippocampal or medial prefrontal cortex lesions produced a marked deficit for all temporal distances with a slight improvement for the longest temporal distance. In this task it is necessary to separate one event from another. Hippocampal-lesioned rats cannot separate events across time because of an inability to inhibit interference that is likely to accompany sequential occurring events. The resultant increase in temporal interference impairs the rat's ability to remember the order of specific events. It appears that the larger the damage to the hippocampus, the greater the temporal interference. It is possible to reduce the presence of temporal interference by presenting the rats with a constant sequence of eight spatial locations followed by temporal distance tests and at the same time reduce the importance of the involvement of the data-based memory system and accentuating the importance of the knowledge-based memory system. The results are shown in Figure 2 and indicate that large or small hippocampal lesions following training did not result in any significant deficits. However, lesions of the medial prefrontal cortex produced a significant deficit (Chiba et al., 1994, 1992).

The events do not have to be based on only spatial location information. Similar temporal distance deficits have been observed with lists of visual objects in rats and lists of spatial locations and words in patients with hippocampal damage due to an hypoxic episode or temporal lobe resection as well as early and middle DAT patients (Hopkins et al., 1995b; Chiba et al., submitted).

These data support the idea that the hippocampus might function to reduce temporal interference between events. Similarly, the temporal interference effect can be observed during the learning of new information. In one study it was shown that hippocampal-lesioned rats do not have a problem in learning (consolidating) a single object-pair discrimination, but have difficulty in learning eight-pair concurrent object discriminations (Shapiro and Olton, 1994). In contrast to the one-pair discrimination, there is a heightened temporal interference in learning eight pairs simultaneously. This increased temporal interference could account for the observed impairment in hippocampal-lesioned rats. Thus, it is postulated that hypoxic and temporal-lobe-resected patients and DAT patients perform more poorly, especially at short distances, because of increased interference in the temporal resolution of events.

In summary, the hippocampus appears to be important in processing spatial and

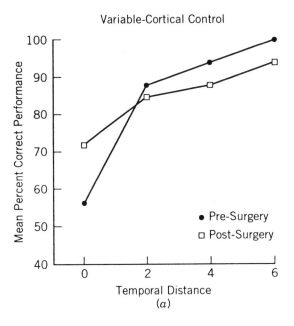

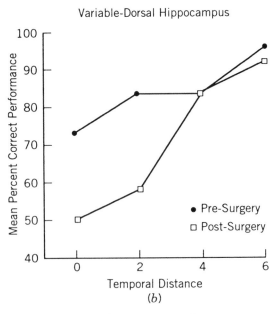

FIGURE 1. Mean percent correct performance pre- and postsurgery as a function of temporal distance for (a) cortical control, (b) dorsal hippocampus. (c) total (dorsal and ventral) hippocampus, and (d) medial prefrontal cortex lesioned rats within a short-term memory for variable temporal order of a spatial location information task.

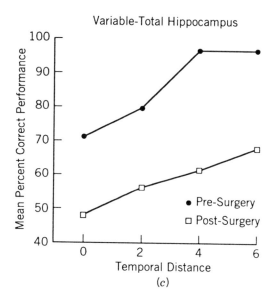

Variable-Total Hippocampus

(c)

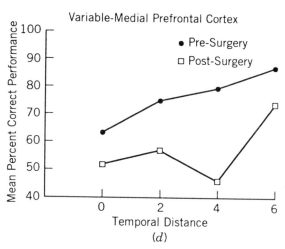

Variable-Medial Prefrontal Cortex

(d)

FIGURE 1. *(Continued)*

temporal information in terms of short-term memory representations and in terms of promoting consolidation of new information. This is accomplished in part by selective attention or filtering of interfering spatial and temporal information and thus accentuating the temporal and spatial resolution of events.

With respect to response, affect, and sensory-perceptual information it has been shown that for rats or humans with hippocampal damage with the use of short-term

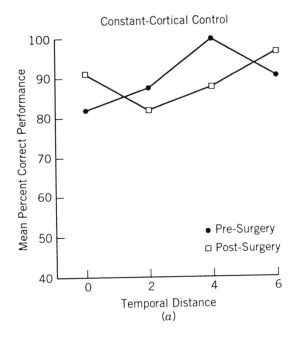

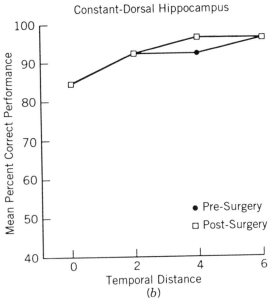

FIGURE 2. Mean percent correct performance pre- and postsurgery as a function of temporal distance for (*a*) cortical control, (*b*) dorsal hippocampus. (*c*) total (dorsal and ventral) hippocampus, and (*d*) medial prefrontal cortex lesioned rats within a short-term memory for a constant temporal order of a spatial location information task.

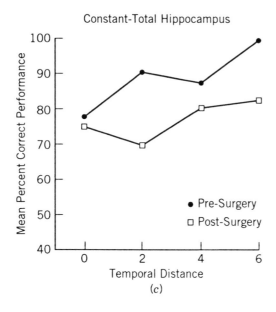

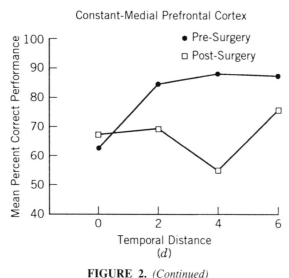

FIGURE 2. *(Continued)*

memory paradigms to measure short-term memory, there are no impairments for remembering (a) a right or left turn response or distance of a motor movement response, (b) magnitude of reward or a liking response based on mere exposure of stimuli, and (c) a visual object or an odor (Kesner et al., 1993; Kesner and Williams, 1995; Chiba et al., 1993; Otto and Eichenbaum, 1992; Leonard and

Milner, 1991), suggesting that the hippocampus does not play a role in short-term memory representations of response, affect, and sensory-perceptual attribute information. Rats and humans with hippocampal lesions are also not impaired in the acquisition (consolidation) of stimulus–response associations or motor skills (mirror reading or pursuit rotor) (McDonald and White, 1993; Squire, 1987).

There are other interference paradigms that emphasize the scaling or discrimination of odors, color, or size of objects. It is assumed, but still needs to be tested, that the hippocampus does not play an important role in these paradigms; rather, one would expect the perirhinal and entorhinal cortex to be of importance. Thus, the role of the hippocampus is specific only to reducing spatial and temporal interference.

With respect to language attribute information, it can be shown that with the use of the above-mentioned paradigms to measure short-term memory there are severe impairments for lists of words for humans with left hippocampal or bilateral hippocampal damage (Kesner et al., 1992), suggesting that the hippocampus plays an important role in short-term memory representation of word information as an important feature of language attribute information.

Response Attribute

With respect to response attribute information, it can be shown that with the use of the above-mentioned paradigms to measure short-term memory for rats with caudate-putamen lesions and humans with caudate-putamen damage due to Huntington's disease, there are profound deficits for a right or left turn response or a list of hand motor movement responses (Cook and Kesner, 1988; Kesner et al., 1993; Duncan-Davis et al., in press), suggesting that the caudate-putamen plays an important role in short-term memory representation for the feedback from a motor response feature of response attribute information. It has also been shown that caudate-putamen lesions in the rat impair acquisition or consolidation of a stimulus (light)–response association within a radial arm maze and that Huntington's patients are impaired in learning motor skills (mirror reading and pursuit-rotor) (McDonald and White, 1993; Heindel et al., 1988; Heindel et al., 1989), suggesting that the caudate-putamen might also be involved in learning stimulus–response associations and motor skill learning requiring the activation of response attribute information. The memory impairments following caudate-putamen lesions are specific to the response attribute, because these same lesions in rats do not impair short-term memory performance or acquisition of spatial location, visual object, or affect attribute information (Kesner et al., 1993; Kesner and Williams, 1995; McDonald and White, 1993).

Affect Attribute

With respect to affect attribute information, it can be shown that with the use of the above-mentioned paradigms to measure short-term memory for rats with amygdala lesions and humans with amygdala damage, there are major deficits for reward value associated with magnitude of reinforcement or for a liking response based on the mere exposure of a novel stimulus (Kesner and Williams, 1995; Chiba et al.,

1993), suggesting that the amygdala plays an important role in short-term memory representation for reward value as a critical feature of the affect attribute. It has also been shown that amygdala lesions in the rat impair acquisition or consolidation of fear conditioning, place or cue preference, and taste aversion (McDonald and White, 1993; Phillips and LeDoux, 1992; Nachman and Ashe, 1974), suggesting that the amygdala might also be involved in learning both positive and negative affect attribute information. The memory impairments following amygdala lesions are specific to the affect attribute, because these same lesions in rats do not impair short-term memory performance or acquisition of spatial location, visual object, response or temporal attribute information (Kesner et al., 1993; McDonald and White, 1993; Olton et al., 1987).

Sensory-Perceptual Attribute

With respect to sensory-perceptual attribute information, we will concentrate on visual object information as an exemplar of memory representation of the sensory-perceptual attribute. It can be shown that with the use of the above-mentioned paradigms to measure short-term memory, there are severe impairments for visual object information for rats and monkeys with extra-striate or perirhinal lesions (Horel et al., 1987; Kesner et al., 1993; Gaffan and Murray, 1992; Mumby and Pinel, 1994; Suzuki et al., 1993), suggesting that the extra-striate and perirhinal cortex play an important role in short-term memory representation for visual object information as an exemplar of the sensory-perceptual attribute. The memory impairments following extra-striate lesions are specific to the visual object component of the sensory-perceptual attribute, because these same lesions in rats do not impair short-term memory performance of spatial location or response attribute information (Kesner et al., 1993).

KNOWLEDGE-BASED MEMORY SYSTEM

The knowledge-based memory system is biased in providing more permanent representations of previously stored information in long-term memory and can be thought of as one's general knowledge of the world. It can operate in the abstract in the absence of incoming data. The emphasis is on top–down processing. The knowledge-based memory system would tend to be of greater importance after a task has been learned given that the situation is invariant and familiar. In most situations, however, one would expect a contribution of both systems with a varying proportion of involvement of one relative to the other.

The knowledge-based memory system is composed of the same set of different independently operating forms or attributes of memory. These attributes include *space, time, response, sensory-perception, and affect*. In humans a *language* attribute is also added. A spatial attribute within this framework involves long-term memory representations of places or relationships between places, which are usually independent of the subject's own body schema. It is exemplified by long-term storage of a spatial cognitive map based on higher-order (global) organization of a number of individual spatial features.

A temporal attribute within this framework involves long-term memory representations of programs for the temporal order of temporally separated events or stimuli, and from a time perspective the memory representation of the future.

A response attribute within this framework involves long-term memory representations of motor programs based on feedback from motor responses (often based on kinesthetic and vestibular cues) that occur in specific situations as well as memory programs for representations of stimulus–response associations and selection of appropriate responses.

A sensory-perceptual attribute within this framework involves long-term memory representations of higher-order organization of a set of sensory stimuli. Each sensory modality (olfaction, auditory, vision, somatosensory, and taste) has its own long-term memory representations and can be considered to be part of the sensory-perceptual attribute component of memory.

An affect attribute within this framework involves long-term memory representations of reward value, positive or negative emotional experiences, and the associations between stimuli and rewards.

A language attribute within this framework involves memory representations of syntax, semantic, and lexicon information.

The organization of these attributes within the knowledge-based memory system can take many forms and are assumed to be organized as a set of cognitive maps or neural nets and their interactions, which are unique for each memory. It is assumed that long-term representations within cognitive maps are more abstract and less dependent on specific features. Some interactions between attributes are important and can aid in identifying specific neural regions that might subserve a critical interaction. For example, the interaction between sensory-perceptual attributes and the spatial attribute can provide for the long-term memory representation of a spatial cognitive map or spatial schemas, the interaction between temporal and spatial attributes can provide for the long-term memory representation of scripts, the interaction between temporal and affect attributes can provide for the long-term memory representation of moods, and the interaction between sensory-perceptual and response attributes can provide for the long-term memory of skills.

Within the knowledge-based memory system there are operational characteristics associated with each attribute, which include a number of processes: (a) selective attention and selective filtering associated with permanent memory representations of familiar information, (b) long-term memory storage, (c) selection of strategies and rules ("executive functions"), and (d) retrieval of familiar information based on flexibility and action.

Based on a series of experiments, it can be shown that within the knowledge-based memory system, different neural structures and circuits mediate different forms or attributes of memory. The most extensive data set is based on the use of paradigms that measure the acquisition of new information, discrimination performance, executive functions, strategies, and rules to perform in a variety of tasks including skills and the operation of a variety of long-term memory programs.

Spatial Attribute

With respect to spatial attribute information it can be shown that rats with parietal cortex lesions display deficits in both the acquisition and retention of spatial navigation tasks that are presumed to measure the operation of a spatial cognitive map (Di-Mattia and Kesner, 1988a; Kesner et al., 1992). Furthermore, rats with parietal lesions are impaired in the acquisition and retention of a spatial location plus object discrimination but show no deficits for only spatial or object discriminations (Long et al., 1996). These rats are also not impaired in discrimination of single spatial features including allocentric and egocentric spatial distance (Long and Kesner, in press; Long and Kesner, 1994). Similar deficits have been reported in humans with parietal cortex damage in that they display topographical amnesia (DeRenzi, 1982), spatial neglect, and deficits in spatial attention (Heilman et al., 1993). Using positron emission tomography (PET) scan and functional magnetic resonance imaging (MRI) data, it can be shown that spatial information results in activation of the parietal cortex (Ungerleider, 1995). The parietal cortex is probably not the only neural region that mediates long-term memory for spatial information. For example, topographical amnesia has also been reported for patients with parahippocampal lesions, and spatial navigation deficits have also been found following retrosplenial and entorhinal cortex lesions (Sutherland and Hoesing, 1993; Habib and Sirigu, 1987). Thus, other neural regions (e.g., parahippocampal cortex, entorhinal cortex, and retrosplenial cortex) may also contribute to the long-term representation of a spatial cognitive map.

Temporal Attribute

With respect to temporal attribute information it can be shown that rats with anterior cingulate cortex lesions and humans with dorsolateral prefrontal cortex lesions display deficits in tasks that measure memory for temporal order (Kesner and Holbrook, 1987; Kesner et al., 1994), suggesting deficits in mediating temporal programs. This temporal order deficit also manifests itself in rats and humans as a deficit in planning, problem solving, thinking logically, and the inability to use prospective coding strategies as well as an inability to shift strategies to solve specific problems (Kesner and Jackson-Smith, 1992; Baddeley, 1986). It has been suggested that these problems reflect the operation of a defective executive control mechanism.

Language Attribute

With respect to language attribute information it can be shown that humans with left parietal cortex damage have word finding difficulties (Caramazza and Berndt, 1978), suggesting that the parietal cortex might mediate the lexicon feature of the language attribute. In other subjects, damage to Wernicke's area and Broca's area results in difficulties with semantic and syntactic processing of language information (Caramazza and Berndt, 1978), suggesting that these areas might mediate syntax and semantic featues of the language attribute.

Response Attribute

With respect to response attribute information, it can be shown that the premotor, supplementary, and motor cortex in conjunction with the cerebellum mediate motor programs dealing with stimulus–response associations (Karni et al., 1995; Roland, 1985; Thompson, 1986) and that the dorsolateral frontal cortex in humans and anterior cingulate and precentral motor cortex in rats mediate long-term memory programs associated with response feedback in the form of egocentric localization as indicated by lesion-induced deficits in tasks that measure egocentric localization (Pohl, 1973; Semmes et al., 1963; Passingham, 1978).

Affect Attribute

With respect to affect attribute information, it can be shown that lesions of the orbital frontal cortex in humans can result in euphoria, lack of responsibility, and lack of affect (Hecaen and Albert, 1978); in monkeys there are emotional changes such as decreased aggression and a reduced tendency to reject certain foods like meat (Butter et al., 1970); and in rats there are also reductions in aggressive behavior (Kolb, 1974). Orbitofrontal-cortex-damaged animals have difficulty changing their behavior when the value or rewards are not consistent with expectations based on prior experiences. Thus, monkeys with orbitofrontal cortex lesions display prolonged extinction of a previously rewarded response (Butter, 1969), and they are impaired in visual and spatial discrimination reversal tasks (Butter, 1969; Iversen and Mishkin, 1970; Jones and Mishkin, 1972). Also, Thorpe and co-workers (1983) have found cells in orbitofrontal cortex that respond differentially to the expectation of a reward or a punishment. These data suggest that the orbital frontal cortex may subserve the affect attribute within the knowledge-based memory system.

Sensory-Perceptual Attribute

With respect to sensory-perceptual attribute information, we will concentrate on visual object information as an exemplar of memory representation of the sensory-perceptual attribute. It can be shown that inferotemporal cortex lesions in monkeys and humans and temporal cortex (TE2) in rats result in visual object discrimination problems (Gross, 1973; McCarthy and Warrington, 1990; Dean, 1990; Fuster, 1995; Weiskrantz and Saunders, 1984), suggesting that the inferotemporal or TE2 may play an important role in mediating long-term representations of visual object information. Additional support comes from PET scan and functional MRI data, where it can be shown that visual object information results in activation of inferotemporal cortex (Ungerleider, 1995).

Even though the two systems have different neural substrates and different operating characteristics, suggesting that the two systems can operate independent of each other, there are also important interactions between the two systems, especially during the consolidation of new information and retrieval of previously stored information. It is thus likely to be very difficult to separate the contribution of each system in new learning tasks, since each system supports one component of the consolidation process.

ALZHEIMER'S DISEASE

What are the neural substrates associated with mnemonic impairments in DAT? In an extensive review Van Hoesen and Damasio (1987; see also Chapter 7) have pointed to a number of neural regions that develop a high density of senile or neuritic plaques and neurofibrillary tangles and neuronal loss. The brain regions that develop a high density of senile plaques, neurofibrillary tangles, and cell loss include the hippocampus, amygdala, entorhinal cortex, parasubicular cortex, parahippocampal gyrus, perirhinal cortex, anterior cingulate, orbital frontal cortex, peristriate cortex, association cortex including the temporal, and parietal and frontal cortex with relative sparing of the sensory and motor cortical areas. There are also changes, especially cell loss in the basal forebrain, locus coeruleus, and raphe nuclei, whose cells provide for cholinergic, adrenergic, and serotonergic innervation, respectively, to cortex and limbic system. The exact order of progression in the development of these cytoskeletal changes is difficult to determine because the varied time course of the disease, differences in the age of onset, and individual differences among the patients. It has been suggested that the hippocampus, entorhinal cortex, and amygdala regions are the first to develop the anatomical changes associated with DAT, followed by parietal and prefrontal cortex association areas, and finally specific sensory and motor cortical areas (Van Hoesen and Damasio, 1987; Van Hoesen and Hyman, 1990). Given this anatomical distribution of DAT makers, it becomes readily apparent that there is an extensive overlap between the above-mentioned neural regions and the neural regions that mediate the data-based and knowledge-based memory systems. Based on the idea that the hippocampus, entorhinal cortex, and amygdala develop DAT markers early in the progression of the disease (early stage) and that the association cortical areas including parietal, dorsolateral frontal cortex, orbital frontal cortex, and anterior cingulate cortex develop DAT markers later in the progression of the disease (middle stage), it can be hypothesized that the data-based memory system and its operating characteristics are affected early in the disease progression and that the knowledge-based memory and its operating characteristics are affected later in the disease progression. In support of this idea are the observations that in the early stages of the disease there are memory deficits involving the processing and temporary memory representation of especially new spatial-temporal and affect attribute information, such as not remembering to pay bills, not remembering recent events in the news, and not remembering appointments. Short-term memory is relatively intact for a very short duration followed by rapid forgetting of new attribute information. There are also learning and retention deficits of verbal and nonverbal information over a series of trials requiring consolidation of new information (Bondi et al., 1994). These memory deficits are consistent with reduced function of part of the data-based memory system as a result of compromise of some of the critical neural substrates, including the hippocampus, entorhinal cortex, and amygdala. In the middle stages of the disease additional memory deficits include word finding difficulties, problems in visuospatial processing, spatial disorientation such as a diminished ability of finding places on a map or of estimating distances accurately, and route finding difficulties in the context of a familiar environment (Zec, 1993). There are also problems in executive control functions, including an impairment of judgment, an impairment in future planning, an impairment in memory for temporal programs, an inability to keep track of ongoing activities, and an impairment in the ability to solve problems (Van Hoesen and Damasio, 1987). These memory deficits are consistent with reduced function of part of the knowledge-based memory system due to compromise of some of the critical neural substrates, including the parietal and prefrontal association cortical areas.

In order to test the DAT early- versus middle-stage hypothesis, a spatial location list learning task was selected because this task can be shown to be sensitive to hippocampal dysfunction and should be representative of temporary processing of spatial attribute information within the data-based memory system and because it provides a human analogue to comparable studies that had been carried out with normal and hippocampal-damaged rats. It is well known that both animals and humans show better memory for the first and last items compared to the middle items within a list, that is, they display serial position curves. Subjects with early and middle DAT, normal elderly subjects with no intellectual impairment, normal college students, and subjects that had experienced an hypoxic episode that resulted in bilateral hippocampal damage were tested for item recognition memory on a spatial location task. In this task subjects were presented with X's on sheets of paper or a computer screen that was divided into a grid including 16 possible spaces. For each trial during the study phase, a subject encountered a subset of six stimulus locations (X's) randomly selected from a set of 16 and presented in a sequential manner. Each stimulus was presented for a period of 5 s. Immediately following the study phase, the test phase was presented. During the test phase, two items were presented simultaneously on the screen, one which occurred in the study sequence and one which did not. The subject was asked to choose the item he or she saw in the previous list. Twenty-four trials were presented per test session, which allowed for four observations for each serial position. The results are shown in Figure 3 and indicate that college students and healthy elderly adults performed very well for all serial positions. Patients diagnosed with early DAT and hypoxic patients showed intact memory performance for the last item within the list (recency effect), but were impaired for all the other serial positions. These findings are consistent with the results obtained by Gibson (1981) and Wilson et al. (1983), who also showed that demented patients display a deficit only for the early items of lists of nonspatial events. Patients diagnosed with middle DAT showed a deficit for all spatial locations within the list (Kesner et al., 1989; Adelstein et al., 1992; Hopkins et al., 1995a). These data indicate that early DAT, but not middle DAT, parallels deficits observed in hippocampal-damaged patients, suggesting a potential critical involvement of the hippocampus in early DAT patients.

In order to further search for a possible correspondence in pattern of memory performance between DAT patients and animals with hippocampal or parietal cortex lesions, rats were trained on a spatial location list learning task that was procedurally similar to the experiment described for the DAT patients. In this experiment each rat is allowed to visit a pseudorandom sequence of five arms on each trial (one per day) on an eight-arm maze. This constituted the study phase. Immediately after the animal had received reinforcement from the last of the five arms, the test phase began. Only one test was given for each trial and consisted of opening two doors si-

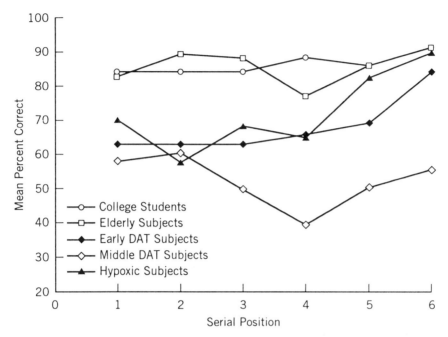

FIGURE 3. Mean percent correct performance as a function of serial position for college students, elderly subjects, early DAT subjects, middle DAT subjects, and hypoxic subjects within a spatial location item recognition task.

multaneously, with one door representing an arm previously visited for that trial and the other door representing a novel arm for that trial. The rule to be learned, leading to an additional reinforcement, was to choose the arm that had been previously visited during the study phase. After reaching criterion performance, the rats either received small dorsal hippocampal, large dorsal hippocampal lesions, large parietal cortex lesions, or cortical control lesions dorsal to the hippocampus. The results are shown in Figure 4 and indicate that control rats perform well for all serial positions. In contrast, the small dorsal hippocampal-lesioned rats showed intact memory performance for the last item within the list (recency effect) but were impaired for all the other serial positions. Finally, rats with large dorsal hippocampal or large parietal cortex lesions were impaired on all serial positions (DiMattia and Kesner, 1998a; Kesner et al., 1988). These data further confirm that partial hippocampal damage in rats and humans parallels the memory deficit pattern observed in early DAT. Middle DAT, however, could be mediated either by more complete hippocampal damage or hippocampal plus parietal cortex damage in that both large hippocampal lesions and parietal cortex lesions paralleled the memory function observed in middle DAT subjects.

In order to further test the DAT early- versus middle-stage hypothesis, a temporal order memory task was selected because this task is sensitive to hippocampal dysfunction and should be representative of temporary processing of temporal at-

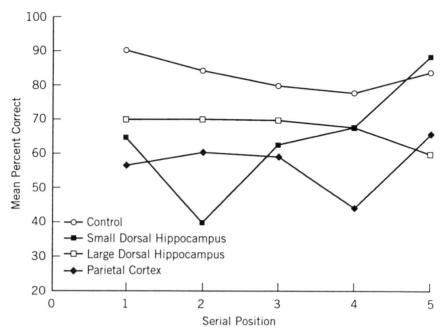

FIGURE 4. Mean percent correct performance as a function of serial position for control, small dorsal hippocampus, large dorsal hippocampus, and parietal cortex lesioned rats within a spatial location item recognition task.

tribute information for spatial location within the data-based memory system and because it provides a human analogue to comparable studies that had been carried out using a temporal order memory task for spatial locations with normal hippocampal and medial prefrontal cortex damaged rats (see Figure 1). In this series of studies, patients with early and middle DAT, hypoxics with bilateral damage to the hippocampus, patients with right temporal lobe resection including the hippocampus, patients with right prefrontal cortex lesions, elderly controls, and college students were presented one at a time with a list of eight spatial locations (X's) on a grid on a Macintosh computer and tested for memory for temporal distances (Chiba et al., submitted; Hopkins et al., 1995b; Johnson and Kesner, in press).

In the spatial task during the study phase a series of random (novel) sequences of eight X's appeared on the screen, for a period of 5 s each. Subjects were instructed to pay attention to the locations of the X's as well as to the order in which they occurred. In the test phase subjects were presented with two X's and were asked to determine which one occurred earlier in the study phase. Unlimited time was allowed for the subjects to make their choices. Temporal distances of 0, 2, 4, and 6 were assessed with eight observations for each distance. Temporal distance is determined by the number of items in the study phase that occur between the two test items. For each study phase, four tests were given, one for each temporal distance. The results are shown in Figure 5 and indicate that relative to college students, the elderly subjects showed a slightly lower level of performance; the early DAT, right temporal lobe resected, and hypoxic subjects performed the task accurately only at the longest temporal distances; the middle DAT and right prefrontal cortex damaged subjects performed at chance level for all temporal distances. These results are similar to what was found in rats (see Figure 1) and suggest that patients with early DAT or bilateral hippocampus dysfunction or rats with dorsal hippocampal lesions have difficulty in encoding or remembering temporal contexts for spatial information due to increased interference in the temporal resolution of

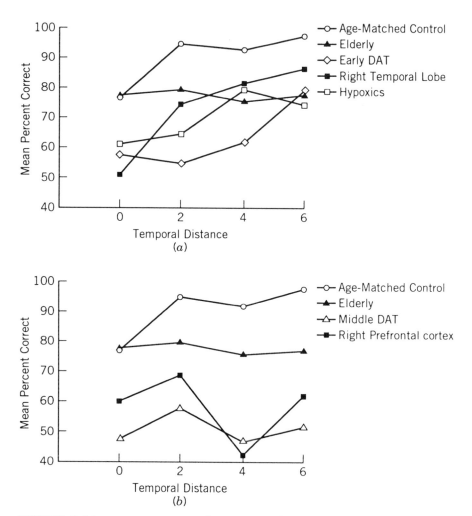

FIGURE 5. Mean percent correct performance as a function of temporal distance for (*a*) age-matched controls, elderly, early DAT subjects, right temporal lobe resected subjects, and hypoxic subjects and (*b*) age-matched controls, elderly, middle DAT subjects, and right prefrontal cortex damaged subjects within a novel, unstructured spatial location task.

specific spatial locations. Furthermore, patients with middle DAT or right prefrontal cortex damage and rats with large hippocampal or medial prefrontal cortex lesions have a more complete and severe deficit with very little ability to utilize temporal order information. These data further confirm that partial hippocampal damage in rats and humans parallels the memory deficit pattern observed in early DAT. Middle DAT, however, could be mediated either by more complete hippocampal damage or hippocampal plus prefrontal cortex damage in that in rats both large hippocampal lesions and prefrontal cortex lesions paralleled the memory function observed in middle DAT subjects.

Thus far, two tests were selected that were sensitive to hippocampal dysfunction and appeared to reflect the memory disturbance observed in early, but not middle, DAT patients. It had been shown that familiarity with a situation based on past experience or the ability to use a well-known strategy can attenuate interference and might therefore not involve the hippocampus, but rather temporal distance performance might be supported by prefrontal cortex. Therefore, a new test was constructed and administered to early and middle DAT, hypoxic subjects with bilateral hippocampal damage, right temporal lobe resected patients with hippocampal damage, right prefrontal cortex damaged subjects, and age-matched control subjects. These subjects were given sequences where the X's appeared in a meaningful geometric pattern. An example of a meaningful and familiar pattern would be the presentation of the locations in the pattern of a large X. The first X would be presented in the top left corner of the grid and then in each subsequent square down the diagonal ending in the bottom right corner. The next X would be presented in the bottom left corner of the grid and in each subsequent square up the diagonal ending in the top right corner. In the test phase subjects were presented with two X's and were asked to determine which one occurred earlier in the study phase. Unlimited time was allowed for the subjects to make their choices. Temporal distances of 0, 2, 4, and 6 were assessed with eight observations for each distance. For each study phase, four tests were given, one for each temporal distance (Chiba et al., submitted; Hopkins et al., 1995b; Johnson and Kesner, in press). There were no significant differences between the age-matched controls and elderly subjects, so that the two groups were combined into a single control group. The results are shown in Figure 6 and indicate that age-matched controls, right temporal lobe damaged subjects, and hypoxic subjects performed very well for all spatial distances. In contrast, the early DAT and middle DAT and right prefrontal cortex damaged subjects performed the task accurately only at the longest temporal distances, and the middle DAT had a greater impairment relative to the early DAT subjects only for the shortest temporal distance. These results are similar to what was found in rats (see Figure 2) and suggest that patients with right or bilateral hippocampal dysfunction or rats with total or dorsal hippocampal lesions have only mild difficulty in encoding or remembering temporal contexts that are aided by familiarity for the material to be studied aided by knowledge-based strategies. However, patients with early and middle DAT or right prefrontal cortex damage and rats with medial prefrontal cortex damage show impairments primarily for the short, but not for the long-distances. These data further confirm that for a knowledge-based temporal distance task, medial pre-

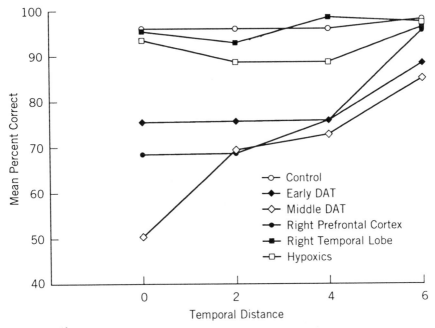

FIGURE 6. Mean percent correct performance as a function of temporal distance for controls, early DAT, middle DAT, right prefrontal cortex damaged subjects, right temporal lobe resected subjects, and hypoxic subjects within a familiar, structured spatial location task.

frontal cortex in rats and right prefrontal cortex in humans parallels the memory deficit pattern observed in middle DAT. However, there is also a deficit for early DAT, even though hippocampal damage in rats and humans do not produce a memory deficit pattern. This latter result suggests that even in early DAT there might be some damage in prefrontal cortex that is detectable only in a task that measures primarily the involvement of the knowledge-based memory system. Combining the results of the three experiments with rats and humans, it appears that there is strong support for an involvement of the hippocampus with early DAT indicating an involvement of the data-based memory system in early DAT with perhaps some mild dysfunction of the parietal and prefrontal cortex and good support for additional extensive involvement of cortical association areas including prefrontal and parietal cortex with middle DAT indicating the involvement of the knowledge-based memory system later in the progression of the disease.

MODELS OF ALZHEIMER'S DISEASE

The most frequently employed animal model to study DAT has been to lesion the basal forebrain. The focus on understanding the basal forebrain in relation to learning and memory has evolved out of studies indicating a loss of basal forebrain cholinergic neurons and decrease of hippocampal and cortical cholinergic markers in DAT (Davies and Maloney, 1976; Coyle et al., 1983; Whitehouse et al., 1982). The importance of the forebrain cholinergic systems in cognitive function is suggested by studies demonstrating a correlation between dementia severity and decrease in cholinergic markers (Perry et al., 1978; Wilcock et al., 1982).

The basal forebrain contains separate cholinergic nuclei with different target areas (Mesulam et al., 1983). In the rodent, the nucleus basalis magnocellularis (NBM) projects to the neocortical, mesocortical, and amygdaloid regions. The medial septum/vertical nucleus of the diagonal band (MS/VNDB) area projects predominantly to the hippocampus. The horizontal nucleus of the diagonal band (HNDB) projects to the olfactory bulb, piriform cortex, and entorhinal cortex.

The main purpose for developing the basal forebrain model has been to understand the functional organization of this system, which may render treatments that prevent or ameliorate the clinical symptoms. The focus for this research has been on unraveling the mnemonic function of the basal forebrain cholinergic systems. One difficulty that has arisen is in drawing parallels between the memory tests applied in the animal models and those used in DAT. However, some tasks have been developed in rodents that assess memory attributes that are similar in humans. Thus, memory impairments revealed in animal models of DAT may prove useful in understanding some of the cognitive deficits found in early and middle stages of DAT. Because the research focus has been on the mnemonic function of the NBM and MS/VNDB and not the HNDB, the discussion will be limited to experiments on the NBM and MS/VNDB cholinergic systems.

As discussed earlier in this chapter, the prominent memory impairment exhibited in early stages of DAT is an inability to remember new information. This deficit is consistent with the type of memories represented in the data-based memory system. MS/VNDB lesions consistently impair spatial tasks using a short-term or working-memory paradigm (Walsh et al., 1984; Hepler et al., 1985). In our laboratory using order and item list learning for spatial location information tasks, small MS/VNDB lesions only produce a primacy impairment for item and order memory (Kesner et al., 1986; Kesner, 1988). These results are comparable to those following dorsal hippocampal lesions (see Figure 1) (Kesner, 1988). A recent study examined the effects of the selective cholinergic neurotoxin, (IgG-) immunoglobin G-saporin (Baxter et al., 1995). IgG-saporin lesions of the MS/VNDB produce no deficits on the consolidation of new spatial information in the water maze. However, on a delay match-to-place task, MS/VNDB lesions do result in a short-term memory impairment. These findings suggest that the MS/VNDB cholinergic system may only be involved in modulating some aspects of the data-based memory system. More importantly, the memory impairments following MS/VNDB lesions are similar to those exhibited by individuals with early-stage DAT (Kesner et al., 1989).

Several studies have examined the effects of NBM lesions in tasks that require the data-based memory system. In some experiments, NBM lesions impair performance in tasks requiring win-shift and delayed nonmatch-to-sample (DNMS) for spatial locations (Dubois et al., 1985; Hepler et al., 1985; Knowlton et al., 1985; Markowska et al., 1990). However in other cases, NBM lesions produce minimal or no deficits in these tasks (Bartus et al., 1985; Murray and Fibiger, 1985; Markowska et al., 1990). In contrast to the effects of the MS/VNDB lesions, small NBM lesions produce only a recency deficit for order memory (Kesner et al., 1986), while small or large NBM lesions result in no reduction of item memory (Kesner et al., 1987a). Even though the order memory results with NBM lesions are consistent with the results observed in early DAT patients in a comparable spatial location list learning task, the item memory results with NBM lesions are inconsistent with the results observed in early DAT patients, in that early DAT patients have a primacy deficit, whereas NBM lesioned rats show no impairments (Adelstein et al., 1992). In more recent studies IgG-saporin lesions of the NBM do not impair spatial DNMS (Wenk et al., 1994) and produce minor impairments in operant DNMS and match-to-place in the water maze (Torres et al., 1994; Baxter et al., 1995).

The different behavioral outcomes following lesions of the NBM may result from factors such as the extent of preoperative training and/or the method to destroy NBM cells. For example, the neurotoxin, quisqualic acid (QUIS) produces a greater reduction in cortical choline acetyltransferase activity than ibotenic acid (IBO) when injected into the NBM, but IBO lesions cause a more severe behavioral deficit than QUIS lesions (Dunnett et al., 1987; Markowska et al., 1990). The findings suggest that other NBM neurons, besides cholinergic, are important for memory as assessed in the tasks mentioned above. As an alternative, recent reports suggest that the NBM cholinergic system is more important for modulating the selective attention process rather than the short-term memory or consolidation process associated with data-based memories (Chiba et al., 1995; Stoehr and Wenk, in press; see also Chapter 10).

The varied behavioral results following NBM lesions may alternatively arise because the NBM cholinergic system projects to cortical areas, proposed to mediate knowledge-based information, but also projects to the amygdala, which may be involved in data-based memory. Thus, the NBM cholinergic system may be involved in modulating both data-based and knowledge-based memories. In support of this hypothesis, inactivation of the amygdala just prior to a 1-day retention test in inhibitory avoidance impairs performance but does not impair when inactivated prior to a 21-day retention test. In contrast, inactivation of the frontal cortex before the 21-day retention task decreases retention but does not impair retention when testing occurs 1 day after training (Liang and Liao, 1995). Furthermore, phthalic acid lesions of the NBM preferentially decrease choline acetyltransferase (ChAT) activity in the amygdala. QUIS lesions primarily reduce ChAT activity in the cortex (Mallet et al., 1995). NBM lesions induced by phthalic acid result in data-based memory deficits; however, QUIS lesions do not produce a data-based memory impairment (Mallet et al., 1995). In comparison, intraamygdala injections of scopolamine, a muscarinic cholinergic antagonist, produce similar memory deficits as phthalic acid lesions of the NBM (Ingles et al., 1993). The findings suggest that the NBM cholinergic projection to the amygdala is important for modulating data-based memories.

Interestingly, there are parallels between lesions of the NBM and the parietal cortex. Lesions of the NBM and parietal cortex both cause impairments in learning a place navigation task in a water maze and cheese board (Whishaw et al., 1985; Dunnett et al., 1987; DiMattia and Kesner, 1988a). In these tasks, rats must locate a place in the testing environment that remains constant. This form of learning involves both the data-based and knowledge-based memory systems. In another experiment using a radial arm maze, NBM lesions and parietal cortex lesions produce knowledge-based memory impairments but do not result in data-based memory deficits (Kesner et al., 1987b). The results connote that the NBM cholinergic system may modulate different types of memory dependent on its cortical and subcortical targets.

Althought the memory deficits following MS/VNDB lesions more closely mimic the deficits observed in early stage DAT than those following NBM lesions, damage to either basal forebrain area may not represent an ideal model for early stages of DAT. Despite a degree of heterogeneous pathology in brain regions, there is accumulating evidence that the primary degeneration occurs in cortical areas whereas subcortical damage appears secondary (Braak and Braak, 1991; Simonian et al., 1994). Furthermore, the brains of individuals with DAT is marked by several neurochemical deficits, with acetylcholine representing only one of them (Gottfries, 1990). Moreover, basal forebrain lesions in rodents do not mimic the neurochemical changes in cortical areas that are seen in DAT (Gaykema et al., 1989). Finally, basal forebrain lesions lead to anterograde cell death in certain cortical areas that are not affected in early- or middle-stage DAT (Braak and Braak, 1991; Simonian et al., 1994).

In conclusion, it appears that the cholinergic system may play an important modulatory role in mediating both data-based memory functions dependent on the MS/VNDB and NBM cholinergic projections to, for example, the hippocampus and amygdala and knowledge-based functions dependent on NBM and HNDB cholinergic projections to neocortex including parietal and prefrontal cortex. However, it should be noted that the primary modulatory influence of the cholinergic system could be on the selective attention and selective filtering of attribute information operating characteristic of the data-based and knowledge-based memory systems.

We have not presented other models of DAT in part because of space limitations and because none of the other animal models, that is, the glutaminergic, adrenergic, serotonergic, nerve growth factor models is currently as well developed as the cholinergic model. Our recommendation is first to develop tasks for both animals and humans that directly involve (a) neural regions (i.e., hippocampus and amygdala that not only subserve the data-based memory system but can also be shown to be affected in early DAT) and (b) neural regions (i.e., prefrontal and parietal cortex association areas that not only subserve the knowledge-based memory system but can also be shown to be affected in middle DAT). Second, we recommend the development of therapeutic agents that can directly target neocortical and limbic brain structures.

In summary, in this chapter an updated version of the neurobiology of multiple attribute model was presented. It was then shown that the assumptions of the model have utility in describing the neural bases of mnemonic dysfunction in various stages of DAT. Data were presented in rats with hippocampal or neocortical lesions and humans with hippocampal or neocortical lesions as well as humans with early- or middle-stage DAT in two tasks that measured the operation of the data-based memory system and one task that measured the operation of the knowledge-based memory system to support the utility of the multiple attribute model. Finally, one animal model, namely the basal forebrain cholinergic model, was analyzed and evaluated within the context of the attribute model and the stages of DAT.

REFERENCES

Adelstein TB, Kesner RP, Strassberg DS (1992): Spatial recognition and spatial order memory in patients with dementia of the Alzheimer's type. Neuropsychologia 30:59–67.

Baddeley A (1986): "Working Memory." Oxford: Oxford University Press.

Bartus RT, Flicker C, Dean RL, Pontecorvo M, Figueiredo JC, Fisher SK (1985): Selective memory loss following nucleus basalis lesions: Long term behavioral recovery despite persistent cholinergic deficiencies. Pharmacol Biochem Behav 23:125–135.

Baxter MG, Bucci DJ, Gorman LK, Wiley RG, Gallagher M (1995): Selective immunotoxic lesions of basal forebrain cholinergic cells: Effects on learning and memory in rats. Behav Neurosci 109:714–722.

Bondi MW, Salmon DP, Butters N (1994): Neuropsychological features of memory disorders in Alzheimer disease. In Terry RD, Katzman R, Bick KL (eds): "Alzheimer Disease." New York: Raven Press.

Braak H, Braak E (1991): Neuropathological staging of Alzheimer-related changes. Acta Neuropathol 82:239–259.

Butter CM (1969): Perseveration in extinction and in discrimination reversal tasks following selective frontal ablations in Macaca mulatta. Physiol Behav 4:163–171.

Butter CM, Snyder DR, McDonald JA (1970): Effects of orbitofrontal lesions on aversive and aggressive behaviours in rhesus monkeys. J Comp Physiol Psychol 72:132–144.

Caramazza A, Berndt RS (1978): Semantic and syntactic processes in aphasia: A review of the literature. Psychol Bull 85:898–918.

Chiba AA, Kesner RP, Matsuo F, Heilbrun MP, Plumb S (submitted): A double dissociation between the right and left hippocampus in processing the temporal order of spatial and verbal information.

Chiba AA, Bushnell PJ, Oshiro WM, Gallagher M (1995): Altered selective attention in rats with cholinergic lesions of the substantia innominata. Soc Neurosci Abst 21:936.

Chiba AA, Kesner RP, Reynolds AM (1994): Memory for spatial location as a function of temporal lag in rats: Role of hippocampus and medial prefrontal cortex. Behav Neural Biol 61:123–131.

Chiba AA, Kesner RP, Matsuo F, Heilbrun MP (1993): A dissociation between affect and recognition following unilateral temporal lobectomy including the amygdala. Soc Neurosci Abst 19:792.

Chiba AA, Johnson DL, Kesner RP (1992): The effects of lesions of the dorsal hippocampus or the ventral hippocampus on performance of a spatial location order recognition task. Soc Neurosci Abst 18:1422.

Cohen NJ, Eichenbaum HB (1993): "Memory, Amnesia, and the Hippocampal System." Cambridge, MA: MIT Press.

Cook D, Kesner RP (1988): Caudate nucleus and memory for egocentric localization. Behav Neural Biol 49:332–343.

Coyle JT, Price DL, DeLong MR (1983): Alzheimer's disease: A disorder of cortical cholinergic innervation. Science 219:1184–1190.

Dakis M, Martinez JS, Kesner RP, Jackson-Smith P (1992): Effects of phencyclidine and naloxone on learning of a spatial navigation task and performance of a spatial delayed non-matching to sample task. Soc Neurosci Abst 18:1220.

Davies P, Maloney AFJ (1976): Selective loss of cerebral cholinergic neurones in Alzheimer's disease. Lancet 2:1403.

Dean P (1990): Sensory cortex: Visual perceptual functions. In Kolb B, Tees RC (eds): "Cerebral Cortex of the Rat." Cambridge, MA: MIT Press, pp 275–308.

DeRenzi E (1982): "Disorders of Space Exploration and Cognition." New York: Wiley.

DiMattia BV, Kesner RP (1988a): Spatial cognitive maps: Differential role of parietal cortex and hippocampal formation. Behav Neurosci 102:471–480.

DiMattia BV, Kesner RP (1988b): The role of the posterior parietal association cortex in the processing of spatial event information. Behav Neurosci 102:397–403.

Dubois B, Mayo W, Agid Y, Le Moal M, Simon H (1985): Profound disturbances of spontaneous and learned behaviors following lesions of the nucleus basalis magnocellularis in the rat. Brain Res 338:249–258.

Duncan-Davis J, Filoteo V, Kesner RP (in press): Memory impairment for spatial location and motor movements in patients with Huntington's disease. Cogn Neurosci Soc Abst.

Dunnett SB, Whishaw IQ, Jones GH, Bunch ST (1987): Behavioural, biochemical and histochemical effects of different neurotoxic amino acids injected into nucleus basalis magnocellularis of rats. Neuroscience 20:653–699.

Eichenbaum H, Stewart C, Morris RGM (1990): Hippocampal representation in spatial learning. J Neurosci 10:331–339.

Fuster JM (1995): "Memory in the Cerebral Cortex: An Empirical Approach to Neural Networks in the Human and Nonhuman Primate." Cambridge, MA: MIT Press.

Gaffan DG, Murray EA (1992): Monkeys with rhinal cortex ablations succeed in object discrimination learning despite 24-hr intertrial intervals and fail at matching to sample despite double sample presentations. Behav Neurosci 106:30–38.

Gaykema RPA, Compaan JC, Nyakas C, Horvath E, Luiten PGM (1989): Long-term effects of cholinergic basal forebrain lesions on neuropeptide Y and somatostatin immunoreactivity in rat neocortex. Brain Res 489:392–396.

Gibson AJ (1981): A further analysis of memory loss in dementia and depression in the elderly. Br J Clin Psychol 20:179–185.

Gottfries CG (1990): Disturbance of the 5-hydroxytryptamine metabolism in brains from patients with Alzheimer's dementia. J Neural Trans 30:33–43.

Gross CG (1973): Inferotemporal cortex and vision. In Stellar E, Sprague JM (eds): "Progress in Physiological Psychology, Vol. 5." New York: Academic, pp 77–123.

Habib M, Sirigu A (1987): Pure topographic disorientation: A definition and anatomical basis. Cortex 23:73–85.

Hecaen H, Albert ML (1978): "Human Neuropsychology." New York: Wiley.

Heilman KM, Watson RT, Valenstein E (1993): Neglect and related disorders. In Heilman KM, Valenstein E (eds): "Clinical Neuropsychology," 3rd ed. New York: Oxford University Press.

Heindel W, Salmon D, Shults C, Walicke P, Butters N (1989): Neuropsychological evidence for multiple implicit memory systems: A comparison of Alzheimer's, Huntington's and Parkinson's disease patients. J Neurosci 9:582–587.

Heindel W, Butters N, Salmon D (1988): Impaired learning of a motor skill in patients with Huntington's disease. Behav Neurosci 102:141–147.

Hepler DJ, Olton DS, Wenk GL, Coyle JT (1985): Lesions in nucleus basalis magnocellularis and medial septal area of rats produce qualitatively similar memory impairments. J Neurosci 5:866–873.

Hopkins RO, Kesner RP (1994): Short-term memory for duration in hypoxic subjects. Soc Neurosci Abst 20:1075.

Hopkins RO, Kesner RP (1993): Memory for temporal and spatial distances for new and previously learned geographical information in hypoxic subjects. Soc Neurosci Abst 19:1284.

Hopkins RO, Kesner RP, Goldstein M (1995a): Item and order recognition memory for words, pictures, abstract pictures, spatial locations, and motor responses in subjects with hypoxic brain injury. Brain Cogn 27:180–201.

Hopkins RO, Kesner RP, Goldstein M (1995b): Memory for novel and familiar spatial and linguistic temporal distance information in hypoxic subjects. J Int Neuropsychol Soc 1:454–468.

Horel JA, Pytko-Joiner DE, Voytko ML, Salsbury K (1987): The performance of visual tasks while segments of the inferotemporal cortex are suppressed by cold. Behav Brain Res 23:29–42.

Hunt ME, Kesner RP, Evans RB (1994): Memory for spatial location: Functional dissociation of entorhinal cortex and hippocampus. Psychobiology 22:186–194.

Ingles JL, Beninger RJ, Jhamandas K, Boegman RJ (1993): Scopolamine injected into the rat amygdala impairs working memory in the double Y-maze. Brain Res Bull 32:339–344.

Iversen SD, Mishkin M (1970): Perseverative interference in monkey following selective lesions of the inferior prefrontal convexity. Exp Brain Res 11:376–386.

Jackson-Smith P, Kesner RP, Amann K (1994): Effects of hippocampal and medial prefrontal lesions on discrimination of duration in rats. Soc Neurosci Abst 20:1210.

Johnson DL, Kesner RP (in press): Comparison of temporal order memory in early and middle stage Alzheimer's disease J Clin Exp Neuropsych.

Jones B, Mishkin M (1972): Limbic lesions and the problem of stimulus-reinforcement associations. Exp Neurol 36:362–377.

Karni A, Meyer G, Jezzard P, Adams MM, Turner R, Ungerleider LG (1995): Functional MRI evidence for adult motor cortex plasticity during motor skill learning. Nature 377: 155–158.

Kesner RP (1990): Learning and memory in rats with an emphasis on the role of the hippocampal formation. In Kesner RP, Olton DS (eds): "Neurobiology of Comparative Cognition." Hillsdale, NJ: Erlbaum, pp 179–204.

Kesner RP (1988): Reevaluation of the contribution of the basal forebrain cholinergic system to memory. Neurobiol Aging 9:609–616.

Kesner RP, Hopkins RO (in preparation): Memory for duration and spatial distance in hypoxic subjects.

Kesner RP (in preparation): Spatial recognition memory: Role of entorhinal cortex, pre- and parasubiculum and pre- and infralimbic cortex.

Kesner RP, Dakis M (1995): Phencyclidine injections into the dorsal hippocampus disrupt long- but not short-term memory within a spatial learning task. Psychopharmacology, 120:203–208.

Kesner RP, DiMattia BV (1987): Neurobiology of an attribute model of memory. In Morrison AR, Epstein AN (eds): "Progress in Psychobiology and Physiological Psychology." New York: Academic, pp 207–277.

Kesner RP, Holbrook T (1987): Dissociation of item and order spatial memory in rats following medial prefrontal cortex lesions. Neuropsychologia 25:653–664.

Kesner RP, Jackson-Smith P (1992): Neurobiology of an attribute model of memory: Role of prefrontal cortex. In Gormezano I, Wasserman EA (eds): "Learning and Memory: Behavioral and Biological Processes." Hillsdale, NJ: Lawrence Erlbaum, pp 251–273.

Kesner RP, Williams JM (1995): Memory for magnitude of reinforcement: Dissociation between the amygdala and hippocampus. Neurobiol Learn Mem 64:237–244.

Kesner RP, Hopkins RO, Fineman B (1994): Item and order dissociation in humans with prefrontal cortex damage. Neuropsychologia 32:881–891.

Kesner RP, Bolland BL, Dakis M (1993): Memory for spatial locations, motor responses, and objects: Triple dissociation among the hippocampus, caudate nucleus, and extrastriate visual cortex. Exp Brain Res 93:462–470.

Kesner RP, Hopkins RO, Chiba AA (1992): Learning and memory in humans with an emphasis on the role of the hippocampus. In Squire L, Butters N (eds): "Neuropsychology of Memory," 2nd ed. New York: Guilford, pp 106–121.

Kesner RP, Farnsworth G, Kametani H (1991): Role of parietal cortex and hippocampus in representing spatial information. Cereb Cortex 1:367–373.

Kesner RP, Adelstein TB, Crutcher KA (1989): Equivalent spatial location memory deficits in rats with medial septum or hippocampal formation lesions and patients with dementia of the Alzheimer's type. Brain Cogn 9:289–300.

Kesner RP, Crutcher K, Beers D (1988): Serial position curves for item (spatial location) information: Role of the dorsal hippocampus and medial septum. Brain Res 454:219–226.

Kesner RP, Adelstein TB, Crutcher KA (1987a): Rats with nucleus basalis lesions mimic mnemonic symptomatology of Alzheimer's disease. Behav Neurosci 101:451–456.

Kesner RP, DiMattia BV, Crutcher KA (1987b): Evidence for neocortical involvement in reference memory. Behav Neural Biol 47:40–53.

Kesner RP, Crutcher K, Meason M (1986): Medial septal and nucleus basalis magnocellularis lesions produce order memory deficits in rats which mimic symptomatology of Alzheimer's disease. Neurobiol Aging 7:287–295.

Knowlton BJ, Wenk GL, Olton DS, Coyle JT (1985): Basal forebrain lesions produce a dissociation of trial-dependent and trial-independent memory performance. Brain Res 345:315–321.

Kolb B (1974): Social behavior of rats with chronic prefrontal lesions. Physiol Psychol 87:466–474.

Kubie JL, Ranck JB (1983): Sensory-behavioral correlates in individual hippocampal neurons in three situations: Space and context. In Seifert W (ed): "Neurobiology of the Hippocampus." New York: Academic, pp 433–447.

Leonard G, Milner B (1991): Contribution of the right frontal lobe to the encoding and recall of kinesthetic distance information. Neuropsychologia 29:47–58.

Liang KC, Liao WL (1995): Pretest infusion of lidocaine into the insular or medial prefrontal cortex impairs retrieval of remote memory in an inhibitory avoidance task. Soc Neurosci Abst 21:1448.

Long JM, Mellen J, Kesner RP (in press): The effects of total and partial parietal cortex lesions on memory for an object/spatial location paired associate task in rats. Soc Neurosci Abst.

Long JM, Kesner RP (1996): The effects of dorsal vs. ventral hippocampal, total hippocampal, and parietal cortex lesions on memory for allocentric distance in rats. Behav Neurosci 22:682.

Long JM, Kesner RP (1994): The effects of parietal cortex and hippocampal lesions on memory for allocentric distance, egocentric distance, and spatial location in rats. Soc Neurosci Abst 20:1210.

Mallet PE, Beninger RJ, Flesher SN, Jhamandas K, Boegman RJ (1995): Nucleus basalis lesions: Implication of basoamygdaloid cholinergic pathways in memory. Brain Res Bull 36:51–56.

Markowska AL, Wenk GL, Olton DS (1990): Nucleus basalis magnocellularis and memory: Differential effects of two neurotoxins. Behav Neural Biol 54:13–26.

McCarthy RA, Warrington EK (1990): "Cognitive Psychology: A Clinical Introduction." London: Academic.

McDonald RJ, White NM (1995): Hippocampal and nonhippocampal contributions to place learning in rats. Behav Neurosci 109:579–593.

McDonald RJ, White NM (1993): A triple dissociation of systems: Hippocampus, amygdala, and dorsal striatum. Behav Neurosci 107:3–22.

McNaughton BL, Barnes CA, O'Keefe J (1983): The contributions of position, direction and velocity to single unit activity in the hippocampus of freely-moving rats. Exp Brain Res 52:41–49.

Mesulam MM, Mufson EJ, Wainer BH, Levey Al (1983): Central cholinergic pathways in the rat: An overview based on an alternative nomenclature (Ch1–Ch6). Neuroscience 10:1185–1201.

Mizumori SJY, Williams JD (1993): Directionally selective mnemonic properties of neurons in the lateral dorsal nucleus of the thalamus of rats. J Neurosci 13:4015–4028.

Morris RGM, Garrud JNP, Rawlins JNP, O'Keefe J (1982): Place navigation impaired in rats with hippocampal lesions. Nature 297:681–683.

Mumby DG, Pinel JPJ (1994): Rhinal cortex lesions and object recognition in rats. Behav Neurosci 108:11–18.

Murray CL, Fibiger HC (1985): Learning and memory deficits after lesions of the nucleus basalis magnocellularis: Reversal by physostigmine. Neuroscience 14:1025–1032.

Myers CE, Gluck MA, Granger R (1995): Dissociation of hippocampal and entorhinal function in associative learning: A computational approach. Psychobiology 23:116–138.

Nachman M, Ashe JH (1974): Effects of basolateral amygdala lesions on neophobia, learned taste aversions, and sodium appetite in rats. J Comp Physiol Psychol 87:622–643.

O'Keefe J (1983): Spatial memory within and without the hippocampal system. In Seifert W (ed): "Neurobiology of the Hippocampus." London: Academic, pp 375–403.

O'Keefe J, Nadel L (1978): "The Hippocampus as a Cognitive Map." Oxford: Clarendon.

O'Keefe J, Speakman A (1987): Single unit activity in the rat hippocampus during a spatial memory task. Exp Brain Res 68:1–27.

Olton DS (1986): Hippocampal function and memory for temporal context. In Isaacson RL, Pribram KH (eds): "The Hippocampus, Vol. 3." New York: Plenum.

Olton DS (1983): Memory functions and the hippocampus. In Seifert W (ed): "Neurobiology of the Hippocampus." New York: Academic.

Olton DS, Meck WH, Church RM (1987): Separation of hippocampal and amygdaloid involvement in temporal memory dysfunctions. Brain Res 404:180–188.

Otto T, Eichenbaum H (1992): Complementary roles of the orbital prefrontal cortex and the perirhinal-entorhinal cortices in an odor-guided delayed-nonmatching-to-sample task. Behav Neurosci 106:762–775.

Parkinson JK, Murray EA, Mishkin M (1988): A selective mnemonic role for the hippocampus in monkeys: Memory for the location of objects. J Neurosci 8:4159–4167.

Passingham R (1978): Information about movements in monkeys (Macaca mulatta) with lesions of dorsal prefrontal cortex. Brain Res 152:313–328.

Perry EK, Tomlinson BE, Blessed G, Bergmann K, Gibson P, Perry RH (1978): Correlation of cholinergic abnormalities with senile plaques and mental test scores in senile dementia. Br Med J 2:1457–1459.

Phillips RG, LeDoux JE (1992): Differential contribution of amygdala and hippocampus to cued and contextual fear conditioning. Behav Neurosci 106:274–285.

Pohl W (1973): Dissociation of spatial discrimination deficits following frontal and parietal lesions in monkeys. J Comp Physiol Psychol 82:227–239.

Quirk GJ, Muller RU, Kubie JL, Ranck JB Jr. (1992): The positional firing properties of medial entorhinal neurons: Description and comparison with hippocampal place cells. J Neurosci 12:1945–1963.

Roland PE (1985): Cortical organization of voluntary behavior in man. Hum Neurobiol 4:155–167.

Rolls ET, Miyashita Y, Cahusac PMB, Kesner RP, Niki H, Feigenbaum J, Bach L (1989): Hippocampal neurons in the monkey with activity related to the place in which a stimulus is shown. J Neurosci 9:1835–1844.

Schacter DL (1987): Implicit memory: History and current status. J Exp Psychol: Learn Mem Cogn 13:501–518.

Semmes J, Weinstein S, Ghent L, Teuber HL (1963): Correlates of impaired orientation in personal and extrapersonal space. Brain 86:747–772.

Shapiro ML, Olton DS (1994): Hippocampal function and interference. In Schacter DL, Tulving E (eds): "Memory Systems 1994." Cambridge, MA: MIT Press.

Simonian NA, Rebeck GW, Hyman BT (1994): Functional integrity of neural systems related to memory in Alzheimer's disease. Prog Brain Res 100:245–254.

Smith ML, Milner B (1981): The role of the right hippocampus in the recall of spatial location. Neuropsychologia 19:781–793.

Squire LR (1994): Declarative and nondeclarative memory: Multiple brain systems supporting learning and memory. In Schacter DL, Tulving E (eds): "Memory Systems 1994." Cambridge, MA: MIT Press.

Squire LR (1987): "Memory and Brain." New York: Oxford University Press.

Stoehr JD, Wenk GL (in press): The effects of basal forebrain lesions upon expectancy in the rat. Behav Neurosci.

Sutherland RJ, Hoesing JM (1993): Posterior cingulate cortex and spatial memory: A microlimnology analysis. In Vogt BA, Gabriel M (eds): "Neurobiology of Cingulate Cortex and Limbic Thalamus: A Comprehensive Handbook." Boston: Birkhauser.

Suzuki WA, Zola-Morgan S, Squire LR, Amaral DG (1993): Lesions of the perirhinal and parahippocampal cortices in the monkey produce long-lasting memory impairment in the visual and tactual modalities. J Neurosci 13:2430–2451.

Taube JS (1995): Place cells recorded in the parasubiculum of freely moving rats. Hippocampus 5:569–583.

Thompson RF (1986): The neurobiology of learning and memory. Science 233:941–947.

Thorpe SJ, Rolls ET, Maddison S (1983): The orbitofrontal cortex: Neuronal activity in the behaving monkey. Exp Brain Res 49:93–115.

Torres EM, Perry TA, Blokland A, Wilkinson LS, Wiley RG, Lappi DA, Dunnett SB (1994): Behavioral, histochemical and biochemical consequences of selective immunolesions in discrete regions of the basal forebrain cholinergic system. Neuroscience 63:95–122.

Tulving E (1983): "Elements of Episodic Memory." Oxford: Clarendon Press.

Ungerleider LG (1995): Functional brain imaging studies of cortical mechanisms of memory. Science 270:769–775.

Van Hoesen GW, Damasio AR (1987): Neural correlates of cognitive impairment in Alzheimer's disease. In Plum F (ed): "Higher Functions of the Nervous System, the Handbook of Physiology." Baltimore: Williams and Wilkins, pp 871–898.

Van Hoesen GW, Hyman BT (1990): Hippocampal formation: Anatomy and the patterns of pathology in Alzheimer's disease. Prog Brain Res 83:445–457.

Walsh TJ, Tilson HA, DeHaven DL, Mailman RB, Fisher A, Hanin I (1984): AF64A, a cholinergic neurotoxin, selectively depletes acetylcholine in hippocampus and cortex, and produces long-term passive avoidance and radial-arm maze deficits in the rat. Brain Res 321:91–102.

Weiskrantz L, Saunders C (1984): Impairments of visual object transforms in monkeys. Brain 107:1033–1072.

Wenk GL, Stoehr JD, Quintana G, Mobley S, Wiley RG (1994): Behavioral, biochemical, histological, and electrophysiological effects of 192 IgG-Saporin injections into the basal forebrain of rats. J Neurosci 14:5986–5995.

Whishaw IQ, O'Connor WT, Dunnett ST (1985): Disruption of central cholinergic systems in the rat by basal forebrain lesions: Effects on feeding, sensorimotor behaviour, locomotor activity and spatial navigation. Behav Brain Res 17:103–115.

Whitehouse PJ, Price DL, Struble RG, Clark AW, Coyle JT, DeLong MR (1982): Alzheimer's disease and senile dementia: A quantitative study. Science 215:1237–1239.

Wilcock GK, Esiri MM, Bowen DM, Smith CCT (1982): Alzheimer's disease: Correlation of cortical choline acetyltransferase activity with the severity of dementia and histological abnormalities. J Neurol Sci 57:407–417.

Wilson RS, Bacon LD, Fox JH, Kaszniak AW (1983): Primary memory and secondary memory in dementia of the Alzheimer type. J Clin Neuropsychol 5:337–344.

Zec RF (1993): Neuropsychological functioning in Alzheimer's disease. In Parks RW, Zec RF, Wilson RS (eds): "Neuropsychology of Alzheimer's Disease and Other Dementias." New York: Oxford University Press, pp 3–80.

CHAPTER 2

Interaction of Neuromodulatory Systems Regulating Memory Storage

JOHN F. GUZOWSKI and JAMES L. McGAUGH

Center for the Neurobiology of Learning and Memory (J.F.G. and J.L.M.) and
Departments of Psychobiology and Pharmacology (J.L.M.),
University of California, Irvine, California 92697-3800

INTRODUCTION

Our view of how the brain processes information to form long-term memories is rapidly changing. Within the past few years, once-foreign disciplines such as molecular biology and molecular genetics have joined with more traditional neuroscience approaches in efforts to unravel the mysteries of the mammalian brain. However, although neuroscience is clearly multidisciplinary at a technical level, it is not yet truly integrative at a theoretical or conceptual level. In an effort to bridge approaches to the study of memory formation, this chapter considers the concept of memory consolidation from the level of interacting brain systems to the molecular and cellular processes underlying neuronal plasticity. As a comprehensive review of current research at each of these levels is beyond the scope of this chapter, we will focus on research from our laboratory using an integrative research strategy designed to provide increased understanding of long-term memory storage mechanisms at the system, cellular, and molecular level. Fundamental, multiple-level understanding of the neurobiological basis of memory is, of course, essential for advances in the diagnosis, treatment and, ultimately, prevention of memory disorders.

Extensive systems-level pharmacological research in our laboratory has investigated the role of the amygdala as a component of an endogenous memory modulatory system in rodents; this research is briefly discussed in the following section. A central hypothesis of this research is that the amygdala modulates the

Pharmacological Treatment of Alzheimer's Disease: Molecular and Neurobiological Foundations,
Edited by Brioni and Decker
ISBN 0-471-16758-4   © 1997 Wiley-Liss, Inc.

storage of memory at other brain sites in accordance with the affective importance of the experience. This premise predicts functional interactions between
the amygdala and other structures known to be important in memory formation
and storage; recent findings suggesting such interactions are next discussed. The
conceptual core of memory consolidation is that molecular processes that alter
synaptic function within individual neurons are initiated during training and mature in the subsequent hours. The electrophysiological phenomena of long-term
potentiation (LTP) and long-term depression (LTD) in mammalian systems, and
long-term facilitation (LTF) in invertebrate systems provide the most plausible
known cellular substrates of behavioral memory. Research in these systems
has identified specific molecular pathways important for neuronal plastic responses. Recent investigations using molecular genetic approaches have begun
to analyze the role of these molecular pathways in learning and memory in animals. These strategies and initial findings from our laboratory are then discussed. Next, we briefly discuss how molecular and systems-level approaches
will necessarily converge to contribute to our understanding of how the brain encodes memories. And lastly, we consider how the findings of integrative neuroscience research may help in the development of treatments for neurological diseases of memory.

MODULATION OF MEMORY STORAGE:
THE ROLE OF THE AMYGDALA

Amygdala as Critical Component of Endogenous Memory Modulation System

Memory formation is a temporally dependent process that requires the functional interaction of many types of neurons in several different brain structures.
Extensive research findings indicate that the amygdala serves as a critical component of a neuromodulatory system that serves to regulate the strength of newly
acquired memories. This research and the general approaches used will be
briefly discussed here [for more comprehensive reviews see McGaugh et al.,
(1992, 1993a, 1995a)]. A working model of the neuromodulatory influences on
memory storage that are at least in part mediated by the amygdala is shown in
Figure 1.

The involvement of the amygdala in the regulation of memory storage was first
suggested by studies using posttraining electrical stimulation of the amygdala
(Kesner and Wilburn, 1974; McGaugh and Gold, 1976). Depending on the intensity
of foot shock used in inhibitory avoidance training, the same posttraining electrical
stimulation either enhanced or impaired retention performance: When low foot
shock intensities were used, retention was enhanced; in contrast, when high foot
shock intensities were used, retention was impaired (Gold et al., 1975). Furthermore, stimulation of the amygdala, which impaired retention in naive rats, enhanced retention performance of adrenal demedullated rats (Bennett et al., 1985;
Liang et al., 1985). Other investigators have reported that posttraining reversible in-

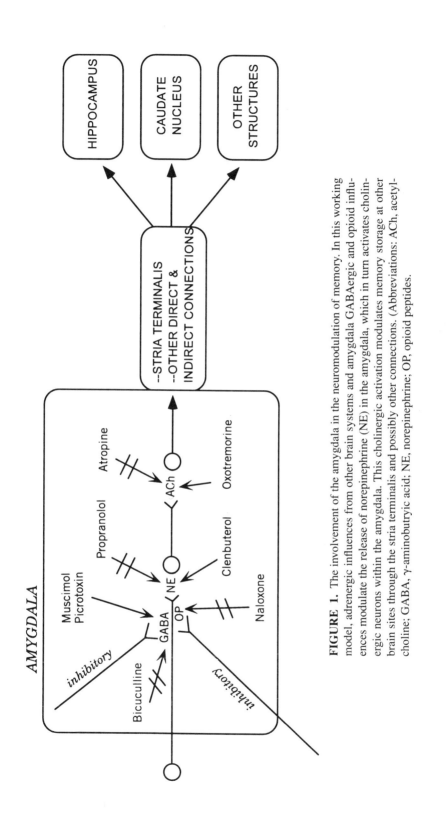

FIGURE 1. The involvement of the amygdala in the neuromodulation of memory. In this working model, adrenergic influences from other brain systems and amygdala GABAergic and opioid influences modulate the release of norepinephrine (NE) in the amygdala, which in turn activates cholinergic neurons within the amygdala. This cholinergic activation modulates memory storage at other brain sites through the stria terminalis and possibly other connections. (Abbreviations: ACh, acetylcholine; GABA, γ-aminobutryic acid; NE, norepinephrine; OP, opioid peptides.

activation of the amygdala using tetrodotoxin produced retrograde amnesia in rats trained in an inhibitory avoidance task (Bucherelli et al., 1992). Additionally, findings from our laboratory indicated that, in an appetitively motivated task, posttraining reversible inactivation of the amygdala with lidocaine following a decrease in food award impaired rats' memory for this "disappointing" event (Salinas et al., 1993). Together, these and numerous other studies provide strong evidence that the amygdala is critically involved in modulating the storage of memory for affective experiences [reviewed in McGaugh et al. (1992, 1993a, 1995a) and Roozendaal et al. (In press)].

Amygdala Noradrenergic, Opioid Peptidergic, and GABAergic Influences on Memory Storage

It is well established that posttraining systemic administration of the adrenomedullary hormone epinephrine can enhance long-term memory of recently acquired information (Borrell et al., 1983; Gold and van Buskirk 1975; Gold et al., 1977; Introini-Collison and McGaugh, 1986; Liang et al., 1985; Sternberg et al., 1985). Moreover, animals given memory-enhancing doses of epinephrine achieve plasma levels comparable to those of untreated animals given training that results in good retention (Gold and McCarty, 1981). Such findings suggest that endogenous release of epinephrine and possibly other stress hormones following behavioral training modulates the storage of recently acquired memories.

Extensive evidence supports the view that epinephrine influences on memory are due, at least in part, to activation of the central noradrenergic systems mediated through stimulation of peripheral β-adrenergic receptors on visceral afferents (Gold and van Buskirk, 1978a, b; Introini-Collison et al., 1992; Weil-Malherbe et al., 1959). Moreover, the memory-enhancing effects of systemic treatments of epinephrine can be blocked by: (1) excitotoxic lesions of the amygdala (Cahill and McGaugh, 1991); (2) intra-amygdala infusions of the β-adrenergic antagonist propranolol (Liang et al., 1986); and (3) lesions of the stria terminalis, a major afferent/efferent pathway of the amygdala (Liang and McGaugh, 1983). Also, intra-amygdala infusion of propranolol impairs retention performance (Gallagher et al., 1981). Further, concurrent intra-amygdala administration of norepinephrine and propranolol block the enhancement of memory seen when norepinephrine is administered alone (Liang et al., 1986). These experiments strongly suggest that release of norepinephrine in the amygdala regulates memory storage. In support of this view, the findings of a recent study from our laboratory using microdialysis and high-performance liquid chromatography (HPLC) indicate that norepinephrine levels in the amygdala increase markedly after rats receive foot shock stimulation comparable in intensity and duration to that typically used in inhibitory avoidance training (McGaugh et al., 1995b).

It is well established that systemic administration of opioid peptidergic and γ-amino-butyric-acid-related (GABAergic) drugs also modulate memory storage [Brioni and McGaugh (1988); and reviewed in Castellano et al. (1990, Gallagher et al. (1985), Izquierdo et al. (1991), and McGaugh et al. (1993b)]. Furthermore, extensive experimental evidence indicates that the amygdala mediates the memory-modulating effects of such drugs [Brioni et al. (1989); and reviewed in McGaugh et al. (1992, 1993a)]. Other findings strongly argue that intra-amygdala opioid and GABAergic drug effects on memory are mediated by the amygdala noradrenergic system. For example, intra-amygdala infusion of the opiate antagonist naloxone alone enhances memory, whereas concurrent infusion of naloxone and propranolol blocks the enhancement (Gallagher et al., 1981; Introini-Collison et al., 1989). Similarly, the memory-enhancing effects of intra-amygdala infusions of the $GABA_A$ antagonist bicuculline are attenuated when bicuculline is administered concurrently with propranolol (Introini-Collison et al., 1994). The evidence indicating that the memory-modulating effects of intra-amygdala GABAergic and opioid peptidergic drugs can be overridden by noradrenergic influences strongly suggests that these systems function within the amygdala to modulate norepinephrine release in the amygdala. Such a role for opioid peptides in the brain has been reported (Werling et al., 1989).

Two additional findings from our laboratory indicate that amygdala norepinephrine release exerts its effects on memory by activating cholinergic receptors within the amygdala. First, concurrent intra-amygdala infusion of the cholinergic antagonist atropine and the adrenergic agonist clenbuterol blocks the memory-enhancing effects seen when clenbuterol is administered alone (Introini-Collison et al., 1996). Second, intra-amygdala infusion of propranolol does not block the memory-enhancing effects of systemically administered oxotremorine, a muscarinic cholinergic agonist (Introini-Collison et al., 1996). Again, these results suggest that amygdala noradrenergic systems subsequently activate cholinergic receptors within the amygdala (see Figure 1).

Basolateral Nucleus of Amygdala Mediates Several Memory Modulatory Effects

Recent work in this laboratory suggests that the basolateral nucleus of the amygdala plays an especially important role in modulating memory stage. As was noted, inactivation of the amygdala following inhibitory avoidance training impairs retention (Bucherelli et al., 1992). The findings of a recent study from our laboratory using lidocaine to functionally and transiently inactivate specific amygdala nuclei suggest that the basolateral nucleus of the amygdala plays a critical role in memory consolidation. Rats implanted with cannulae aimed at either the central nucleus or the basolateral complex of the amygdala were trained in one-trial inhibitory avoidance, and lidocaine or vehicle infusions were administered at different delays after training (Parent and McGaugh, 1994). As shown in Figure 2, infusion of lidocaine immediately after training into the basolateral, but not central, nucleus significantly impaired retention performance 2 days later relative to controls. Additionally, infusion of lidocaine into the basolateral nucleus 6 h, but not 24 h, after training also impaired retention of the task; these data clearly indicate the importance of the basolateral nucleus of the amygdala for consolidation of this aversive task.

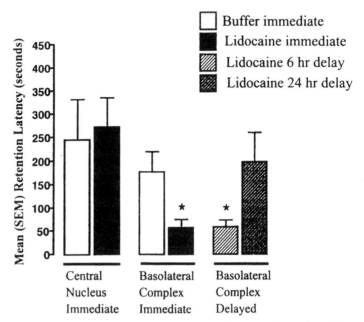

FIGURE 2. Posttraining infusion of lidocaine into the basolateral complex of the amygdala impairs memory of inhibitory avoidance training. Lidocaine hydrochloride was infused into the basolateral complex immediately, 6 h, or 24 h after training in one trial inhibitory avoidance, or into the central nucleus immediately after training. Infusion of lidocaine into the basolateral complex immediately or up to 6 h after training impaired retention performance 48 h later (*, $P < 0.05$ compared to vehicle infusion group; from Parent and McGaugh, 1994).

It is well established that benzodiazepines impair memory (Lister, 1985; Thiebot, 1985). Our finding that lesions of the amygdala block the amnestic effects of diazepam in an inhibitory avoidance task suggest that benzodiazepine effects on memory are mediated at least in part through influences involving the amygdala (Tomaz et al., 1991). To localize the site of action within the amygdala mediating the benzodiazepine effect on memory, rats with excitotoxic-induced lesions of either the central, lateral, or basolateral nuclei or sham lesions were given systemic injections of diazepam or vehicle prior to training in a continuous multiple-trial inhibitory avoidance task. The lesions and drug treatments did not affect acquisition of this task. Diazepam impaired retention performance in sham-, central-nucleus-, and lateral-nucleus-lesioned rats, but did not affect retention performance of the basolateral-lesioned group (Tomaz et al., 1992). These findings suggest that the benzodiazepine effect on memory is mediated by the basolateral nucleus. Interestingly, an intact basolateral nucleus is not required for acquisition of this task. But, as noted above, inactivation of this nucleus after training (i.e., during the consolidation process) interferes with memory formation (Parent and McGaugh, 1994).

Adenocortical hormones such as glucocorticoids are released in stressful conditions and are known to modulate memory storage in animals [reviewed in Bohus (1994) and McEwen and Sapolsky (1995). Glucocorticoids readily cross the blood–brain barrier, and because of their lipophilic properties, cross cellular membranes to bind their intracellular receptors. Glucocorticoid receptors are ligand-modulated transcription factors that regulate gene expression through specific DNA sequences, hormone response elements, in the promoters of individual responsive genes [reviewed in Beato et al. (1995)]. As synaptic activity-dependent changes in gene expression are critical to the formation of long-term memory, regulation of transcriptional processes provides an important mechanism for the modulation of memory storage. Several recent experiments from within out laboratory demonstrate that the basolateral complex mediates the memory modulatory effects of glucocorticoids in inhibitory avoidance and spatial water maze tasks (Roozendaal and McGaugh, 1996; Roozendaal et al., in press). These experiments show that the memory-modulating effects of systemically or centrally administered glucocorticoid receptor agonists or antagonists are blocked by lesions of the basolateral, but not central, amygdaloid nucleus. Moreover, and as discussed in further detail later, recent evidence suggests that basolateral nucleus neuronal activity functions as a cofactor for the neuroplastic changes in the hippocampus and possibly other brain structures (Roozendaal and McGaugh, in press).

EVIDENCE FOR AMYGDALA MODULATION OF MEMORY STORAGE AT OTHER BRAIN SITES

As discussed, extensive evidence indicates that the amygdala modulates the storage of memories at other sites within the brain and that the basolateral nucleus plays an important role in this modulation. Recent experimental evidence indicates that hippocampal and caudate nucleus processes involved in memory storage may be targets of this amygdala-mediated modulation. The findings of a recent series of experiments by Ikegaya and colleagues indicate that the basolateral nucleus is involved in modulating *in vivo* LTP in the medial perforant path. Lesions, or functional inactivation using the local anesthetic tetracaine, of the basolateral, but not central, nucleus of the amygdala significantly attenuated the induction of perforant path LTP without affecting baseline synaptic responses (Ikegaya et al., 1994, 1995a). Additionally, they reported that LTP was induced in the dentate gyrus by high-frequency stimulation of the basolateral nucleus of the amygdala paired with weak tetanic stimulation of the perforant path; weak tetanic stimulation of the perforant path alone was not sufficient to induce LTP (Ikegaya et al., 1995). Together, these results suggest that the basolateral nucleus of the amygdala modulates neuroplastic changes in the dentate gyrus.

It is well established that the water maze spatial task, in which an animal has to learn the location of a submerged platform in a pool of water by utilizing extramaze cues, is critically dependent on hippocampal, but not caudate nucleus, function (Morris et al., 1982; Moser et al., 1993; Packard and McGaugh, 1992). In contrast, cued learning, in which an animal swims to a variably positioned visible platform, is dependent on caudate nucleus, and not hippocampal, function (Packard and Mc-Gaugh, 1992). Recent findings from our laboratory indicate that the amygdala can modulate memory of both tasks, but that amygdala function is not required for the retention performance of either (Packard et al., 1994). Immediately after animals were trained in either the spatial or cued water maze tasks, amphetamine or vehicle was infused into the hippocampus, the caudate nucleus, or the amygdala via implanted cannulae. In the spatial learning task, the posttraining amphetamine enhanced retention performance when infused into either the hippocampus or amygdala, whereas in the cued learning task, caudate nucleus and amygdala infusions enhanced retention performance. Thus, although the memory-enhancing effects of posttraining intracaudate or intrahippocampal infusions of amphetamine were specific to the tasks known to be dependent on their respective functions, the intra-amygdala amphetamine effect was not task dependent. To determine whether the memory-enhancing effect of intra-amygdala amphetamine was based on neural changes within the amygdala, additional animals were trained in the two tasks and, as in the prior experiment, given either vehicle or amphetamine infusions into the amygdala following training. However, these animals were then given intra-amygdala infusions of the local anesthetic lidocaine immediately prior to the retention test. As in the initial experiment, intra-amygdala amphetamine enhanced retention performance of both tasks. Importantly, however, intra-amygdala lidocaine infusions administered prior to the retention test did not block the memory-enhancing effects of intra-amygdala amphetamine. These experiments indicate that a functional amygdala is not critical for the expression of the enhanced memory and provide further support for the view that amygdala activity modulates memory storage at other brain sites.

Recent experiments within our laboratory provide additional evidence for a functional interaction between the basolateral nucleus of the amygdala and the hippocampus. As described earlier, the basolateral nucleus of the amygdala mediates the memory-modulating effects of systemically administered dexamethasone, a potent glucocorticoid receptor agonist (Roozendaal and McGaugh, 1996; Roozendaal et al., in press). To examine possible interactions between the basolateral nucleus and the hippocampus in glucocorticoid modulation of memory, sham-, central-nucleus-, or basolateral-nucleus-lesioned rats were given intrahippocampal infusions of the glucocorticoid receptor antagonist RU 38486 or vehicle prior to training in the spatial water maze task (Figure 3; Roozendaal and McGaugh, in press). Two days later animals were given a retention test consisting of three trials. RU 38486 did not affect the acquisition of the task for any of the groups. Also, none of the lesions affected acquisition or retention in the vehicle-treated groups. In sham- and central-nucleus-lesioned animals, however, RU 38486 impaired retention performance. Strikingly, the memory-impairing effects of intrahippocampal infusions of the glucocorticoid receptor antagonist were completely blocked in the basolateral-lesioned animals.

Taken together, the experiments discussed strongly support the hypothesis that the amygdala is involved in modulating the storage of information in other brain regions. The finding that lesions of the basolateral nucleus of the amygdala block the

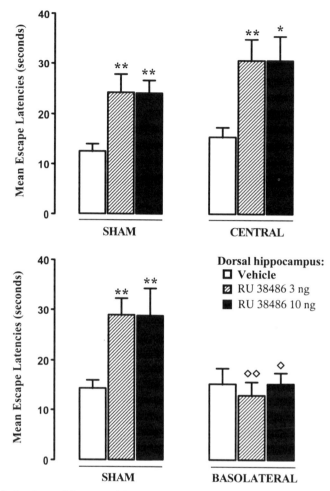

FIGURE 3. Lesions of the amygdala basolateral complex block the memory-impairing effects of intrahippocampal infusion of RU 38486. Prior to training in a spatial water maze task, rats with central nucleus, basolateral complex, or sham lesions were infused with the glucocorticoid receptor antagonist RU 38486 or vehicle. RU 38486 impaired 48-h retention of the task in sham- and central-nucleus-lesioned, but not basolateral-complex-lesioned, rats relative to the appropriate vehicle control (from Roozendaal and McGaugh, in press). Shown are retention escape latencies (mean ± SEM). *, $P < 0.05$; **, $P < 0.01$ as compared to corresponding vehicle group. ◇, $P < 0.05$; ◇◇, $P < 0.01$ as compared with the corresponding sham lesion-RU 38486 group.

memory-modulating influence of a glucocorticoid receptor antagonist administered directly into the hippocampus clearly suggests that amygdala activity enables the induction of neuroplasticity in the hippocampus. Again, these findings are consistent with evidence that the basolateral nucleus modulates LTP in the dentate gyrus (Ikegaya et al., 1994, 1995a).

SEARCH FOR CELLULAR AND MOLECULAR PATHWAYS OF MEMORY CONSOLIDATION

Cellular Models and Molecular Pathways

It is generally believed that memories are created by experience-induced changes in synaptic strengths. The predominant cellular models of such input-specified synaptic alterations are LTF in aplysia neurons and LTP and LTD in mammalian systems [for reviews see Alberini et al. (1995), Malenka (1994), and Maren and Baudry (1995)]. A central commonality of these cellular phenomena is the critical importance of localized changes in intracellular Ca^{2+} and adenosine $3',5'$-monophosphate (cyclic-AMP, or cAMP) concentrations in both pre- and postsynaptic sites (Alberini et al., 1995; Huang et al., 1994; Malenka, 1991; Otani and Ben-Ari, 1993; Weisskopf et al., 1994). These cellular second messengers and associated systems modulate the activity of kinases and phosphatases, which have a wide range of substrates ranging from synaptic proteins to nuclear transcription factors. Short-term modification of synaptic function, which may provide a basis for short-term memory, is most likely due to transient changes in phosphorylation state of synaptic components rather than to alterations in cellular transcriptional or translational processes.

The formation or consolidation of long-term memory requires additional mechanisms. There are several parallels between behavioral memory consolidation and the maintenance phases of LTF, LTD, and LTP. These parallels involve a number of common biochemical pathways including, but not necessarily limited to, alteration of kinase and phosphatase activities, redistribution of kinases within the cell, glycosylation of synaptic components, modulation of proteins involved in neuronal adhesion properties, and alterations in transcriptional programs of cells [reviewed in Abraham et al. (1991), Alberini et al. (1995), Cole et al. (1990), Kaczmarek (1993), Malenka (1991, 1994), Maren and Baudry (1995), Matthies (1989), Otani and Ben-Ari (1993), Rose (1991, 1995a), and Worley et al. (1990a, b)]. Of these many biochemical changes that comprise the cellular correlates of consolidation, it is the behaviorally driven changes in transcription patterns within individual neurons that may be of the greatest utility in providing a bridge between cellular and systems-level understanding of memory. A simple diagram of proposed molecular pathways leading to the formation of long-term memory with an emphasis on the transcriptionally mediated events is shown in Figure 4.

Transient administration of inhibitors of RNA and protein synthesis during a critical period following either behavioral training or direct neuronal stimulation is known to impair long-term memory, LTF, and LTP (Davis and Squire, 1984; Huang et al., 1994; Nguyen et al., 1994; Tully et al., 1994). The effect of RNA and protein synthesis inhibitors on long-term plasticity could be due either to interruption of steady-state gene expression or disruption of an inducible program of gene expression or a combination of the two. We now know that the transcriptional programs of neurons can be readily altered after periods of synaptic activity driven by behavioral, pharmacological, or electrical influences (Cole et al., 1990; Hess et al., 1995;

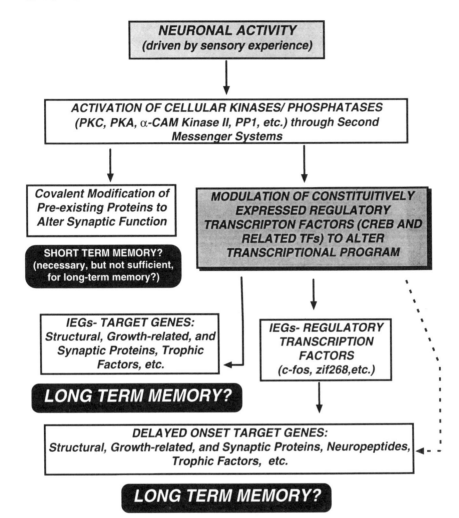

FIGURE 4. A proposed molecular pathway leading to the formation of long-term memory, with an emphasis on transcriptionally mediated events. Synaptic activity driven by information processing in the brain leads to localized alterations in intraneuronal pools of Ca^{2+} and cAMP, which in turn activate cellular kinases and phosphatases. These enzymes modulate the activity of a wide range of preexisting cellular proteins including synaptic components and nuclear localized transcription factors. In the nucleus, activation of CREB and related transcription factors initiates a cascade of gene expression, which is required for the formation of long-term memory.

Kaczmarek, 1993; Konradi et al., 1994; Lyford et al., 1995; Nikolaev et al., 1992; Popovici et al., 1990; Worley et al., 1990b; Yamagata et al., 1993). The transcription of immediate-early genes (IEGs) occurs rapidly after neuronal stimulation and is not dependent on protein synthesis; the transcription factors required to express these genes are constituitively present and need only to be posttranslationally modified for high activity (Armstrong and Montminy, 1993). While many of the first identified IEGs were shown to encode transcription factors such as c-Fos and zif268 (also known as egrl, Krox24, and NGFI-A), recently identified IEGs have been shown to encode cytoplasmic and dendritic proteins with both known and unknown functions (Lyford et al., 1995; Yamagata et al., 1993). In contrast to IEGs, delayed-onset genes require the expression of transcription factor encoding IEGs before their expression can commence. These genes can encode trophic factors, neuropeptides, synaptic components, structural proteins, and so forth. The regulation of this transcriptional cascade and the relevance of specific transcription factors in long-term memory processes is considered below.

Correlational Studies: Use of IEGs as Markers of Plastic Responses

Because the steady-state levels of IEGs within individual neurons are extremely low but can be rapidly and transiently induced, IEGs have quickly gained utility as markers of neuronal plasticity. For such studies, antibodies or antisense riboprobes are typically used to detect the cellular localization of the protein or the RNA, respectively, of the IEG of interest in brain slices. Recent studies have almost exclusively used probes for regulatory transcription factor IEGs such as c-Fos and zif268 (Beck and Fibiger, 1995; Bialy et al., 1992; Duncan et al., 1993; Hess et al., 1995; Kaczmarek, 1993; Mello et al, 1995; Nikolaev et al., 1992). By the very complex nature of eukaroytic transcriptional regulation, regulatory transcription factors are likely to have pleiotropic effects in different neurons; thus, transient induction of c-Fos in "neuron A" may initiate a completely different transcriptional cascade than the transient induction of c-Fos in neighboring "neuron B." Stated simply, transcription factor IEGs are of little diagnostic value as markers of *specific* plastic changes, but only indicate the likelihood of plastic change. The further discovery and characterization of neuronal IEGs with defined roles in cellular physiology such as those described by Worley and colleagues (Lyford et al., 1995; Yamagata et al., 1993) will be of great utility as markers of specific plastic responses in behavioral studies.

Correlational studies in which molecular changes of trained animals are compared to control groups (as described earlier) face two fundamental problems. First, such experiments confront the nearly intractable problem of the appropriate "learning controls." That is, although a training-induced change in the levels of a specific mRNA or protein may be detected, it is impossible to know if that change reflects memory formation per se and is not a general response related to sensory stimulation, novelty, stress, or changes in physical activity. Second, it is the underlying assumption that a large percentage of cells will undergo a change in expression levels of the studied gene, thus allowing detection above a background threshold; it remains possible that such critical, memory-related biochemical change may occur in only a small percentage of neurons precluding detection by current techniques. In this case, a negative result might be interpreted inappropriately. So, while correlative data are a necessary part of an experimental investigation into the molecular basis of memory formation, such data gain much more power when applied in conjunction with a functional demonstration of the role of the molecule of interest in a specific aspect of behavior. Our recent efforts to establish a functional role for two specific gene products in learning and memory are discussed below.

Transcription Factors CREB and c-Fos in Hippocampally Mediated Memory Storage

Our investigation of the role of transcriptional plasticity, the changing of the cellular transcriptional program in response to extracellular signals, in the formation of long-term memory in the rat has focused on two specific regulatory transcription factors, the cAMP response element binding protein (CREB) and c-Fos. As will be described, both of these have been implicated in modulating neuronal plasticity in the central nervous system. For these experiments, we used intrahippocampal infusion of antisense oligonucleotides to disrupt the expression of these two transcription factors and examine the effect on learning and memory of different tasks. The hippocampus was chosen as an anatomical site for these studies because of its well-established role in the time-limited storage and/or retrieval of memories (Jarrard, 1993; Zola-Morgan and Squire, 1993).

Antisense oligonucleotide strategies provide an approach that circumvents many of the limitations of genetically modified "knockout" mice for use in behavioral studies (Routtenberg 1995; Takahashi et al., 1994; Wahlestedt, 1994). Importantly, antisense approaches allow anatomical specificity of protein function to be assessed and provide precise temporal control. The acute nature of administration obviates problems associated with molecular compensatory mechanisms (Bourtchuladze et al., 1994; Hummler et al., 1994; Rudnicki et al., 1992) or developmental defects (Grant et al., 1992; Johnson et al., 1992; Paylor et al., 1994) seen in knockout mice. Also, the use of sense and mismatch oligonucleotide control groups allows careful assessment of the specificity of antisense oligonucleotide-mediated effects on learning and memory.

Oligonucleotides are readily taken up by cells in the brain; cellular uptake of oligonucleotides may occur via receptor-mediated endocytosis (Loke et al., 1989; Yakubov et al., 1989). For use in antisense experiments, a modified form of oligonucleotides, termed phosphorothioate oligonucleotides (S-oligos), are frequently used. S-oligos replace one of the nonbridging oxygen atoms in the phosphodiester backbone of DNA with a sulfur atom; this conservative modification makes S-oligos much more resistant to the action of intracellular nucleases. Inside the cell, antisense oligodeoxynucleotides, both unmodified (phosphodiester) and phosphorothioate, are thought to decrease the levels of a particular protein by base pairing to the mRNA encoding it to form a partially duplex structure that can act as a substrate for cellular RNases to increase the turnover of the message, or block translation of the mRNA (translation arrest) or both [reviewed in Ghosh and Cohen (1992)]. CREB and c-Fos antisense S-oligos of the same base composition as used in our studies have previously been shown to specifically decrease the levels of their respective proteins in the rat striatum (Konradi et al., 1994; Konradi and Heckers, 1995).

The regulatory transcription factor CREB is expressed throughout the brain and can be phosphorylated both by protein kinase A and α-calcium/calmodulin kinase II, which are activated by cAMP and Ca^{2+}, respectively [reviewed in Vallejo and Habener (1994)]. Phosphorylated CREB activates transcription of genes containing calcium/cAMP response elements (Ca^{2+}/CREs) in their promoters [reviewed in Montminy et al. (1990)]. Thus, CREB and related transcription factors provide the link between changes in second messenger levels to changes in the cell's transcriptional program. Recent studies suggest that transcriptional regulation by CREB and other Ca^{2+}/CRE binding transcription factors plays an important role in neuronal plasticity *in vitro* and in long-term memory in animals (Bourtchuladze et al., 1994; Dash et al., 1990; Yin et al., 1994).

In a recent series of experiments, we used antisense oligonucleotides to acutely alter CREB protein levels in the hippocampus and determine the effect on learning and memory in a water maze spatial task (Guzowski and McGaugh, submitted). In experiment 1 (see Figure 5a), CREB antisense or "scrambled" sequence control S-oligos (2 nmol/side in a volume of 1 µL) were infused bilaterally into the dorsal hippocampus approximately 20 h prior to training in a water maze spatial task. On the day of training, animals were given two training sessions consisting of five trials each. The AM and PM training sessions were separated by 4 h. Two days later, a retention test consisting of three trials was given. The antisense treatment did not affect acquisition performance: Antisense CREB and scrambled S-oligo groups learned to swim to and mount the submerged platform at similar rates. In contrast, the retention performance of the CREB antisense group was significantly worse than the random group. Although the antisense group showed significant "forgetting" relative to the scrambled group in the retention test, the antisense group readily relearned the location of

---

FIGURE 5. Intrahippocampal administration of antisense oligonucleotides to the transcription factor CREB impairs memory consolidation of a spatial water maze task. (*a*) 18–20 h prior to training in a spatial water maze task, rats were infused with 2 nmol of either CREB antisense S-oligos or control "scrambled" S-oligos. Two training sessions of five trials each were given, separated by 4 h; 48-h retention performance of the CREB antisense group was significantly impaired for retention trials 1 and 2 and for the retention session as a whole (ANOVA; **, $P < 0.01$; $\diamond$, $P < 0.001$, respectively), while no significant differences between the groups were observed for the training trials or sessions. (Guzowski and McGaugh, submitted). (*b*) Three experiments examining the temporal specificity of the CREB antisense S-oligo effects on retention performance (unpublished data). Experiment 1 is described above. For experiment 2, rats were trained exactly as described for experiment 1, except S-oligo infusions were given the day after training. Retention performance was tested 3 days after infusions. In experiment 3, rats were given two infusions of either CREB antisense S-oligos or scrambled S-oligos 5 and 6 days before training. A single training session of 6 trials was given and retention was tested 2 days later. Of these experiments, only CREB antisense infusions one day prior to training (experiment 1) led to significant retention deficits indicating a specific effect on memory consolidation.

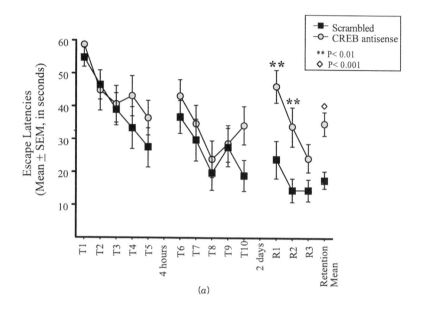

(a)

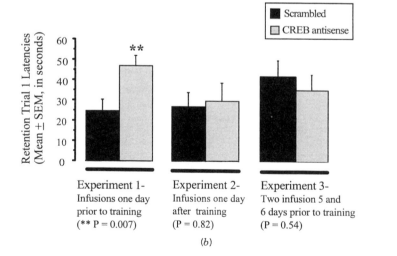

(b)

the platform during the three retention trials, demonstrating that hippocampal function was intact in these animals at the time of the retention test. These findings support the view that CREB regulates the expression of genes involved in the process of memory consolidation. Additionally, the findings indicate that memory up to 4 h after training is not critically dependent on CREB-mediated processes.

Two additional experiments were performed to address the temporal specificity of the observed antisense of oligonucleotide effect on retention performance. In experiment 2 (Figure 5*b*), rats were trained exactly as described for experiment 1. The day following training, animals were counterbalanced, based on acquisition performance, and divided into two groups for bilateral antisense or scrambled oligonucleotide infusion (2 nmol in 1 μL per hemisphere). Three days later, a retention test consisting of three trials was given. For both experiments 1 and 2, the time from oligonucleotide infusions to retention test was 3 days. The infusions of the CREB antisense S-oligos one day after training did not affect retention performance. This result indicates that the antisense oligonucleotide-mediated impairment of retention performance in experiment 1 was not due to a generalized impairment of retrieval mechanisms, but rather, was due to impairment in the consolidation of the memory of the training experience.

For experiment 3 (Figure 5*b*), hippocampally cannulated rats were given two bilateral infusions (1 nmol in 1 mL per hemisphere per day) of either CREB antisense or scrambled S-oligos separated by 1 day, 5 and 6 days prior to training in the water maze. Training consisted of one session of six trials. Two days later, a retention test of three trials was given. No differences were observed in acquisition or retention performance of the two groups. The fact that infusions 1 day (experiment 1), but not 5 days, prior to training impaired memory was expected in view of the fairly rapid turnover of S-oligos in the brain (unpublished observations). Other investigators have reported that, in a sequence-specific fashion, the same CREB antisense S-oligo sequences applied to the striatum blocked the induction of c-Fos in striatal neurons when infused 18, 26, and 46, but not 70, hours prior to systemic administration of haloperidol (Konradi and Heckers, 1995). Thus, the time course of recovery from CREB antisense S-oligos is consistent when examined at biochemical or behavioral levels. Taken together, the data from experiments 1, 2, and 3 provide the most direct evidence to date that CREB plays a critical role in mediating cellular events required for long-term memory storage in the mammalian brain.

One of the genes CREB regulates is yet another transcription factor, the IEG c-Fos (Armstrong and Montminy, 1993; Konradi et al., 1994; Robertson et al., 1995). c-Fos interacts with members of the Jun transcription factor family to form the functional transcription factor AP-1; AP-1 activates transcription of genes containing AP-1 binding sites within their promoters (Curran and Vogt, 1992; Morgan and Curran, 1989). In formulating these experiments, CREB and c-Fos were chosen for study because they represent interrelated primary and secondary links, respectively, from activation of second messenger systems to changes in genomic expression. As noted above, c-Fos protein and RNA levels can be rapidly induced in the brain in response to behavioral training and as such have been used as markers of "neuronal activity" by many. Despite this, there has not yet been a clear demonstration that c-Fos induction in any particular brain structure is related to processes critical to long-term memory formation. For example, while c-Fos knockout mice have been generated, the severe developmental defects seen in these mice preclude any straightforward interpretation of behavioral data (Johnson et al., 1992; Paylor et al., 1994).

Recent findings indicate that, following active avoidance training, hippocampal c-Fos RNA levels are elevated in comparison with those of caged control rats (Nikolaev et al., 1992). Using quantitative Western blot analysis, we have observed an approximately 50% increase in hippocampal c-Fos protein levels 90 min after training in the continuous multiple-trial inhibitory avoidance (CMIA) task (Guzowski and McGaugh, unpublished results). To examine whether this induction plays a role in memory of this task, rats received bilateral intrahippocampal infusions of either c-Fos antisense S-oligos or random sequence S-oligos (1 nmol in 1 µL per hemisphere) 3–4 h prior to training in CMIA; retention was tested 2 days later. The infusions of c-Fos antisense S-oligos did not affect acquisition. In contrast, the retention performance of the c-Fos antisense group was significantly worse than that of the random control group; several animals in the c-Fos antisense group showed almost complete amnesia, while no such animals were observed in the random group (Figure 6; Guzowski and McGaugh, unpublished results). These results strongly suggest a functional role for c-Fos protein expression in memory consolidation of this task.

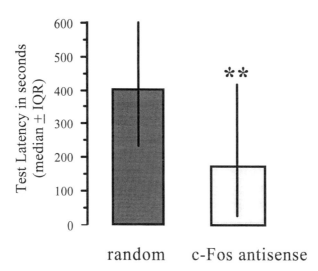

FIGURE 6. Intrahippocampal administration of antisense oligonucleotides to the immediate early transcription factor c-Fos impairs retention in an inhibitory avoidance task. 3–4 h prior to training in continuous multiple-trial inhibitory avoidance (CMIA), rats received infusion of either c-Fos antisense S-oligos or random sequence control S-oligos. No differences were observed between the groups for acquisition of the task. Retention was tested 2 days later; relative to the random control group, the c-Fos antisense group exhibited significant memory impairment for this task. (**, $P < 0.05$, Mann-Whitney U test; Guzowski and McGaugh, unpublished findings).

INTEGRATION OF MOLECULAR AND SYSTEM APPROACHES TO MEMORY

As the relevant molecular pathways integral to memory formation become well defined, it will be possible to exploit this information to learn more about the interactions between different systems within the brain. Future experiments may be designed to examine the consequences of known memory-modulating drugs and hormones on defined molecular pathways within specific neurons of particular structures. Additionally, the effect of lesions, reversible inactivation, or neurotransmitter stimulation of specific neuromodulatory structures, such as the basolateral complex of the amygdala, on these same defined molecular pathways in distal structures will help elucidate functionally interacting systems involved in memory storage. Such integrative approaches will become necessary to lead toward a more complete understanding of brain function and dysfunction.

CONCLUDING REMARKS: TOWARD NEW CLINICAL APPROACHES

Because the research being done in our laboratory has focused on animal models, we can only speculate how its implications might translate into clinical applications for the treatment of memory disorders such as Alzheimer's disease. Although it may seem a simplistic and obvious statement, cellular physiology is the net result of the genes expressed within a cell; the results of aging and the development of neurodegenerative conditions are the products of altered cellular physiology due to changes in the control of gene expression and the predisposing influences of genetic background. Many of these degenerative changes in genomic control may be the result of cumulative oxidative damage to cellular components and changes in the levels of critical regulatory factors. If these can be forestalled, the onset and severity of neurodegenerative disorders might be controlled.

While this is easily said, the hard question of "How?" remains. Certainly, antioxidant compounds may have a number of beneficial applications in the prevention of disease, including memory disorders associated with aging. Also, if we know how the "regulators" of basic brain function are regulated, perhaps we can stimulate these pathways that are waning in the aging individual. Toward this end, and as discussed in Chapter 22 of this volume, hormonal replacement therapies may prove beneficial in reducing the incidence of Alzheimer's disease. Although such treatments undoubtedly affect many systems and molecular pathways, a recent study demonstrates that CREB levels can be regulated by hormones (Walker et al., 1995). As demonstrated (in Figure 5a), acute disruption of hippocampal CREB levels can have dramatic effects on memory. While it is not known whether CREB levels change in the aging individual, it can be easily imagined that aging-related chronic down-regulation of CREB within the brain could lead to degenerative conditions and memory impairment. Again, it is our hope that a detailed basic knowledge of the critical pathways important in different aspects of brain function will lead to earlier diagnosis of brain disease and more effective treatments.

Gene therapy offers an alternative approach to correcting imbalances in the levels of specific gene products and may prove useful in the future for the treatment of Alzheimer's disease. These strategies involve the use of vector delivery systems or grafts of genetically modified cells to either replace a defective allele or increase expression of a limiting factor [reviewed in Suhr and Gage (1993)]. As opposed to hormonal replacement therapies that may help prevent neurological disease, the invasive nature of gene therapy approaches will limit their use to the treatment of disease states. While these techniques currently have limitations for use in the treatment of neurological disease, this is an extremely active field of research and given time, these limitations will likely be overcome.

ACKNOWLEDGMENTS

This research was supported by an Institutional NRSA T32A600096 (JFG) and USPHS Research Grant MH12526 from the National Institute of Mental Health and the National Institute on Drug Abuse (JLM).

REFERENCES

Abraham WC, Dragunow M, and Tate WP (1991): The role of immediate early genes in the stabilization of long-term potentiation. Mol Neurobiol 5:297–313.

Alberini CM, Ghirardi M, Huang Y-Y, Nguyen PV, Kandel ER (1995): A molecular switch for the consolidation of long-term memory: cAMP-inducible gene expression. Ann N Y Acad Sci 758:261–286.

Armstrong RC, Montminy MR (1993): Transsynaptic control of gene expression. Ann Rev Neurosci 16:17–29.

Beato M, Herrlich P, Schutz G (1995): Steroid hormone receptors: Many actors in search of a plot. Cell 83:851–857.

Beck, CHM, Fibiger HC (1995): Condition fear-induced changes in behavior and in the expression of the immediate early gene c-fos: With and without diazepam pretreatment. J Neurosci 15(1):709–720.

Bennett C, Liang KC, McGaugh JL (1985): Depletion of adrenal catecholamines alters the amnestic effect of amygdala stimulation. Beh Brain Res 15:83–91.

Bialy M, Nikolaev E, Beck J, Kaczmarek L (1992): Delayed c-fos expression in sensory cortex following sexual learning in male rats. Mol Brain Res 14:352–356.

Bohus B (1994): Humoral modulation of learning and memory process: Physiological significance of brain and peripheral mechanisms. In Delacour J (ed): The Memory Systems of the Brain. Advanced Series in Neuroscience, Vol. 4. Singapore: World Scientific, pp 337–364.

Borrell J, de Kloet ER, Versteeg DHG, Bohus B (1983): Inhibitory avoidance deficit following short-term adrenalectomy in the rat: The role of adrenal catecholamines. Beh Neural Biol 39:241–258.

Bourtchuladze R, Frenguelli B, Blendy J, Cioffi D, Shutz G, Silva AJ (1994): Deficient long-term memory in mice with a targeted mutation of the cAMP-responsive element-binding protein. Cell, 79:59–68.

Brioni JD, McGaugh JL (1988): Posttraining administration of GABAergic antagonists enhance retention of aversively motivated tasks. Psychopharmacology 96:505–510.

Brioni JD, Nagahara AH, McGaugh JL (1989): Involvement of the amygdala GABAergic system in the modulation of memory storage. Brain Res 487:105–112.

Bucherelli C, Tassoni G, Bures J (1992): Time-dependent disruption of passive avoidance acquisition by posttraining intra-amygdala injection of tetrodotoxin in rats. Neurosci Lett 140:231–234.

Cahill L, McGaugh JL (1991): NMDA-induced lesions of the amygdaloid complex block the retention enhancing effect of posttraining epinephrine. Psychobiology, 19:206–210.

Castellano C, Brioni JD, McGaugh JL (1990): GABAergic modulation of memory. In Squire L, Lindenlaub E (eds): "Biology of Memory." Stuttgart: F. K. Schattauer Verlag, pp 361–378.

Cole AJ, Saffen DW, Baraban JM, Worley PF (1990): Synaptic regulation of transcription factor mRNA in the rat hippocampus. In Wurtman, RJ et al. (eds): "Advances in Neurology: Alzheimer's Disease." New York: Raven, pp 103–108.

Curran T, Vogt PK (1992): Dangerous liasons: Fos and Jun, oncogenic transcription factors. In McKnight SL, Yamamoto KR (eds): "Transcriptional Regulation." Cold Spring Harbor, NY: Cold Spring Harbor Laboratory Press, pp 797–831.

Dash PK, Hochner B, Kandel ER (1990): Injection of the cAMP-responsive element into the nucleus of Aplysia sensory neurons blocks long-term facilitation. Nature 345:718–721.

Davis H, Squire LR (1984): Protein synthesis and memory: A review. Psychol Bull 96(3):518–559.

Duncan GE, Johnson KB, Breese GR (1993): Topographic patterns of brain activity in response to swim stress: Assessment by 2-deoxyglucose uptake and expression of Fos-like immunoreactivity. J Neurosci 13(9):3932–3943.

Gallagher M, Fanelli RJ, Bostock E (1985): Opioid peptides: Their position among other neuroregulators of memory. In McGaugh JL (ed): "Contemporary Psychology: Biological Processes and Theoretical Issues." Amsterdam: North Holland, pp 69–94.

Gallagher M, Kapp BS, Pascoe JP, Rapp PR (1981): A neuropharmacology of amygdaloid systems which contribute to learning and memory. In Ben-Ari Y (ed): "The Amygdaloid Complex." Amsterdam: Elsevier-N. Holland, pp 343–354.

Ghosh MK, Cohen JS (1992): Oligodeoxynucleotides as antisense inhibitors of gene expression. Prog Nucleic Acid Res Mol Biol 42:79–126.

Gold PE, McCarty R (1981): Plasma catecholamines: Changes after footshock and seizure-producing frontal cortex stimulation. Beh Neural Biol 31:247–260.

Gold PE, van Buskirk R (1978a): Effects of alpha and beta adrenergic receptor antagonists on post-trial epinephrine modulation of memory: Relationship to posttraining brain norepinephrine concentrations. Beh Biol 24:168–184.

Gold PE, van Buskirk R (1978b): Postttaining brain norepinephrine concentrations: Correlation with retention performance of avoidance training with peripheral epinephrine modulation of memory processing. Beh Biol 23:509–520.

Gold PE, van Buskirk R (1975): Facilitation of time-dependent memory processes with postrial amygdala stimulation: Effect on memory varies with footshock level. Brain Res 86:509–513.

Gold PE, van Buskirk R, Haycock J (1977): Effects of posttraining epinephrine injections on retention of avoidance training in mice. Beh Biol 20:197–207.

Gold PE, Hankins L, Edwards RM, Chester J, McGaugh JL (1975): Memory interference and facilitation with posttrial amygdala stimulation: Effect on memory varies with footschock level. Brain Res 86:509–513.

Grant SGN, O'Dell TJ, Karl KA, Stein PL, Soriano P, Kandel ER (1992): Impaired long-term potentiation, spatial learning, and hippocampal development in *fyn* mutant mice. Science 258:1093–1910.

Guzowski, JF, McGaugh JL: Antisense oligodeoxynucleotide-mediated disruption of hippocampal CREB protein levels impairs memory of a water maze task (submitted).

Hess US, Lynch G, Gall CM (1995): Changes in *c-fos* mRNA expression in rat brain during odor discrimination learning: Differential involvement of hippocampal subfields CA1 and CA3. J Neurosci 15(7):4786–4795.

Huang, Y-Y, Li X-C, Kandel ER (1994): cAMP contributes to mossy fiber LTP by initiating both a covalently mediated early phase and macromolecular synthesis-dependent late phase. Cell 79:69–79.

Hummler E, Cole TJ, Blendy JA, Ganss R, Aguzzi A, Schmid W, Beerman F, Schutz G (1994): Targeted mutation of the CREB gene: Compensation within the CREB/ATF family of transcription factors. Proc Natl Acad Sci (U S A) 91:5647–5651.

Ikegaya Y, Saito H, Abe K (1995a): Requirement of basolateral amygdala neuron activity for the induction of long-term potentiation in the dentate gyrus *in vivo*. Brain Res 671:351–354.

Ikegaya Y, Sait0 H, Abe K (1995b): High-frequency stimulation of the basolateral amygdala facilitates the induction of long-term potentiation in the dentate gyrus *in vivo*. Neurosci Res 22:203–207.

Ikegaya Y, Saito H, Abe K (1994): Attenuated hippocampal long-term potentiation in basolateral amygdala-lesioned rats. Brain Res 656:157–164.

Introini-Collison IB, McGaugh, JL (1986): Epinephrine modulates long-term retention of an aversively motivated discrimination task. Beh Neural Biol 45:358–365.

Introini-Collison IB, Dalmaz C, McGaugh JL (1996): Amygdala β-noradrenergic influences on memory storage involve cholinergic activation. Neurobiol Learn Mem 65:57–64.

Introini-Collison IB, Castellano C, McGaugh JL (1994): Interaction of GABAergic and β-noradrenergic drugs in the regulation of memory storage. Beh Neural Biol 61(2):150–155.

Introini-Collison IB, Saghafi D, Novack G, McGaugh JL (1992): Memory-enhancing effects of posttraining dipivefrin and epinephrine: Involvement of peripheral and central adrenergic receptors. Brain Res 572:81–86.

Introini-Collison IB, Nagahara AH, McGaugh JL (1989): Memory-enhancement with intra-amygdala posttraining naloxone is blocked by concurrent administration of propranolol. Brain Res 476:94–101.

Izquierdo I, Medine JH, Netto CA, Pereira ME (1991): Peripheral and central effects on memory of peripherally and centrally administered opiods and benzodiazepines. In Frederickson RCA, McGaugh JL, Felten DL (eds): "Peripheral Signaling of the Brain: Role in Neural-Immune Interactions, Learning and Memory." Toronto: Hogrefe & Huber, pp 303–314.

Jarrard LE (1993): On the role of the hippocampus in learning and memory. Beh Neural Biol 60:9–26.

Johnson RS, Spiegelman BM, Papaioannou V (1992): Pleiotropic effects of a null mutation in the *c-fos* proto-oncogene. Cell 71(4):577–586.

Kaczmarek L (1993): Molecular biology of vertebrate learning: Is *c-fos* a new beginning? J Neurosci Res 34:377–381.

Kesner RP, Wilburn MW (1974): A review of electrical stimulation of the brain in the context of learning and retention. Behav Biol 10:259–293.

Konradi C, Heckers S (1995): Haloperidol-induced fos expression in striatum is dependent upon transcription factor cyclic AMP response element binding protein. Neuroscience 65(4):1051–1061.

Konradi C, Cole RL, Heckers S, Hyman SE (1994): Amphetamine regulates gene expression in rat striatum via transcription factor CREB. J Neurosci 14(9):5623–5634.

Liang KC, McGaugh JL (1983): Lesions of the stria terminalis attenuate the enhancing effect of posttraining epinephrine on retention of an inhibitory avoidance response. Beh Brain Res 9:49–58.

Liang KC, Juler R, McGaugh JL (1986): Modulating effects of posttraining epinephrine on memory: Involvement of the amygdala noradrenergic system. Brain Res 368:125–133.

Liang, KC, Bennett C, McGaugh JL (1985): Peripheral epinephrine modulates the effects of posttraining amygdala stimulation on memory. Beh Brain Res 15:93–100.

Lister RG (1985): The amnesic action of benzodiazepines in man. Biobehav Rev 9:87–94.

Loke SL, Stein, CA, Zhang, XH, Mori K, Nakanishi M, Subasinghe C, Cohen JS, Neckers, LM (1989): Characterization of oligonucleotide uptake transport into living cells. Proc Natl Acad Sci (U S A) 86:3474–3478.

Lyford GL, Yamagata K, Kaufmann WE, Barnes CA, Sanders LK, Copeland NG, Worley PF (1995): Arc, a growth factor and activity-regulated gene, encodes a novel cytoskeleton-associated protein that is enriched in neuronal dendrites. Neuron 14:433–445.

Malenka RC (1991): The role of postsynaptic calcium in the induction of long-term potentiation. Mol Neurobiol 5:289–295.

Malenka RC (1994): Synaptic plasticity in the hippocampus: LTP and LTD. Cell 78:535–538.

Maren S, Baudry M (1995): Properties and mechanisms of long-term synaptic plasticity in the mammalian brain: Relationships to learning and memory. Neurobiol Learn Mem 63:1–18.

Matthies H (1989): In search of cellular mechanisms of memory storage. Prog Neurobiol 32:277–349.

McEwen BS, Sapolsky RM (1995): Stress and cognitive function. Curr Opin Neurobiol 5:205–216.

McGaugh JL, Gold PE (1976): Modulation of memory by electrical stimulation of the brain. In Rosenzweig MR, Bennett EL (eds): "Neural Mechanisms of Learning and Memory." Cambridge: MIT Press, pp 549–560.

McGaugh JL, Cahill L, Parent MB, Mesches MH, Coleman-Mesches K, Salinas J (1995a): Involvement of the amygdala in the regulation of memory storage. In McGaugh JL, Bermudez-Rattoni F, Prado-Alcala RA (eds): "Plasticity in the Central Nervous System: Learning and Memory." Hillsdale, NJ: Lawrence Erlbaum Associates, pp 17–39.

McGaugh JL, Galvez R, Mesches MH (1995b): Norepinephrine release in the amygdala in response to footshock stimulation used in inhibitory avoidance training. Soc Neurosci Abst 481.14.

McGaugh JL, Introini-Collison IB, Cahill LF, Castellano C, Dalmaz C, Parent MB, Williams CL (1993a): Neuromodulatory systems and memory storage: Role of the amygdala. Behav Brain Res 58:81–90.

McGaugh JL, Introini-Collison IB, Castellano C (1993b): Involvement of opioid peptides in learning and memory. In Herz A, Akil H, Simon EJ (eds): "Handbook of Experimental Pharmacology, Opioids, Part II." Heidelberg: Springer-Verlag, pp 429–447.

McGaugh JL, Introini-Collison IB, Cahill L, Kim M, Liang KC (1992): Involvement of the amygdala in neuromodulatory influences on memory storage. In Aggleton J (ed): "The Amygdala." New York: Wiley, pp 431–451.

Mello C, Nottehohm F, Clayton D (1995): Repeated exposure to one song leads to a rapid and persistent decline in an immediate early gene's response to that song in zebra finch telencephalon. J Neurosci 15(10):6919–6925.

Montminy MR, Gonzalez GA, Yamamoto KK (1990): Regulation of cAMP-inducible genes by CREB. Trends Neurosci 13(5):184–188.

Morgan J, Curran T (1989): Stimulus-transcription coupling in neurons: Role of cellular immediate-early genes. Trends Neurosci 12(11):459–462.

Morris RGM, Garrud P, Rawlins JNP, O'Keefe J (1982): Place navigation impaired in rats with hippocampal lesions. Nature 297:681–683.

Moser E, Moser M-B, Andersen P (1993): Spatial learning impairment parallels the magnitude of dorsal hippocampal lesions, but is hardly present following ventral lesions. J Neurosci 13:3916–3925.

Nguyen PV, Abel T, Kandel ER (1994): Requirement of a critical period of transcription for induction of a late phase of LTP. Science 265:1104–1107.

Nikolaev E, Kaminska B, Tischmeyer W, Matthies H, Kaczmarek L (1992): Induction of expression of genes encoding transcription factors in the rat brain elicited by behavioral training. Behav Brain Res 28:479–484.

Otani S, Ben-Ari Y (1993): Biochemical correlates of long-term potentiation in hippocampal slices. Int Rev Neurobiol 35:1–41.

Packard MG, McGaugh JL (1992): Double dissociation of fornix and caudate nucleus lesions on acquisition of two water maze tasks: Further evidence for multiple memory systems. Behav Neurosci 106:439–446.

Packard MG, Cahill L, McGaugh JL (1994): Amygdala modulation of hippocampal-dependent and caudate nucleus-dependent memory processes. Proc Natl Acad Sci (U S A) 91:8477–8481.

Parent MB, McGaugh JL (1994): Posttraining infusion of lidocaine into the amygdala basolateral complex impairs retention of inhibitory avoidance training. Brain Res 661:97–103.

Paylor R, Johnson RS, Papaioannou V, Spiegelman, BM, Wehner JM (1994): Behavioral assessment of *c-fos* mutual mice. Brain Res 651:275–282.

Popovici T, Represa A, Crepel V, Barbin G, Beaudoin M, Ben-Ari Y (1990): Effects of kainic acid induced seizures and ischemia on *c-fos*-like proteins in rat brain. Brain Res 536:183–194.

Robertson LM, Kerpola TK, Vendrell M, Luk D, Smeyne RJ, Bocchiaro C, Morgan JI, Curran T (1995): Regulation of *c-fos* expression in transgenic mice requires multiple interdependent transcription control elements. Neuron 14:241–252.

Roozendaal B, McGaugh JL (in press): Basolateral amygdala lesions block the memory-enhancing effect of glucocorticoid administration in the dorsal hippocampus. Eur J Neurosci

Roozendaal B, McGaugh JL (1996): Amygdaloid nuclei lesions differentially affect glucocorticoid-induced memory enhancement in an inhibitory avoidance task. Neurobiol Learn Mem 65:1–8.

Roozendaal B, Portillo-Marquez G, McGaugh JL (in press): Basolateral amygdala lesions block glucocorticoid-induced modulation of memory for spatial learning. Behav Neurosci

Roozendaal B, Cahill L, McGaugh JL (in press): Interaction of emotionally activated neuro-modulatory systems in regulating memory storage. In "Excerpta Medica International Congress Series." Amsterdam: Elsevier.

Rose SPR (1995a): Cell-adhesion molecules, glucocorticoids and long-term memory formation. Trends Neurosci 18(11):502–506.

Rose SPR (1995b): Time-dependent biochemical and cellular processes in memory formation. In McGaugh JL, Bermudez-Rattoni F, Prado-Alcala RA (eds): "Plasticity in the Central Nervous System: Learning and Memory." Mahwah, NJ: Lawrence Erlbaum Assoc., pp 171–184.

Rose SPR (1991): How chicks make memories: The cellular cascade from *c-fos* to dendritic remodeling. Trends Neurosci 9:390–397.

Routtenberg A (1995): Knockout mouse fault lines. Nature 374:314–315.

Rudnicki MA, Braun T, Hinuma S, Jaenisch R (1992): Inactivation of MyoD in mice leads to up-regulation of the myogenic HLH gene Myf-5 and results in apparently normal muscle development. Cell 71(3):383–390.

Salinas JA, Packard MG, McGaugh JL (1993): Amygdala modulates memory for changes in reward magnitude: Reversible posttraining inactivation with lidocaine attenuates the response to a reduction in reward. Behav Brain Res 59:153–159.

Sternberg DB, Isaacs K, Gold PE, McGaugh JL (1985): Epinephrine facilitation of appetitive learning: Attenuation with adrenergic receptor antagonists. Behav Neural Biol 44:447–453.

Suhr ST, Gage FH (1993): Gene therapy for neurologic disease. Arch Neurol 50:1252–1268.

Takahashi JS, Pinto LH, Vitaterna MH (1994): Forward and reverse genetic approaches to behaior in the mouse. Science 264:1724–1739.

Thiebot M-H (1985): Some evidence for amnesic-like effects of benzodiazepines in animals. Neurosci Biobehav Rev 9:95–100.

Tomaz C, Dickinson-Anson, H, McGaugh JL (1992): Basolateral amygdala lesions block diazepam-induced amnesia in an inhibitory avoidance task. Proc Natl Acad Sci (U S A) 89:3615–3619.

Tomaz C, Dickinson-Anson H, McGaugh JL (1991): Amygdala lesions block the amnesic effects of diazepam. Brain Res 568:85–91.

Tully T, Preat T, Boynton SC, Del Vecchio M (1994): Genetic dissection of consolidated memory in Drosophila. Cell 79:35–47.

Vallejo M, Habener JF (1994): Mechanisms of transcriptional regulation by cAMP. In Conaway RC, Weliky Conaway J (eds): "Transcription: Mechanisms and Regulation." New York: Raven, pp 353–368.

Wahlestedt C (1994): Antisense oligonucleotide strategies in neuropharmacology. Trends Pharmacol Sci 15(2):42–46.

Walker WA, Fucci L, Habener JF (1995): Expression of the gene encoding transcription factor cyclic adenosine 3′,5′-monophosphate (cAMP) response element-binding protein (CREB): Regulation by follicle-stimulating hormone-induced cAMP signaling in primary rat Setoli cells. Endocrinol 136(8):3534–3545.

Weil-Malherbe H, Axelrod J, Tomchick R (1959): Blood-brain barrier for adrenalin. Science 129:1226–1228.

Weisskopf MG, Castillo PE, Zalutsky RA, Nicoll RA (1994): Mediation of hippocampal mossy fiber long-term potentiation by cyclic AMP. Science 265:1878–1882.

Werling LL, McMahon PN, Portoghese PS, Takemori AE, Cox BM (1989): Selective opioid antagonist effects on opioid-induced inhibition of release of norepinephrine in guinea pig cortex. Neuropharmacology 28:103–107.

Worley PF, Cole AJ, Murphy TH, Christy BA, Nakabeppu Y, Baraban JM (1990a): Synaptic regulation of immediate-early genes in brain. In "Cold Spring Harbor Symposia on Quantitative Biology." Cold Spring Harbor, NY: Cold Spring Harbor Laboratory Press, pp 213–223.

Worley PF, Cole AJ, Saffen DW, Baraban JM (1990b): Regulation of immediate early genes in brain: Role of NMDA receptor activation. In Coleman P, Higgins G, Phelps C (eds): "Progress in Brain Research." Amsterdam: Elsevier, pp 277–285.

Yakubov LA, Deeva EA, Zarytova VF, Ivanova EM, Ryte AS, Yurchenko LV, Vlassov VV (1989): Mechanism of oligonucleotide uptake by cells: Involvement of specific receptors? Proc Natl Acad Sci U S A, 86:6454–6458.

Yamagata K, Andreasson KI, Kaufmann WE, Barnes CA, Worley PF (1993): Expression of mitogen inducible cyclooxygenase in brain neurons: Regulation by synaptic activity and glucocorticoids Neuron 11:371–386.

Yin JCP, Wallach JS, Del Vecchio M, Wilder EL, Zhou, H, Quinn WG, Tully T (1994): Induction of a dominant negative CREB transgene specifically blocks long-term memory in Drosophila. Cell 79:49–58.

Zola-Morgan S, Squire LR (1993): Neuroanatomy of memory. Ann Rev Neurosci 16:547–563.

CHAPTER 3

Monoamine and Acetylcholine Influences on Higher Cognitive Functions in Nonhuman Primates: Relevance to the Treatment of Alzheimer's Disease

AMY F. T. ARNSTEN and CHRISTOPHER H. VAN DYCK

Section of Neurobiology (A.F.T.A.) and Department of Psychiatry (C.H.V.D.), Yale Medical School, New Haven, Connecticut 06510-8001

INTRODUCTION

Nonhuman primates provide an excellent model for examining the efficacy of potential cognitive enhancers. Monkeys possess a highly developed neocortex and a parallel elaboration of cognitive abilities. Furthermore, the pattern and organization of monoaminergic and cholinergic projections to cortex in nonhuman primates appears analogous to that observed in humans. Finally, monkeys and humans often exhibit similar responses to drugs. For example, effective doses (milligrams/kilograms) and side effect profiles in monkeys are generally comparable to those in humans. Recently, a number of seminal findings have emerged from nonhuman primate studies that may guide the development of cognitive enhancing compounds for disorders such as Alzheimer's disease (AD).

OVERVIEW OF NEUROPSYCHOLOGICAL FINDINGS IN MONKEYS

Among the advantages of nonhuman primate research is the opportunity to produce circumscribed lesions to elucidate the contributions of individual cortical regions to

Pharmacological Treatment of Alzheimer's Disease: Molecular and Neurobiological Foundations,
Edited by Brioni and Decker
ISBN 0-471-16758-4 © 1997 Wiley-Liss, Inc.

specific cognitive functions. Over the last 60 years a rich literature has emerged, demonstrating that interconnected cortical circuits subserve distinct cognitive abilities. A few of the relevant findings are reviewed briefly here and in Table 1 to provide a background for the pharmacological studies presented later.

Studies of the primate neocortex have revealed a surprising degree of segregation of cortical functions. Cortical circuits are specialized to perform distinct cognitive duties. For example, a ventral circuit (ventral occipital cortex and inferior temporal cortex) performs feature analysis of visual information (e.g., color, shape), while a dorsal circuit (dorsal occipital cortex and parietal association cortex) analyzes spatial position of a visual stimulus (Ungerleider, 1985). These parallel circuits are found in both monkey (Ungerleider, 1985) and human [e.g., Haxby et al. (1991)] cortex, again emphasizing the appropriateness of the monkey as a model for higher-order cognitive functions.

TABLE 1. Tasks Used to Assess Cognitive Function in Monkeys

Cognitive Function Tested	Cognitive Tests	Most Reliant On	References
Working memory	Spatial delayed response, delayed alternation, delayed match- or nonmatch-to-sample (repeated stimuli)	Dorsolateral PFC, head of caudate[a]	Jacobsen, 1936; Divac et al., 1967; Goldman and Rosvold, 1970; Goldman-Rakic, 1987; Fuster and Bauer, 1974; Mishkin and Manning, 1978
Behavioral inhibition	Reversal of visual discrimination	Orbital PFC	Mishkin, 1964; Ridley et al., 1993
Recognition memory	Delayed match- or nonmatch-to-sample (trial unique stimuli)	Medial temporal cortex, orbital cortex?	Bachevalier and Mishkin, 1986; Mishkin, 1978; Mishkin, 1982; Squire and Zola-Morgan, 1991; Zola-Morgan and Squire, 1985
Visuospatial attention	Route-finding, covert orientation	Parietal cortex (area 7)	Petrides and Iversen, 1979; Goldberg and Bruce, 1985
Visuofeature analysis (associative memory)	Visual pattern or object discrimination	Inferior temporal cortex, tail of caudate	Cowey and Gross, 1970; Divac et al., 1967; Horel and Misantone, 1976

[a]Performance also impaired by medial temporal lesions if delay greater than 10 s (Zola-Morgan and Squire, 1985).

Memory and attentional abilities are also segregated in both monkey and human cortex. For example, monkeys with lesions to the inferior temporal cortex (Cowey and Gross, 1970; Doyon and Milner, 1991) or the tail of the caudate (Divac et al., 1967) are impaired on a visual discrimination task in which the animal must learn to associate one of several visual patterns or objects with food reward. In contrast, habit memory for visuospatial information relies on parietal association cortex (area 7) and its striatal connections, as illustrated by the route-finding task in monkeys (Petrides and Iversen, 1979). The parietal association cortex and its connections with the pulvinar have also been shown to be critical to covert movement of visuospatial attention in monkeys (Goldberg and Bruce, 1985; Robinson and Petersen, 1987) and humans (Posner et al., 1984). These abilities are spared in monkeys or people with lesions of the medial temporal lobe who are amnesic (Squire and Zola-Morgan, 1991). Monkeys with large medial temporal lobe lesions are unable to recognize a previously viewed object after delays of only 15–30 s when tested on the delayed nonmatch-to-sample task with trial unique stimuli (DNMS-TU) (Mishkin, 1978, 1982; Zola-Morgan and Squire, 1985), while lesions to the striatum have no effect on this task (Wang et al., 1990). The mnemonic abilities of the medial temporal lobe are utilized by the prefrontal cortex (PFC) to guide behavior by working memory (Goldman-Rakic, 1987). In monkeys, lesions to the dorsolateral PFC produce dramatic impairments on the spatial delayed response task, in which the memory of the location of a hidden reward must be constantly updated (Goldman and Rosvold, 1970; Jacobsen, 1936). Similarly, PFC lesions can induce deficits on nonspatial working-memory tasks such as delayed match- or nonmatch-to-sample when repeated stimuli are used (Fuster and Bauer, 1974). The cognitive abilities of the PFC are particularly evident when memory must be used to overcome interference from irrelevant stimuli or prepotent response tendencies (Bartus and Levere, 1977; Malmo, 1942). Inhibition of prepotent response tendencies is particularly apparent during reversals of discrimination problems, and lesions to the orbital and ventromedial PFC produce robust reversal deficits (Mishkin et al., 1969; Ridley et al., 1993).

Much of the focus of pharmacological studies has been on the working-memory functions of the PFC as (1) working-memory tasks are particularly amenable to repeated designs needed for drug testing, and (2) working memory is especially vulnerable to the effects of normal aging.

COGNITIVE DEFICITS ASSOCIATED WITH NORMAL AGING IN MONKEYS

Studies of aged nonhuman primates agree that PFC functions decline with advancing age. This observation was first made by Bartus (Bartus, 1979) and has been supported by all researchers since. Thus, marked deficits on the delayed response task emerge early in the aging process (Bachevalier et al., 1991; Bartus et al., 1978; Rapp and Amaral, 1989; Walker et al., 1988), and these deficits are particularly pronounced in the presence of distracting stimuli (Bartus and Dean, 1979). In general, aged monkeys are impaired under conditions of high, but not low, interference [e.g., see Bartus and Dean, 1979, Rapp and Amaral (1989)]. In contrast, they are not impaired on the Posner test of covert orienting of visuospatial attention subserved by the parietal cortex (Voytko, personal communication), although difficult visuospatial abilities of the parietal cortex do appear vulnerable to the aging process (Walker et al., 1988). Similarly, recognition memory and feature discrimination are only impaired in a subset of elderly monkeys (Bartus et al., 1979; Rapp and Amaral, 1992).

Aged humans also show signs of PFC dysfunction [reviewed in Hochanadel and Kaplan (1984)], including an increased susceptibility to interference [e.g., Hoyer et al. (1979)]. For example, Knight reported age-related changes in auditory even-related potentials that resemble those produced by PFC lesions (Chao and Knight, 1994). Also consistent with PFC dysfunction, Davis et al. (1990) observed progressive deficits on the Wisconsin Card Sorting and Stroop tasks with increasing age. Perseverative errors were significantly increased on the Wisconsin card sorting task, reminiscent of the perseverative thinking described by Hebb (1978). In contrast, recognition memory remained quite stable across the life span (Davis et al., 1990). Elderly human subjects did not show deficits on the "Posner task" of covert attentional shifting, suggesting that the visuospatial attentional abilities of the parietal lobe are less affected by the aging process (Greenwood et al., 1993; Robinson and Kertzman, 1990). Thus, the cognitive abilities of the PFC appear preferentially affected by the aging process in both human and nonhuman primates.

Although aged monkeys appear to provide an excellent model of normal aging, these animals may have serious limitations when used as a model for AD. Aged monkeys do not develop global cognitive impairment constituent of dementia. Furthermore, although senile plaques are evident in the aged monkey cortex, monkeys show little evidence of neurofibrillary tangle formation (Walker et al., 1988). Thus the application of pharmacological findings in aged monkeys to patients with AD must be viewed with caution. Nevertheless, the nonhuman primate has offered a valuable opportunity to examine how monoaminergic and cholinergic mechanisms influence higher cortical function.

DOPAMINE

Although many studies of aging and AD have focused on the cholinergic system, sutdies indicate that the dopamine (DA) system may be especially vulnerable to the processes of normal aging. Biochemical analysis of aged rat (Luine et al., 1990) or monkey (Goldman-Rakic and Brown, 1981; Wenk et al., 1989) cortex has shown as marked loss of DA from the PFC, and depletion is evident quite early in the aging process (Goldman-Rakic and Brown, 1981; Wenk et al., 1989). In aged rats, impairment on a spatial working-memory task correlated best with loss of DA metabolites from the PFC (Luine et al., 1990), indicating that the degeneration of this system has functional significance. In monkey cortex, DA loss with age is also prominent in the temporal pole (Goldman-Rakic and Brown, 1981), but other cortical and subcortical areas are more modestly affected (Goldman-Rakic and Brown, 1981; Wenk et al., 1989). Levels of the catecholamine precursor, L-dopa, are also markedly reduced in the PFC (Goldman-Rakic and Brown, 1981), suggesting that turnover of both DA and norepinephrine (NE) would be impaired with age. The very low levels of NE and DA in cortex have precluded accurate measurement of NE and DA levels from human postmortem tissue. Levels are also too low to be detected using modern imaging techniques, which can visualize age-related loss of DA uptake sites in the striatum of living individuals [e.g., van Dyck et al., (1995)]. The effects of age on DA cell bodies projecting to the PFC from the ventral tegmental area and other midbrain areas have not been examined in monkey or human tissue, as they are scattered throughout the midbrain, and thus would require labeling from the PFC for identification. However, there is a substantial age-related loss of cells from the ventral tegmental area in monkeys, and preliminary results suggest a relationship between cell loss in this region and age-related cognitive decline (Siddiqi et al., 1995).

Why might DA in the PFC be so vulnerable to the aging process? The DA neurons projecting to the PFC in rodents are known to have many special properties: They fire faster, have fewer autoreceptors regulating cell firing and DA synthesis, and are uniquely sensitive to stress exposure (Deutch and Roth, 1990; Thierry et al., 1976). Thus, exposure to mild (e.g., psychological) stress selectively increases DA turnover in the PFC, but no other cortical or subcortical DA fields. The effects of stress are blocked by pretreatment with anxiolytics, such as lorazepam, and mimicked by anxiogenic beta carbolines, such as FG7142 (Roth et al., 1988). This sensitivity to stress is thought to arise from differential regulation of PFC-projecting DA neurons [see Deutch and Roth (1990) for review] and may contribute to a preferential "burnout" of the meso-PFC DA system over the life span.

Research in young adult monkeys indicates that DA is critical to the proper functioning of the PFC, thus suggesting that age-related loss of DA from the PFC may contribute to cognitive deficits in the elderly. Marked depletion of DA from the PFC (Brozoski et al., 1979) or infusion of DA D1 receptor antagonists into the PFC (Sawaguchi and Goldman-Rakic, 1991) produces profound impairment of spatial working memory. Spatial working memory is similarly impaired by systemic treatment with DA D1 receptor antagonists (Arnsten et al., 1994) or by presynaptic doses of a D2 agonist that inhibits DA release (Arnsten et al., 1995). With advancing age, these agents lose their ability to impair spatial working memory, consistent with a loss of endogenous DA stimulation in the PFC of elderly monkeys (Arnsten et al., 1994; Arnsten et al., 1995). In contrast, these agents retain their ability to induce sedation (Arnsten et al., 1994) or impair fine motor performance (Arnsten et al., 1995), consistent with a preferential loss of DA from the PFC relative to other brain regions.

Given the importance of DA mechanisms to proper PFC function, and the loss of DA from the PFC, might DA agonist replacement therapy restore PFC function in aged monkeys? This hypothesis has been tested with both D1 and D2 receptor agonists. The D2 agonist, quinpirole, has been found to improve working-memory performance through actions at postsynaptic receptors (Arnsten et al., 1995). However, the preponderance of side effects (hypotension, sedation, agitation, dyskinesias, "hallucinatory-like" behaviors) would limit clinical utility (Arnsten et al., 1995). In contrast, the D1 partial agonist, SKF38393, was found to produce a small but significant improvement in spatial working-memory performance in aged monkeys with no side effects [Figure 1; (Arnsten et al., 1994)]. However, with increasing dose, several animals showed marked cognitive impairment (Arnsten et al., 1994). A similar profile was found with the full D1 agonist, dihydrexidine, which was even more potent in producing cognitive impairment (Arnsten et al., 1994). These findings are in keeping with recent studies in monkeys and rodents demonstrating that excessive DA stimulation is as harmful to PFC function as is insufficient DA stimulation (Arnsten and Goldman-Rakic, 1990b; Murphy et al., 1996; Murphy et al., 1994). However, the development of superior D1 agonists with greater selectivity and/or brain penetration suggest that this mechanism may show promise. Preliminary evidence with more selective full D1 agonists suggest that very low doses can improve working memory in aged monkeys, while much higher doses are needed to induce impairment (Cai, personal communication; Arnsten, preliminary results). Thus, these more selective D1 agonists may provide a strategy for improving working memory in the elderly with few evident side effects.

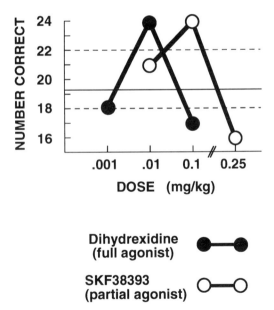

FIGURE 1. Effects of a partial (SKF38393) and full (dihydrexidine) DA D1 receptor agonist on spatial working-memory performance in an aged monkey. The horizontal line indicates mean performance on saline; the dashed lines represent the range of performance on saline. The D1 agonists improved performance following low doses but impaired performance at higher doses. The full agonist was more potent than the partial agonist. (Adapted from Arnsten et al., 1994).

Might DA D1 agonists also be useful in treating PFC cognitive deficits in AD? These agents are just entering human trials; thus their potential as cognitive enhancers remains to be evaluated. However, the discovery of a dopaminergic deficit in AD has provided a rationale for developing DA replacement therapies in this disease. Although the methodological difficulties in studying the mesocortical DA system have limited its investigation in AD [and most studies have focused on loss of DA in the striatum, e.g., Gottfries et al., (1983)], a few, careful studies have shown evidence that the mesocortical DA system is affected in AD relative to age-matched controls. German and colleagues have observed neurofibrillary tangles in the ventral tegmental area in addition to the locus coeruleus and raphe (German et al., 1987), and Reinikainen colleagues have measured decreased levels of DA in cortex and hippocampus (Reinikainen et al., 1990).

Several dopaminergic agents have been tested in AD patients, including the catecholamine precursor L-dopa [e.g., Jellinger et al. (1980), Kristensen et al. (1977) and Lewis et al. (1978)], the DA D2 agonist bromocriptine (Adolfsson et al., 1978), and the indirectly acting DA agonists amantadine (Schubert and Fleischhacker, 1979) and memantine (Fleischhacker et al., 1986). These studies have shown mixed results, which is not surprising given their presynaptic actions and side effects (bromocriptine) or their reliance on the integrity of the endogenous DA system for their actions (indirectly acting agents). Several trials have also been completed with L-deprenyl, an irreversible inhibitor of B-type monoamine oxidase which also possesses antioxidant and catecholamine reuptake-blocking properties. Contradictory results have been reported with short-term (1–3 months) administration of L-deprenyl (Burke et al., 1993; Mangoni et al., 1991; Piccinin et al., 1990; Tariot et al., 1987). Longer trials have subsequently been undertaken to resolve these inconsistencies and to elucidate purported neuroprotective effects. It is important to note that most of these agents enhance noradrenergic, as well as DA transmission.

NOREPINEPHRINE

Increasing evidence demonstrates that NE, as well as DA, has a vital influence on PFC cognitive functioning [see Arnsten et al. 1996 for review]. The NE system is vulnerable to both normal aging and AD: there is a marked (60%) loss of NE locus coeruleus (LC) neurons in aged rodents (e.g. Leslie et al., 1985), monkeys (Sladek and Sladek, 1979) and humans [e.g., German et al. (1988); Iversen et al. (1983), and Vijayashankar and Brody (1979)], and this loss is significantly exaggerated in AD [e.g., German et al. (1992); and Tomlinson et al. (1981)]. Norepinephrine itself is not significantly reduced with age in monkey PFC (Goldman-Rakic and Brown, 1981; Wenk et al., 1989), although rat studies have found a decrease in PFC NE with age (Luine et al., 1990) and further suggest that NE turnover can be decreased even when NE levels are normal (Hadfield and Milio, 1990). In humans, immunocytochemical analysis of catecholamine synthetic enzymes has shown a prominent loss of NE fibers from the PFC with advancing age (Gaspar et al., 1989, 1991), and NE levels in cortex are significantly reduced in AD [e.g., Adolfsson et al. (1979) and Gottfries et al. (1983)].

Interestingly, the NE projection from the LC to the PFC appears to be reciprocal; the dorsolateral and dorsomedial PFC may provide the sole cortical inputs to the LC (Arnsten and Goldman-Rakic, 1984). These anatomical findings suggest a special relationship between the PFC and LC, whereby PFC dysfunction may impair regulation of the LC and vice versa. Indeed, recent evidence indicates that PFC dysfunction results in disinhibition of LC firing (Hervé and Sara, 1994), a state that diminishes LC responsivity to appropriate stimuli (Kubiak et al., 1995). Thus, in aged individuals a vicious circle may develop in which LC degeneration impairs PFC function, which further disrupts LC function, and so on.

Research in aged monkeys has shown that PFC cognitive functions can be improved by α-2 agonists. Clonidine, UK14304, BHT920, and guanfacine can improve delayed response performance (Arnsten et al., 1988; Arnsten and Goldman-Rakic, 1985; Arnsten and Leslie, 1991), and these improvements are blocked by the α-2 antagonists yohimbine and idazoxan, but not by the α_1 antagonist, prazosin (Arnsten et al., 1988; Arnsten and Goldman-Rakic, 1985). Conversely, yohimbine by itself impairs delayed response performance, while prazosin is without effect (Arnsten and Goldman-Rakic, 1985). This pharmacological profile is consistent with an α_2 mechanism, but not an $\alpha1$ or imidazoline site of drug action. The varying potency of α_2 agonists further indicates the subtype of α_2 receptor underlying these beneficial effects. Three α_2 subtypes have now been cloned in primates: the α_{2A}, α_{2B}, and α_{2C}, the genes for which reside on chromosomes 10, 2, and 4, respectively (Kobilka et al., 1987; Lomasney et al., 1990; Regan et al., 1988). The ability of an α_2 agonist to improve PFC function without side effects was found to correspond to its selectivity for the α_{2A} site: guanfacine $>$ UK14304 $>$ clonidine $>$ BHT920 (Arnsten et al., 1988; Arnsten and Leslie, 1991; Uhlen and Wikberg, 1991). Thus, low doses of guanfacine are able to improve delayed response performance without inducing sedation or hypotension, while clonidine's beneficial effects require higher doses, which are accompanied by marked sedative and hypotensive side effects (Arnsten et al., 1988). An α_{2A} mechanism is also supported by the prazosin data. In addition to its α_1 receptor blocking properties, prazosin has quite high affinity for the α_{2B} and α_{2C} subtypes but has low affinity for the α_{2A} receptor (Marjamäki et al., 1993; Uhlen and Wikberg, 1991). In contrast, idazoxan has high affinity for the α_{2A} site (Marjamäki et al., 1993; Uhlen and Wikberg, 1991). Thus, the ability of idazoxan, but not prazosin, to block clonidine's beneficial effects is consistent with actions at α_{2A} receptors.

Additional data suggest actions at *post*synaptic receptors, that is, receptors on non-NE cells. Although most researchers have focused on the autoreceptor actions of α_2 agonists, inhibiting NE release and decreasing LC firing, a very large portion of α_2 receptors are localized on non-NE cells that receive NE input (Aoki et al., 1994; Scheinin et al., 1994; U'Prichard et al., 1979). Indeed, Aoki et al. (1994) have used electron microscopy to demonstrate postjunctional α_{2A} immunoreactivity over postsynaptic membranes in the monkey PFC. Evidence from several labs indicates that α_{2A} agonists improve spatial working memory through actions at postsynaptic receptors. Clonidine becomes more, rather than less effective, in young monkeys in whom the presynaptic element is destroyed or depleted with 6-hydroxydopamine

(6-OHDA) (Arnsten and Goldman-Rakic, 1985), 1-methy 1-4-phenyl-1,2,3,6-tetra hydropyridine (MPTP) (Schneider and Kovelowski, 1990), or chronic reserpine (Cai et al., 1993). Thus, the cognitive-enhancing actions of α_2 agonists result from actions at postsynaptic receptors with an α_{2A} pharmacological profile.

At least some of these drug actions occur directly in the PFC. In young monkeys with 6-OHDA lesions restricted to the PFC, clonidine's potency directly relates to the degree of NE depletion in this region, a result consistent with drug actions as supersensitive, postsynaptic receptors in the PFC (Arnsten and Goldman-Rakic, 1985). Importantly, α_2 agonists lose their efficacy when the PFC is ablated (Arnsten and Goldman-Rakic, 1985), suggesting that an intact cortex is necessary for α_2 agonists to have their beneficial effects. Findings from an aged monkey support this interpretation: Although monkey 445 showed robust improvement with clonidine treatment prior to a PFC lesion, clonidine lost its cognitive-enhancing properties after the monkey sustained a bilateral lesion of the PFC (Figure 2). Interestingly, the sedative effects of clonidine were retained postlesion (Figure 2), consistent with a thalamic (Buzsaki et al., 1991) or LC mechanism (Berridge and Foote, 1991) underlying the sedative actions of these compounds. The loss of cognitive-enhancing properties in monkeys with cortical ablations may have particular relevance to AD, as the damage to cortical neurons in this illness may remove the substrate needed for the beneficial effects of α_2 agonists.

Intracortical infusion studies also indicate that α_2 agents alter cognitive function through actions in the PFC. Direct infusion of clonidine or guanfacine into the PFC, but not the nearby premotor cortex, improves delayed response performance in aged monkeys (Arnsten, unpublished results). Conversely, infusion of the α_2 antagonist, yohimbine, directly into the PFC impairs delayed response performance under delay, but no delay (0 s) control conditions (Li and Mei, 1994b). Comparable infusions of the α_1 antagonist, prazosin, or the β antagonist, propranolol, do not impair performance (ibid), again indicating that the α_2 adrenergic system has a special role in PFC function. It is noteworthy that yohimbine infusions into the PFC significantly increased errors of commission (Li and Mei, 1994b), suggesting that endogenous α_2 stimulation is important for regulating the inhibitory abilities of the PFC. Electrophysiological studies have shown that either systemic or iontophoretic application of clonidine enhances delay-related firing of PFC neurons, while yohimbine has the reverse effect (Li and Mei, 1994a). Most recently, iontophoresis of yohimbine onto PFC pyramidal neurons has been found to suppress the memory fields exhibited by these neurons (Sawaguchi, personal communication).

In contrast, the functions subserved by posterior cortical regions appear less responsive to α_2 adrenergic treatment. For example, clonidine or guanfacine have little effect on reference memory [Figure 3; (Arnsten and Goldman-Rakic, 1985)] or recognition memory (Arnsten and Goldman-Rakic, 1990a), tasks which depend on the inferior or medial temporal cortex, respectively. Similar negative effects have been seen when guanfacine is administered to rats performing a reference memory task (Sirviö et al., 1991). In contrast, α_2 agonists administered to rats or monkeys have been shown to improve a variety of working-memory tasks that utilize PFC abilities: for example, delayed response [Figure 3; (Arnsten et al., 1988)], delayed

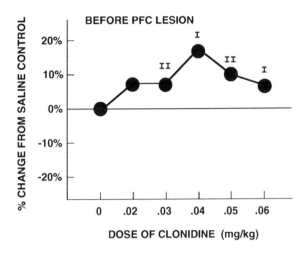

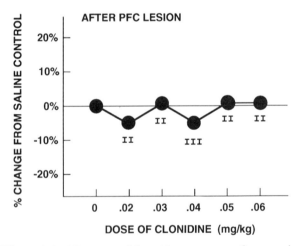

FIGURE 2. Effects of clonidine on spatial working-memory performance in an aged monkey before (top graph) and after (bottom graph) sustaining a bilateral, dorsolateral PFC lesion. Clonidine no longer improved performance following the PFC lesion. Results represent percent change from performance on saline; a 20% improvement represents near perfect performance on the task. Sedation scores are indicated whereby I = quieter than usual, II = sedated (slowed movements, drooping eyelids) and III = intermittent sleeping. No sedation score indicates a normal level of arousal.

alternation (Arnsten and Goldman-Rakic, 1985; Carlson et al., 1992), and delayed match-to-sample with repeated stimuli (Jackson and Buccafusco, 1991). α_2 Agonists are most effective under conditions of high interference or distraction when the PFC is challenged (Arnsten and Contant, 1992; Jackson and Buccafusco, 1991). Indeed, even very low doses of guanfacine can protect the performance of aged monkeys from the deleterious effects of irrelevant stimulation (Arnsten and Contant, 1992). Thus, the monkey research has shown tht α_2 agonists are especially effective in enhancing working-memory performance under distracting conditions, and they have these effects through actions as postjunctional, α_{2A} receptors in the PFC.

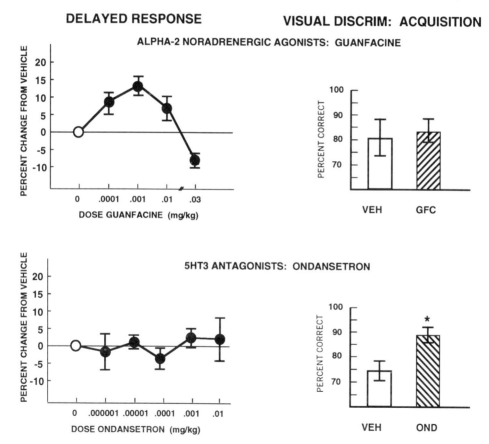

FIGURE 3. Effects of the α_{2A} receptor NE agonist, guanfacine, and the 5-HT$_3$ receptor antagonist, ondansetron, on the performance of two cognitive tasks in aged monkeys. The delayed response task is a spatial working memory task that depends on the cognitive functioning of the dorsolateral PFC, while acquisition of a visual object discrimination problem is especially dependent on the inferior temporal cortex. Results represent mean ± SEM number correct. Guanfacine significantly improved performance of the delayed response task but did not improve discrimination performance; ondansetron exhibited the converse profile of improvement. (Results adapted from Arnsten et al., 1988 and Arnsten et al., in press).

α_2 Agonists have been shown to improve PFC functioning in human patients with symptoms of PFC cognitive dysfunction. For example, clonidine improved the performance of Korsakoff's patients on PFC tasks such as the Stroop Interference Test (Mair and McEntree, 1986) and word fluency (Moffoot et al., 1994), and the improvement in word fluency correlated with increased regional cerebral blood flow in the left PFC, the cortical region most affiliated with performance of this task (Moffoot et al., 1994). Clonidine also increased regional cerebral blood flow in the anterior cingulate cortex in these patients (Moffoot et al., (1994). Clonidine's beneficial effects in Korsakoff's patients appeared to result from actions at postjunctional receptors, as the drug was most efficacious in those patients with greatest NE loss (McEntee and Mair, 1990). Thus, α_2 agonists can mimic NE at postjunctional α_2 receptors and improve PFC function in both monkeys and humans with PFC dysfunction and signs of NE loss. Clonidine has also been used to treat Attention Deficit Hyperactivity Disorder (ADHD), although the sedative and hypotensive side effects of this medication have limited its use (Hunt et al., 1985). Most recently, the more selective α_{2A} agonist, guanfacine has been tested in ADHD subjects based on the successful results in nonhuman primates. Open trials of guanfacine in ADHD children have shown significant improvement on parents ratings of inattention and disinhibited behaviors (Chappell et al., 1995; Horrigan and Barnhill, 1995; Hunt et al., 1995), as well as improved performance of continuous performance tasks (Chappell et al., 1995). Double-blind, placebo-controlled trials are currently in progress and are examining the effects of guanfacine on PFC vs. non-PFC cognitive functions.

Although α_2 agonists have demonstrated clinical benefit in several patient populations with prominent PFC cognitive deficits, they have not proven helpful in the treatment of AD. Neither clonidine (Mohr et al., 1989) nor guanfacine (Crook et al., 1992; Schlegel et al., 1989) has yielded cognitive benefit in this patient population, although small improvements in mood have been noted with guanfacine (Schlegel et al., 1989). These negative results ae not unexpected given that nonhuman primate studies have shown that α_2 agonists fail to improve: (1) medial temporal lobe memory function and (2) PFC cognitive function in the presence of cortical damage. The recall and recognition memory functions of the medial temporal lobe are most affected in AD and are central to most neuropsychological batteries used to assess drug efficacy in AD [e.g., the Alzheimer's Disease Assessment Scale (Rosen et al., 1984)]. Furthermore, although α_2 agonists might improve PFC cognitive deficits early in the disease process, they would not be efficacious at later stages when cortical degeneration is prominent. Thus the negative results with these agents in AD patients are in keeping with basic studies and provide a cautionary note that replacement therapy may not provide an effective strategy for treating AD.

SEROTONIN

As with the other monoaminergic systems projecting to the cortex, the serotonergic system is affected by AD. Serotonin is depleted from cortex [e.g., Bowen et al. (1983) and Gottfries et al. (1983)], and the serotonergic cell bodies in the raphe nuclei exhibit tangles and prominent cell loss (Curcio and Kemper, 1984). However, it seems unlikely that degeneration of the serotonergic system contributes substantially to the cognitive deficits observed in AD, as serotonin depletion or blockade in animals is either without effect (Brozoski et al., 1979) or is associated with cognitive enhancement, not impairment [see Altman and Normile (1988), Gower (1992), and McEntee and Crook (1991) for reviews]. Interestingly, rodent studies indicate that reference memory functions may be most sensitive to manipulations of the serotonergic system (Altman and Normile, 1988; Gower, 1992; McEntee and Crook, 1991).

Studies of the serotonin's effects on cognitive function in nonhuman primates have focused on 5-HT_3 receptor antagonists, and these agents are currently being considered as potential cognitive enhancers for use in the treatment of dementia. 5-HT_3 receptors are concentrated in limbic and cortical areas (Bachevalier and Mishkin, 1986; Kilpatrick et al., 1987; Waeber et al., 1988, 1989), and studies in rodents have demonstrated that 5-HT_3 receptor antagonists such as ondansetron can enhance cognitive function (Barnes et al., 1990; Hodges and Fletcher, in press) and central acetylcholine release (Barnes et al., 1989; Robinson, 1983). 5-HT_3 receptor antagonists may also influence cognitive function in scopolamine-treated (Carey et al., 1992) and untreated (Domeney et al., 1991) marmosets. Domeney et al. (1991) reported that repeated daily treatment with low doses of ondansetron (0.000001–0.0001 mg/kg) could improve visual object discrimination performance in young adult marmosets. This study showed improved acquisition (initial performance), and reversal of the visual object discrimination problem with repeated ondansetron treatment. Recently, we have replicated improved acquisition of visual object discrimination performance in aged rhesus monkeys [Figure 3; (Arnsten et al., in press)], although ondansetron had no significant effect on the spatial working-memory functions subserved by the PFC. (Arnsten et al., in press). Thus, in contrast to α_2 NE agents, 5-HT_3 receptor antagonists may have little effect on PFC functions while enhancing those cognitive abilities subserved by the posterior cortices such as the inferior temporal cortex.

Ondansetron has recently been tested in AD patients in multicenter trials in the United States and abroad. These studies have failed to demonstrate that this drug is an effective treatment for AD (Glaxo, Inc., personal communication). As with α_2 agents, negative results with 5-HT_3 receptor antagonists in AD patients may ensue from the cortical damage inherent in AD. Moreover, the types of cognitive tasks shown to be sensitive to treatment with 5-HT_3 receptor antagonists in animal studies are not well represented in the outcome measures commonly employed in investigational AD drug trials (Rosen et al., 1984).

ACETYLCHOLINE

Drug development in AD has focused on cholinergic agents, based in part on the cholinergic hypothesis of age-related cognitive decline described by Bartus and colleagues (1982). Bartus's pioneering research demonstrated that the muscarinic antagonist, scopolamine, could induce working-memory deficits in young monkeys that resembled the impairment that developed naturally in aged monkeys (Bartus, 1982; Bartus and Johnson, 1976). Learning and memory deficits were also observed in humans treated with scopolamine [e.g., Drachman (1981)], leading to the supposition that cholinergic loss underlay cognitive decline in normal aging. The marked degeneration of the basal forebrain cholinergic system in AD (Whitehouse et al., 1982) was thus hypothesized to produce the prominent deficits of learning and memory that constitute the hallmarks of this disease. Research in rodents and lower primates (e.g., marmosets) has, in general, supported this view, as lesions to the medial septum and basal forebrain often result in predicted cognitive impairment that can be markedly improved by cholinergic agonists [e.g., Ridley et al. (1985) and Roberts et al. (1992)]. However, further research in higher primates with more developed neocortices has seriously challenged this view.

Studies of aged rhesus monkeys have revealed very small changes in the cholinergic projections to cortex. Age-related changes in the nucleus basalis and medial septum are subtle (Stroessner-Johnson et al., 1992; Voytko et al., 1995), and there is only a small decline in cholinergic uptake sites in cortex (Wenk et al., 1989). Similarly, indirectly acting cholinergic agonists such as physostigmine and tacrine have only small and inconsistent effects on working-memory performance in aged monkeys (Bartus and Dean, 1988). Most importantly, lesions to the basal forebrain have surprisingly little effect on learning and memory performance (Aigner et al., 1987; Voytko et al., 1994), although they do increase susceptibility to scopolamine treatment (Aigner et al., 1987; Voytko et al., 1994). In their landmark study, Voytko et al. (1994) produced extensive lesions of the medial septum, diagonal band of Broca, and nucleus basalis of Meynert in cynomolgus monkeys and observed little effect on performance of the delayed response, delayed nonmatch-to-sample, visual discrimination, spatial discrimination, or discrimination reversal tasks. These findings were particularly surprising, as scopolamine is known to impair performance of many of these tasks (Aigner and Mishkin, 1986; Bartus and Johnson, 1976). These results suggest that the marked deficits observed with scopolamine on learning and memory tasks may result from the drugs actions on other cholinergic systems, for example, profound effects on thalamic physiology and thus on thalamocortical activation.

An additional surprising finding from the Voytko et al. study (Voytko et al., 1994) was that basal forebrain lesions did produce significant impairment of the Posner visuospatial attention task (Posner, 1980). This task measures the covert orienting of visuospatial attention and is especially sensitive to parietal lobe lesions in humans (Posner et al., 1984). Studies in rhesus monkeys have demonstrated an abundance of cholinergic neurons projecting from basal forebrain to parietal cortex (Kievit and Kuypers, 1975), which may be particularly important for the proper functioning of this region.

The finding of Voytko et al. (1994) may have direct relevance to AD, raising important questions about a link between the cholinergic system and the parietal lobes in this disease. The parietal association cortex is among the brain regions with the greatest abnormalities of both cholinergic innervation (measured by the activity of the marker enzyme choline acetyltransferase, ChAT) (Najlerahim and Bowen, 1988; Procter et al., 1988), as well as regional cerebral blood flow (rCBF) and metabolism [e.g., Holman et al. (1992), Johnson et al. (1990) and Kumar et al. (1991)]. Moreover, central cholinergic drugs have frequently been shown to produce a relatively selective increase of rCBF in the parietal association cortex of AD patients (Battistin et al., 1989; Geaney et al., 1990; Gustafson et al., 1987; van Dyck et al., 1995a).

Numerous studies have now been conducted testing the efficacy of cholinergic compounds in the treatment of AD (extensively reviewed elsewhere in this volume). Tacrine has emerged as the first agent approved by the Food and Drug Administration for the treatment of AD but demonstrates only modest efficacy in large-scale clinical trials (Davis et al., 1992; Farlow et al., 1992; Knapp et al., 1994). Although the outcome measures commonly employed in these and other investigational AD drug trials (Rosen et al., 1984) preferentially assess memory and language abilities, some preliminary research has shown that "parietal" visuospatial abilities, such as constructional praxis, are strongly enhanced by cholinergic therapies in AD (Muramoto et al., 1984, 1979). The results of primate studies argue strongly that, in the development of cholinergic drug therapies for AD, greater utilization should be made of tasks subserved by the parietal lobes.

SUMMARY

Research in nonhuman primates provides several cautionary notes for the development of cognitive enhancers to treat AD. Most importantly, evidence to date indicates that different cortical areas have distinct neurochemical needs. Therefore, a single agent is unlikely to produce global cognitive improvement. Rather, catecholaminergic, serotonergic, and cholinergic drugs may preferentially affect specific domains of cognitive functioning. This specificity of drug actions must be considered in the selection of appropriate patient populations and neuropsychological assessment batteries. Finally, research in nonhuman primates cautions that drug replacement therapy may require an intact cortical substrate for beneficial drug actions. Thus many cognitive enhancers may have little effect in AD beyond its earliest stages.

REFERENCES

Adolfsson R, Gottfries CG, Roos BE, Winblad B (1979): Changes in brain catecholamines in patients with dementia of Alzheimer type. Br J Psychiatry 135:216–223.

Adolfsson R, Gottfries CG, Oreland L, Roos BE, Winblad B (1978): Reduced levels of catecholamines in the brain and increased activity of monoamine oxidase in platelets in Alzheimer's disease: Therapeutic implications. In Katzmann R, Terry RD, Bick KL (eds): "Alzheimer's Disease: Senile Dementia and Related Disorders, Aging, Vol. 7. New York: Raven pp 441–451.

Aigner TG, Mishkin M (1986): The effects of physostigmine and scopolamine on recognition memory in monkeys. Behav Neural Biol 45:81–87.

Aigner TG, Mitchell SJ, Aggleton JP, DeLong MR, Struble RG, Price DL, Wenk GL (1987): Effects of physostigmine and scopolamine on recognition memory in monkeys with ibotinic-acid lesions of the nucleus basalis of Meynert. Psychopharmacology 92:292–300.

Altman HJ, Normile HJ (1988): What is the nature of the role of the serotonergic nervous system in the learning and memory: Prospects for development of and effective treatment strategy for senile dementia. Neurobiol Aging 9:627–638.

Aoki C, Go C-G, Venkatesan C, Kurose H (1994): Perikaryal and synaptic localization of alpha-2A-adrenergic receptor-like immunoreactivity. Brain Res 650:181–204.

Arnsten AFT, Contant TA (1992): Alpha-2 adrenergic agonists decrease distractability in aged monkeys performing a delayed response task. Psychopharmocology 108:159–169.

Arnsten AFT, Goldman-Rakic PS (1990a): Analysis of alpha-2 adrenergic agonist effects on the delayed nonmatch-to-sample performance of aged rhesus monkeys. Neurobiol Aging 11:583–590.

Arnsten AFT, Goldman-Rakic PS (1990b): Stress impairs prefrontal cortex cognitive function in monkeys: Role of dopamine. Soc Neurosci Abstr 16:164.

Arnsten AFT, Goldman-Rakic PS (1984): Selective prefrontal cortical projections to the region of the locus coeruleus and raphe nuclei in the rhesus monkey. Brain Res 306:9–18.

Arnsten AFT, Goldman-Rakic PS (1985): Alpha-2 adrenergic mechanisms in prefrontal cortex associated with cognitive decline in aged nonhuman primates. Science 230: 1273–1276.

Arnsten AFT, Leslie FM (1991): Behavioral and receptor binding analysis of the alpha-2 adrenergic agonist, UK-14304 (5 bromo-6 [2-imidazoline-2-yl amino] quinoxaline): Evidence for cognitive enhancement at an alpha-2 adrenoceptor subtype. Neuropharmocology 30:1279–1289.

Arnsten AFT, Steere JC, Hunt RD (1996): The contribution of α-2 noradrenergic mechanisms to prefrontal cortical cognitive function: Potential significance to Attention Deficit Hyperactivity Disorder. Arch Gen Psychiatry, 53:448–455.

Arnsten AFT, Lin, CH, van Dyck CH, Stanhope KJ (1996): The effects of 5-HT$_3$ receptor antagonists on cognitive performance in aged monkeys. Neurobiol Aging, in press.

Arnsten AFT, Cai JX, Steere JC, Goldman-Rakic PS (1995): Dopamine D2 receptor mechanisms contribute to age-related cognitive decline: The effects of quinpirole on memory and motor performance in monkeys. J Neurosci 15:3429–3439.

Arnsten AFT, Cai JX, Murphy BL, Goldman-Rakic PS (1994): Dopamine D1 receptor mechanisms in the cognitive performance of young adult and aged monkeys. Psychopharmacology 116:143–151.

Arnsten AFT, Cai JX, Goldman-Rakic PS (1988): The alpha-2 adrenergic agonist guanfacine improves memory in aged monkeys without sedative or hypotensive side effects. J Neurosci 8:4287–4298.

Bachevalier J, Mishkin M (1986): Visual recognition impairment follows ventromedial but not dorsolateral prefrontal lesions in monkeys. Behav Brain Res 20:249–261.

Bachevalier J, Landis LS, Walker LC, Brickson M, Mishkin M, Price DL, Cork LC (1991): Aged monkeys exhibit behavioral deficits indicative of widespread cerebral dysfunction. Neurobiol Aging 12:99–111.

Barnes JM, Costall B, Coughlin J, Domeney AM, Gerrard PA, Kelly ME, Naylor RJ, Onaivi ES, Tomkins DM, Tyers MB (1990): The effects of ondansetron, a 5-HT$_3$ receptor antagonist on cognition in rodents and primates. Pharmacol Biochem Behav 35:955–962.

Barnes JM, Barnes NM, Costall B, Naylor RJ, Tyers MB (1989): 5-HT$_3$ receptors mediate inhibition of acetylcholine release in cortical tissue. Nature 338:762–763.

Bartus RT (1982): Effects of cholinergic agents on learning and memory in animal models of aging. In Corkin S, Growden JH, Davis KL, Usdin E, Wurtman RJ (eds): "Alzheimer's Disease: A Report of Progress in Research," Aging, Vol. 19. New York: Raven, pp 271–280.

Bartus RT (1979): "Effects of aging on visual memory, sensory processing and discrimination learning in a nonhuman primate." In Ordy JM, Brizzee K (eds): "Aging, Vol. 10." New York: Raven, pp 85–114.

Bartus RT, Dean RL (1988): Tetrahydroaminoacridine, 3,4 diaminopyridine and physostigmine: Direct comparisons of effects on memory in aged primates. Neurobiol Aging 9:351–356.

Bartus RT, Dean RL (1979): Recent memory in aged non-human primates: Hypersensitivity to visual interference during retention. Exp Aging Res 5:385–400.

Bartus RT, Johnson HR (1976): Short-term memory in the rhesus monkey: Disruption from the anti-cholinergic scopolamine. Pharmacol Biochem Behav 5:39–46.

Bartus RT, Levere TE (1977): Frontal decortication in rhesus monkeys: A test of the interference hypothesis. Brain Res 119:233–248.

Bartus RT, Dean RL, Beer B, Lippa AS (1982): The cholinergic hypothesis of geriatric memory dysfunction. Science 217:408–417.

Bartus RT, Dean RL, Fleming DL (1979): Aging in the rhesus monkey: Effects on visual discrimination learning and reversal learning. J Gerontol 34:209–219.

Bartus RT, Fleming D, Johnson HR (1978): Aging in the rhesus monkey: Debilitating effects on short-term memory. J Gerontol 33:858–871.

Battistin L, Pizzolato G, Dam M, Da Col C, Perlotto N, Saitta B, Borsato N, Calvani M, Ferlin G (1989): Single-photon emission computed tomography studies with ^{99m}Tc-hexamethylpropyleneamine oxime in dementia: Effects of acute administration of l-acetylcarnitine. Eur Neurol 29:261–265.

Berridge CW, Foote SL (1991): Effects of locus coeruleus activation on electroencephalographic activity in neocortex and hippocampus. J Neurosci 11:3135–3145.

Bowen DN, Allen SJ, Benton JS, Goodhardt MJ, Hann EA, Palmer AM, Sims NR, Smith CCT, Spillane JA, Esiri MM, Neary D, Snowden JS, Wilcock GK, Davison AN (1983): Biochemical assessment of serotonergic and cholinergic dysfunction and cerebral atrophy in Alzheimer's Disease. J Neurochem 41:266–272.

Brozoski T, Brown RM, Rosvold HE, Goldman PS (1979): Cognitive deficit caused by regional depletion of dopamine in prefrontal cortex of rhesus monkey. Science 205: 929–931.

Burke WJ, Ranno AE, Roccaforte WH, Wengel SP, Bayer BL, Willcockson NK (1993): L-Deprenyl in the treatment of mild dementia of the Alzheimer type: Preliminary results. J Am Geriatr Soc 41:367–370.

Buzsaki G, Kennedy B, Solt VB, Ziegler M (1991): Noradrenergic control of thalamic oscillation: The role of alpha-2 receptors. Eur J Neuro 3:222–229.

Cai JX, Ma Y, Xu L, Hu X (1993): Reserpine impairs spatial working memory performance in monkeys: Reversal by the alpha-2 adrenergic agonist clonidine. Brain Res 614: 191–196.

Carey GJ, Costell B, Domeney AM, Gerrard PA, Jones DNC, Naylor RJ, Tyers MB (1992): Ondansetron and arecoline prevent scopolamine-induced cognitive deficits in the marmoset. Pharmacol Biochem Behav 42:75–83.

Carlson S, Ranila H, Rama P, Mecke E, Pertovaara A (1992): Effects of medetomidine, an alpha-2 adrenoceptor agonist, and atipamezole, an alpha-2 antagonist, on spatial memory performance in adult and aged rats. Behav Neural Biol 58:113–119.

Chao LL, Knight RT (1994): Age-related prefrontal changes during auditory memory. Abst Soc Neurosci 20:1003.

Chappell PB, Riddle MA, Scahill L, Lynch KA, Schultz R, Arnsten A, Leckman JF, Cohen DJ (1995): Guanfacine treatment of comorbid attention deficit hyperactivity disorder and Tourette's Syndrome: Preliminary clinical experience. J Am Acad Child Adol Psychiatry 34:1140–1146.

Cowey A, Gross CG (1970): Effects of foveate prestriate and inferotemporal lesions on visual discrimination by rhesus monkeys. Exp Brain Res 11:128–144.

Crook T, Wilner E, Rothwell A, Winterling D, McEntee W (1992): Noradrenergic intervention in Alzheimer's disease. Psychopharmacol Bull 28:67–70.

Curcio CA, Kemper T (1984): Nucleus raphe dorsalis in dementia of the Alzheimer type; neurofibrillary changes and neuronal packing density. J Neuropathol Exp Neurol 43: 359–368.

Davis HP, Cohen A, Gandy M, Colombo P, Van Dusseldorp G, Simolke N, Romano J (1990): Lexical priming deficits as a function of age. Behav Neurosci 104:286–295.

Davis KL, Thal LJ, Gamzu ER, Davis CS, Woolson RF, Gracon SI, Drachman DA, Schneider LS, Whitehouse PJ, Hoover TM, Morris JC, Kawas CH, Knopman DS, Earl NL, Kumar V, Doody RS (1992): A double-blind, placebo-controlled multicenter study of tacrine for Alzheimer's disease. N Engl J Med 327:1253–1259.

Deutch AY, Roth RH (1990): The determinants of stress-induced activation of the prefrontal cortical dopamine system. Prog Brain Res 85:367–403.

Divac I, Rosvold HE, Szwarcbart MK (1967): Behavioral effects of selective ablation of the caudate nucleus. J Comp Physiol 63:184–190.

Domeney AM, Costall B, Garrard PA, Jones DNC, Naylor RJ, Typers MB (1991): The effect of ondansetron on cognitive performance in the marmoset. Pharmacol Biochem Behav 38:169–175.

Doyon J, Milner B (1991): Role of the right temporal lobe in visual-cue learning during repeated pattern discriminations. Neuropsychologia 29:861–876.

Drachman DA (1981): The cholinergic system, memory and aging. In Enna SJ, Samorajski T, Beer B (eds): "Brain Neurotransmitters and Receptors in Aging and Age-related Disorders, Aging, Vol. 17." New York: Raven, pp 255–268.

Farlow M, Gracon SI, Hershey LA, Lewis KW, Sadowsky CH, Dolan-Ureno J (1992): A controlled trial of tacrine in Alzheimer's disease. JAMA 268:2523–2529.

Fleischhacker WW, Buchgeher A, Schubert H (1986): Memantine in the treatment of senile dementia of the Alzheimer's type. Cog Neuro-Psychopharmacol Biol Psychiatry 10: 87–93.

Fuster JM, Bauer RH (1974): Visual short-term memory deficit from hypothermia of frontal cortex. Brain Res 81:393–400.

Gaspar P, Duyckaerts C, Alvarez C, Javoy-Agid F, Berger B (1991): Alterations of dopaminergic and noradrenergic innervations in motor cortex in Parkinson's disease. Ann Neurol 30:365–374.

Gaspar P, Berger B, Febvret A, Vigny A, Henry JP (1989): Catecholamine innervation of the human cerebral cortex as revealed by comparative immunohistochemistry of tyrosine hydroxylase and dopamine-beta-hydroxylase. J Comp Neurol 279:249–271.

Geaney DP, Soper N, Shepstone BJ, Cowen PJ (1990): Effect of central cholinergic stimulation on regional cerebral blood flow in Alzheimer disease. Lancet 335:1484–1487.

German DC, Manaye KF, White CLI, Woodward DJ, McIntire DD, Smith WK, Kalaria RN, Mann DMA (1992): Disease-specific patterns of locus coeruleus cell loss. Ann Neurol 32:667–676.

German DC, Walker BS, Manaye K, Smith WK, Woodward DJ, North AJ (1988): The human locus coeruleus: Computer reconstruction of the cellular distribution. J Neurosci 8:1776–1788.

German DC, White CLI, Sparkman DR (1987): Alzheimer's disease: Neurofibrillary tangles in nuclei that project to the cerebral cortex. Neuroscience 21:305–312.

Goldberg ME, Bruce CJ (1985): Cerebral cortical activity associated with the orientation of visual attention in the rhesus monkey. Vision Res 25:471–481.

Goldman PS, Rosvold HE (1970): Localization of function within the dorsolateral prefrontal cortex of the rhesus monkey. Exp Neurol 27:291–304.

Goldman-Rakic PS (1987): Circuitry of the primate prefrontal cortex and the regulation of behavior by representational memory. In Plum F (eds): "Handbook of Physiology, The Nervous System, Higher Functions of the Brain." Bethesda: American Physiological Society, pp 373–417.

Goldman-Rakic PS, Brown RM (1981): Regional changes of monoamines in cerebral cortex and subcortical structures of aging rhesus monkeys. Neuroscience 6:177–187.

Gottfries C-G, Adolfsson R, Aquilonius S-M, Carlsson A, Eckernas S-A, Nordberg A, Oreland L, Svennerholm L, Wiberg A, Winblad B (1983): Biochemical changes in dementia disorders of Alzheimer's type (AD/SDAT). Neurobiol Aging 4:261–271.

Gower AJ (1992): 5-HT receptors and cognitive function. In Marsden CA, Heal DJ (eds): "Frontiers in pharmacology and therapeutics: Central serotonin receptors and psychotropic drugs." Oxford: Blackwell Scientific, pp 239–259.

Greenwood PM, Parasuraman R, Haxby JV (1993): Changes in visuospatial attention over the adult lifespan. Neuropsychologia 31:471–485.

Gustafson I, Edvinsson L, Dahlgren N, Hagberg B, Risberg J, Rosén I, Fernö H (1987): Intravenous physostigmine treatment of Alzheimer's disease evaluated by psychometric testing, regional cerebral blood flow (rCBF) measurement, and EEG. Psychopharmacology 93:31–35.

Hadfield MG, Milio C (1990): Regional brain monoamine levels and utilization in middle-aged rats. Life Sci 46:295–299.

Haxby JV, Grady CL, Horwitz B, Ungerleider L, Mishkin M, Carson RE, Herscovitch P, Schapiro MB, Rapoport SI (1991): Dissociation of object and spatial visual processing pathways in human extrastriate cortex. Proc Natl Acad Sci 88:1621–1625.

Hebb DO (1978): On watching myself get old. Psychol Today 12:15–23.

Hervé A, Sara SJ (1994): Inhibitory influences of frontal cortex on locus coeruleus activity. Soc Neurosci Abs 20:806.

Hochanadel G, Kaplan E (1984): Neuropsychology of normal aging. In Albert ML (eds): "Clinical Neurology of Aging." New York: Oxford University Press, pp 231–244.

Hodges H, Fletcher A (in press): Comparison of the 5-HT$_3$ receptor antagonists WAY-100579 and ondansetron on spatial learning in the water maze in rats with excitotoxic lesions of the forebrain cholinergic system. Psychopharmacology, in press.

Holman BL, Johnson KA, Gerada B, Carvalho PA, Satlin A (1992): The scintigraphic appearance of Alzheimer's disease: A prospective study using technetium-99m-HMPAO SPECT. J Nucl Med 33:181–185.

Horel JA, Misantone LJ (1976): Visual discrimination impaired by cutting temporal lobe connections. Science 193:336–338.

Horrigan JP, Barnhill LJ (1995): Guanfacine for treatment of attention-deficit-hyperactivity disorder in boys. J Child Adolesc Psychopharmacol 5:215–223.

Hoyer WJ, Rebok GW, Sved SM (1979): Effects of varying irrelevant information on adult age differences in problem solving. J Gerontol 34:553–560.

Hunt RD, Arnsten AFT, Asbell MD (1995): An open trial of guanfacine in the treatment of attention deficit hyperactivity disorder. J Am Acad Child Adolesc Psychiatry 34:50–54.

Hunt RD, Mindera RB, Cohen DJ (1985): Clonidine benefits children with attention deficit disorder and hyperactivity: Reports of a double-blind placebo-crossover therapeutic trial. J Am Acad Child Psychiatry 24:617–629.

Iversen LL, Rossor MN, Reynolds GP, Hills R, Roth M, Mountjoy CQ, Foote SL, Morrison JH, Bloom FE (1983): Loss of pigmented dopamine beta hydroxylase positive cells from locus coeruleus in senile dementia of Alzheimer's type. Neurosci Lett 39:95–100.

Jackson WJ, Buccafusco JJ (1991): Clonidine enhances delayed matching-to-sample performance by young and aged monkeys. Pharmacol Biochem Behav 39:79–84.

Jacobsen CF (1936): Studies of cerebral function in primates. Comp Psychol Monogr 13:1–68.

Jellinger K, Flament H, Riederer P, Schmid H, Ambrozi L (1980): Levodopa in the treatment of (pre) senile dementia. Mech Ageing Dev 14:253–264.

Johnson KA, Holman BL, Rosen TJ, Nagel JS, English RJ, Growdon JH (1990): Iofetamine I 123 single photon emission computed tomography is accurate in the diagnosis of Alzheimer's disease. Arch Intern Med 150:752–756.

Kievit J, Kuypers HGJM (1975): Basal forebrain and hypothalamic connections to frontal and parietal cortex in the rhesus monkey. Science 187:660–662.

Kilpatrick GJ, Jones BJ, Typers MB (1987): Identification and distribution of 5HT3 receptors in rat brain using radioligand binding. Nature 330:746–748.

Knapp MJ, Knopman DS, Solomon PR, Pendlebury WW, Davis CS, Gracon SI (1994): A 30-week randomized controlled trial of high-dose tacrine in patients with Alzheimer's disease. JAMA 271:985–991.

Kobilka BK, Matsui H, Kobilka TS, Yang-Feng TL, Francke U, Caron MG, Lefkowitz RJ, Regan JW (1987): Cloning, sequencing, and expression of the gene encoding for the human platelet alpha-2-adrenergic receptor. Science 238:650–656.

Kristensen V, Olsen M, Theilgaard A (1977): Levodopa treatment of presenile dementia. Acta Psychiatry Scand 55:41–51.

Kubiak P, Ivanova S, Rajkowski J, Aston-Jones G (1995): Contrasting responses of monkey locus coeruleus neurons to conditioned vs. unconditioned stimuli: Relationship to arousal, performance and vigilance. Soc Neurosci Abst 21:2092.

Kumar A, Schapiro MB, Grady C, Haxby JV, Wagner E, Salerno JA, Friedland RP, Rapoport SI (1991): High-resolution PET studies in Alzheimer's disease. Neuropsychopharmacology 4:35–46.

Leslie FM, Loughlin SE, Sternberg DB, McGaugh JL, Young LE, Zornetzer SF (1985): Noradrenergic changes in senescent memory loss. Brain Res 359:292–299.

Lewis C, Ballinger BR, Presly AS (1978): Trial of levo-dopa in senile dementia. Br Med J 1:550.

Li B-M, Mei Z-T (1994a): Alpha-2 adrenergic modulation of prefrontal neuronal activity related to working memory in monkeys. Abstracts of the 3rd Congress of Federation of Asian and Oceanian Physiological Societies 96.

Li B-M, Mei Z-T (1994b): Delayed response deficit induced by local injection of the alpha-2 adrenergic antagonist yohimbine into the dorsolateral prefrontal cortex in young adult monkeys. Behav Neural Biol 62:134–139.

Lomasney JW, Lorenz W, Allen LF, King K, Regan JW, Yang-Feng TL, Caron M, Lefkowitz RJ (1990): Expansion of the alpha-2-adrenergic family: Cloning and characterization of a human alpha-2-adrenergic receptor subtype, the gene for which is located on chromosome 2. Proc Natl Acad Sci U S A 87:5094–5098.

Luine V, Bowling D, Hearns M (1990): Spatial memory deficits in aged rats: Contributions of monoaminergic systems. Brain Res 537:271–278.

Mair RG, McEntree WJ (1986): Cognitive enhancement in Korsakoff's psychosis by clonidine: A comparison with L-dopa and ephedrine. Psychopharmacology 88:374–380.

Malmo RB (1942): Interference factors in delayed response in monkeys after removal of frontal lobes. Neurophysiology 5:295–308.

Mangoni A, Grassi MP, Frattola L, Piolti R, Bassi S, Motta A, Marcone A, Smirne S (1991): Effects of a MAO-B inhibitor in the treatment of Alzheimer disease. Eur Neurol 31: 100–107.

Marjamäki A, Luomala K, Ala-Uotila S, Scheinin M (1993): Use of recombinant human alpha-2-adrenoceptors to characterize subtype selectivity of antagonist binding. Eur J Pharmacol 246:219–226.

McEntee WJ, Crook TH (1991): Serotonin, memory, and the aging brain. Psychopharmacology 103:143–149.

McEntee WJ, Mair RG (1990): The Korsakoff syndrome: A neurochemical perspective. Trends Neurosci 13:340–344.

Mishkin M (1964): Perseveration of central sets after frontal lesions in monkeys. In: The Frontal Granular Cortex and Behavior, JM Warren and K Akert, Eds., pp 219–241, McGraw-Hill, New York.

Mishkin M, Manning FJ (1978): Non-spatial memory after selective prefrontal lesions in monkeys. Brain Res 143:313–323.

Mishkin M (1982): A memory system in the monkey. Phil Trans R Soc Lond B298:85–95.

Mishkin M (1978): Memory in monkeys severely impaired by combined but not by separate removal of amygdala and hippocampus. Nature 273:297–298.

Mishkin M, Vest B, Morris M, Rosvold HE (1969): A re-examination of the effects of frontal lesions on object alternation. Neuropsychology 7:357–363.

Moffoot A, O'Carroll RE, Murray C, Dougall N, Ebmeier K, Goodwin GM (1994): Clonidine infusion increases uptake of Tc-exametazime in anterior cingulate cortex in Korsakoff's psychosis. Psychol Med 24:53–61.

Mohr E, Schlegel J, Fabbrini G, Williams J, Mouradian M, Mann UM, Claus JJ, Fedio P, Chase NC (1989): Clonidine treatment of Alzheimer's disease. Arch Neurol 46:376–378.

Muramoto O, Sugishita M, Ando K (1984): Cholinergic system and constructional praxis: A further study of physostigmine in Alzheimer's disease. J Neurol Neurosurg Psychiatry 47:485–491.

Muramoto O, Sugishita M, Sugita H, Toyokura Y (1979): Effect of physostigmine on constructional and memory tasks in Alzheimer's disease. Arch Neurol 36:501–503.

Murphy BL, Arnsten AFT, Goldman-Rakic PS, Roth RH (1996): Increased dopamine turnover in the prefrontal cortex impairs spatial working memory performance in rats and monkeys. Proc Natl Acad Sci U S A, in press. 93:1325–1329.

Murphy BL, Roth RH, Arnsten AFT (1994): The effects of FG7142 on prefrontal cortical dopamine and spatial working memory in rat and monkey. Soc Neurosci Abst 20:1018.

Najlerahim A, Bowen DM (1988): Biochemical measurements in Alzheimer's disease reveal a necessity for improved neuroimaging techniques to study metabolism. Biochem J 251: 305–308.

Petrides M, Iversen SD (1979): Restricted posterior parietal lesions in the rhesus monkey and performance on visuospatial tasks. Brain Res 161:63–77.

Piccinin GL, Finali G, Piccirilli M (1990): Neuropsychological effects of L-deprenyl in Alzheimer's type dementia. Neuropharmacology 13:147.

Posner MI (1980): Orienting of attention: The Seventh Sir F. C. Bartlett Lecture. Q J Exp Psychol 32:3–25.

Posner MI, Walker JA, Friedrich FJ, Rafal RD (1984): Effects of parietal injury on covert orienting of visual attention. J Neurosci 4:1863–1874.

Procter AW, Lowe SL, Palmer AM, Francis PT, Esiri MM, Stratmann GC, Najlerahim A, Patel AJ, Hunt A, Bowen DM (1988): Topographical distribution of neurochemical changes in Alzheimer's disease. J Neurol Sci 84:125–140.

Rapp PR, Amaral DG (1992): Individual differences in the cognitive and neurobiological consequences of normal aging. TINS 15:340–345.

Rapp PR, Amaral DG (1989): Evidence for task-dependent memory dysfunction in the aged monkey. J Neurosci 9:3568–3576.

Regan JW, Kobilka TS, Yang-Feng TL, Caron MG, Lefkowitz RJ, Kobilka BK (1988): Cloning and expression of a human kidney cDNA for an alpha-2 adrenergic receptor subtype. PNAS 85:6301–6305.

Reinikainen KJ, Soininen H, Riekkinen PJ (1990): Neurotransmitter changes in Alzheimer's disease: Implications to diagnostics and therapy. J Neurosci Res 27:576–586.

Ridley RM, Durnford LJ, Baker JA, Baker HF (1993): Cognitive inflexibility after archicortical and paleocortical prefrontal lesions in marmosets. Brain Res 628:56–64.

Ridley RM, Baker HF, Drewett B, Johnson JA (1985): Effects of ibotinic acid lesions of the basal forebrain on serial reversal learning in marmosets. Psychopharmacology 86: 438–443.

Roberts AC, Robbins TW, Everitt BJ, Muir JL (1992): A specific form of cognitive rigidity following excitotoxic lesions of the basal forebrain in marmosets. Neuroscience 47: 251–264.

Robinson DL, Kertzman C (1990): Visuospatial attention: Effects of age, gender and spatial reference. Neuropsychologia 28:291–301.

Robinson DL, Petersen SE (1987): Contributions of the pulvinar to visual spatial attention. Neuropsychologia 25:97–105.

Robinson SE (1983): Effect of specific serotonergic lesions on cholinergic neurons in the hippocampus, cortex and striatum. Life Sci 32:345–353.

Rosen WG, Mohs RC, Davis KL (1984): A new rating scale for Alzheimer's disease. Am J Psychiatry 141:1356–1364.

Roth RH, Tam S-Y, Ida Y, Yang J-X, Deutch AY (1988): Stress and the mesocorticolimbic dopamine systems. Ann N Y Acad Sci 537:138–147.

Sawaguchi T, Goldman-Rakic PS (1991): D1 dopamine receptors in prefrontal cortex: Involvement in working memory. Sci 251:947–950.

Scheinin M, Lomasney JW, Hayden-Hixson DM, Schambra UB, Caron MG, Leflowitz RJ, Fremeau RT (1994): Distribution of alpha-2-adrenergic receptor subtype gene expression in rat brain. Brain Res 21:133–149.

Schlegel J, Mohr E, Williams J, Mann U, Gearing M, Chase TN (1989): Guanfacine treatment of Alzheimer's disease. Clin Neuropharmacol 12:124–128.

Schneider JS, Kovelowski CJ (1990): Chronic exposure to low doses of MPTP. I. Cognitive deficits in motor asymptomatic monkeys. Brain Res 519:122–128.

Schubert H, Fleischhacker W (1979): Therapeutische Ansätze bei dementiellen Syndromen. ergebnisse mit Amantadin-Sulfat unter stationären Bedingungen. Ärztl Praxis 46: 2157–2160.

Siddiqi ZA, Kemper TL, Rosene DL, Feldman M (1995): Age related changes in the rhesus monkey: Neuronal loss in subsantia nigra-pars compacta and ventral tegmental area. Soc Neurosci Abst 21:1565.

Sirviö J, Riekkinen P, Vajanto I, Koivisto E, Riekkinnen PJ (1991): The effects of guanfacine, alpha-2 agonist, on the performance of young and aged rats in spatial navigation task. Behav Neural Biol 56:101–107.

Sladek JR, Sladek CD (1979): Relative quantification of monoamine histofluorescence in young and old nonhuman primates. In Finch CE, Potter DE, Kenny AD (eds): "Parkinson's Disease II." New York: Plenum, pp 231–239.

Squire LR, Zola-Morgan S (1991): The medial temporal lobe memory system. Science 253: 1380–1386.

Stroessner-Johnson HM, Rapp PR, Amaral DG (1992): Cholinergic cell loss and hypertrophy in the medial septal nucleus of the behaviorally characterized aged monkey. J Neurosci 12:1936–1944.

Tariot PN, Cohen RM, Sunderland T, Newhouse PA, Young D, Mellow AM, Weingartner H, Mueller EA, Murphy DL (1987): L-Deprenyl in Alzheimer's disease. Arch Gen Psychiatry 44:427–433.

Thierry AM, Tassin JP, Blanc G, Glowinski J (1976): Selective activation of the mesocortical DA system by stress. Nature 263:242–244.

Tomlinson BE, Irving D, Blessing G (1981): Cell loss in the locus coeruleus in senile dementia of Alzheimer type. J Neurol Sci 49:419–428.

Uhlen S, Wikberg JES (1991): Delineation of rat kidney alpha 2A and alpha 2B-adrenoceptors with [^{3}H]RX821002 radioligand binding: Computer modeling revels that guanfacine is an alpha-2A-selective compound. Eur J Pharmacol 202:235–243.

Ungerleider LA (1985): The corticocortical pathways for object recognition and spatial perception. In Chagas C, Gattass R, Gross C (eds): "Pattern Recognition Mechanisms." Pontifical Academy of Sciences, pp 21–37.

van Dyck CH, Lin CH, Robinson R, Cellar J, Narayan M, Arnsten AFT, Hoffer PB (1995a): Effects of the acetylcholine releaser linopirdine on SPECT rCBF and cognitive function in Alzheimer's disease. Soc Neurosci Abst 21:1976.

van Dyck CH, Seibyl JP, Malison RT, Wallace E, Zoghbi SS, Zea-Ponce Y, Baldwin RM, Charney DS, Hoffer PB, Innis RB (1995b): Age-related decline in dopamine transporter binding in human striatum with [^{123}I]β-CIT SPECT. J Nucl Med 36:1175–1181.

Vijayashankar N, Brody H (1979): A quantitative study of the pigmented neurons in the nuclei locus coeruleus and subcoeruleus in man as related to aging. J Neuropathol Exp Neurol 38:490–497.

Voytko ML, Sukhov RR, Walker LC, Breckler SJ, Price DL, Koliatsos VE (1995): Neuronal number and size are preserved in the nucleus basalis of aged rhesus monkeys. Dementia 6:131–141.

Voytko ML, Olton DS, Richardson RT, Gorman LK, Tobin JT, Price DL (1994): Basal forebrain lesions in monkeys disrupt attention but not learning and memory. J Neurosci 14:167–186.

Waeber C, Hoyer D, Palacios JM (1989): 5-HT$_3$ receptors in the human brain: Autoradiographic visualization using ^{3}[H]ICS 205-930. Neuroscience 31:393–400.

Waeber C, Dixon K, Hoyer D, Palacios JM (1988): Localization by autoradiography of neuronal 5-HT$_3$ receptors in the mouse CNS. Eur J Pharmacol 151:351–352.

Walker LC, Kitt CA, Struble RG, Wagster MV, Price DL, Cork LC (1988): The neural basis of memory decline in aged monkeys. Neurobiol Aging 9:657–666.

Wang J, Aigner T, Mishkin M (1990): Effects of neostriatal lesions on visual habit formation in rhesus monkeys. Abst Soc Neurosci 16:617.

Wenk GL, Pierce DJ, Struble RG, Price DL, Cork LC (1989): Age-related changes in multiple neurotransmitter systems in the monkey brain. Neurobiol Aging 10:11–19.

Whitehouse PJ, Price DL, Struble RG, Clark AW, Coyle JT, DeLong MR (1982): Alzheimer's disease and senile dementia: Loss of neurons in the basal forebrain. Science 215:1237–1239.

Zola-Morgan S, Squire LR (1985): Medial temporal lesions in monkeys impair memory on a variety of tasks sensitive to human amnesia. Behav Neurosci 99:22–34.

CHAPTER 4

Cognitive Effects of Selective Loss of Basal Forebrain Cholinergic Neurons: Implications for Cholinergic Therapies of Alzheimer's Disease

MARK G. BAXTER and MICHELA GALLAGHER

Curriculum in Neurobiology (M.G.B.) and Department of Psychology (M.G.),
University of North Carolina, Chapel Hill, North Carolina

INTRODUCTION

The development of 192 IgG-saporin (192 immunoglobulin G-saporin) as a selective immunotoxin for basal forebrain cholinergic neurons has ushered in a new era of studies on the behavioral role of the basal forebrain cholinergic system (BFCS). Recent data with this selective toxin suggest that the BFCS may be involved in regulation of attention, rather than learning and memory as was previously thought. The present chapter aims to review briefly the evidence linking the BFCS to cognitive function. Originally, the "cholinergic hypothesis of memory" directed the search for pharmacological treatments of Alzheimer's disease (AD). More recent findings on the role of the BFCS in attentional processes (but not learning and memory) have implications for therapies of AD based on enhancement of cholinergic function. We discuss these newer findings and their implications for pharmacological therapy of AD.

CHOLINERGIC HYPOTHESIS OF MEMORY

The cholinergic hypothesis states that neurons that utilize acetylcholine as a neurotransmitter play a critical role in the formation or retrieval of memories, and that disorders of memory that occur in normal aging or pathological conditions such as

Pharmacological Treatment of Alzheimer's Disease: Molecular and Neurobiological Foundations,
Edited by Brioni and Decker

AD result from cholinergic deficiency. Several different lines of evidence converged to suggest a cholinergic basis for memory impairment in aging and AD; a comprehensive historical review by Bartus et al. (1985) provides an excellent summary of the evidence leading to the formulation of this hypothesis. We will briefly summarize some of these lines of research here.

Early pharmacological studies demonstrating modulation of learning and memory following administration of cholinergic drugs supported a role for central cholinergic systems in cognitive function (e.g., Meyers et al., 1964; Deutsch et al., 1966). Drachman and Leavitt (1974) first proposed that loss of cholinergic function in aging contributed to age-related memory deficits, based on correspondence between the pattern of memory impairment seen in normal aging and in young volunteers treated with the cholinergic antagonist scopolamine. Experiments in nonhuman primates demonstrated a similar pattern: A striking correspondence was noted between memory impairments in aged rhesus monkeys and memory impairments induced in young monkeys by administration of scopolamine (Bartus and Johnson, 1976; Bartus et al.,1978).

A preliminary finding of reduced cortical choline acetyltransferase (ChAT) activity in patients with senile dementia (Bowen et al., 1976) was quickly replicated by several investigators; reductions were largest in neocortical areas, the amygdala, and hippocampus (Davies and Maloney, 1976; Perry et al., 1977). This finding appeared to be relatively specific for cholinergic markers and not a reflection of generalized degeneration in multiple neurochemical systems (Bowen et al., 1976; Davies and Maloney, 1976; Perry et al., 1977). The demonstration of cholinergic projections from the basal forebrain to the hippocampus and neocortex (e.g., Lewis et al., 1967; Johnston et al., 1979) prompted studies of neurodegeneration within the basal forebrain in patients with Alzheimer's disease (AD). Severe neuronal loss throughout the basal forebrain was demonstrated (Whitehouse et al., 1981; Nakano and Hirano, 1982; Whitehouse et al., 1982; Wilcock et al., 1983). A more modest reduction in the integrity of the basal forebrain cholinergic system seemed to take place in normal aging (Lippa et al., 1980; Strong et al., 1980; reviewed in Bartus et al., 1982).

The consistent and dramatic reduction in cholinergic markers in brain areas critical for cognitive function, combined with the evidence for the involvement of cholinergic systems in learning and memory, informed the formulation of the cholinergic hypothesis of memory (Bartus et al., 1982; Coyle et al., 1983). The implication of this hypothesis was that treatments that enhance or restore cholinergic function should ameliorate cognitive impairments associated with aging and AD. Indeed, age-related cognitive impairments could be ameliorated by treatments with drugs that enhance cholinergic function (Bartus, 1979; Bartus et al., 1980; Bartus et al., 1981). Similarly, drugs that enhance cholinergic functions have produced modest benefits in cognition in patients with AD [e.g., physostigmine (Thal et al., 1989) and tacrine (Davis et al., 1992)].

Development of models for cognitive impairment in AD would naturally facilitate the study of the relationship between cholinergic loss and cognitive impairment and would provide a setting for evaluation of potential therapies for AD. We now turn to such models developed to study this relationship. Particular interest has focused on animals with experimentally induced lesions of the basal forebrain that reduce cholinergic innervation of cortical and limbic areas, reproducing the putative cause of cognitive impairment in AD.

LESION MODELS OF CHOLINERGIC DEFICIENCY IN ALZHEIMER'S DISEASE

A large number of studies have investigated effects of neurotoxic basal forebrain lesions on cognitive function in the laboratory rat. The basal forebrain of the rat contains groups of cholinergic neurons that can be distinguished according to their efferent targets (Wainer and Mesulam, 1990). One major system of cholinergic neurons in the medial septum (MS) and vertical limb of the diagonal band (VDB) provides input to the hippocampal formation; cholinergic neurons in the VDB also innervate cingulate and infralimbic cortex. However, the majority of cholinergic innervation of cortex in the rat derives from neurons located in the sublenticular substantia innominata (SI) and nucleus basalis magnocellularis (nBM).

Cholinergic neurons within basal forebrain nuclei are intermingled with a variety of noncholinergic neurons. Figure 1A shows cholinergic neurons in the medial septum/vertical limb of the diagonal band (MS/VDB) identified with immunohistochemistry using a selective monoclonal antibody directed against ChAT, the synthetic enzyme for acetylcholine and a phenotypic marker of cholinergic neurons. A Nissl-stained section at the same level of the MS/VDB is shown for comparison in Figure 1B, demonstrating the presence of other neurons that do not express ChAT. A similar set of sections is shown in Figures 1C and 1D, at the level of the nucleus basalis magnocellularis/substantia innominata (nBM/SI). The primary method of producing lesions in these areas is by microinjection of glutamate analogs (excitotoxins). Although different excitotoxins produce different degrees of damage to cholinergic neurons as compared to noncholinergic neurons (e.g., Dunnett et al., 1987), the dispersion of cholinergic neurons within the basal forebrain makes it impossible to produce anatomically discrete lesions that will damage only cholinergic neurons with these toxins.

Lesions of the MS/VDB, removing both cholinergic and noncholinergic projections to the hippocampus, result in relatively consistent disruptions in learning and memory. For example, these lesions impair spatial learning in the water maze, reproducing the effects of lesions of the hippocampus on this task (Hagan et al., 1988; Marston et al., 1993).

In contrast, studies of effects of lesions of the nBM have produced discrepant effects on learning and memory. Learning and memory impairments following excitotoxic lesions of the nBM vary depending on the specific toxin used, and do not correlate with the degree of loss of cholinergic neurons produced by the lesion. For example, lesions of the nBM with ibotenic acid produce deficits in learning and memory (Dunnett et al., 1987). However, lesions of the nBM with quisqualic acid, which result in similar or greater depletion of markers of cortical

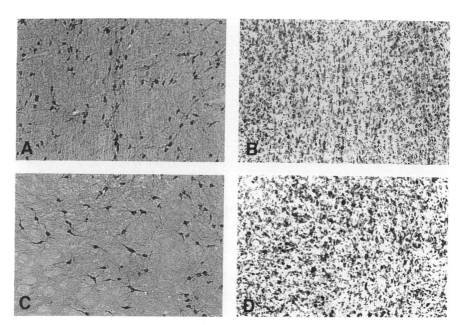

FIGURE 1. Neurons in the basal forebrain at the level of the medial septum/vertical limb of the diagonal band (MS/VDB) (A, B) and nucleus basalis magnocellularis/substantia innominata (nBM/SI) (C, D). (A, C) Immunohistochemistry for choline acetyltransferase (ChAT) demonstrates large cholinergic neurons in both regions. (B, D) Thionin-stained sections demonstrate the density of neurons in the region: large numbers of noncholinergic neurons are interspersed within these regions.

cholinergic innervation, do not produce deficits in learning and memory (Dunnett et al., 1987; Markowska et al., 1990). The discrepancies between results with different neurotoxins, and the implications of these data for the cholinergic hypothesis, have been debated extensively in the literature (Dunnett et al., 1991; Fibiger, 1991; Gallagher and Colombo, 1995). The consensus in these reviews is that damage to cholinergic neurons in the nBM is not the cause of learning and memory deficits, based on a lack of correspondence between reductions in cortical ChAT activity and impairment in these behavioral domains. Efforts to identify populations of noncholinergic neurons in the nBM/SI that might be more closely linked to learning and memory thus far have been largely unsuccessful (Wenk et al., 1992).

Although evidence linking loss of septohippocampal cholinergic systems to memory is more consistent than evidence linking loss of corticopetal cholinergic systems to memory, the data from these experiments remain inconclusive. Neurotoxic basal forebrain lesions invariably result in considerable destruction of noncholinergic neurons in the lesion area, preventing dissociation of the contribution of the cholinergic system from other neurochemical systems.

EFFECTS OF SELECTIVE BASAL FOREBRAIN CHOLINERGIC LESIONS ON LEARNING AND MEMORY

A new lesion method for basal forebrain cholinergic neurons has made possible direct investigations of the effects of selective destruction of these neurons on behavior. In contrast to the learning deficits observed following neurotoxic basal forebrain lesions, the overall conclusion from studies with selective lesions of basal forebrain cholinergic neurons is that despite dramatic reductions in cholinergic innervation of limbic and cortical regions (often exceeding deficits observed even in AD patients), learning and memory remains remarkably unimpaired. A summary of these recent studies follows.

The immunotoxin 192 IgG-saporin is composed of a monoclonal antibody to the low-affinity nerve growth factor receptor (LNGFR), coupled to a ribosome-inactivating cytotoxin, saporin (Wiley et al., 1991). Injections of 192 IgG-saporin into the cerebral ventricles, basal forebrain nuclei, and into target areas of the basal forebrain all produce damage to basal forebrain cholinergic neurons, sparing noncholinergic basal forebrain neurons (Heckers et al., 1994; Holley et al., 1994). Intracerebroventricular (i.c.v.) infusions have the unfortunate side effect of destroying LNGFR-bearing cerebellar Purkinje cells, making it difficult to interpret behavioral deficits consequent to i.c.v. infusions of 192 IgG-saporin as specific to loss of basal forebrain cholinergic neurons (Heckers et al., 1994).

An initial study with i.c.v. infusions of 192 IgG-saporin reported that immunolesions of basal forebrain cholinergic neurons resulted in spatial learning deficits (Nilsson et al., 1992), but, as previously mentioned, the loss of cerebellar Purkinje neurons following this lesion could produce motor deficits that would disrupt water maze performance in the absence of a learning deficit; a nonspatial cue-learning task was not included for comparison in this study. A subsequent study by Berger-Sweeney et al. (1994) confirmed that i.c.v. infusions of 192 IgG-saporin disrupt performance in both spatial and nonspatial versions of the water maze task.

Several later experiments utilizing injections of 192 IgG-saporin directly into the basal forebrain suggested that learning and memory impairments produced by selective lesions of basal forebrain cholinergic neurons were considerably less severe than would be expected, based on the hypothesized role of the cholinergic system in cognitive function. The initial study by Berger-Sweeney et al. (1994) examined rats with site-specific infusions of the immunotoxin into the medial septal area (MSA) or nucleus basalis magnocellularis (nBM). Rats with immunolesions of the MSA were nearly as good as controls in the spatial water maze task, despite the near-complete loss of cholinergic projections to the hippocampus. Rats with nBM lesions showed spatial learning impairments but were also somewhat impaired in the nonspatial task. Moreover, Berger-Sweeney et al. did not interpret the effects of lesions in this group as being specific to loss of corticopetal cholinergic projections because of the loss of striatal cholinergic interneurons produced by the toxin injections into the nBM. These results presented a significant challenge to the cholinergic hypothesis of learning and memory: Selective damage to the cholinergic input to the hippocampus failed to result in a profound learning impairment, as would have been predicted based on previous studies with less selective lesions. Torres et al. (1994) demonstrated completely intact spatial learning in rats with immunolesions of the medial septum (MS), diagonal band of Broca (DBB), or nBM; however, nBM lesions produced deficits in passive avoidance retention, and MS lesions produced a small delay-dependent deficit in a delayed nonmatching-to-position (DNMTP) task. Wenk et al (1994) produced relatively small lesions of the nBM and found no deficits in passive avoidance acquisition or in spatial alternation in a T-maze.

To summarize, these initial behavioral studies with 192 IgG-saporin found either no effect or a very small effect of selective lesions of basal forebrain cholinergic neurons on learning and memory in behavioral tests commonly employed to assess these cognitive functions in rats. This is in stark contrast to effects of nonselective neurotoxic lesions (e.g., those made with ibotenic acid) of the same areas that do produce substantial behavioral impairments. More recently, we have examined immunolesions of the medial septum/vertical limb of the diagonal band (MS/VDB) and nucleus basalis magnocellularis/substantia innominata (nBM/SI) in an attempt to produce nearly complete destruction of cholinergic projections to hippocampus or neocortex (respectively) and to evaluate the behavioral effects of these lesions in a testing protocol employed by our laboratory to determine age-related deficits in spatial learning (Gallagher et al., 1993). We found that neither lesion produced significant disruption of spatial learning ability despite reduction of ChAT activity by 90% in the hippocampus of MS/VDB-lesioned rats and by 63% in the cortex of nBM/SI-lesioned rats (Baxter et al., 1995a). Lesions of both this extent and specificity have proven impossible to obtain with excitotoxic lesion techniques.

The lack of effect of lesions of basal forebrain cholinergic neurons on spatial learning is striking in view of the central role hypothesized for the basal forebrain cholinergic system in learning and memory. It is of note that severe behavioral impairments have only been observed following i.c.v. infusions of 192 IgG-saporin (Nilsson et al., 1992; Waite et al., 1995). These deficits could be due to cerebellar damage, but could also be the result of conjoint damage to both hippocampal and cortical cholinergic afferents, producing more severe deficits than loss of either one alone. Waite et al. (1995) only observed behavioral deficits following i.c.v. doses of 192 IgG-saporin that resulted in near-complete loss of cholinergic neurons throughout the basal forebrain. Unfortunately, these doses of 192 IgG-saporin also produced cerebellar damage, making it impossible to dissociate spatial learning deficits from motor deficits. Consistent with this view, those groups with apparent spatial learning impairment also exhibited increased latencies in a nonspatial cue-learning task, suggestive of motoric impairment. We have recently produced basal forebrain lesions with injections of 192 IgG-saporin into the MS/VDB and nBM/SI, destroying both cortical and hippocampal cholinergic projections but sparing cerebellar Purkinje neurons. These rats demonstrate completely normal spatial learning ability in the water maze [Figure 2; Baxter et al. (1996)].

It is relatively clear from the results with selective cholinergic immunolesions that near-total destruction of basal forebrain cholinergic neurons largely spares learning and memory in these behavioral procedures. This result is surprising, given other data that indicate a correlation between cholinergic cell loss and degree of cognitive im-

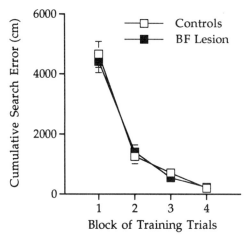

FIGURE 2. Effects of combined lesions of the MS/VDB and nBM/SI [basal forebrain (BF) lesion] on spatial learning in the water maze (Baxter et al., 1996). The dependent measure, cumulative search error, is based on a calculation of average distance from the platform every second during the training trial (Gallagher et al., 1993). Higher scores indicate poorer spatial learning and less accurate search. Both control and lesioned rats show comparable learning. Reproduced by permission of Rapid Science Publishers, London.

pairment (specifically, spatial learning impairment) in aging (e.g., Fischer et al., 1991; Gallagher et al., 1995). This raises the possibility that aged animals may differentially rely on the cholinergic system for learning and memory, perhaps to compensate for other neurobiological changes throughout the brain that also occur with aging. Hence, effects of selective cholinergic lesions in aged animals may differ from effects of those lesions in young animals. Indeed, aged animals provide additional utility as a model system because AD pathology is associated with aging.

Based on the central role of the hippocampus in spatial learning and the correspondence between indices of septohippocampal cholinergic function and age-related spatial learning impairment [for review, see Gallagher et al. (1995)], we hypothesized that destruction of cholinergic neurons in the MS/VDB (which fails to affect spatial learning in young rats) might produce an impairment in aged rats with relatively preserved spatial learning ability. To examine this directly we produced immunolesions of the MS/VDB in young and aged rats that had been prescreened for spatial learning ability: Only aged rats with relatively intact spatial learning ability were included to prevent a possible floor effect. Spatial learning was assessed again after the lesion, in a different environment so that acquisition of new spatial information was required to solve the task. Immunolesions of the MS/VDB producing 90% depletion of hippocampal ChAT activity also failed to produce spatial learning deficits in aged rats [Figure 3; Baxter and Gallagher (1996)]. These data suggest that cholinergic loss, even against a background of other neurobiological changes that occur with aging, is insufficient to produce learning and memory deficits in these testing procedures.

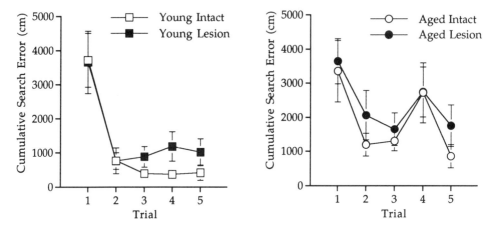

FIGURE 3. Effects of MS/VDB immunolesions in young and aged rats on spatial learning. All rats were tested in a standard water maze protocol (Gallagher et al., 1993) prior to assignment to lesion or control groups; rats within an age group were matched for preoperative spatial learning ability and aged rats with severely impaired spatial learning were excluded. Following surgery, spatial learning was tested in a new maze with different extra-maze cues. There was no significant effect of the MS/VDB immunolesion on spatial learning in either young or aged rats (Baxter and Gallagher, 1996).

EFFECTS OF SELECTIVE BASAL FOREBRAIN CHOLINERGIC LESIONS ON ATTENTION

The absence of significant learning impairment following extensive damage to basal forebrain cholinergic neurons suggests that these neurons do not play as central a role in learning and memory as was previously believed. Despite this lack of effect on learning and memory, selective removal of basal forebrain cholinergic neurons in young rats is sufficient to produce substantial behavioral impairments in tasks that primarily assess the regulation of attention. Moreover, the findings we will summarize have indicated that lesions of corticopetal and septohippocampal cholinergic projections disrupt attentional processing in distinctive ways. These findings are also in agreement with several reports indicating that less selective neurotoxic lesions of nBM/SI alter the performance of rats in tests of attention (e.g., Robbins et al., 1989; Muir et al., 1994).

The term "attention" refers to cognitive processes that control the selection of incoming sensory information to be processed by the animal. Attention can be directed by "bottom–up" processes, involving filtering of selected sensory events from a large number of competing simultaneous stimuli, or by "top–down" processes, such as cognitive set or memory for the significance of stimuli (Desimone and Duncan, 1995).

Previous studies of the effects of neurotoxic basal forebrain lesions on attention have generally employed performance-based assessments that are sensitive to disruption of bottom–up processes, for example, the ability of an animal to detect and respond to a briefly presented visual stimulus that can appear in any of several different locations (the five-choice serial reaction time task). Neurotoxic lesions of the nBM/SI and blockade of cholinergic neurotransmission decrease choice accuracy in this procedure; however, these deficits can be overcome by increasing target duration, suggesting that the nature of the impairment is attentional in nature (e.g., Muir et al., 1992; Muir et al., 1994). Attentional impairments following nBM/SI lesions directly correspond to the degree of loss of cholinergic projections (Muir et al., 1994): injections of toxins that produce relatively greater damage to cholinergic neurons compared to noncholinergic neurons [e.g., α-amino-3-hydroxy-5-methyl-4-isoxazole propionic acid (AMPA)] still produce severe attentional deficits, in contrast to impairments in learning and memory following excitotoxic lesions of nBM/SI that do not correspond to the degree of cholinergic loss. Based on these earlier findings, it would be predicted that attentional processing (unlike spatial learning) is sensitive to selective loss of basal forebrain cholinergic neurons.

We have examined effects of selective cholinergic lesions of the nBM/SI on attention in a performance-based procedure designed to assess spatial orienting of attention (Chiba et al., 1995b), similar in design to that employed by Voytko et al. (1994) in their assessment of attentional function in basal forebrain-lesioned monkeys and based on human studies by Posner and colleagues (e.g., Posner et al., 1984). In this procedure, rats are trained to respond to a target that can appear in one of two locations. The target is preceded by a visual cue at one of the possible target locations that either accurately or inaccurately predicts the location of the subsequent target. In this procedure, response time on trials when the cue accurately predicts the location of the target ("valid" trials) is more rapid than response time on trials when the cue inaccurately predicts the location of the target ("invalid" trials). Similarly, accuracy on valid trials is slightly greater compared to accuracy on invalid trials. Hence, the subjects use the cue to optimize performance on the task (responding faster and more accurately to the target). Trials with no cue preceding the target ("neutral" trials) are also included for comparison.

Rats were trained on this task and then given immunotoxic lesions of the nBM/SI or a control surgery. Following surgery, rats were given a brief reacclimation to the operant procedure and then reassessed in the attention task. Rats with nBM/SI lesions exhibited an enhanced sensitivity to the disruptive effects of invalid trials: The cost of an invalid trial (manifested by both reduced accuracy and increased reaction time) was disproportionately larger in lesioned rats (Figure 4A). This effect gradually diminished with continued postsurgical testing until the lesioned rats were performing at comparable levels to controls (Figure 4B). However, the lesion effect could be reinstated by reducing the target duration, thereby making the target more difficult to detect and increasing the demand on attention (Figure 4C). This lesion effect resembles the effect of basal forebrain lesions in monkeys (Voytko et al., 1994) and is strikingly similar to deficits of AD patients on this task (Parasuraman et al., 1992).

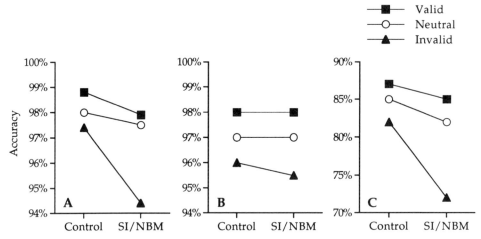

FIGURE 4. Effect of nBM/SI immunolesions on attention in a spatially cued reaction time task (Chiba et al., 1995b). Rats are to respond to a target in one of two spatial locations. The target can be preceded by a cue in the same spatial location as the target ("valid" trials), a cue in the opposite spatial location ("invalid" trial), or no cue ("neutral" trial). Accuracy is increased on valid trials and decreased on invalid trials relative to neutral trials, reflective of the orienting of attention to the cue. (A) After a brief reacclimation to the operant procedure following surgery, nBM/SI-lesioned rats show an increased cost of invalid trials, manifested by a disproportionately larger decrease in accuracy following invalid cues. (B) This lesion effect recovers following several weeks of post-lesion testing. (C) Increasing attention demands by decreasing target duration reinstates the lesion effect after it recovers under baseline test parameters. (Note the overall decrease in accuracy in both groups following the reduction in target duration, as evidenced by the difference in scale on the y-axis.)

These data indicate that cholinergic projections from nBM/SI to cortex are involved in regulation of attention in a performance-based assessment, effects that are manifested over very brief time intervals (less than a second). As mentioned previously, another process that controls attention is the learned significance of events. In this context, it is interesting to note that neurons in the nBM register associations between stimuli during learning. These neurons display firing correlates to events associated with rewarding or aversive stimuli (Richardson and DeLong, 1986, 1990, 1991). Therefore, cholinergic neurons in the nBM/SI (and the MS/VDB as well) might also be involved in directing attention based on the learned significance of stimuli. These effects of attention could manifest themselves over much longer time periods to optimize performance.

Our studies of this function of the basal forebrain cholinergic system have examined attentional processing of conditioned stimuli in Pavlovian conditioning paradigms, based on the Pearce and Hall (1980) model of associative learning. A serial conditioning procedure originally designed by Wilson et al. (1992) was used to produce increased attention to a target cue. A predictive relationship of that cue with another event is established in the conditioning procedure and is subsequently altered ("shifted"). The violation of expectations about the predictive relationship between events produces enhanced attention to the target cue, an effect that is apparent in more rapid conditioning to the target cue when it is paired directly with a reward. A summary of data from a study of effects of nBM/SI immunolesions on this phenomenon appears in Figure 5. Compared to rats in which the relationship between stimuli remains consistent, rats that receive the shift in predictive relationship show greater conditioning to that stimulus. Rats with immunolesions of nBM/SI fail to show this increment in attentional processing (Chiba et al., 1995a).

Based on this finding, we sought to determine if these lesions would also disrupt decreases in processing of conditioned stimuli ("decremental" attention), which reduce attentional allocation. One assessment of decremental attentional processing can be made in a latent inhibition procedure. One of two visual stimuli is exposed alone for several sessions. Subsequently, both the pre-exposed stimulus and the novel stimulus are (independently) paired with food. The decreased attention to the pre-exposed stimulus results in reduced conditioning to that stimulus as compared to the novel stimulus.

Rats with immunolesions of either the nBM/SI or MS/VDB were tested in this latent inhibition procedure (Figure 6; Baxter et al., 1995b; Chiba et al., 1995a). Control rats show reduced conditioning to the pre-exposed stimulus. Interestingly, nBM/SI-lesioned rats also show this decrement in attention to the pre-exposed stimulus. Hence, destruction of corticopetal basal forebrain projections does not disrupt

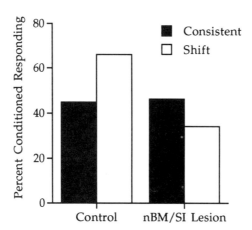

FIGURE 5. Effects of nBM/SI immunolesions on increments in attentional processing (Chiba et al., 1995a). Data presented are average levels of conditioned responding (food cup behavior during the presentation of the conditioned stimulus) during the final phase of the conditioning procedure (direct pairing of the target cue with food reward). Control rats in the SHIFT condition (that increments attention to the target stimulus) show greater conditioned responding than control rats in the CONSISTENT condition, indicative of an increase in attentional processing of the target cue. In contrast, nBM/SI-lesioned rats in the SHIFT condition fail to show this increase in attention. Data adapted from Chiba et al., 1995a, by permission of the Society for Neuroscience.

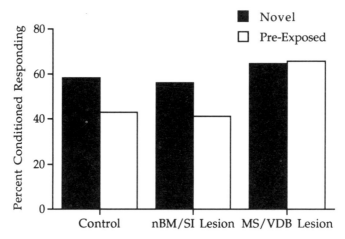

FIGURE 6. Effects of nBM/SI and MS/VDB immunolesions on decrements in attentional processing in a latent inhibition procedure (Baxter et al., 1995b; Chiba et al., 1995a). Data presented are average levels of conditioned responding (food cup behavior during the presentation of the conditioned stimulus) during the conditioning phase. Control rats demonstrate greater conditioning to a novel stimulus compared to a preexposed stimulus, indicative of a decrement in attentional processing of the pre-exposed cue. nBM/SI-lesioned rats also show this decrement in attention. In contrast, MS/VDB-lesioned rats fail to show this decrement in attention: conditioning to the preexposed stimulus occurs at equivalent levels to conditioning to the novel stimulus. nBM/SI lesion data adapted from Chiba et al., 1995a, by permission of the Society for Neuroscience.

the ability to decrease attentional processing. However, MS/VDB-lesioned rats *do* show a disruption of decremental attentional processing: These rats demonstrate equivalent conditioning to both novel and pre-exposed stimuli, indicating a failure to reduce attention to the pre-exposed stimulus. It is important to note that the failure to exhibit latent inhibition is not attributable to an effect of the lesion on associative learning, because formation of the association between the novel cue and food is comparable between the lesion and control groups.

The results with the selective cholinergic immunotoxin provide evidence that learning and memory functions remain intact following near-total removal of basal forebrain cholinergic neurons, confirming impressions from studies with less selective toxins that cholinergic loss alone may be insufficient to produce learning and memory impairment. However, the absence of learning and memory impairments following selective lesions of basal forebrain cholinergic neurons do not indicate that this system is uninvolved in cognitive function or that loss of these neurons can be rapidly and completely compensated. Reliable attentional impairments emerge following selective cholinergic lesions, and these deficits are in agreement with results from less selective lesion methods.

IMPLICATIONS FOR CHOLINERGIC THERAPIES OF ALZHEIMER'S DISEASE

What is the significance of these results for pharmacological therapy of Alzheimer's disease? The studies with selective cholinergic immunolesions provide fairly conclusive evidence that loss of basal forebrain cholinergic neurons does not result in impaired learning and memory, at least in the procedures employed to model human cognitive functions in laboratory animals. Cholinergic depletion produced by these lesions is often greater than that seen even in advanced cases of AD. Instead, loss of these neurons results in disruption of attentional processes. Indeed, regulation of attention may represent the primary function of the BFCS (Muir et al., 1993; Voytko, 1996).

In terms of an animal model of AD, selective cholinergic basal forebrain lesions fail to reproduce the entire spectrum of cognitive deficits observed in AD. However, they do mimic a specific feature of AD, namely, deficits in attention (Parasuraman et al., 1992; Parasuraman and Haxby, 1993; Sahakian et al., 1993). Thus, animals with selective cholinergic basal forebrain lesions may be useful as a model system for attentional deficits in AD and may provide the most relevant setting for assessing effectiveness of treatments of these types of deficits in AD.

The lesion results also suggest that treatments aimed at enhancing cholinergic function would produce improvements in attentional function, as opposed to memory per se, based on the hypothesis that the cholinergic deficit is specifically involved in attentional dysfunction rather than mnemonic deficits in AD. Treatment with tacrine produces amelioration of attentional deficits in AD patients, as assessed in a human version of the five-choice serial reaction time task employed by Robbins and colleagues (Sahakian et al., 1993); this study also failed to find effects of tacrine on tests of memory. Hence, direct assessments of attention are likely to be more useful for revealing beneficial effects of cholinergic therapies for AD.

REFERENCES

Bartus RT (1979): Physostigmine and recent memory: Effects in young and aged nonhuman primates. Science 206:1087–1089.

Bartus RT, Johnson HR (1976): Short-term memory in the rhesus monkey: Disruption from the anticholinergic scopolamine. Pharmacol Biochem Behav 5:31–39.

Bartus RT, Dean RL, Pontecorvo MJ, Flicker C (1985): The cholinergic hypothesis: A historical overview, current perspective, and future directions. Ann N Y Acad Sci 444:332–358.

Bartus RT, Dean RL, Beer B, Lippa AS (1982): The cholinergic hypothesis of geriatric memory dysfunction. Science 217:408–417.

Bartus RT, Dean RL, Sherman KA, Friedman E, Beer B (1981): Profound effects of combining choline and piracetam on memory enhancement and cholinergic function in aged rats. Neurobiol Aging 2:105–111.

Bartus RT, Dean RL, Beer B (1980): Memory deficits in aged Cebus monkeys and facilitation with central cholinomimetics. Neurobiol Aging 1:145–152.

Bartus RT, Fleming D, Johnson HR (1978): Aging in the rhesus monkey: Debilitating effects on short-term memory. J Gerontol 33:858–871.

Baxter MG, Gallagher M (1996): Intact spatial learning in both young and aged rats following selective removal of hippocampal cholinergic input. Behav Neurosci 110:460–467.

Baxter MG, Bucci DJ, Sobel TJ, Williams MJ, Gorman LK, Gallagher M (1996): Intact spatial learning following lesions of basal forebrain cholinergic neurons. Neuro Report 7:1417–1420.

Baxter MG, Gallagher M, Holland PC (1995b): Disruption of decremental attentional processing by selective removal of hippocampal cholinergic input. Soc Neurosci Abst 21:935.

Baxter MG, Bucci DJ, Gorman LK, Wiley RG, Gallagher M (1995a): Selective immunotoxic lesions of basal forebrain cholinergic cells: Effects on learning and memory in rats. Behav Neurosci 109:714–722.

Berger-Sweeney J, Heckers S, Mesulam M-M, Wiley RG, Lappi DA, Sharma M (1994): Differential effects on spatial navigation of immunotoxin-induced cholinergic lesions of the medial septal area and nucleus basalis magnocellularis. J Neurosci 14:4507–4519.

Bowen DM, Smith CB, White P, Davison AN (1976): Neurotransmitter-related enzymes and indices of hypoxia in senile dementia and other abiotrophies. Brain 99:459–496.

Chiba AA, Bucci DJ, Holland PC, Gallagher M (1995a): Basal forebrain cholinergic lesions disrupt increments but not decrements in conditioned stimulus processing. J Neurosci 15:7315–7322.

Chiba AA, Bushnell PJ, Oshiro WM, Gallagher M (1995b): Altered selective attention in rats with cholinergic lesions of the substantia innominata. Soc Neurosci Abstr 21:936.

Coyle JT, Price DL, DeLong MR (1983): Alzheimer's disease: A disorder of cortical cholinergic innervation. Science 219:1184–1190.

Davies P, Maloney AJF (1976): Selective loss of central cholinergic neurons in Alzheimer's disease. Lancet 2:1403.

Davis KL, Thal LJ, Gamzu ER, Davis CS, Woolson RF, Gracon SI, Drachman DA, Schneider LS, Whitehouse PJ, Hoover TM, Morris JC, Kawas CH, Knopman DS, Earl NL, Kumar V. Doody RS (1992): A double-blind, placebo-controlled multicenter study of tacrine for Alzheimer's disease. New Engl J Med 327:1253–1259.

Desimone R, Duncan J (1995): Neural mechanisms of selective visual attention. Ann Rev Neurosci 18:193–22.

Deutsch JA, Hamburg MD, Dahl H (1966): Anticholinesterase-induced amnesia and its temporal aspects. Science 151:221–223.

Drachman D, Leavitt JL (1974): Human memory and the cholinergic system: A relationship to aging? Arch Neurol 30:113–121.

Dunnett SB, Everitt BJ, Robbins TW (1991): The basal forebrain-cortical cholinergic system: Interpreting the functional consequences of excitotoxic lesions. Trends Neurosci 14:494–501.

Dunnett SB, Whishaw IQ, Jones GH, Bunch ST (1987): Behavioural, biochemical and histochemical effects of different neurotoxic amino acids injected into nucleus basalis magnocellularis of rats. Neuroscience 20:653–669.

Fibiger HC (1991): Cholinergic mechanisms in learning, memory, and dementia: A review of recent evidence. Trends Neurosci 14:220–223.

Fischer W, Chen KS, Gage FH, Björklund A (1991): Progressive decline in spatial learning and integrity of forebrain cholinergic neurons in rats during aging. Neurobiol Aging 13:9–23.

Gallagher M, Colombo PJ (1995): Ageing: The cholinergic hypothesis of cognitive decline. Curr Opin Neurobiol 5:161–168.

Gallagher M, Nagahara AH, Burwell RD (1995): Cognition and hippocampal systems in aging: Animal models. In McGaugh JL, Weinberger NM, Lynch G (eds) "Brain and Memory: Modulation and Mediation of Neuroplasticity." New York: Oxford, pp 103–126.

Gallagher M, Burwell R, Burchinal M (1993): Severity of spatial learning impairment in aging: Development of a learning index for performance in the Morris water maze. Behav Neurosci 107:618–626.

Hagan JJ, Salamone JD, Simpson J, Iversen SD, Morris RGM (1988): Place navigation in rats is impaired by lesions of medial septum and diagonal band but not nucleus basalis magnocellularis. Behav Brain Res 27:9–20.

Heckers S, Ohtake T, Wiley RG, Lappi DA, Geula C, Mesulam M-M (1994): Complete and selective cholinergic denervation of rat neocortex and hippocampus but not amygdala by an immunotoxin against the p75 NGF receptor. J Neurosci 14:1271–1289.

Holley LA, Wiley RG, Lappi DA, Sarter M (1994): Cortical cholinergic deafferentation following the intracortical infusion of 192 IgG-saporin: A quantitative histochemical study. Brain Res 663:277–286.

Johnston MV, McKinney M, Coyle JT (1979): Evidence for a cholinergic projection to neocortex from neurons in basal forebrain. Proc Natl Acad Sci U S A 76:5392–5396.

Lewis PR, Shute CCD, Silver A (1967): Confirmation from choline acetylase analyses of a massive cholinergic innervation to the rat hippocampus. J Physiol 191:215–224.

Lippa AS, Pelham RW, Beer B, Critchett DJ, Dean RL, Bartus RT (1980): Brain cholinergic dysfunction and memory in aged rats. Neurobiol Aging 1:13–19.

Markowska AL, Wenk GL, Olton DS (1990): Nucleus basalis magnocellularis and memory: Differential effects of two neurotoxins. Behav Neural Biol 54:13–26.

Marston HM, Everitt BJ, Robbins TW (1993): Comparative effects of excitotoxic lesions of the hippocampus and septum/diagonal band on conditional visual discrimination and spatial learning. Neuropsychologia 31:1099–1118.

Meyers B, Roberts KH, Riciputi RH, Domino EF (1964): Some effects of muscarinic cholinergic blocking drugs on behavior and the electrocorticogram. Psychopharmacologia 5:289–300.

Muir JL, Everitt BJ, Robbins TW (1994): AMPA-induced excitotoxic lesions of the basal forebrain: A significant role for the cortical cholinergic system in attentional function. J Neurosci 14:2313–2326.

Muir JL, Page KJ, Sirinathsinghji DJS, Robbins TW, Everitt BJ (1993): Excitotoxic lesions of basal forebrain cholinergic neurons: Effects on learning, memory, and attention. Behav Brain Res 57:123–131.

Muir JL, Dunnett SB, Robbins TW, Everitt BJ (1992): Attentional functions of the forebrain cholinergic systems: Effects of intraventricular hemicholinium, physostigmine, basal forebrain lesions and intracortical grafts on a multiple-choice serial reaction time task. Exp Brain Res 89:611–622.

Nakano I, Hirano A (1982): Loss of large neurons of the medial septal nucleus in an autopsy case of Alzheimer's disease. J Neuropathol Exp Neurol 41:341.

Nilsson OG, Leanza G, Rosenblad C, Lappi DA, Wiley RG, Björklund A (1992): Spatial learning impairments in rats with selective immunolesion of the forebrain cholinergic system. NeuroReport 3:1005–1008.

Parasuraman R, Haxby JV (1993): Attention and brain function in Alzheimer's disease: A review. Neuropsychology 7:242–272.

Parasuraman R, Greenwood PM, Haxby JV, Grady CL (1992): Visuospatial attention in dementia of the Alzheimer type. Brain 115:711–733.

Pearce JM, Hall G (1980): A model for Pavlovian learning: Variations in the effectiveness of conditioned but not of unconditioned stimuli. Psychol Rev 106:532–552.

Perry EK, Perry RH, Blessed G, Tomlinson BE (1977): Necropsy evidence of central cholinergic deficits in senile dementia. Lancet i:189.

Posner MI, Walker JA, Friedrich FJ, Rafal RD (1984): Effects of parietal injury on covert orienting of attention. J Neurosci 4:1863–1874.

Richardson RT, DeLong MR (1991): Electrophysiological studies of the functions of the nucleus basalis in primates. Adv Exp Med Biol 295:233–252.

Richardson RT, DeLong MR (1990): Context-dependent responses of primate nucleus basalis neurons in a go/no-go task. J Neurosci 10:2528–2540.

Richardson RT, DeLong MR (1986): Nucleus basalis of Meynert neuronal activity during a delayed response task in monkey. Brain Res 399:364–368.

Robbins TW, Everitt BJ, Marston HM, Wilkinson J, Jones GH, Page KJ (1989): Comparative effects of ibotenic acid- and quisqualic acid-induced lesions of the substantia innominata on attentional function in the rat: Further implications for the role of the cholinergic neurons of the nucleus basalis in cognitive processes. Behav Brain Res 35:221–240.

Sahakian BJ, Owen AM, Morant NJ, Eagger SA, Boddington S, Crayton L, Crockford HA, Crooks M, Hill K, Levy R (1993): Further analysis of the cognitive effects of tetrahydroaminoacridine (THA) in Alzheimer's disease: Assessment of attentional and mnemonic function using CANTAB. Psychopharmacology 110:395–401.

Strong R, Hicks P, Hsu L, Bartus RT, Enna SJ (1980): Age-related alterations in the rodent brain cholinergic system and behavior. Neurobiol Aging 1:59–63.

Thal LJ, Masur DM, Blau AD, Fuld PA, Klauber MR (1989): Chronic oral physostigmine without lecithin improves memory in Alzheimer's disease. J Am Geriat Soc 37:42–48.

Torres EM, Perry TA, Blokland A, Wilkinson LS, Wiley RG, Lappi DA, Dunnett SB (1994): Behavioural, histochemical and biochemical consequences of selective immunolesions in discrete regions of the basal forebrain cholinergic system. Neuroscience 63:95–122.

Voytko ML (1996): Cognitive functions of the basal forebrain cholinergic system in monkeys: Memory or attention? Behav Brain Res 75:13–25.

Voytko ML, Olton DS, Richardson RT, Gorman LK, Tobin JR, Price DL (1994): Basal forebrain lesions in monkeys disrupt attention but not learning and memory. J Neurosci 14:167–186.

Wainer BH, Mesulam M-M (1990): Ascending cholinergic pathways in the rat brain. In Steriade M, Biesold D (eds): "Brain Cholinergic Systems." Oxford: Oxford University Press, pp 65–119.

Waite JJ, Chen AD, Wardlow ML, Wiley RG, Lappi DA, Thal LJ (1995): 192 immunoglobulin G-saporin produces graded behavioral and biochemical changes accompanying the loss of cholinergic neurons of the basal forebrain and cerebellar Purkinje cells. Neuroscience 65:463–476.

Wenk GL, Stoehr JD, Quintana G, Mobley S, Wiley RG (1994): Behavioral, biochemical, histological and electrophysiological effects of 192 IgG-saporin injections into the basal forebrain of rats. J Neurosci 14:5986–5995.

Wenk GL, Harrington CA, Tucker DA, Rance NE, Walker LC (1992): Basal forebrain lesions and memory: A biochemical histological, and behavioral study of differential vulnerability to ibotenate and quisqualate. Behav Neurosci 106:909–923.

Whitehouse PJ, Price DL, Struble RG, Clark AW, Coyle JT, DeLong MR (1982): Alzheimer's disease and senile dementia: Loss of neurons in the basal forebrain. Science 215:1237–1239.

Whitehouse PJ, Price DL, Clark AW, Coyle JT, DeLong MR (1981): Alzheimer disease: Evidence for selective loss of cholinergic neurons in the nucleus basalis. Ann Neurol 10:122–126.

Wilcock GK, Esiri MM, Bowen DM, Smith CCT (1983): The nucleus basalis in Alzheimer's disease: Cell counts and cortical biochemistry. Neuropath Appl Neurobiol 9:175–179.

Wiley RG, Oeltmann TN, Lappi DA (1991): Immunolesioning: Selective destruction of neurons using immunotoxin to rat NGF receptor. Brain Res 562:149–153.

Wilson PN, Boumphrey P, Pearce JM (1992): Restoration of the orienting response to a light by a change in its predictive accuracy. Q J Exp Psychol 44B:17–36.

CHAPTER 5

Cortical Acetylcholine and Attention: Neuropharmacological and Cognitive Principles Directing Treatment Strategies for Cognitive Disorders

MARTIN SARTER, JOHN P. BRUNO, and ANNE MARIE HIMMELHEBER

Department of Psychology and Neuroscience Program, Ohio State University, Columbus, Ohio 43210

BEHAVIORAL AND COGNITIVE FUNCTIONS OF CORTICAL ACETYLCHOLINE

The functions of cortical acetylcholine (ACh) have remained a major research topic in biopsychology for over 50 years. Contemporary reviews of biopsychological research on forebrain ACh usually begin by pointing to the early studies on the behavioral effects of muscarinic antagonists (e.g., Hearst, 1959; Herz, 1960). Furthermore, a considerable increase in research activity in this area was stimulated by the finding that forebrain cholinergic systems degenerate in senile dementia (Pope et al., 1964; Bowen et al., 1976; Perry et al., 1977; Whitehouse et al., 1982) and that decreases in cortical ACh, but not in the activity of other cortical inputs, correlate with the severity of the dementia (e.g., Sims et al., 1983; DeKosky et al., 1992; Palmer et al., 1987a,b). However, attempts to measure cortical ACh and to determine its functions date back to the 1940s. Feldberg and Vogt reported in 1948 that cortical ACh content "is comparatively uniform even in areas functionally and architecturally as different as area 4 (motor), area 3 (somaesthetic), area 17 (visual) and area 51 (olfactory)" (p. 374). Richter and Crossland (1949) undertook original research into the role of ACh in arousal by assessing the effects of, for example, sleeping and emotional excitement on ACh content. As would be expected based on

Pharmacological Treatment of Alzheimer's Disease: Molecular and Neurobiological Foundations,
Edited by Brioni and Decker
ISBN 0-471-16758-4   © 1997 Wiley-Liss, Inc.

present knowledge, they found that ACh content (essentially the opposite of extracellular levels) "vary inversely with the degree of functional activity of the brain" (p. 253). Studies by Phillis and Chong (1965; Phillis, 1968) and Collier and Mitchell (1966) stressed the fact that stimulation of a sensory modality elicited widespread increases in cortical ACh *release* and attributed arousal-like and augmenting functions to cortical ACh [see also Celesia and Jasper (1966) and Szerb (1967)]. These authors assumed that an ascending reticular, cholinergic system mediates the effects of arousal on the cortex. Finally, in view of recent discussions centering around the speculation about the role of cortical ACh in consciousness and in cognitive functions, which are instrumental for the state of consciousness (Posner, 1994; Sarter, 1994), it is noteworthy that Collier and Mitchell in 1967 had already linked cortical ACh with "the maintenance of consciousness" (p. 97). Thus, these early studies have provided a fertile ground for biopsychological research on forebrain ACh.

In the 1960s, the dominating role of operant conditioning theory in biopsychological research strongly influenced the development of hypotheses about the functions of the cholinergic system. Carlton's (1965) hypothesis that the "cholinergic system acts selectively by preferentially antagonizing the effects of activation on unrewarded behavior" (p. 19) represents a major example of such a highly specific, behavioral-theory-driven hypothesis. Carlton's theory, however, did not attempt to incorporate or benefit from the early studies that suggested a more fundamental role of ACh in behavior and cortical information processing.

The investigation of the effects of scopolamine or of basal forebrain lesions on performance in various behavioral paradigms, specifically spatial tasks, has dominated the research on the cholinergic system over the last 20 years (e.g., Olton and Wenk, 1987). Numerous methodological reasons may be held responsible for the view that progress toward the elucidation of the functions of forebrain ACh has been surprisingly slow during this period of time [for a critical review see Fibiger (1991)]. The focus of an enormous number of studies on the behavioral effects of lesions of the cholinergic system resulted in impressive lists of behavioral deficits produced by such lesions [for review see Collerton (1986), Olton and Wenk (1987), Kesner (1988), and Dekker et al. (1991)]. However, this research, while considerably productive, apparently did not readily translate into unifying theories about the functions of cortical ACh. Generally, conclusions from these studies rarely extended beyond notions about the cholinergic system as "being involved in learning and memory." Additionally, the assertion that lesion-induced behavioral deficits solely reflected decreases in cortical ACh or choline acetyltransferase (ChAT) activity was difficult to interpret given the nonselectivity of the excitotoxic amino acids used to lesion the basal forebrain [for review of this issue see Dunnett et al. (1991)].

Considering the almost uniform innervation of the cortex by cholinergic neurons (see Sarter and Bruno, 1996b, for this discussion), attempts to develop a unifying hypothesis about the functions of the cholinergic system have been considered ill-advised (Fibiger, 1991). The widespread telencephalic target areas of the basal forebrain cholinergic projection system have suggested to some that assumptions about single *behavioral* functions of cortical ACh (such as the activational effects of non-reward) are unlikely to account for the role of ACh in all cortical areas.

However, the very same reasons that, on the one hand, form the basis for the rejection of unitary theories in terms of the *behavioral* functions of cortical ACh (e.g., largely uniform innervation of all cortical areas and layers; limited topographic organization of the afferent projections of the cholinergic neurons in the basal forebrain etc.; see Sarter and Bruno, 1996), on the other hand, are considered to suggest a general, global function of ACh on cortical information processing. The effects of ACh on cortical information processing may be independent from the type of cortical region (e.g., neo- vs. allocortex; primary sensory vs. associational cortex), modality (e.g., auditory vs. visual), and so forth. Early (see above) and more recent studies have attempted to describe such a general function of cortical ACh, similar to functions attributed to ascending projections originating in brainstem areas, in terms of "arousal" (e.g., Buzsaki and Gage, 1991; Semba, 1991). However, the usefulness of a generalization of arousal concepts to forebrain ascending systems appears questionable. Robbins and Everitt (1994) provided an ardent account of the usefulness and, more importantly, the limitations of arousal-like constructs in the investigation of the functions of ascending systems. Clearly, a useful, testable theory about the general role of ACh in cortical information processing requires a more precise cognitive framework and terminology than provided by the phrases used to describe concepts of arousal. Furthermore, such a theory would be expected to be sufficiently specific to foster conceptual dissociations between the functions of cortical cholinergic inputs and brainstem ascending projections to the cortex (Robbins, 1986; Robbins and Everitt, 1994).

We have recently attempted to describe the major elements of such a theory (Sarter and Bruno, 1996b). This attempt was inspired primarily by (1) the anatomy of the cholinergic system, (2) electrophysiological studies on the effects of ACh on cortical sensory information processing (e.g., Weinberger, 1993), (3) recent behavioral studies on the effects of cholinergic lesions on attentional functions (Robbins et al., 1989; Muir et al., 1992, 1994; Voytko et al., 1994; see also Chapter 4, this volume), (4) our own studies on the effects of various manipulations of cortical ACh and noradrenaline on sustained and divided attention (McGaughy and Sarter, 1995; McGaughy et al., 1994, 1996; Holley et al., 1995; Ruland et al., 1995; Turchi et al., 1995), and (5) our studies on in situ ACh release in animals while they perform operant tasks designed to tax attentional functions (Himmelheber et al., 1995; Sarter et al., 1996). In brief, cortical ACh is generally hypothesized to modulate the efficacy of the cortical processing of sensory or associational information. The integrity of cortical cholinergic inputs is required for the subjects' ability to detect and select stimuli and associations for extended processing, and for the appropriate allocation of processing resources to these functions. In addition to evidence from electrophysiological and behavioral studies on the role of cortical ACh in sensory information processing and attention, this hypothesis is consistent with the proposed functions of the limbic and paralimbic networks, which regulate the activity of the basal forebrain cholinergic neurons. Furthermore, this theory implies that changes in activity in cortical ACh occur in widespread cortical areas, and that the selectivity and precision of the functions of cortical ACh are largely due to interactions with the activity of converging sensory or associational inputs. Based on this theory, the dynamic, escalating consequences of alterations in the activity of cortical ACh (hypo- and hyperactivity) represent an adequate basis to describe the development of major cognitive disorders such as dementia and schizophrenia (Sarter, 1994).

PREVALENT POINTS OF CRITIQUE

The general view about the crucial role of aberrations in the functions of cortical cholinergic inputs for the development of cognitive dysfunctions and the associated focus on the development of pharmacological treatments acting via cholinergic mechanisms have been discussed critically in recent years (e.g., Holttum and Gershon, 1992). These criticisms have been primarily based on (1) the limited potency of muscarinic antagonists to produce the symptoms of dementia; (2) the failure of conventional cholinomimetic drugs to enhance cognitive functions or to attenuate age- or dementia-related cognitive impairments; (3) in this context the rejection of the idea that attentional abnormalities, which represent the primary consequence of cholinergic dysfunction, are sufficiently potent to account for the emergence of clinical syndromes; and (4) the exclusive focus on symptomatic therapy by cholinomimetic drugs.

Muscarinic Antagonists and Dementia

Cholinergic receptor blockade in humans, while producing various impairments in cognitive functions, does not readily result in retrograde amnesia and does not robustly produce impairments in lexical-semantic functions (e.g., Kopelman and Corn, 1988; Huff et al., 1988; Beatty et al., 1986; but see Aarsland et al., 1994). Consequently, the effects of muscarinic antagonists in intact humans have been considered to provide a model for the attentional disorders and the anterograde amnesia in senile dementia. However, language-related dysfunctions and retrograde amnesia have been assumed to be due to degeneration in noncholinergic systems in the brain of demented patients. Although evidence to reject this possibility is not available, it appears quite inadequate to assume that the *acute* effects of scopolamine or atropine in intact humans are capable of modeling the consequences of *years* of escalating cognitive impairments [for a particularly disturbing misunderstanding of this issue, based on the results of a single dose study using diphenhydramine as an anticholinergic compound, see Oken et al. (1994)]. Thus, theoretically, the validity of the pharmacological model should be determined on the basis of the effects of chronically (over years) administered muscarinic antagonists. The prediction that chronic cholinergic receptor blockade yields the full range of symptoms of dementia appears readily acceptable considering the dynamic relationships between attentional functions, learning and rehearsal and memory (see the discussion on attention and cognition). Persistent impairments in executive functions undoubtedly yield memory impairments in the long term (e.g., Grober et al., 1989). Thus, it is safe to predict that long-term administration of muscarinic antagonists would robustly produce retrograde amnesia as well as impairments in language functions. Therefore, the impressive fact that acute muscarinic receptor blockade actually produces *some* of the cardinal symptoms of a chronic, accelerating cognitive dysfunction based on multiple generative processes, strongly supports the crucial role of the cholinergic system in cognition.

Limited Potency of Cholinomimetic Drugs

As previously discussed (Sarter et al., 1990), the assumption that the cognitive effects of cholinergic cell loss can be treated by direct transmitter replacement (i.e., by muscarinic receptor agonists or cholinesterase inhibitors) has been modeled in accordance to the dopamine replacement therapy in Parkinson's disease. This assumption implies that cortical cholinergic inputs, similar to striatal dopamine, are characterized by a predominantly tonic acitivity [see Zigmond and Stricker (1989) for a discussion of striatal dopamine]. The loss of largely tonically active inputs can be functionally replaced by the administration of direct receptor agonists. However, it seems generally unlikely that neuronal systems mediating complex cognitive and behavioral functions act on the basis of largely tonic activity. As phasic or stimulus-bound activity presumably represents an essential component of cortical cholinergic transmission, the effects of direct muscarinic agonists would not be expected to replace the functions of presynaptic neurons but may actually worsen the ability of this system to modulate meaningfully cortical information processing [see also Drachman (1978)]. The same argument holds basically true for cholinesterase inhibitors, as the increases of ACh in the synaptic cleft eventually result in a stimulation of postsynaptic receptors that is dissociated from presynaptic activity and thus is expected to impair cognitive function (e.g., Bowers et al., 1964; Sarter, 1994). Additionally, increases in ACh in the synaptic cleft may further antagonize the ability of presynaptic neurons to transmit appropriately because of excessive autoreceptor stimulation (Becker and Giacobini, 1988a,b). Therefore, conventional cholinomimetic drugs, particularly muscarinic agonists, are not expected to improve the functions of an impaired cholinergic system, and their lack of beneficial effects on cognitive functions does not contradict the crucial role of cortical ACh in cognition but is, in fact, predicted by the nature of neurotransmission in this system (see also Sarter and Bruno, 1996a).

Attention and Cognition

As already mentioned, several lines of empirical evidence and theoretical conceptualization have characterized the crucial role of cortical ACh in attentional processes. Generally, the rather isolated, static assessments of cognitive functions by standard neuropsychological tests (e.g., Butters and Delis, 1995) have impeded our understanding of the dynamic and devastating effects of persistent attentional impairments on learning, memory, and language functions. Also, the limited clinical effects of tetrahydroaminoacridine (THA) on attention (e.g., Sahakian et al., 1993) raised questions about the clinical significance of a therapeutic strategy that focuses on the restoration of attentional capacities. Although psychological or cognitive theories of attention lack the desired clarity of concepts and paradigms, they indicate that the integrity of input functions, that is, of the ability to detect and select stimuli (including associations), to submit them to perceptual and postperceptual processing, and to assign processing capacity to these "pipeline functions," determine the efficacy of learning and the ability to rehearse information and form memory (e.g., Hunt and Lansman, 1986; Nissen and Bullemer, 1987; Cowan, 1988; Kinchla, 1992; Posner, 1994). Consequently, the decreases in input functions associated with normal aging (Craik and Byrd, 1982; Light, 1991) and dementia (Sahakian et al., 1990; Baddeley et al., 1991; Foldi et al., 1992; Parasuraman et al., 1992; Parasuraman and Haxby, 1993; Parasuraman and Nestor, 1993), or the hyperattentional impairments resulting from filter dysfunctions in psychosis (Venables, 1964; McGhie and Chapman, 1961; Gray et al., 1991; Sarter, 1994; Mar et al., 1996), do not only represent symptoms but rather the primary variables propelling the development of the respective cognitive disorder. Thus, a therapeutic focus on the attenuation of the different attentional impairments appears productive, specifically when considering the fact that our understanding of the neuronal mechanisms mediating memory formation is poor, and that clinically relevant approaches to treat memory disorders appear unavailable. In contrast, the cognitive and pharmacological concepts that define the constraints for a pharmacological treatment of input dysfunctions, and its significance for general cognitive abilities, are maturing (Sarter and Bruno, 1996a,b; Sarter et al., 1996).

However, preclinical and clinical assessment of the usefulness of such a focus implies many problems and requires new research approaches, including the development of new methods for the evaluation of the dynamic, long-term implications of attentional impairments on learning and memory. As will be pointed out further below, such an approach, in conjunction with neuropharmacological criteria for a rational pharmacological therapy, also requires adequate training of cognitive functions in drug-treated patients to achieve beneficial drug effects—a request that is not incorporated in presently accepted strategies for the development of treatments for age- and dementia-associated cognitive disorders (see Sarter and Bruno, 1996a; see also discussion on the implications for the design of clinical studies).

Treatment of Symptoms versus Ameliorating the Disease Process

Considering the heterogeneity of the brain pathology in dementia, the focus on the development of treatments directed to a singular neurotransmitter system, that is, the cholinergic system, has been criticized and a search for etiological therapies has been favored [e.g., Fibiger (1991); see also several chapters in Part II of this volume]. However, it seems increasingly likely that the changes in the cholinergic system in dementia play a major role in the manifestation of the classical neuropathological symptoms of this disease, and that pro-cholinergic treatments act via symptomatic as well as neuroprotective mechanisms (e.g., Perry et al., 1994). One of the classic hallmarks of dementia, amyloid deposition, may be closely related to, or even a result of, dysfunctions in cholinergic systems. Presuming that the increased frequency of apolipoprotein E (apoE) ϵ4 allele accelerates sequestration of β-amyloid and thus amyloid deposition (e.g., Younkin, 1995), the finding that demented patients carrying multiple ϵ4 allele show lower levels of cortical choline acetyltransferase (ChAT) suggests links between ChAT levels and amyloid deposition (Soininen et al., 1995). This assumption is further substantiated when considering the potential role of apoE in the phospholipid homeostasis of cholinergic neurons and the potential, devastating consequences of increases in the number of copies of ϵ4 allele on the integrity of these neurons (Poirier, 1994; Wurtman et al., 1985; Dresse et al., 1994). Finally, accumulating evidence suggests that β-amyloid precursor protein is regulated by cholinergic mechanisms and that cholinomimetic treatments possibly inhibit amyloid deposition (Buxbaum et al., 1992; Felder et al., 1993; Francis et al., 1993; Giacobini, 1994; Lahiri et al., 1994; Nitsch et al., 1992; Eckols et al., 1995).

TRANS-SYNAPTIC REGULATION OF CORTICAL ACh AND ATTENTION

As stressed earlier (Sarter and Bruno, 1994, 1996a), the investigation of the functions of cortical ACh as well as the development of pharmacological therapies of dysfunctional cholinergic systems require a focus on presynaptic cholinergic activity. Therefore, several questions guide our research on cortical ACh: (1) What behavioral and/or cognitive stimuli activate cortical ACh? (2) How can the activity of cortical cholinergic inputs be manipulated within relatively physiological ranges and, if possible, bidirectionally (i.e., hypoactive and hyperactive), so that the functions of this system can be studied in intact subjects and the usefulness of pharmacological treatment strategies focusing on presynaptic mechanisms can be evaluated? (3) How can the activity of a residual cholinergic system be augmented in a way that avoids presynaptic activity-*in*dependent stimulation of cholinergic receptors in the cortex? Lessons learned from studying these issues are expected to provide insight into the elementary functions of this system and to advance the development of treatment for the cognitive impairments associated with dysfunctional cholinergic systems.

Cognitive Correlates of Cortical ACh

Using the microdialysis technique for the measurement of cortical ACh release, the conclusions from the early studies on ACh release (see above) have been considerably refined by recent investigations. Furthermore, the more recent experiments have revealed a tremendous complexity inherent in the design of studies intended to attribute function to changes in neurotransmitter release. Specifically, the requirement for exhaustive control studies in order to specify and validate relationships between behavior/cognition and cortical ACh has become evident.

As previously demonstrated (see also Imperato et al., 1992), "arousal"-inducing manipulations generally increase cortical ACh release (e.g., anticipation/consumption of palatable food; transfer of animals between environments; Moore et al., 1992, 1993; Inglis et al., 1994; Sarter et al., 1996). However, both Inglis and co-workers and we observed that the increases in ACh release were more robust in animals trained to associate stimuli or procedures with the presentation of palatable food compared with untrained animals. These data suggested that the anticipation of palatable food and food consumption per se do not represent the critical variables associated with increases in cortical ACh release.

A similar complication applies to the conclusion that locomotor activity generally correlates with cortical ACh release (Day et al., 1991). Our own data demonstrated that increases in locomotor activity are not necessarily associated with increases in cortical ACh increase (Moore et al., 1993, 1995a). As assumed by Day et al. (1991), locomotor activity may represent a correlate of an ongoing process that is mediated via increases in cortical ACh. However, increases in locomotor activity may not represent a primary correlate of ACh release.

The size and complexity of these interpretative problems have been revealed even more clearly by a recent experiment intended to assess cortical (medial prefrontal) ACh release in animals performing in a task designed to measure sustained attention (Himmelheber et al., 1995; Sarter et al., 1996). Increases in attentional demands were produced by increases in background "noise," resulting in a decrease in vigilance level and an augmentation in the vigilance decrement [see McGaughy and Sarter (1995) for a validation of the effects of flashing houselight]. Increases in background noise were produced by presenting a flashing houselight in the operant boxes (0.5 Hz) during one out of four blocks of trials per session. Compared to the performance in blocks with constantly lit houselight, the overall vigilance performance decreased by approximately 44%. Simultaneously, ACh efflux increased by approximately 250% relative to the efflux recorded during performance under standard task conditions [see Sarter et al (1996) for details]. These findings suggested that cortical ACh efflux mediates increased demands on attentional functions.

However, several issues prohibited the definitive conclusion that the increase in ACh efflux was a specific correlate of the increases in demands on attentional functions. While the number of omitted trials was not affected by flashing houselight, the animals received less reward (because of the impairment in performance), a new sensory stimulus (flashing houselight) was introduced, and their overall behavior in the operant chambers presumably changed in response to flashing houselight. Any or all of these events potentially stimulated cortical ACh release. Therefore, the role of such variables was systematically studied.

We conducted two sets of experiments in order to assess the effects of bar pressing behavior, reward density, sensory stimulation, and other variables (Himmelheber et al., 1995). First, animals were trained in a simple visual discrimination task requiring the animals to press the lever (one of two) above which a panel light was illuminated for 3 s. This task did not explicitly tax attentional functions. Animals were generally well trained before surgery and were pre-exposed to flashing houselight for two sessions (one of four blocks of trials in each session) before guide cannula were implanted in the medial prefrontal cortex. The animals' performance accuracy was expectedly high (almost 100%) and did not change throughout 4 blocks of 12 min. The number of omissions increased from about 20% in the first block to about 90% of all trials in the last block. However, ACh efflux did not change throughout the four blocks of trials. Presentation of flashing houselight did not affect performance accuracy and did not increase cortical ACh efflux. We also tested the effects of extinction by terminating reinforcement delivery during the last three blocks of trials. This manipulation augmented the increase in omissions but did not affect response accuracy. Again, cortical ACh efflux remained unchanged in response to this manipulation.

In a second series of experiments, Himmelheber et al. (1995) trained animals in a VI 12 ± 3 s schedule of reinforcement. While lever-pressing behavior in this task obviously is independent from sensory stimuli, panel lights were presented similar to the visual discrimination task described earlier to maintain comparable sensory stimulation. This schedule produces relatively high levels of lever-pressing rates but comparable levels of reinforcements as in the visual discrimination task (see Figure 1).

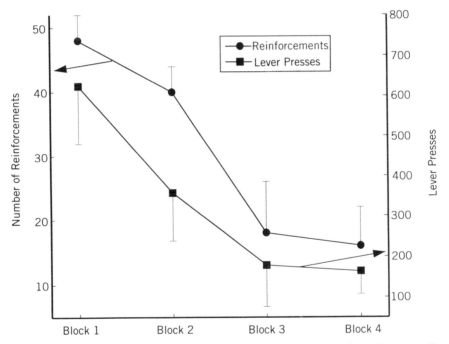

FIGURE 1. Performance of rats in a simple VI 12 ± 3 s schedule of reinforcement (for water; 40–45 μL per reinforcement). This experiment was designed to control for the effects of several behavioral variables on cortical ACh release [motor activity, extinction, sensory stimuli; see text and Himmelheber et al. (1995); data are from six test sessions]. Each block consisted of 12 min, and each daily session of four blocks. Note the relatively high number of lever presses (filled squares, right ordinate), which decreased over blocks. Similarly, the number of reinforcements (filled circles; left ordinate) also decreased over blocks. Flashing houselight was presented during the third block and did not affect performance. Termination of water delivery (blocks 2–4) augmented the decrease in lever presses and reinforcements (not shown).

Consequently, both the lever-pressing rate and the reinforcement rate declined over time (see Figure 1). However, ACh efflux remained stable (see Figure 2). Similar to the findings from the first series of experiments, presentation of flashing houselight did not affect performance or ACh efflux. Finally, termination of reward (i.e., extinction), while increasing the negative slope of the lever-pressing rate, again failed to affect ACh efflux.

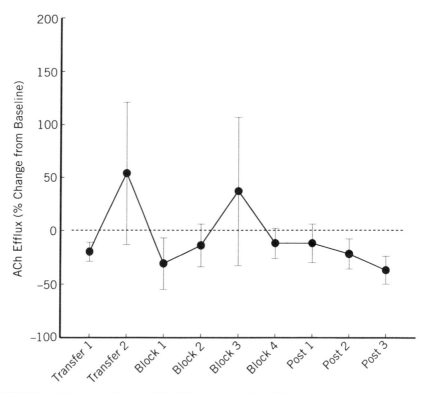

FIGURE 2. Medial prefrontal ACh efflux in animals while they performed as shown in Figure 1. The ordinate depicts ACh efflux as a percent change from baseline. The two collection intervals following transfer of the animals to the operant box, prior to task onset, (transfer 1 and transfer 2) were relative to basal efflux measured while the animals rested in clear parabolic test bowls. Efflux from collection intervals during the performance of the operant task (blocks 1–4) and after task (post 1–3) were relative to basal efflux determined during transfer 2. Transfer into the operant boxes increased the variability of ACh release in the second collection period. ACh release during the four blocks of trials remained essentially stable, that is, neither the high levels of lever presses and reinforcements at the beginning of the session nor the decrease in lever presses and reinforcements over blocks was correlated with changes in ACh efflux. Flashing houselight and extinction (not shown) also failed to affect ACh. As neither variable interval nor visual conditional discrimination performance (see text) affected cortical ACh efflux, the increase in ACh efflux observed when demands on vigilance performance were increased (Sarter et al., 1996) are considered a specific correlate of attentional processes.

These data suggest that lever-pressing activity, sensory stimulation, and reward loss are not sufficient to produce changes in cortical ACh efflux. It is necessary to reiterate the fact that these animals were extremely well habituated to the testing environments and procedures, and that they were pre-exposed to flashing houselight (but not to extinction sessions). If flashing houselight was not previously presented, the novelty of the stimulus would have been expected to increase ACh (see also Inglis and Fibiger, 1995).

These data support the hypothesis that the increase in ACh efflux in animals performing a sustained attention task while being challenged by a distractor were due to the increased demands in attentional functions and not to the secondary behavioral effects of this manipulation. However, it is evident that further studies are required to affirm this conclusion by data that extend beyond a solely correlational analysis of the relationships between attentional and cortical ACh. Experiments intended to systematically vary cortical ACh efflux and to simultaneously assess the effects on attention will generate such data. For this purpose, neuropharmacological means to manipulate cortical ACh are needed.

GABA-cholinergic Interactions

The anatomical, physiological, and neuropharmacological bases of basal forebrain γ-aminobutyric acid (GABA)-cholinergic interactions have been summarized before (e.g., Sarter et al., 1990; Decker and McGaugh, 1991; Sarter and Bruno, 1994; Bruno and Miller 1995; Sarter et al., 1995). It seems necessary, however, to reiterate one crucial aspect of this approach. As the goal of this approach is to modulate the excitability of basal forebrain neurons without producing major distortions of the function of basal forebrain circuits, the use of benzodiazepine receptor (BZR) ligands to manipulate allosterically GABAergic transmission represents an essential aspect of this strategy. As would be expected, blockade of GABAergic transmission by using direct GABA$_A$ receptor antagonists, or direct receptor stimulation by agonists, produces behavioral and neuropharmacological effects that are not reproduced by the effects of BZR ligands (see Givens and Sarter, 1996). Modulation of GABAergic transmission by BZR ligands modulates the excitability of target neurons but, in contrast to direct modulation by GABA$_A$ receptor ligands, does not block or initiate GABAergic transmission.

We have previously demonstrated that systemic administration, or infusions into the basal forebrain, of BZR agonists and inverse agonists block and augment, respectively, *increased* (or *activated*) cortical ACh efflux (Moore et al., 1993, 1995a,b; Bruno and Miller, 1995; Sarter and Bruno, 1994). As would be expected considering the role of the chloride equilibrium potential in determining the resting potential of neurons, BZR agonists and selective inverse agonists do not robustly affect *basal* or resting cortical ACh efflux. As discussed, various, often seemingly trivial experimental manipulations, which are associated with novelty, stress, or arousal, stimulate cortical ACh efflux. Therefore, we have assumed that several previous reports demonstrating decreases in cortical ACh efflux following the administration of BZR agonists inadvertently assessed the effects of such compounds on activated release [that was due to, e.g., the transfer of the animals into the test environment; see Bruno and Miller (1995) and Sarter and Bruno (1994) for discussion].

As the effects of infusions of BZR ligands into the basal forebrain are based on interactions with the state of activity of basal forebrain neurons, the efficacy of BZR ligands is expected to be restricted to situations in which the basal forebrain system is activated. In other words, BZR ligands can be used to determine the behavioral functions that involve basal forebrain activation (Givens and Sarter, 1996). For example, performance in a conditional visual discrimination task (which does not entail explicit demands on attentional functions) is insensitive to the effects of BZR agonists infused into the basal forebrain [but is sensitive to the effects of muscimol; see Dudchenko and Sarter (1991, 1992)]. Similarly, McNamara and Skelton (1993) showed that water maze performance is not affected by infusions of chlordiazepoxide into the basal forebrain.

In contrast, the performance of animals in the behavioral vigilance task (similar to that used in the microdialysis experiments described earlier) is highly sensitive to the effects of BZR ligands. As performance in this task is assumed to activate cortical ACh efflux (see above), BZR agonists were expected to impair performance, as they block increases in ACh efflux. Administration of BZR inverse agonists in intact animals were also expected to produce detrimental effects on performance because drug-induced augmentation of neuronal excitability (and cortical ACh efflux) in intact, optimally performing animals appears unlikely to facilitate performance. The available data show, however, that the impairments of the two types of BZR ligands differ qualitatively. Similar to the effects of systemically administered BZR agonists (McGaughy and Sarter, 1995), infusions of a BZR agonist into the basal forebrain resulted in a selective decrease in the relative number of hits and an augmentation of the vigilance decrement (Holley et al., 1995). The fact that the relative number of correct rejections (or its inverse, the relative number of false alarms) were completely spared indicated the absence of effects on well-trained response rules (i.e., on reference memory) and motor biases. Notably, this pattern of effect was identical to the effects of 192 IgG-saporin-induced lesions of the basal forebrain cholinergic system on vigilance performance (McGaughy et al., 1996).

Infusions of the BZR inverse agonist β-carboline-methyl beta carboline-3-carboxylate (β-CCM) produced a very different pattern of effects on vigilance performance. While the animals' ability to correctly respond to signals was unchanged, the animals demonstrated more false alarms following the infusion of β-CCM. In other words, the inverse agonist increased the number of claims for signals while no signals were presented. As infusions of similar doses of β-CCM into the basal forebrain increase activated cortical ACh efflux (Moore et al., 1995a), it is hypothesized that cortical cholinergic hyperactivity mediates the type of attentional "overprocessing" observed in this experiment. Evidence for detrimental stimulus overprocessing following the administration of inverse agonists was also found in psychophysiological studies (Quigley et al., 1994) and demonstrated to depend on the integrity of the cholinergic basal forebrain (Berntson et al., 1996). Future studies will employ these trans-synaptic modulations of cortical ACh efflux and attentional performance to assess both variables simultaneously to test their interrelationships.

Enhancement of Activated ACh Efflux and Attenuation of Attentional Impairments

In subjects suffering from attentional impairments due to cholinergic cell loss, BZR inverse agonist-induced increases in the excitability of cholinergic neurons are expected to alleviate these symptoms. The validity of this prediction, however, hinges on several important assumptions. While the focus on such a trans-synaptic approach and on attentional functions is well justified (see above), it is less clear whether the remaining cholinergic neurons in dementia or in basal forebrain-lesioned animals maintain the capacity to respond to increased demands on ACh synthesis and release. Secondarily, it is also not clear whether drug-induced increases in presynaptic cholinergic excitability affects the integrity of these neurons, particularly if these effects interact with an ongoing neurodegenerative process.

Information about the status and capacity of residual cholinergic terminals in dementia is rare. Decreases in conventional markers of presynaptic cholinergic activity (including high-affinity choline uptake and ACh synthesis) usually reflect the loss of presynaptic sites and do not inform about the ability of the remaining terminals to synthesize and release ACh (e.g., Bowen et al., 1983; Rylett et al., 1983; Sims et al., 1983). This information is critically needed.

Many studies in basal forebrain-lesioned animals revealed a recovery of ChAT activity in the cortex that was not associated with obvious signs of sprouting (e.g., Cossette et al., 1993). While the relevance of these findings for dementia is unclear, they suggest that the residual terminals in lesioned animals have increased their capacity for ACh synthesis. This conclusion was corroborated by our finding that cortical vesamicol binding returned to normal 100 days after ibotenic acid-induced lesion of the basal forebrain (Holley et al., 1993). As vesamicol is thought to bind to sites incorporating ACh into recycling vesicles (e.g., Suszkiw and Toth, 1986), unchanged vesamicol binding in combination with loss of terminals (as was indicated by decreased hemicholinium binding), suggests an increased potency of residual terminals to store and release ACh. Interestingly, unchanged vesamicol binding was also documented in the cortex of patients with Alzheimer's disease (Kish et al., 1990), providing some validity to the data from lesioned animals and permitting the speculation that the remaining cholinergic neurons in dementia are capable of releasing more ACh in response to increased activity.

In lesioned animals, the prediction made on the basis of the vesamicol data has gained some support from studies assessing cortical ACh efflux in vivo. Similar to the effects of basal forebrain lesions, aged animals also show decreases in markers of cortical cholinergic activity [for review see Gallagher and Colombo, (1995); but see Abdulla et al. (1995)]; however, cortical ACh efflux in aged rats remains unchanged (Fischer et al., 1991; Moore et al., 1992). More direct evidence for the capacity of residual cholinergic neurons to respond to stimulation was found in a recent series of experiments by Fadel et al. (1996). Using the technique of multiple intracortical infusions of the immunotoxin 192 IgG-saporin to partially deafferent cortical cholinergic afferents [see Holley et al., (1994) for this method], about 40–70% of all cholinergic inputs to the cortex were lesioned. The degree of this loss corresponds well with the decrease in cortical ChAT activity in aged and demented humans (e.g., Perry et al., 1992). Baseline ACh efflux in the frontoparietal cortex of these animals was decreased by an average of 47% compared with sham-lesioned controls. However, activation of cortical ACh in animals trained to associate darkness with the presentation of palatable food [see above and Moore et al. (1992, 1993)] was normal in lesioned animals in terms of relative increases in ACh efflux. Similarly, administration of the BZR partial inverse agonist FG 7142, which is known to increase baseline cortical ACh release (Moore et al., 1995c), produced comparable relative increases in ACh efflux in lesioned and sham-lesioned animals (Fadel et al., 1996). These data indicate that, in animals with compromised cholinergic systems, this system remains capable of responding to behavioral activation and trans-synaptic stimulation of cortical ACh efflux. The question of whether *chronic* stimulation of a residual cholinergic system involves unwelcome effects on the integrity of these neurons remains to be studied. If it is true that, in senile dementia, basal forebrain cholinergic neurons are subject to excessive inhibition as a result of the early loss of basal forebrain excitatory afferents originating in the temporal lobe (Procter and Bowen, 1988), trans-synaptic stimulation with BZR inverse agonists would seem beneficial by counteracting the long-term detrimental effects of excessive inhibition on the general status of residual cholinergic neurons. Moreover, as discussed above, evidence for neuroprotective effects of pro-cholinergic pharmacological therapies is accumulating.

A series of studies from various laboratories has demonstrated that the behavioral effects of basal forebrain lesions are attenuated by the treatment with certain BZR inverse agonists, specifically by the BZR selective inverse agonist ZK 93426 [see Table 4 in Sarter et al. (1995) for an overview of these studies]. We attempted to test the effects of unusually small doses of the BZR partial inverse agonist FG 7142 on the attentional impairments in animals with lesions of the basal forebrain produced by infusions of 192 IgG-saporin. The selection of this compound and doses was motivated by reports about the cognition enhancing doses of this BZR partial inverse agonist in intact rats (Smith et al., 1994; Cole and Hillman, 1994). Administration of this compound, however, did not significantly improve the performance of lesioned animals in the vigilance task (McGaughy et al., 1996). As the histological analysis showed that the dose of 192 IgG-saporin used in this study depleted more than 90% of cortical cholinergic inputs in most cortical areas, it was speculated that the potential potency of FG 7142 to produce beneficial effects was limited by the completeness of the lesion. This speculation was substantiated by a post hoc analysis showing a significant, negative correlation between the loss of cholinergic inputs and the ability of FG 7142 to increase the relative number of hits. In other words, the less complete the lesion, the more beneficial the effects of this compound. Current experiments intend to test this hypothesis in animals with partial lesions of the cholinergic sysem produced by intracortical infusions of 192 IgG-saporin [similar to the animals in the study by Fadel et al. (1996) described earlier]. It cannot be excluded, however, that the speculation that small doses of FG 7142 act similar to the ligands with weaker or more selective efficacy such as ZK 93426 or MDL 26,479 (Holley et al., 1993; Sarter et al., 1995; Miller, 1995) is invalid, or that FG 7142 may be working via other neuronal mechanisms [e.g., stimulation of mesolimbic dopamine; (Brose et al., 1987; Brad-berry et al., 1991; McCullough and Salamone, 1992)]. As discussed, the beneficial cognitive effects of these compounds in animals and humans [for a review see Sarter et al. (1995) and Duka and Dorow (1995)] are hypothesized to be due to their interactions with an activated cholinergic system.

IMPLICATIONS FOR DESIGN OF CLINICAL STUDIES

This chapter summarizes the behavioral and neuropharmacological aspects of a trans-synaptic approach to treat the cognitive impairments associated with cholinergic hy-pofunction. Considering the functions of cortical ACh, a drug-induced augmentation of cortical presynaptic cholinergic activity is considered a rational mechanism to alleviate the functional consequences of a loss of cholinergic inputs to the cortex.

Several aspects of this approach have significant clinical implications. Above all, the trans-synaptic stimulation of cortical ACh with BZR inverse agonists is based on an interaction with the activity in the cholinergic system (see above). This concept suggests that drug-induced increases in ACh release occur only when the system is activated. In other words, the neuropharmacological mechanisms underlying this strategy remain "silent" unless cognitive efforts activate the cholinergic system. Such an approach avoids irrelevant activation of the system, which would produce "noise" and thus impairments in cognition (e.g., Drachman, 1978). An important corollary of such an approach is given by the prediction that drug effects cannot be demonstrated in the absence of cognitive activity, as the cholinergic target system would not be sufficiently active to allow BZR inverse agonists to further disinhibit its excitability. If this assumption is correct, the demonstration of beneficial drug effects requires an interaction between drug treatment and cognitive activity. Indeed, MDL 26,479 was found to alleviate the cognitive impairments in basal fore-brain-lesioned animals following chronic administration of the drug *and* concurrent chronic behavioral training. In this study, between 35 and 40 training sessions and days of drug administration were required to reveal beneficial behavioral drug effects in lesioned animals (Holley et al., 1993).

As direct, cognition-independent drug effects on cognition are extremely difficult to imagine, the prediction that the demonstration of efficacy of putative cognition enhancers requires concurrent drug treatment and cognitive training represents a conservative view. Future preclinical efforts to determine novel approaches for the treatment of cognitive dysfunctions need to incorporate this view (see also Sarter et al., 1996). It is not clear, however, whether the typical design of clinical studies in this area provides the basis for the demonstration of drug-induced improvement of cognitive functions. Studies that, in addition to drug treatment, systematically and persistently engage patients in cognitive activity are not considered practical at the present time.

It is quite astonishing to note that many researchers and clinicians consider the development of pharmacological treatments for neuropsychiatric disorders to be a search for "magic bullets," that is, for drugs that are expected to produce beneficial effects irrespective of the patient's cognitive status while being treated with drugs, or the status of his cognitive functions in general (e.g., Traub and Friedman, 1992; Schneider and Tariot, 1994; Bartus, 1990). Similarly, studies that dissociated "responders" from "nonresponders" rarely speculated about cognitive variables contributing to the putative efficacy of drugs assumed to facilitate cognitive functions (e.g., Soncrant et al., 1993). While many medicinal therapies of more peripheral malfunctions (e.g., cardiovascular diseases) have recognized the need for combinations of drug treatment and physical therapy, it appears extremely difficult to conceive therapeutic efforts for the treatment of cognitive dysfunctions that integrate cognitive exercise as a variable in the efficacy of pharmacological treatments (i.e., as a form of "physical" co-therapy). The small number of studies on the effects of mental exercise on cognitive functions in old or demented subjects revealed impressive beneficial effects (e.g., Hanley, 1981; Karlsson et al., 1989; Bird and Luszcz, 1993). As is pointed out in this chapter, evidence is available to support the conclusion that pharmacological approaches to enhance presynaptic cholinergic function will not simply benefit from, but require concurrent cognitive activity. Magic bullets for the treatment of cognitive impairments are difficult to conceive. To the extent this assumption is correct, preclinical and clinical research on treatments for cognitive disorders needs to investigate interactions between the effects of putative therapeutic drugs and cognitive exercise or research will fail to develop useful treatments for cognitive disorders.

ACKNOWLEDGMENT

The authors' research was supported in part by PHS Grants AG10173 (MS and JPB) and NS32938 (MS). MS was supported by a Research Scientist Award (MH01072).

REFERENCES

Aarsland D, Larsen JP, Reinvang I, Aarsland AM (1994): Effects of cholinergic blockade in language in healthy young women. Brain 117:1377–1384.

Abdulla FA, Abu-Bakra MAJ, Calaminici MR, Stephenson JD, Sinden JD (1995): Importance of forebrain cholinergic and GABAergic systems to the age-related deficits in water maze performance of rats. Neurobiol Aging 16:41–52.

Baddeley AD, Bressi S, Della Salla S, Logie R, Spinnler H (1991): The decline of working memory in Alzheimer's disease. Brain 114:2521–2542.

Bartus RT (1990): Drugs to treat age-related neurodegenerative problems. J Am Ger Soc 38:680–695.

Beatty WW, Butters N, Janowski DS (1986): Patterns of memory failure after scopolamine treatment: Implications for cholinergic hypotheses of dementia. Behav Neural Biol 45:196–211.

Becker RE, Giacobini E (1988a): Pharmacokinetics and pharmacodynamics of acetylcholinesterase inhibition: Can acetylcholine levels in the brain be improved in Alzheimer's disease? Drug Dev Res 14:235–246.

Becker RE, Giacobini E (1988b): Mechanisms of cholinesterase inhibition in senile dementia of the Alzheimer type: Clinical, pharmacological, and therapeutic aspects. Drug Dev Res 12:163–195.

Berntson GG, Hart S, Ruland S, Sarter M (1996): A central cholinergic link in the cardiovascular effects of the benzodiazepine receptor partial inverse agonist FG 7142. Behav Brain Res 74:91–103.

Bird M, Luszcz M (1993): Enhancing memory performance in Alzheimer's disease: Acquisition assistance and cue effectiveness. J Clin Exp Neuropsychol 15:921–932.

Bowen DM, Allen SJ, Benton JS, Goodhardt MJ, Haan EA, Palmer AM, Sims NR, Smith CCT, Spillane JA, Esiri MM, Neary D, Snowdon, JS, Wilcock GK, Davison AN (1983): Biochemical assessment of serotonergic and cholinergic dysfunction and cerebral atrophy in Alzheimer's disease. J Neurochem 41:266–272.

Bowen DM, Smith CB, White P, Davidson AN (1976): Neurotransmitter-related enzymes and indices of hypoxia in senile dementia and other abiotrophies. Brain 99:457–496.

Bowers MB, Goodman E, Sim VM (1964): Some behavioral changes in man following anticholinesterase administration. J Nerv Ment Dis 138:383–389.

Bradberry CW, Lory JD, Roth RH (1991): The anxiogenic β-carboline FG 7142 selectively increases dopamine release in rat prefrontal cortex as measured by microdialysis. J Neurochem 56:748–752.

Brose N, O'Neill RD, Boutelle MG, Anderson SMP, Fillenz M (1987): Effects of an anxiogenic benzodiazepine receptor ligand on motor activity and dopamine release in nucleus accumbens and striatum in the rat. J Neurosci 7:2917–2926.

Bruno JP, Miller JA (1995): Inhibition of GABAergic transmission: Interactions with other transmitter systems. In Sarter M, Nutt DJ, Lister RG (eds): "Benzodiazepine Receptor Inverse Agonists." New York: Wiley, pp 41–82.

Butters N, Delis DC (1995): Clinical assessment of memory disorders in amnesia and dementia. Ann Rev Psychol 46:493–523.

Buxbaum JD, Oishi M, Chen HI, Pinkas-Kramarski R, Jaffe EA, Gandy SE, Greengard P (1992): Cholinergic agonists and interleukin 1 regulate processing and secretion of the Alzheimer β/A$_4$ amyloid precursor. Proc Natl Acad Sci U S A 89:10075–10078.

Buzsaki G, Gage FH (1991): Role of the basal forebrain cholinergic system in cortical activation and arousal. In Richardson RT (ed): "Activation to Acquisition. Functional Aspects of the Basal Forebrain Cholinergic System." Boston: Birkhäuser, pp 115–134.

Carlton PL (1965): Cholinergic mechanisms in the control of behavior by the brain. Psychol Rev 70:19–39.

Celesia GG, Jasper HH (1966): Acetylcholine release from cerebral cortex in relation to state of activation. Neurology 16:1053–1063.

Cole BJ, Hillman M (1994): Effects of benzodiazepine receptor ligands on the performance of an operant delayed matching to position task in rats: Opposite effects of FG 7142 and lorazepam. Psychopharmacology 115:350–357.

Collerton D (1986): Cholinergic function and intellectual decline in Alzheimer's disease. Neuroscience 19:1–28.

Collier B, Mitchell JF (1967): The central release of acetylcholine during consciousness and after brain lesions. J Physiol 188:83–98.

Collier B, Mitchell JF (1966): The central release of acetylcholine during stimulation of the visual pathway. J Physiol 184:239–254.

Cossette P, Umbriaco D, Zamar N, Hamel E, Descarries L (1993): Recovery of choline acetyltransferase activity without sprouting of the residual acetylcholine innervation in adult rat cerebral cortex after lesion of the nucleus basalis. Brain Res 630:195–206.

Cowan N (1988): Evolving conceptions of memory storage, selective attention, and their mutual constraints within the human information-processing system. Psychol Bull 104:163–191.

Craik FIM, Byrd M (1982): Aging and cognitive deficits. The role of attentional resources. In Craik FIM, Trehub S (eds): "Aging and Cognitive Processes." New York: Plenum, pp 191–211.

Day J, Damsma G, Fibiger HC (1991): Cholinergic activity in the rat hippocampus, cortex and striatum correlates with locomotor activity: An in vivo microdialysis study. Pharmacol Biochem Behav 38:723–729.

Decker MW, McGaugh JL (1991): The role of interactions between the cholinergic system and other neuromodulatory systems in learning and memory. Synapse 7:151–168.

Dekker JAM, Connor DJ, Thal LJ (1991): The role of cholinergic projections from the nucleus basalis in memory. Neurosci Biobehav Rev 15:299–317.

DeKosky ST, Harbaugh RE, Schmitt FA, Bakay RA, Chui HC, Knopman DS, Reeder TM, Shetter AG, Senter HJ, Markesberry WR (1992): Cortical biopsy in Alzheimer's disease: Diagnostic accuracy and neurochemical, neuropathological, and cognitive correlations. Ann Neurol 32:625–632.

Drachman DA (1978): Central cholinergic system and memory. In Lipton MA, DiMascio A, Killam KF (ed): "Psychopharmacology: A Generation of Progress." New York: Raven, pp 651–661.

Dresse A, Marechal D, Scuvee-Moreau J, Seutin V (1994): Towards a pharmacological approach of Alzheimer's disease based on the molecular biology of the amyloid precursor protein (APP). Life Sci 55:2179–2187.

Dudchenko P, Sarter M (1992): Failure of chlordiazepoxide to reproduce the behavioral effects of muscimol administered into the basal forebrain. Behav Brain Res 47:202–205.

Dudchenko P, Sarter M (1991): GABAergic control of basal forebrain cholinergic neurons and memory. Behav Brain Res 42:33–41.

Duka T, Dorow R (1995): Human experimental psychopharmacology of benzodiazepine receptor inverse agonists and antagonists. In Sarter M, Nutt DJ, Lister RG (eds): "Benzodiazepine Receptor Inverse Agonists." New York: Wiley, pp 243–270.

Dunnett SB, Everitt BJ, Robbins TW (1991): The basal forebrain-cortical cholinergic system: Interpreting the functional consequences of excitotoxic lesions. Trends Neurosci 14:494–501.

Eckols K, Bymaster FP, Mitch CH, Shannon HE, Ward JS, DeLapp W (1995): The muscarinic M1 agonist xanomeline increases soluble amyloid precursor protein release from chinese hamster ovary-1 cells. Life Sci 57:1183–1190.

Fadel J, Sarter M, Bruno JP (1996): Trans-synaptic stimulation of cortical acetylcholine release following partial 192 IgG-saporin-induced loss of cortical cholinergic afferents. J Neurosci, 16:6592–6600.

Feldberg W, Vogt M (1948): Acetylcholine synthesis in different regions of the central nervous system. J Physiol 107:372–381.

Felder CC, Ma AI, Briley EM, Axelrod J (1993): Muscarinic acetylcholine receptor subtypes associated with release of Alzheimer amyloid precursor derivatives activate multiple signal pathways. Ann N Y Acad Sci 695:15–18.

Fibiger HC (1991): Cholinergic mechanisms in learning and dementia: A review of recent evidence. Trends Neurosci 14:220–223.

Fischer W, Nilsson, OG, Björklund A (1991): In vivo acetylcholine release as measured by microdialysis is unaltered in the hippocampus of cognitively impaired aged rats with degenerative changes in the basal forebrain. Brain Res 556:44–52.

Foldi NS, Jutagir R, Davidoff D, Gould T (1992): Selective attention skills in Alzheimer's disease: Performance on graded cancellation tests varying in density and complexity. J Gerontol 47:P146–P153.

Francis PT, Webster MT, Chessell IP, Holmes C, Stratman GC, Procter AW, Cross AJ, Green AR, Bowen DM (1993): Neurotransmitters and second messengers in aging and Alzheimer's disease. Ann N Y Acad Sci 695:19–26.

Gallagher M, Colombo PJ (1995): Ageing: The cholinergic hypothesis of cognitive decline. Curr Opin Neurobiol 5:161–168.

Giacobini E (1994): Therapy of Alzheimer disease: Symptomatic or neuroprotective? J Neural Trans 43:(Suppl), 211–217.

Givens BS, Sarter M (1996): Modulation of cognitive processes by transsynaptic activation of the basal forebrain. Behav Brain Res, in press.

Gray JA, Feldon J, Rawlins JNP, Hemlsey DR, Smith DA (1991): The neuropsychology of schizophrenia. Behav Brain Sci 14:1–84.

Grober E, Leipzig RM, Lipton RB, Wisniewski W, Schroeder M, Davies P, Ritter W, Buschke H (1989): Does scopolamine directly impair memory? J Cogn Neurosci 1: 327–335.

Hanley IG (1981): The use of signposts and active training to modify ward disorientation in elderly patients. J Behav Ther Exp Psychiatry 12:241–247.

Hearst E (1959): Effects of scopolamine on discriminated responding in the rat. J Pharmacol Exp Ther 126:349–358.

Herz A (1960): Die Bedeutung der Bahnung für die Wirkung von Scopolamin und ähnlichen Substanzen auf bedingte Reaktionen. Z Biol 112:104–112.

Himmelheber AM, Moore H, McGaughy J, Givens B, Bruno JP, Sarter M (1995): Cortical acetylcholine efflux and single unit activity in rats performing operant procedures assessing behavioral vigilance, or sensorimotor and motivational task components. Soc Neurosci Abst 21:763.6.

Holley LA, Turchi J, Apple C, Sarter M (1995): Dissociation between the attentional effects of infusions of a benzodiazepine receptor agonist and an inverse agonist into the basal forebrain. Psychopharmacology 120:99–108.

Holley LA, Wiley RG, Lappi DA, Sarter M (1994): Cortical cholinergic deafferentation following the intracortical infusion of 192 IgG-saporin: A quantitative histochemical study. Brain Res 663:277–286.

Holley LA, Miller JA, Chmielewski PA, Dudchenko P, Sarter M (1993): Interactions between the effects of basal forebrain lesions and chronic treatment with MDL 26,479 on learning and markers of cholinergic transmission. Brain Res 610:181–193.

Holttum JR, Gershon S (1992): The cholinergic model of dementia, Alzheimer type: Progression from the unitary transmitter concept. Dementia 3:174–185.

Huff FJ, Mickel SF, Corkin S, Growdon JH (1988): Cognitive functions affected by scopolamine in Alzheimer's disease and normal aging. Drug Dev Res 12:217–278.

Hunt E, Lansman M (1986): Unified model of attention and problem solving. Psychol Rev 93:446–461.

Imperato A, Puglisi-Allegra S, Grazia Scrocco M, Casolini P, Bacchi S, Angelucci L (1992): Cortical and limbic dopamine and acetylcholine release as neurochemical correlates of emotional arousal in both aversive and non-aversive environmental changes. Neurosci 20:265S–270S.

Inglis FM, Fibiger HC (1995): Increases in hippocampal and frontal cortical acetylcholine release associated with presentation of sensory stimuli. Neuroscience 66:81–86.

Inglis FM, Day JC, Fibiger HC (1994): Enhanced acetylcholine release in hippocampus and cortex during the anticipation and consumption of a palatable meal. Neuroscience 62:1049–1056.

Karlsson T, Backman L, Herlitz A, Nilsson LG, Winblad B, Osterlind PE (1989): Memory improvements at different stages of Alzheimer's disease. Neuropsychologia 27:737–742.

Kesner RP (1988): Reevaluation of the contribution of the basal forebrain cholinergic system to memory. Neurobiol Aging 9:609–616.

Kinchla RA (1992): Attention. Ann Rev Psychol 43:711–742.

Kish SJ, Distefano LM, Dozic S, Robitaille Y, Rajput A, Deck JHN, Hornykiewicz O (1990): [^{3}]Vesamicol binding in human brain cholinergic deficiency disorders. Neurosci Lett 117:347–352.

Kopelman MD, Corn TH (1988): Cholinergic "blockade" as a model for cholinergic depletion. Brain 111:1079–1110.

Lahiri DK, Lewis S, Farlow MR (1994): Tacrine alters the secretion of the beta-amyloid precursor protein in cell lines. J Neurosci Res 37:777–787.

Light LL (1991): Memory and aging: Four hypotheses in search of data. Ann Rev Psychol 42:333–376.

Mar CM, Smith AD, Sarter M (1996): Behavioral vigilance in schizophrenia: Evidence for hyperattentional processing. Br J Psychiat, in press.

McCullough LD, Salamone JD (1992): Anxiogenic drugs beta-CCE and FG 7142 increase extracellular dopamine levels in nucleus accumbens. Psychopharmacology 109:379–382.

McGaughy J, Sarter M (1995): Behavioral vigilance in rats: Task validation and effects of age, amphetamine, and benzodiazepine receptor ligands. Psychopharmacology 117: 340–357.

McGaughy J, Kaiser T, Sarter M (1996): Behavioral vigilance following the infusions of 192 IgG-saporin into the basal forebrain: Selectivity of the behavioral impairment and relation to cortical AChE-positive fiber density. Behav Neurosci, 110:247–265.

McGaughy J, Turchi J, Sarter M (1994): Crossmodal divided attention in rats: Effects of chlordiazepoxide and scopolamine. Psychopharmacology 115:213–220.

McGhie A, Chapman J. (1961): Disorders of attention and perception in early schizophrenia. Br J Med Psychol 34:103–116.

McNamara RK, Skelton RW (1993): Effects of intracranial infusions of chlordiazepoxide on spatial learning in the Morris water maze. I. Neuranatomical specificity. Behav Brain Res 59:175–191.

Miller JA (1995): Evidence for a modified model of agonist and inverse agonist actions at the GABA$_A$ receptor. In Sarter M, Nutt DJ, Lister RG (eds): "Benzodiazepine Receptor Inverse Agonists." New York: Wiley, pp 25–41.

Moore H, Sarter M, Bruno JP (1995a): Bidirectional modulation of cortical acetylcholine efflux by infusion of benzodiazepine receptor ligands into the basal forebrain. Neurosci Lett 189:31–34.

Moore H, Sarter M, Bruno JP (1995b): Interactions between benzodiazepine and dopamine receptors in the modulation of cortical acetylcholine release. Soc Neurosci Abst 21:763.2.

Moore H, Stuckman S, Sarter M, Bruno JP (1995c): Stimulation of cortical acetylcholine efflux by FG 7142 measured with repeated microdialysis sampling. Synapse 21:324–331.

Moore H, Sarter M, Bruno JP (1993): Bidirectional modulation of stimulated cortical acetylcholine release by benzodiazepine receptor ligands. Brain Res 627–274.

Moore H, Sarter M, Bruno JP (1992): Age-dependent modulation of in vivo cortical acetylcholine release by benzodiazepine receptor ligands. Brain Res 596:17–29.

Muir JL, Everitt BJ, Robbins TW (1994): AMPA-induced excitotoxic lesions of the basal forebrain; a significant role for the cortical cholinergic system in attentional function. J Neurosci 14:2313–2326.

Muir JL, Dunnett SB, Robbins TW, Everitt BJ (1992): Attentional functions of the forebrain cholinergic systems: Effects of intraventricular hemicholinium, physostigmine, basal forebrain lesions and intracortical grafts on a multiple-choice serial reaction time task. Exp Brain Res 89:611–622.

Nissen MJ, Bullemer P (1987): Attentional requirements of learning: Evidence from performance measures. Cogn Psychol 19:1–32.

Nitsch RN, Slack BE, Wurtman RJ, Growdon JH (1992): Release of Alzheimer amyloid precursor derivatives stimulated by activation of muscarinic acetylcholine receptors. Science 258:304–307.

Oken BS, Kishiyama SS, Kaye JA, Howieson DB (1994): Attention deficit in Alzheimer's disease is not stimulated by an anticholinergic/antihistaminergic drug and is distinct from deficits in healthy aging. Neurology 44:657–662.

Olton DS, Wenk GL (1987): Dementia: Animal models of the cognitive impairments produced by degeneration of the basal forebrain cholinergic system. In Meltzer HY (ed): "Psychopharmacology: The Third Generation of Progress." New York: Raven, pp 941–953.

Palmer AM, Francis PT, Benton SJ, Sims NR, Mann DMA, Neary D, Snowdon JS, Bowen DM (1987a): Presynaptic serotonergic dysfunction in patients with Alzheimer's disease. J Neurochem 48:8–15.

Palmer AM, Francis PT, Bowen DM, Benton JS, Neary D, Mann DMA, Snowdon JS (1987b): Catecholaminergic neurons assessed ante-mortem in Alzheimer's disease. Brain Res 414:365–375.

Parasuraman R, Haxby JH (1993): Attention and brain function in Alzheimer's disease: A review. Neuropsychology 7:242–272.

Parasuraman R, Nestor PG (1993): Preserved cognitive operations in early Alzheimer's disease. In Cerella C, Hoyer W, Rybash J, Commons ML (eds): "Adult Information Processing: Limits on Loss." Orlando FL: Academic, pp 77–111.

Parasuraman R, Greenwood PM, Haxby JV, Grady CL (1992): Visuospatial attention in dementia of the Alzheimer type. Brain 115:711–733.

Perry EK, Haroutunian V, Davis KL, Levy R, Lantos P, Eagger S, Honavar M, Dean A, Griffiths M, McKeith I, Perry RH (1994): Neocortical cholinergic activities differentiate Lewy body dementia from classical Alzheimer's disease. Neuroreport 5:747–749.

Perry EK, Johnson M, Kerwin JM, Piggott MA, Court JA, Shaw PJ, Ince PG, Brown A, Perry RH (1992): Convergent cholinergic activities in aging and Alzheimer's disease. Neurobiol Aging 13:393–400.

Perry EK, Perry RH, Blessed G, Tomlinson BE (1977): Necropsy evidence of central cholinergic deficits in senile dementia. Lancet i:189.

Phillis JW (1968): Acetylcholine release from the cerebral cortex: Its role in cortical arousal. Brain Res 7:378–389.

Phillis JW, Chong GC (1965): Acetylcholine release from the cerebral and cerebellar cortices: Its role in cortical arousal. Nature 207:1253–1255.

Pope A, Hess HH, Lewin E (1964): Studies on the microchemical pathology of human cerebral cortex. In Cohen MM, Snider RS, (eds): "Morphological and Biochemical Correlates of Neural Activity." New York: Hoeber-Harper, pp 98–111.

Poirier J (1994): Apolipoprotein E in animal models of CNS injury and Alzheimer's disease. Trends Neurosci 17:525–530.

Posner MI (1994): Attention: The mechanisms of consciousness. Proc Natl Acad Sci U S A 91:7398–7403.

Procter AW, Bowen DM (1988): β-carbolines for Alzheimer's disease? More evidence, a test of efficacy and some precautions. Trends Neurosci 11:208–209.

Quigley, KS, Sarter MF, Hart SL, Berntson GG (1994): Cardiovascular effects of the benzodiazepine receptor partial inverse agonist FG 7142 in rats. Behav Brain Res 62:11–20.

Richter D, Crossland J (1949): Variation of acetylcholine content of brain with physiological state. Am J Physiol 159:247–255.

Robbins TW (1986): Psychopharmacological and neurobiological aspects of the energetics of information processing. In Hockey GRJ, Gaillard AWK, Coles MGH (eds): "Energetics and Human Information Processing." Dordrecht: Martinus Nijhoff, pp 71–90.

Robbins TW, Everitt BJ (1994): Arousal systems and attention. In Gazzaniga MS (ed): "The Cognitive Neurosciences." Cambridge: MIT Press, pp 703–720.

Robbins TW, Everitt BJ, Marston HM, Wilkinson J, Jones GH, Page KJ (1989): Comparative effects of ibotenic acid- and quisqualic acid-induced lesions of the substantia innominata on attentional function in the rat: Further implications for the role of the cholinergic neurons of the nucleus basalis in cognitive processes. Behav Brain Res 35:221–240.

Ruland S, Ronis V, Bruno JP, Sarter M (1995): Effects of lesions of the dorsal noradrenergic bundle on behavioral vigilance. Soc Neurosci Abst 21:763.3.

Rylett RJ, Ball MJ, Colhoun EH (1983): Evidence for high affinity choline transport in synaptosomes prepared from hippocampus and neocortex of patients with Alzheimer's disease. Brain Res 289:169–175.

Sahakian BJ, Owen AM, Morant NJ, Eagger SA, Boddington S, Crayton L, Crockford HA, Crooks M, Hill K, Levy R (1993): Further analysis of the cognitive effects of tetrahydroaminoacridine (THA) in Alzheimer's disease: Assessment of attentional and mnemonic function using CANTAB. Psychopharmacology 110:395–401.

Sahakian BJ, Downes JJ, Eagger S, Evenden JL, Levy R, Philpot MP, Roberts AC, Robbins TW (1990): Sparing of attentional relative to mnemonic function in a subgroup of patients with dementia of the Alzheimer type. Neuropsychologia 28:1197–1213.

Sarter M (1994): Neuronal mechanisms of the attentional dysfunctions in senile dementia and schizophrenia: Two sides of the same coin? Psychopharmacology 114:539–550.

Sarter M, Bruno, JP (1996b): Cognitive functions of cortical acetylcholine: Toward a unifying hypothesis. Brain Res Rev, in press.

Sarter M, Bruno JP (1996a): Transsynaptic stimulation of cortical acetylcholine and attention: A rational approach for the development of cognition enhancers. Behav Brain Res, in press.

Sarter M, Bruno JP (1994): Cognitive functions of cortical acetylcholine: Lessons from studies on the transsynaptic modulation of activated efflux. Trends Neurosci 17:17–221.

Sarter M, Bruno JP, Givens B, Moore H, McGaughy J, McMahon K (1996): Neuronal mechanisms mediating drug-induced cognition enhancement: Cognitive activity as a necessary intervening variable. Cogn Brain Res, 3:329–343.

Sarter M, McGaughy JA, Holley LA, Dudchenko P (1995): Behavioral facilitation and cognition enhancement. In Sarter M, Nutt DJ, Lister RG (eds): "Benzodiazepine Receptor Inverse Agonists." New York: Wiley, pp 213–243.

Sarter M, Bruno JP, Dudchenko P (1990): Activating the damaged basal forebrain cholinergic system: Tonic stimulation versus signal amplification. Psychopharmacology 101:1–17.

Schneider LS, Tariot PN (1994): Emerging drugs for Alzheimers disease. Med Clin North Am 78:911–934.

Semba K (1991): The cholinergic basal forebrain: A critical role in cortical arousal. In Napier TC, Kalivas PW, Hanin I (eds): "The Basal Forebrain. Anatomy to Function." New York: Plenum, pp 197–218.

Smith CG, Beninger RJ, Mallet PE, Jhamandas K, Boegman RJ (1994): Basal forebrain injections of the benzodiazepine partial inverse agonist FG 7142 enhance memory of rats in the double Y-maze. Brain Res 666:61–67.

Sims NR, Bowen DM, Allen SJ, Smith CCT, Neary D, Thomas DJ, Davison AN (1983): Presynaptic cholinergic dysfunction in patients with dementia. J Neurochem 40:503–509.

Soininen H, Kosunen O, Helisalmi S, Mannermaa A, Paljärvi L, Talasniemi S, Ryynänen M, Riekkinen PSr (1995): A severe loss of choline acetyltransferase in the frontal cortex of Zlzheimer patients carrying apolipoprotein ϵ 4 allele. Neurosci Lett 187:79–82.

Soncrant TT, Raffaele KC, Asthana S, Berardi A, Morris PP, Haxby JV (1993): Memory improvement without toxicity during chronic, low dose intravenous arecoline in Alzheimer's disease. Psychopharmacology 112:421–427.

Suszkiw JB, Toth G (1986): Storage and release of acetylcholine in rat cortical synaptosomes: Effects of D,L-2-(phenylpiperidino)cyclohexanol (AH5183). Brain Res 386:371–378.

Szerb JC (1967): Cortical acetylcholine release and electroencephalographic arousal. J Physiol 192:329–343.

Traub M, Friedman SB (1992): The implication of current therapeutic approaches for cholinergic hypothesis of dementia. Dementia 3:189–192.

Turchi J, Bruno JP, Sarter M (1995): Cortical acetylcholine and processing capacity: Effects of cortical cholinergic deafferentation on crossmodal divided attention in rats. Soc Neurosci Abst 21:763.9

Venables PH (1964): Input dysfunction in schizophrenia. In: Maher BA (ed): "Progress in Experimental Personality Research." New York: Academic, pp 1–47.

Voytko ML, Olton DS, Richardson RT, Gorman LK, Tobin JR, Price DL (1994): Basal forebrain lesions in monkeys disrupt attention but not learning and memory. J Neurosci 14:167–186.

Whitehouse PJ, Price DL, Struble RG, Coyle JT, DeLong MR (1982): Alzheimer's disease and senile dementia: Loss of neurons in the basal forebrain. Science 215:1237–1239.

Weinberger NM (1993): Learning-induced changes of auditory receptive fields. Cur Opin Neurobiol 3:570–577.

Wurtman RJ, Blusztajn JK, Maire JC (1985): "Autocannibalism" of choline-containing membrane phospholipids in the pathogenesis of Alzheimer's disease—a hypothesis. Neurochem Int 7:369–372.

Younkin SG (1995): Evidence that Aβ42 is the real culprit in Alzheimer's disease. Ann Neurol 37:287–288.

Zigmond MJ, Stricker EM (1989): Animal models of parkinsonism using selective neurotoxins: Clinical and basic implications. Int Rev Neurobiol 31:1–79.

CHAPTER 6

Neuropsychological Features of Alzheimer's Disease

DAVID P. SALMON

Department of Neurosciences, School of Medicine,
University of California, San Diego, La Jolla, California 92093-0948

INTRODUCTION

Alzheimer's disease (AD) is a progressive degenerative brain disorder characterized by neocortical atrophy, neuron and synapse loss (Terry et al., 1981, 1991), and the presence of senile plaques and neurofibrillary tangles (Terry and Katzman, 1983). These neurodegenerative changes occur primarily in the hippocampus and entorhinal cortex and in the association cortices of the frontal, temporal, and parietal lobes (Terry and Katzman, 1983; Hyman et al., 1984). Subcortical neuron loss also occurs, largely in the nucleus basalis of Meynert and the nucleus locus coeruleus, resulting in decrements in neocortical levels of cholinergic and noradrenergic neurotransmitters, respectively (Bondareff et al., 1982; Mann et al., 1984; Whitehouse et al., 1982). Although the temporal progression of the neuropathological changes of AD are not fully known, recent studies suggest that the hippocampus and entorhinal cortex are involved in the earliest stage of the disease, and that frontal, temporal, and parietal association cortices become increasingly involved as the disease progresses (Hyman et al., 1984; Pearson et al., 1985; Braak and Braak, 1991; Arriagada et al., 1992; Bancher et al., 1993; DeLacosta and White, 1993).

The primary clinical manifestation of AD is a profound global dementia that is marked by severe amnesia with additional deficits in language, "executive" functions, attention, and visuospatial and constructional abilities (Corkin et al., 1982; Katzman, 1986). Despite the pervasiveness of the cognitive impairments associated with AD, extensive neuropsychological research during the past decade has begun

Pharmacological Treatment of Alzheimer's Disease: Molecular and Neurobiological Foundations,
Edited by Brioni and Decker
ISBN 0-471-16758-4   © 1997 Wiley-Liss, Inc.

to identify the particular cognitive deficits that occur in the earliest stages of the disease, and to delineate a pattern of deficits that may distinguish between the dementias of AD and other neurodegenerative disorders. In addition, recent neuropsychological research has further characterized the relationship between the cognitive and neuropathologic abnormalities associated with AD. Each of these areas of research will be discussed in the present chapter.

CLINICAL-PATHOLOGICAL RELATIONSHIPS IN ALZHEIMER'S DISEASE

A number of studies have shown that there is a strong relationship between the degree of neuropathologic abnormality and the severity of dementia in patients with AD (Blessed et al., 1968; Terry et al., 1991; Dekosky and Scheff, 1990; Mann et al., 1988; Neary et al., 1986). In one of the first of these studies, Blessed and colleagues (1968) found that the number of senile plaques in the neocortex of patients with AD correlated significantly with their performance on the Information–Memory–Concentration (IMC) test, a brief neuropsychological measure of dementia. This correlation was not particularly strong, however, and some investigators were unable to replicate this finding (Neary et al., 1986; Mann et al., 1988).

Cummings and Cotman (1995) recently argued that the lack of a strong correlation between the number of plaques and dementia severity may be due to an inability to accurately detect and count plaques when they occur with a high density and overlap with one another. To overcome this problem, these investigators developed immunolabeling and imaging techniques to quantify the area of brain tissue occupied by deposits of β-amyloid, one of the primary components of the senile plaque. Using these techniques, a high correlation was observed between levels of β-amyloid deposition and severity of cognitive impairment as measured by the IMC test ($r = .93$) and the Mini-Mental State Examination (MMSE; $r = .90$).

Although Mann and colleagues (1988) were unable to find a relationship between senile plaques and severity of dementia in patients with AD, these investigators did note that large neuron counts correlated significantly with dementia severity and that there was a continuing decline in both large neuron counts and cognitive functioning in autopsied patients who had also undergone brain biopsy about 3–7 years prior to death. This observation led Terry and colleagues (1991) to speculate that extensive synapse loss might also be expected and that this loss might be highly correlated with the severity of dementia prior to death [also see Dekosky and Scheff (1990)]. To examine this hypothesis, Terry and colleagues (1991) quantified synaptic density in the midfrontal, inferior parietal, and superior temporal lobe neocortex of patients with AD and determined the degree of its correlation with their performance on three global mental status examinations: the IMC test, the MMSE, and the Dementia Rating Scale (DRS). The degree of correlation between the mental status examinations and the number of neuritic plaques, neurofibrillary tangles, large neurons (>90 μm), and choline acetyltransferase levels in the three cortical regions was also examined. The results of this study revealed that performance on the three mental status examinations was more highly correlated with synaptic density in the midfrontal and inferior parietal regions of the neocortex than with other neuropathological measures. A stepwise multiple regression analysis of the neuropathological factors that might contribute to DRS performance, for example, produced a model with midfrontal synaptic density, inferior parietal synaptic density, and inferior parietal neuritic plaques that accounted for 92% of the variance in test performance. These results led Terry and colleagues (1991) to suggest that the loss of neocortical synapses may be the primary determinant of dementia in AD, and that other neuropathological changes may play a secondary role.

Understanding the relationship between dementia severity and the neuropathological changes that occur in AD has been complicated by the recent discovery that approximately 25% of patients who manifest a syndrome similar to dementia of the Alzheimer type (DAT) during life have concommitant AD and diffusely distributed neocortical and subcortical Lewy bodies [i.e., abnormal intracytoplasmic eosinophilic neuronal inclusion bodies; for review, see Hansen and Galasko (1992)]. This Lewy body variant of AD (LBV; Hansen et al., 1990) is characterized by the typical cortical distribution of senile plaques and neurofibrillary tangles associated with AD, the typical subcortical changes of Parkinson's disease (i.e., Lewy bodies and cell loss) in the substantia nigra and other pigmented brainstem nuclei, and diffusely distributed neocortical Lewy bodies.

Clinically, patients with LBV exhibit insidious and progressive cognitive decline with no other significant neurologic abnormalities and are often diagnosed with probable or possible AD [e.g., Hansen et al. (1990)]. Retrospective studies indicate, however, that a greater proportion of LBV than AD patients have mild Parkinsonian or extrapyramidal motor findings [e.g., bradykinesia, rigidity, masked facies, gait abnormalities, but no resting tremor, Galasko et al. (1996); Hansen et al. (1990)], and are more likely to manifest fluctuating cognitive impairment, visual or auditory hallucinations, and unexplained falls at some point during the course of the disease (McKeith et al., 1992).

Several recent studies indicate that Lewy body pathology is likely to contribute to the severity of cognitive impairment in patients with LBV (Lennox et al., 1989; Salmon et al., 1996; Samuel et al., 1996). Samuel and colleagues found that the number of Lewy bodies observed in the midfrontal, cingulate, and superior temporal cortices of patients with LBV was significantly correlated with their performance on the IMC test ($r = .74$), MMSE ($r = -.63$), and DRS ($r = -.63$). Although it is likely that AD pathology also contributed to the dementia manifested by these patients, numbers of neurofibrillary tangles and senile plaques did not correlate significantly with level of dementia as measured by any of the three mental status tests.

Further evidence of the contribution of Lewy body pathology to the presence and severity of dementia is provided by a recent retrospective study of five patients who at autopsy were found to have diffuse Lewy body disease (DLBD; subcortical and diffusely distributed neocortical Lewy bodies) with little or no AD pathology (Salmon et al., 1996). All five of these patients had exhibited insidious cognitive decline, global impairment on neuropsychological testing, and mild extrapyramidal motor dysfunction, and all had been clinically diagnosed with probable or possible AD or one of its variants (e.g., LBV, mixed AD, and vascular dementia). This association between dementia and Lewy body pathology in the absence of AD pathology provides strong evidence that both types of pathology are contributing to dementia severity in LBV.

Although the precise cause of the dementia associated with AD remains unknown, the studies reviewed above clearly indicate that the cognitive decline inherent in the disease is related to its neuropathologic abnormalities. While synapse loss may be the strongest correlate of dementia severity in patients with AD, recent evidence indicates that β-amyloid deposition may also be highly correlated, and an understanding of the interrelationship between these factors and dementia awaits further scrutiny. In addition, the possible contribution of diffuse Lewy body pathology to dementia in a significant number of patients with AD (i.e., those with LBV) must be taken into consideration.

EARLY NEUROPSYCHOLOGICAL MANIFESTATION OF DEMENTIA OF THE ALZHEIMER TYPE

Given that neuropathologic abnormalities in the hippocampus and entorhinal cortex are likely to be the first and most severe to occur in AD (Braak and Braak, 1991; Hyman et al., 1984), it is not surprising that failure of recent memory is usually the most prominent feature during the early stages of DAT (Huppert and Tym, 1986; Martin, 1987). Evidence from both human and animal studies indicates that these brain structures are critical for the acquisition and retention of new information, and for the recollection of information learned in the past [for review, see Squire (1992)].

Although the onset of DAT is insidious and initially difficult to distinguish from the normal cognitive changes that occur with aging, extensive neuropsychological research during the past decade has shown that measures of the ability to learn new information and retain it over time are quite sensitive in differentiating between mildly demented patients with clinically diagnosed DAT and normal older adults [e.g., Bayles et al. (1989), Delis et al. (1991), Eslinger et al. (1985), Huff et al. (1987), Kaszniak et al. (1986), and Storandt et al. (1984)]. Welsh and colleagues (1991), for example, found that a delayed free-recall measure on a verbal memory task was highly effective (i.e., 90% accuracy) in distinguishing between very mildly demented patients with DAT (all with MMSE scores above 24 out of 30) and elderly normal control subjects, and that this measure was significantly more effective than measures of learning, confrontation naming, verbal fluency, and constructional ability. Similar results have been obtained in other studies (Flicker et al., 1991; Knopman and Ryberg, 1989; Morris et al., 1991; Tröster et al., 1993).

A number of investigators have suggested that the early involvement of the hippocampus and entorhinal cortex in AD may lead to decrements in learning and memory during a "preclinical" phase of the disease (Katzman, 1994). According to this view, subtle cognitive changes become evident before neural degeneration has progressed to a level sufficient to produce the full clinical manifestation of the dementia syndrome. Consistent with this view, a number of studies have demonstrated decrements in learning and memory in individuals who do not meet established criteria for a clinical diagnosis of DAT, but who develop dementia a number of years later (Bayles and Kaszniak, 1987; Bondi et al., 1994; Fuld et al., 1990; Masur et al., 1990, 1994; La Rue et al., 1992; Linn et al., 1995).

In one series of studies, for example, Fuld and colleagues found that poor performance on measures of recall from the Fuld Object Memory Test (Fuld et al., 1990) or the Selective Reminding Test (Masur et al., 1990) was an accurate indication of those nondemented nursing home residents who would develop DAT within the next 5 years. In a longer-term follow-up, a logistic regression model containing performance on a delayed recall measure from the Selective Reminding Test, a recall measure from the Fuld Object Memory Test, the Digit Symbol Substitution subtest from the Wechsler Adult Intelligence Scale (WAIS), and a measure of verbal fluency was moderately effective in identifying individuals who later developed DAT (32/64; 50%) and provided excellent specificity for identifying individuals who remained free of dementia (238/253; 94%) over a subsequent 11-year period (Masur et al., 1994).

With the identification of a common and specific genetic risk factor for AD, the apolipoprotein E (apoE) ∈4 allele (Strittmatter et al., 1993), several recent studies have focused on episodic memory changes in nondemented elderly subjects who possess this risk factor. This approach assumes that the nondemented elderly individuals with the risk factor for AD are more likely to be in the preclinical phase of the disease than those who do not have the risk factor, and therefore are likely to perform worse on sensitive neuropsychological tests.

In an initial study adopting this approach, Reed and colleagues (1994) found that nondemented elderly male individuals with the ∈4 allele exhibited poorer mean performance on a test of visual memory than their dizygotic twin who did not have the ∈4 allele. Bondi and colleagues (Bondi et al., 1995) demonstrated that the verbal learning and memory performance of nondemented subjects with the apoE ∈4 allele was qualitatively (though not quantitatively) similar to that of early-stage patients with DAT. Furthermore, the nondemented subjects with the apoE ∈4 allele recalled fewer items during the learning trials and over delay intervals, and utilized a less effective organizational strategy for learning, than carefully matched nondemented subjects without the apoE ∈4 allele. Follow-up examinations of some of the subjects in the Bondi et al. (1995) study revealed that 6 of 14 subjects with the ∈4 allele subsequently developed either probable or possible DAT or questionable DAT (i.e., cognitive decline without evidence of significant functional impairment), whereas none of 26 subjects without an ∈4 allele demonstrated any cognitive decline.

Two recent studies have demonstrated that the early appearance of learning and memory decrements in conjunction with the presence of the apoE ∈4 allele is highly predictive of the subsequent development of DAT (Petersen et al., 1995; Tierney et al., 1996). Using a Cox regression model technique, Petersen and colleagues (1995) found that the presence of an ϵ4 allele was the strongest predictor of the subsequent development of DAT in a consecutive series of 66 patients who had mild cognitive impairment that was particularly evident in their performance on the learning and retention measures from the Auditory-Verbal Learning Test. In a similar study, Tierney and colleagues (1996) found that the presence of the ϵ4 allele was an effective predictor of those subjects with learning and memory deficits who went on to develop DAT during the subsequent 2 years.

Although the studies reviewed above indicate that decrements in learning and memory are particularly evident in the early stages of DAT and are likely to precede the development of the full dementia syndrome, it should be noted that other neuropsychological deficits often occur early in the course of the disease (Salmon et al., in press) Monsch and colleagues (1992), for example, demonstrated that mildly demented patients with DAT could be effectively differentiated from normal elderly control subjects strictly on the basis of their performances on several types of verbal fluency tasks. The best discriminator, a semantic category fluency task, had greater than 90% sensitivity and specificity for the diagnosis of DAT. Performance on a modified version of the Wisconsin Card Sorting Task, a test of "executive" functions, has also been found to have a high degree of sensitivity (94.3%) and specificity (86.7%) for differentiating between mildly demented DAT patients and normal elderly individuals (Bondi et al., 1993). Despite the effectiveness of these tests for differentiating between mildly demented patients and normal elderly individuals, it should be noted that relatively few patients with DAT have been reported to initially present with cognitive deficits other than learning and memory impairment. Thus, decrements in learning and memory are likely to be the best neuropsychological indicator of the preclinical phase of DAT.

An intriguing recent study does suggest, however, that cognitive competence in areas other than learning and memory during early life may predict the development in cognitive deficits and AD during late life. Snowdon and colleagues (1996) found that measures of idea density and grammatical complexity in the autobiographies written by women entering a convent at about the age of 22 accurately predicted low cognitive test performance and the development of AD in late life (age 75–95). This finding was not likely to be attributable to environmental factors, as all of the women had lived similar lives in the convent since their early twenties, nor was it an effect of differential education since the same relationship was observed when the analyses were limited to a subset of individuals who were all college educated and had been teachers. The authors speculate that the ability to predict future cognitive impairment on the basis of cognitive performance more than 50 years earlier may indicate that the poorer performers may have lacked a cognitive or brain "reserve" (Katzman, 1993) that would have provided some buffer against the neurodegenerative effects of AD or that the AD degenerative processes are very slow acting, and brain abnormalities in these individuals may have begun in the second decades of their lives. In any event, continued research in this area is clearly necessary to enhance our ability to clinically detect AD in its earliest stages when potential neuroprotective agents designed to impede the progression of the disease might be most effective.

NEUROPSYCHOLOGICAL DIFFERENTIATION OF ALZHEIMER DISEASE FROM OTHER DEMENTING DISORDERS

Considerable evidence has been amassed over the past two decades that indicates that dementia is not a unitary disorder. Rather, degenerative diseases that differ in their sites and extent of neuropathology also differ in the predominant cognitive symptoms they engender. The dementia syndromes associated with Alzheimer's disease and Huntington's disease (HD), for example, differ in a number of respects. As mentioned previously, DAT is broadly characterized by prominent amnesia with additional deficits in language and semantic knowledge (ie., aphasia), abstract reasoning, other executive functions, and constructional and visuospatial abilities (Bayles and Kaszniak, 1987; Parks et al., 1993). In contrast, the dementia syndrome associated with HD, a genetically transmitted neurodegenerative disorder that results in a progressive deterioration of the neostriatum (caudate nucleus and putamen; Bruyn et al., 1979; Vonsattel et al., 1985), involves only a moderate memory disturbance, attentional dysfunction, problem-solving deficits, psychomotor slowing, visuoperceptual and constructional deficits, and a deficiency in performing arithmetic (Brandt and Butters, 1986; Butters et al., 1978). Unlike AD, HD results in little or no aphasia, although patients may be dysarthric due to the motor dysfunction inherent in the disease.

The distinctions that have been noted in the behavioral and cognitive features of various dementia syndromes have led some investigators to propose a "cortical–subcortical" framework based upon whether the dementia is associated with predominant neurodegeneration in the cortex or in subcortical nuclei (Albert et al., 1974; Cummings, 1990; McHugh and Folstein, 1975). Within this cortical–subcortical framework, DAT is viewed as a prototypical cortical dementia, and the dementia associated with HD is considered a prototypical form of subcortical dementia. It should be kept in mind that the cortical–subcortical distinction refers to a particular constellation of symptoms and not strictly to the pathology of the diseases, as many neurodegenerative diseases, including AD and HD, involve both cortical and subcortical neuropathologic changes.

Interestingly, patients with LBV appear to exhibit a superimposition of cortical and subcortical neuropsychological impairments (Byrne et al., 1989; Forstl et al., 1993; Gibb et al., 1985; Hansen et al., 1990; McKeith et al., 1992). Hansen and colleagues (1990), for example, found that neuropathologically confirmed LBV patients performed significantly worse than patients with pure AD on tests of attention, phonemically based verbal fluency, and visuospatial and constructional ability, despite equivalently impaired performance on tests of global mental status (i.e., the IMC test), episodic memory, confrontation naming (i.e., the Boston Naming test), and arithmetic. Thus, the two groups demonstrated equivalent deficits in cognitive abilities usually affected by AD (e.g., memory, confrontation naming), but the LBV patients displayed disproportionately severe deficits in some cognitive abilities that are prominently affected in subcortical diseases (e.g., attention, verbal fluency, and visuospatial processing).

Although the results from the Hansen et al. (1990) study were based on neuropathologically confirmed patient groups, it appears that similar results are obtained with patients with clinically diagnosed LBV (or senile dementia of the Lewy body type; Galloway et al., 1992; Sahgal et al., 1992a, b, 1995), and with clinically diagnosed DAT patients who exhibit mild extrapyramidal motor dysfunction that may be indicative of LBV (Girling and Berrios, 1990; Merello et al., 1994; Richards et al., 1993; Soininen et al., 1992).

Because of the prominence of memory impairment in most dementing disorders, many studies comparing cortical and subcortical dementia syndromes have focused on this aspect of cognition. A number of these studies involve the application of concepts and procedures developed in cognitive psychology to an analysis of the memory deficit that occurs in each syndrome. Thus, studies examining differences in the performance of patients with cortical or subcortical dementia on tests of episodic memory (i.e., temporally dated autobiographical episodes that depend on contextual cues for their retrieval), semantic memory (i.e., overlearned facts and concepts that are not dependent on contextual cues for their retrieval), and implicit memory (i.e., the unconscious recollection of knowledge that is expressed indirectly through the performance of the specific operations comprising a task) have been carried out. For the most part, these studies suggest there are a number of fundamental differences in the nature of the memory impairments that occur in cortical and subcortical disorders.

Patients with a cortical dementia such as DAT exhibit a severe episodic memory deficit that appears to result from ineffective consolidation (i.e., storage) of new information. In contrast, the moderate episodic memory impairment of patients with a subcortical dementia, such as HD, most likely reflects a general difficulty in initiating a systematic retrieval strategy when recalling information from either episodic or semantic memory.

Evidence for a consolidation deficit in DAT patients includes their showing little improvement in acquiring information over repeated learning trials (Buschke and Fuld, 1974; Masur et al., 1989; Moss et al., 1986; Wilson et al., 1983), a tendency to recall only the most recently presented information (i.e., a heightened recency effect) in free-recall tasks (Delis et al., 1991; Massman et al., 1993; Miller, 1971; Pepin and Eslinger, 1989;), an inability to benefit normally from effortful or elaborative encoding at the time of acquisition (Knopman and Ryberg, 1989), a failure to demonstrate a normal improvement in performance when memory is tested with a recognition rather than a free-recall format (Delis et al., 1991; Miller, 1971; Wilson et al., 1983), and rapid forgetting of information over time (Butters et al., 1988; Moss et al., 1986; Tröster et al., 1993; Welsh et al., 1991).

Although HD patients also exhibit difficulty in learning and recalling information in free-recall tasks, evidence of a general retrieval deficit is provided by a marked improvement in their performance when memory is tested with a recognition format (Delis et al., 1991; Moss et al., 1986; but see Brandt et al., 1992), and by their ability to retain information over a delay in near normal fashion (Delis et al., 1991; Moss et al., 1986).

A recent study by Delis and colleagues (1991) highlighted these differences in the nature and pattern of the episodic memory impairments associated with cortical and subcortical dementias. In this study, the verbal learning and memory abilities of patients with DAT and HD were compared using the California Verbal Learning Test (CVLT), a rigorous, standardized memory test that assesses rate of learning, retention after short- and long-delay intervals, semantic encoding ability, recognition (i.e., discriminability), intrusion and perseverative errors, and response biases. In the test, individuals are verbally presented 5 presentation/free-recall trials of a list of 16 shopping items (4 items in each of 4 categories) and are then administered a single trial using a second, different list of 16 items. Immediately after this final trial, individuals are administered a free-recall and then a cued-recall test for the items on the first shopping list. Twenty minutes later, the free-recall and cued-recall tests are repeated, followed by a yes–no recognition test consisting of the 16 items on the first shopping list and 28 distractor items.

The results of this study showed that despite comparable immediate and delayed free-recall and cued-recall deficits, DAT and HD patients could be effectively differentiated by several aspects of their performance. A discriminant function model based on (a) the percentage of cued-recall intrusions and (b) the difference between recognition discriminability and recall on trial 5 of the initial learning trials correctly classified 17 out of 20 DAT patients and 16 out of 19 HD patients. The effectiveness of the first measure contained in the model reflects the greater susceptibility to proactive interference of DAT patients relative to HD patients (Fuld et al., 1982; Jacobs et al., 1990; Tröster et al., 1989). The second measure was effective because it assesses both retention over time and any potential benefit of a recognition format over free recall, characteristics that emphasize the differences between consolidation and retrieval deficits.

The distinct patterns of episodic memory impairment exhibited by patients with cortical and subcortical dementia syndromes is not limited to the learning and retention of new information, but is also apparent in their performances on tests of remote memory. While patients with DAT exhibit a severe loss of memory for information acquired prior to the onset of their disease (i.e., retrograde amnesia), the remote memory loss of HD patients is moderate at worst (Albert et al., 1981; Beatty et al., 1988; Hodges et al., 1993; Kopelman, 1989; Sagar et al., 1988; Wilson et al., 1981). In addition, a number of studies indicate that in the early stages of DAT, remote memory loss is temporally graded with memories from the distant past (i.e., childhood and early adulthood) better remembered than memories from the more remote past (i.e., mid and late adulthood) (Beatty and Salmon, 1991; Beatty et al., 1988; Hodges et al., 1993). In contrast, the relatively mild degree of remote memory loss exhibited by patients with HD (Albert et al., 1981; Beatty et al., 1988) is equally severe across all decades of their lives. The pattern of performance of HD patients on remote memory tests is consistent with the notion that they have a general retrieval deficit that equally affects recollection of information from any decade of their lives. The temporally graded remote memory loss of DAT patients, in contrast, most likely reflects a failure to adequately consolidate information through repeated processing, rehearsal, or reexposure [see Zola-Morgan and Squire (1990) for a discussion of the role of consolidation in temporally graded retrograde amnesia.].

Patients with DAT can be further differentiated from patients with HD and other subcortical dementias by the severity and nature of their semantic memory impairment. Patients with DAT are noted for mild anomia and word-finding difficulties in spontaneous speech, and some evidence suggests that this deficit is indicative of a loss of semantic knowledge and a breakdown in the organization of semantic memory (Chertkow and Bub, 1990; Hodges et al., 1991, 1992; Salmon and Chan, 1994).

Some of the earliest and most important evidence supporting the view that DAT patients suffer a breakdown in the organization of semantic memory emanates from studies examining their performance on various tests of verbal fluency. Butters and colleagues (1987), for example, compared the performances of DAT and HD patients on verbal fluency tasks that differ in the demands they place on semantic memory. In the letter fluency task used in this study, subjects orally generated words beginning with the letters F, A, and S, with 1 min allowed per category. In the category fluency task, subjects generated exemplars from the semantic category "animals" for 1 min. The letter fluency task does not place great demands on the organization of semantic memory since it can be performed using phonemic cues to search a very extensive set of appropriate exemplars within the lexicon. In contrast, the category fluency task requires the generation of words from a small and highly related set of exemplars within a single abstract semantic category.

Although the DAT and HD patient groups were matched for overall severity of dementia, the two groups produced different patterns of performance on the two fluency tasks. Patients with HD demonstrated severe deficits (relative to normal control subjects) on both fluency tasks, whereas the mildly demented patients with DAT were impaired *only* on the semantically demanding category fluency task. While the performance of HD patients on the letter and category fluency tasks is consistent with an inability to effectively retrieve information from semantic memory, DAT patients appear to be deficient in their knowledge of the attributes and/or exemplars that define the relevant semantic category and are thus unable to use this knowledge to locate specific category exemplars [see also, Monsch et al. (1994)].

The semantic memory impairment of DAT patients can be further differentiated from that of HD patients by the differences in their performances on tests of confrontation naming. Patients with DAT perform poorly on tests of confrontation naming and tend to produce semantic errors (Bayles and Tomoeda, 1983; Hodges et al., 1991; Huff et al., 1986; Smith et al., 1989). Patients with HD, in contrast, usually perform at near normal levels on tests of confrontation naming and the errors they produce are often visuoperceptually based rather than semantically based (Hodges et al., 1991).

Recent studies using clustering and multidimensional scaling techniques (Romney et al., 1972; Shepard et al., 1972; Tversky and Hutchinson, 1986) to model the organization of the network of related categories, concepts and attributes that comprise semantic memory (Collins and Loftus, 1975) also differentiate between patients with DAT and HD (Chan et al., 1993a, b, 1995a, b). These studies used multidimensional scaling procedures to generate a spatial representation of the degree of association between concepts in the semantic memory of these patient groups. The spatial representation, or cognitive map, generated in this manner clusters concepts along one or more dimensions according to their proximity, or degree of relatedness, in the patient's semantic network. The distance between concepts in the cognitive map reflects the strength of their association.

In one of the studies from this series (Chan et al., 1995a), the cognitive maps reflecting the organization of semantic memory were generated for DAT, HD, and normal control subjects using proximity data derived from a triadic comparison task in which subjects chose, from among three concepts (i.e., among 3 animals), the two that are most alike. Every possible combination of 3 animals, from a total sample of 12 animals, was presented to determine the degree of association between each pair of animals in relation to all other animal names. The results revealed that although the semantic networks of the DAT patients and normal control subjects were best represented by three dimensions (domesticity, predation, and size), they differed significantly in a number of ways. Patients with DAT focused primarily on concrete perceptual information (i.e., size) in categorizing animals, whereas control subjects stressed abstract conceptual knowledge (i.e., domesticity). A number of animals that were highly associated and clustered together for control subjects were not strongly associated for patients with DAT, and DAT patients were less consistent than normal control subjects in utilizing the various attributes of animals in categorization.

In contrast to the DAT patients, the semantic networks of HD patients and their age-matched control subjects were best represented by two dimensions (domesticity and size) and were virtually identical. Domesticity was the most salient dimension for categorizing animals for HD and normal control subjects, and the groups did not differ in the importance they applied to the various dimensions or in their reliance on a particular dimension for categorization.

A final major neuropsychological distinction between DAT and HD patients is the different patterns of spared and impaired abilities they exhibit on various implicit memory tasks [for reviews, see Bondi et al. (1994) and Butters et al. (1995)]. As mentioned earlier, implicit memory refers to a form of memory in which an individual's performance is facilitated "unconsciously" simply by prior exposure to stimulus material. It has been described as a distinct memory "system" independent from the conscious, episodic memory system (Schacter, 1987; Schacter and Tulving, 1994; Squire, 1987) and is thought to be invoked during classical conditioning, lexical and semantic priming, motor skill learning, and perceptual learning (Squire, 1987). Numerous studies have demonstrated that implicit memory is preserved in patients with severe, circumscribed episodic memory deficits [for review, see Squire (1987)], providing some neuropsychological and neurobiological evidence that it is a distinct form of memory.

Studies comparing the performances of DAT and HD patients have shown that DAT patients, but not HD patients, are significantly impaired on lexical (Bondi and Kaszniak, 1991; Shimamura et al., 1987; Salmon et al., 1988), semantic (Salmon et al., 1988), and pictorial (Heindel et al., 1990) priming tasks. In two of these studies, for example, Shimamura and colleagues (Shimamura et al., 1987; Salmon et al., 1988) demonstrated that DAT patients exhibited significantly less priming on a word stem completion task (Graf et al., 1984) than normal control subjects, patients with circumscribed amnesia, and patients with HD. Although the latter two groups had episodic memory deficits that were equally severe as that of the DAT patients, they performed as well as normal control subjects on the word stem completion task.

In contrast to the pattern of results observed on the implicit priming tasks, HD patients, but not patients with DAT, are impaired on motor skill learning (Eslinger and Damasio, 1986; Heindel et al., 1988, 1989), prism adaptation (Paulsen et al., 1993), and weight biasing (Heindel et al., 1992) tasks that involve the generation and refinement (i.e., learning) of motor programs to guide behavior. For example, Heindel and colleagues (1989) demonstrated that HD patients were impaired in their ability to learn the motor skills necessary to perform a pursuit rotor task, a task in which subjects must learn to maintain contact between a stylus held in their preferred hand and a small metallic disk on a rotating turntable (Heindel et al., 1988). Patients with DAT or circumscribed amnesia, in contrast, demonstrated the same systematic and equivalent improvement in performance across blocks of trials as normal control subjects. It should be noted that the motor skill learning deficit in HD patients was not correlated with their general motor impairment (i.e., chorea) and was confirmed with other tasks that have little, if any, motor component (e.g., weight biasing and prism adaptation).

The contrasting patterns of normal and impaired abilities exhibited by DAT and HD patients provides a double dissociation between the various implicit priming and motor skill learning tasks. This dissociation suggests that different forms of implicit memory, all of which are intact in patients with amnesic syndromes, are not mediated by a single neurological substrate. Rather, forms of priming may be dependent on the functional integrity of the neocortical association areas damaged in patients with DAT, whereas motor skill learning, prism adaptation, and the biasing of weight perception may all be mediated by a corticostriatal and basal ganglia system that is severely compromised in HD

SUMMARY

Considerable progress has been made over the past decade in elucidating the neuropsychological features of AD. Research has identified the specific neuropsychological deficits that occur in the earliest stages of DAT and is beginning to uncover those cognitive changes that may presage the development of dementia by a number of years. Research has also clearly shown that dementia is not a unitary disorder, but that different patterns of relatively preserved and impaired cognitive abilities can be identified among dementing diseases that have different etiologies and sites of neuropathology. These findings have occurred against the backdrop of clinico-pathological research that has begun to identify the relationship between cognitive impairment and the regional neuropathologic abnormalities associated with AD.

ACKNOWLEDGMENTS

Preparation of this chapter was supported in part by funds from NIA grants AG-05131 and AG-12963, and NIMH grant MH-48819.

REFERENCES

Albert MS, Butters N, Brandt J (1981): Development of remote memory loss in patients with Huntington's disease. J Clin Neuropsychol 3:1–12.

Albert ML, Feldman RG, Willis AL (1974): The "subcortical dementia" of progressive supranuclear palsy. J Neurol Neurosurg Psychiatry 37:121–130.

Arriagada PV, Growdon JH, Hedley-Whyte ET, Hyman BT (1992): Neurofibrillay tangles but not senile plaques parallel duration and severity of Alzheimer's disease. Neurology 42:631–639.

Bancher C, Braak H, Fischer P, Jellinger KA (1993): Neuropathological staging of Alzheimer lesions and intellectual status in Alzheimer's and Parkinson's disease patients. Neurosci Lett 162:179–182.

Bayles KA, Boone DR, Tomoeda CK, Slauson TJ, Kaszniak AW (1989): Differentiating Alzheimer's patients from the normal elderly and stroke patients with aphasia. J Speech Hear Disorders 54:74–87.

Bayles KA, Kaszniak AW (1987): "Communication and Cognition in Normal Aging and Dementia." Boston: College-Hill/Little, Brown.

Bayles KA, Tomoeda CK (1983): Confrontation naming impairment in dementia. Brain Lang 19:98–114.

Beatty WW, Salmon DP (1991): Remote memory for visuospatial information in patients with Alzheimer's disease. J Geriatr Psychiatry Neurol 4:14–17.

Beatty WW, Salmon DP, Butters N, Heindel WC, Granholm EL (1988): Retrograde amnesia in patients with Alzheimer's disease or Huntington's disease. Neurobiol Aging 9:181–186.

Blessed G, Tomlinson BE, Roth M (1968): The association between quantitative measures of dementia and of senile change in the cerebral grey matter of elderly subjects. Br J Psychiatry 114:797–811.

Bondareff W, Mountjoy CQ, Roth M (1982): Loss of neurons of origin of the adrenergic projection to cerebral cortex (nucleus locus ceruleus) in senile dementia. Neurology 32:164–167.

Bondi MW, Kaszniak AW (1991): Implicit and explicit memory in Alzheimer's disease and Parkinson's disease. J Clin Exp Neuropsychol 13:339–358.

Bondi MW, Salmon DP, Monsch AU, Galasko D, Butters N, Klauber MR, Thal LJ, Saitoh T (1995): Episodic memory changes are associated with the ApoE-ϵ4 allele in nondemented older adults. Neurology 45:2203–2206.

Bondi MW, Monsch AU, Galasko D, Butters N, Salmon DP, Delis DC (1994): Preclinical cognitive markers of dementia of the Alzheimer type. Neuropsychology 8:374–384.

Bondi MW, Monsch AU, Butters N, Salmon DP, Paulsen JS (1993): Utility of a modified version of the Wisconsin Card Sorting Test in the detection of dementia of the Alzheimer type. Clin Neuropsychol 7:161–170.

Braak H, Braak E (1991): Neuropathological staging of Alzheimer-related changes. Acta Neuropath 82:239–259.

Brandt J, Butters N (1986): The neuropsychology of Huntington's disease. Trends Neurosci 9:118–120.

Brandt J, Corwin J, Krafft L (1992): Is verbal recognition memory really different in Huntington's and Alzheimer's disease? J Clin Exp Neuropsychol 14:773–784.

Bruyn GW, Bots G, Dom R (1979): Huntington's chorea: Current neuropathological status. In Chase T, Wexler N, Barbeau A (eds): "Advances in Neurology, Vol. 23: Huntington's Disease." New York: Raven, pp 83–94.

Buschke H, Fuld PA (1974): Evaluating storage, retention, and retrieval in disordered memory and learning. Neurology 24:1019–1025.

Butters N, Salmon DP, Heindel WC (1995): Specificity of the memory deficits associated with basal ganglia dysfunction. Rev Neurol 150:580–587.

Butters N, Salmon DP, Cullum CM, Cairns P, Tröster AI, Jacobs D, Moss MB, Cermak LS (1988): Differentiation of amnesic and demented patients with the Wechsler Memory Scale-Revised. Clin Neuropsychol 2:133–144.

Butters N, Granholm E, Salmon DP, Grant I, Wolfe J (1987): Episodic and semantic memory: A comparison of amnesic and demented patients. J Clin Exp Neuropsychol 9:479–497.

Butters N, Sax DS, Montgomery K, Tarlow S (1978): Comparison of the neuropsychological deficits associated with early and advanced Huntington's disease. Arch Neurol 35:585–589.

Byrne EJ, Lennox G, Lowe J, Godwin-Austen RB (1989): Diffuse Lewy body disease: Clinical features in 15 cases. J Neurol Neurosurg Psychiatry 52:709–717.

Chan AS, Butters N, Salmon DP, Johnson SA, Paulsen JS, Swenson MR (1995b): Comparison of the semantic networks in patients with dementia and amnesia. Neuropsychology 9:177–186.

Chan AS, Butters N, Paulsen JS, Salmon DP, Swenson MR, Maloney LT (1993a): An assessment of the semantic network in patients with Alzheimer's disease. J Cogn Neurosci 5:254–261.

Chan AS, Butters N, Salmon DP, McGuire KA (1993b): Dimensionality and clustering in the semantic network of patients with Alzheimer's disease. Psychol Aging 8:411–419.

Chan AS, Salmon DP, Butters N, Johnson SA (1995a): Semantic network abnormality predicts rate of cognitive decline in patients with probable Alzheimer's disease. J Int Neuropsychol Soc 1:297–303.

Chertkow H, Bub D (1990): Semantic memory loss in dementia of Alzheimer's type. Brain 118:397–417.

Collins AM, Loftus EF (1975): A spreading activation theory of semantic processing. Psychol Rev 82:407–428.

Corkin S, Davis KL, Growdon JH, Usdin E, Wurtman RJ (1982): "Alzheimer's Disease: A Report of Progress in Research. Aging, Vol. 19." New York: Raven.

Cummings BJ, Cotman CW (1995): Image analysis of β-amyloid load in Alzheimer's disease and relation to dementia severity. Lancet 346:1524–1528.

Cummings JL (1990): "Subcortical Dementia." New York: Oxford University Press.

DeKosky ST, Scheff SW (1990): Synapse loss in frontal cortex biopsies in Alzheimer's disease: Correlation with cognitive severity. Ann Neurol 27:457–464.

DeLacoste M, White CL (1993): The role of cortical connectivity in Alzheimer's disease pathogenesis: A review and model system. Neurobiol Aging 14:1–16.

Delis DC, Massman PJ, Butters N, Salmon DP, Kramer JH, Cermak L (1991): Profiles of demented and amnesic patients on the California Verbal Learning Test: Implications for the assessment of memory disorders. Psychol Assessment 3:19–26.

Eslinger PJ, Damasio AR (1986): Preserved motor learning in Alzheimer's disease: Implications for anatomy and behavior. J Neurosci 6:3006–3009.

Eslinger PJ, Damasio AR, Benton AL, Van Allen M (1985): Neuropsychologic detection of abnormal mental decline in older persons. JAMA 253:670–674.

Flicker C, Ferris SH, Reisberg B (1991): Mild cognitive impairment in the elderly: Predictors of dementia. Neurology 41:1006–1009.

Forstl H, Burns A, Luthert P, Cairns N, Levy R (1993): The Lewy-body variant of Alzheimer's disease: Clinical and pathological findings. Br J Psychiatry 162:385–392.

Fuld PA, Masur DM, Blau AD, Crystal H, Aronson MK (1990): Object-memory evaluation for prospective detection of dementia in normal functioning elderly: Predictive and normative data. J Clin Exp Neuropsychol 12:520–528.

Fuld PA, Katzman R, Davies P, Terry RD (1982): Intrusions as a sign of Alzheimer dementia: Chemical and pathological verification. Ann Neurol 11:155–159.

Galasko D, Katzman R, Salmon DP, Thal LJ, Hansen LA (1996): Clinical and neuropathological findings in Lewy body dementias. Brain Cogn 31:166–175.

Galloway PH, Sahgal A, McKeith IG, Lloyd S, Cook JH, Ferrier IN, Edwardson JA (1992): Visual pattern recognition memory and learning deficits in senile dementias of Alzheimer and Lewy body types. Dementia 3:101–107.

Gibb WRG, Esiri MM, Lees AJ (1985): Clinical and pathological features of diffuse cortical Lewy body disease (Lewy body dementia). Brain 110:1131–1153.

Girling DM, Berrios GE (1990): Extrapyramidal signs, primitive reflexes and frontal lobe function in senile dementia of the Alzheimer type. Br J Psychiatry 157:888–893.

Graf P, Squire LR, Mandler G (1984): The information that amnesics do not forget. J Exp Psychol: Learn Mem Cogn 10:164–178.

Hansen LA, Galasko D (1992): Lewy body disease. Curr Opin Neurol Neurosurg 5:889–894.

Hansen L, Salmon DP, Galasko D, Masliah E, Katzman R, DeTeresa R, Thal LJ, Pay MM, Hofstetter R, Klauber MR, Rice V, Butters N, Alford M (1990): The Lewy body variant of Alzheimer's disease: A clinical and pathologic entity. Neurology 40:1–8.

Heindel WC, Salmon DP, Butters N (1992): The biasing of weight judgments in Alzheimer's and Huntington's disease: A priming or programming phenomenon? J Clin Exp Neuropsychol 13:189–203.

Heindel WC, Salmon DP, Butters N (1990): Pictorial priming and cued recall in Alzheimer's and Huntington's disease. Brain Cogn 13:282–295.

Heindel WC, Salmon DP, Shults C, Walicke P, Butters N (1989): Neuropsychological evidence for multiple implicit memory systems: A comparison of Alzheimer's, Huntington's and Parkinson's disease patients. J Neurosci 9:582–587.

Heindel WC, Butters N, Salmon DP (1988): Impaired learning of a motor skill in patients with Huntington's disease. Behav Neurosci 102:141–147.

Hodges JR, Salmon DP, Butters N (1993): Recognition and naming of famous faces in Alzheimer's disease: A cognitive analysis. Neuropsychologia 31:775–788.

Hodges JR, Salmon DP, Butters N (1992): Semantic memory impairment in Alzheimer's disease: Failure of access or degraded knowledge? Neuropsychologia 30:301–314.

Hodges JR, Salmon DP, Butters N (1991): The nature of the naming deficit in Alzheimer's and Huntington's disease. Brain 114:1547–1558.

Huff FJ, Becker JT, Belle SH, Nebes RD, Holland AL, Boller F (1987): Cognitive deficits and clinical diagnosis of Alzheimer's disease. Neurology 37:1119–1124.

Huff FJ, Corkin S, Growdon JH (1986): Semantic impairment and anomia in Alzheimer's disease. Brain Lang 28:235–249.

Huppert FA, Tym E (1986): Clinical and neuropsychological assessment of dementia. Br Med Bull 42:11–18.

Hyman BT, Van Hoesen GW, Damasio A, Barnes C (1984): Alzheimer's disease: Cell-specific pathology isolates the hippocampal formation. Science 225:1168–1170.

Jacobs D, Salmon DP, Tröster AI, Butters N (1990): Intrusion errors in the figural memory of patients with Alzheimer's and Huntington's disease. Arch Clin Neuropsychol 5:49–57.

Kraszniak AW, Wilson RS, Fox JH, Stebbins GT (1986): Cognitive assessment in Alzheimer's disease: Cross-sectional and longitudinal perspectives. Can J Neurol Sci 13:420–423.

Katzman R (1994): Apolipoprotein E and Alzheimer's disease. Curr Opin Neurobiol 4:703–707.

Katzman R (1986): Alzheimer's disease. N Engl J Med 314:964–973.

Katzman R (1993): Education and the prevalence of dementia and Alzheimer's disease. Neurology 43:13–20.

Knopman DS, Ryberg S (1989): A verbal memory test with high predictive accuracy for dementia of the Alzheimer type. Arch Neurol 46:141–145.

Kopelman MD (1989): Remote and autobiographical memory, temporal context memory and frontal atrophy in Korsakoff and Alzheimer patients. Neuropsychologia 27:437–460.

La Rue A, Matsuyama SS, McPherson S, Sherman J, Jarvik LF (1992): Cognitive performance in relatives of patients with probable Alzheimer disease: An age at onset effect? J Clin Exp Neuropsychol 14:533–538.

Lennox G, Lowe J, Landon M, Byrne EJ, Mayer RJ, Godwin-Austen RB (1989): Diffuse Lewy body disease: Correlative neuropathology using anti-ubiquitin immunocytochemistry. J Neurol Neurosurg Psychiatry 52:1236–1247.

Linn RT, Wolf PA, Bachman DL, Knoefel JE, Cobb JL, Belanger AJ, Kaplan EF, D'Agostino RB (1995): The "preclinical phase" of probable Alzheimer's disease: A 13-year prospective study of the Framingham cohort. Arch Neurol 52:485–490.

Mann DMA, Marcyniuk B, Yates PO, Neary D, Snowden JS (1988): The progression of the pathological changes of Alzheimer's disease in frontal and temporal neocortex examined both at biopsy and at autopsy. Neuropath App Neurobiol 14:177–195.

Mann DMA, Yates PO, Marcyniuk B (1984): A comparison of changes in the nucleus basalis and locus ceruleus in Alzheimer's disease. J Neurol Neurosurg Psychiatry 47:201–203.

Martin A (1987): Representation of semantic and spatial knowledge in Alzheimer's patients: Implications for models of preserved learning in amnesia. J Clin Exp Neuropsychol 9:191–224.

Massman PJ, Delis DC, Butters N (1993): Does impaired primacy recall equal impaired long-term storage?: Serial position effects in Huntington's disease and Alzheimer's disease. Dev Neuropsychol 9:1–15.

Masur DM, Sliwinski M, Lipton RB, Blau AD, Crystal HA (1994): Neuropsychological prediction of dementia and the absence of dementia in healthy elderly persons. Neurology 44:1427–1432.

Masur DM, Fuld PA, Blau AD, Crystal H, Aronson MK (1990): Predicting development of dementia in the elderly with the selective reminding test. J Clin Exp Neuropsychol 12:529–538.

Masur DM, Fuld PA, Blau AD, Thal LJ, Levin HS, Aronson MK (1989): Distinguishing normal and demented elderly with the selective reminding test. J Clin Exp Neuropsychol 11:615–630.

McHugh PR, Folstein MF (1975): Psychiatric symptoms of Huntington's chorea: A clinical and phenomenologic study. In Benson DF, Blumer D (eds): 'Psychiatric Aspects of Neurological Disease." New York: Raven, pp 267–285.

McKeith IG, Perry RH, Fairbairn AF, Jabeen S, Perry EK (1992): Operational criteria for senile dementia of Lewy body type (SDLT). Psychol Med 22:911–922.

Merello M, Sabe L, Teson A, Migliorelli R, Petracchi M, Leiguarda R, Starkstein S (1994): Extrapyramidalism in Alzheimer's disease: Prevalence, psychiatric, and neuropsychological correlates. J Neurol Neurosurg Psychiatry 57:1503–1509.

Monsch AU, Bondi MW, Paulsen JS, Brugger P, Butters N, Salmon DP, Swenson M (1994): A comparison of category and letter fluency in Alzheimer's disease and Huntington's disease. Neuropsychology 8:25–30.

Monsch AU, Bondi MW, Butters N, Salmon DP, Katzman R, Thal LJ (1992): Comparisons of verbal fluency tasks in the detection of dementia of the Alzheimer type. Arch Neurol 49:1253–1258.

Morris JC, McKeel DW, Storandt M, Rubin EH, Price JL, Grant EA, Ball MJ, Berg L (1991): Very mild Alzheimer's disease: Informant-based clinical, psychometric, and pathologic distinction from normal aging. Neurology 41:469–478.

Moss MB, Albert MS, Butters N, Payne M (1986): Differential patterns of memory loss among patients with Alzheimer's disease, Huntington's disease and alcoholic Korsakoff's syndrome. Arch Neurol 43:239–246.

Neary D, Snowden JS, Mann DMA, Bowen DM, Sims NR, Northen B, Yates PO, Davison AN (1986): Alzheimer's disease: A correlative study. J Neurol Neurosurg Psychiatry 49:229–237.

Paulsen JS, Butters N, Salmon DP, Heindel WC, Swenson MR (1993): Prism adaptation in Alzheimer's and Huntington's disease. Neuropsychology 7:73–81.

Parks RW, Zec RF, Wilson RS (1993): "Neuropsychology of Alzheimer's Disease and Other Dementias." New York: Oxford University Press.

Pearson RCA, Esiri MM, Hiorns RW, Wilcock GK, Powell TPS (1985): Anatomical correlates of the distribution of the pathological changes in the neocortex in Alzheimer disease. Proc Natl Acad Sci 82:4521–4534.

Pepin EP, Eslinger PJ (1989): Verbal memory decline in Alzheimer's disease: A multiple-processes deficit. Neurology 39:1477–1482.

Petersen RC, Smith GE, Ivnik RJ, Tangalos EG, Schaid DJ, Thibodeau SN, Kokmen E, Waring SC, Kurland LT (1995): Apolipoprotein E status as a predictor of the development of Alzheimer's disease in memory-impaired individuals. JAMA 273:1274–1278.

Reed T, Carmelli D, Swan GE (1994): Lower cognitive performance in normal older adult male twins carrying the apolipoprotein E ϵ4 allele. Arch Neurol 51:1189–1192

Richards M, Bell K, Dooneief G, Marder K, Sano M, Mayeux R, Stern Y (1993): Patterns of neuropsychological performance in Alzheimer's disease patients with and without extrapyramidal signs. Neurology 43:1708–1711.

Romney AK, Shepard RN, Nerlove SB (1972): "Multidimensional Scaling: Theory and Applications in the Behavioral Sciences, Vol. II." New York: Seminar.

Sagar JJ, Cohen NJ, Sullivan EV, Corkin S, Growdon JH (1988): Remote memory function in Alzheimer's disease and Parkinson's disease. Brain 111:525–539.

Sahgal A, McKeith IG, Galloway PH, Tasker N, Steckler T (1995): Do differences in visuospatial ability between senile dementias of the Alzheimer and Lewy body types reflect differences solely in mnemonic function? J Clin Exp Neuropsychol 17:35–43.

Sahgal A, Galloway PH, McKeith IG, Lloyd S, Cook JH, Ferrier N, Edwardson JA (1992a): Matching-to-sample deficits in patients with senile dementias of the Alzheimer and Lewy body types. Arch Neurol 49:1043–1046.

Sahgal A, Galloway PH, McKeith IG, Edwardson JA, Lloyd S (1992b): A comparative study of attentional deficits in senile dementias of Alzheimer and Lewy body types. Dementia 3:350–354.

Salmon DP, Chan AS (1994): Semantic memory deficits associated with Alzheimer's disease. In Cermak LS (ed): "Neuropsychological Explorations of Memory and Cognition: Essays in Honor of Nelson Butters." New York: Plenum, pp 61–76.

Salmon DP, Butters N, Thal LJ, Jeste DV (in press): Alzheimer's disease: Analysis for the DSM-IV task force. In Widiger TA, Frances A, Pincus H (eds): "DSM-IV Sourcebook, Vol. IV." Washington, DC: American Psychiatric Association.

Salmon DP, Galasko D, Hansen LA, Masliah E, Butters N, Thal LJ, Katzman R (1996): Neuropsychological deficits associated with diffuse Lewy body disease. Brain Cogn 31:148–165.

Salmon DP, Shimamura A, Butters N, Smith S (1988): Lexical and semantic priming deficits in patients with Alzheimer's disease. J Clin Exp Neuropsychol 10:477–494.

Samuel W, Galasko D, Masliah E, Hansen LA (1996): Neocortical Lewy body counts correlate with dementia in the Lewy body variant of Alzheimer's disease. J Neuropathol Exp Neurol 55:44–52.

Schacter DL (1987): Implicit memory: History and current status. J Exp Psychol: Learn Mem Cogn 13:501–518.

Schacter DL, Tulving E (1994): "Memory Systems 1994." Cambridge, MA: MIT Press.

Shepard RN, Romney AK, Nerlove SB (1972): "Multidimensional Scaling: Theory and Applications in the Behavioral Sciences, Vol. I." New York: Seminar.

Shimamura AP, Salmon DP, Squire LR, Butters N (1987): Memory dysfunction and word priming in dementia and amnesia. Behav Neurosci 101:347–351.

Smith SR, Murdoch BE, Chenery HJ (1989): Semantic abilities in dementia of the Alzheimer type: 1. Lexical semantics. Brain Lang 36:314–324.

Snowdon DA, Kemper SJ, Mortimer JA, Greiner LH, Wekstein DR, Markesbery WR (1996): Linguistic ability in early life and cognitive function and Alzheimer's disease in late life. JAMA, 275:528–532.

Soininen H, Helkala EL, Laulumaa V, Soikkeli R, Hartikainen P, Riekkinen PJ (1992): Cognitive profile of Alzheimer patients with extrapyramidal signs: A longitudinal study. J Neural Trans 4:241–254.

Squire LR (1992): Memory and the hippocampus: A synthesis from findings with rats, monkeys and humans. Psycho Rev 99:195–231.

Squire LR (1987): "Memory and Brain." New York: Oxford University Press.

Storandt M, Botwinick J, Danziger WL, Berg L, Hughes CP (1984): Psychometric differentiation of mild senile dementia of the Alzheimer type. Arch Neurol 41:497–499.

Strittmatter WJ, Saunders AM, Schmechel D, Pericak-Vance M, Enghild J, Salvesen GS, Roses AD (1993): Apolipoprotein-E—High-avidity binding to β-amyloid and increased frequency of type 4 allele in late-onset familial Alzheimer disease. Proc Natl Acad Sci 90:9649–9653.

Terry RD, Katzman R (1983): Senile dementia of the Alzheimer type. Ann Neurol 14:497–506.

Terry RD, Masliah E, Salmon DP, Butters N, DeTeresa R, Hill R, Hansen LA, Katzman R (1991): Physical basis of cognitive alterations in Alzheimer's disease: Synapse loss is the major correlate of cognitive impairment. Ann Neurol 30:572–580.

Terry RD, Peck A, DeTeresa R, Schecter R, Horoupian DS (1981): Some morphometric aspects of the brain in senile dementia of the Alzheimer type. Ann Neurol 10:184–192.

Tierney MC, Szalai JP, Snow WG, Fisher RH, Tsuda T, Chi H, McLachlan DR, St. George-Hyslop PH (1996): A prospective study of the clinical utility of APOE genotype in the prediction of outcome in patients with memory impairment. Neurology 46:149–154.

Tröster AI, Butters N, Salmon DP, Cullum CM, Jacobs D, Brandt J, White RF (1993): The diagnostic utility of savings scores: Differentiating Alzheimer's and Huntington's diseases with the logical memory and visual reproduction tests. J Clin Exp Neuropsychol 15:773–788.

Tröster AI, Jacobs D, Butters N, Cullum CM, Salmon DP (1989): Differentiating Alzheimer's disease from Huntington's disease with the Wechsler Memory Scale–Revised. Clin Geriat Med 5:611–632.

Tversky A, Hutchinson JW (1986): Nearest neighbor analysis of psychological spaces. Psychol Rev 93:3–22.

Vonsattel JP, Myers RH, Stevens TJ, Ferrante RJ, Bird ED, Richardson EP (1985): Neuropathological classification of Huntington's disease. J Neuropath Exp Neurol 44:559–577.

Welsh K, Butters N, Hughes J, Mohs R, Heyman A (1991): Detection of abnormal memory decline in mild cases of Alzheimer's disease using CERAD neuropsychological measures. Arch Neurol 48:278–281.

Whitehouse PJ, Price DL, Struble RG, Clark AW, Coyle JT, DeLong MR (1982): Alzheimer's disease and senile dementia: Loss of neurons in the basal forebrain. Science 215:1237–1239.

Wilson RS, Bacon LD, Fox JH, Kaszniak AW (1983): Primary and secondary memory in dementia of the Alzheimer type. J Clin Neuropsychol 5:337–344.

Wilson RS, Kaszniak AW, Fox JH (1981): Remote memory in senile dementia. Cortex 17:41–48.

Zola-Morgan S, Squire LR (1990): The primate hippocampal formation: Evidence for a time-limited role in memory storage. Science 250:288–290.

PART II

MOLECULAR ASPECTS OF ALZHEIMER'S DISEASE

CHAPTER 7

Neuropathology and Functional Anatomy of Alzheimer's Disease

ANA SOLODKIN and GARY W. VAN HOESEN

Departments of Anatomy and Neurology, University of Iowa, Iowa City, Iowa 52242

INTRODUCTION

With an ever-increasing life expectancy, by the year 2050, 25% of the population worldwide will be over 65 years of age (Olshansky et al., 1993). Since the prevalence of Alzheimer's disease (AD) in the population over this age increases exponentially until about age 90 (Katzman and Kawas, 1994), Alzheimer's disease will be the major disorder among this population taxing health providers to limits that can hardly be envisioned in either humanistic or fiscal terms.

The first neuropathological diagnosis of AD, described by its namesake Alois Alzheimer in 1907, was based on the presence of two types of lesions. Even though he attributed the presence of these neuropathological lesions to a case of dementia praecox, it is now clear that they are also the hallmarks for sporadic as well as familial AD. The lesions observed by Alzheimer are of two main types (Figure 1).

1. *Neurofibrillary tangles (NFTs)*

Neurofibrillary tangles are intracellular fibrils formed mainly by paired helical filaments linked together by hyperphosphorylated tau protein [for reviews see Goedert et al. (1991a) and Lee and Trojanowski (1992)]. These fibrils are also found in the neurites (axons and dendrites) commonly found in the extracellular space in the form of neuropil threads, and they are associated with the plaques containing β-amyloid deposits (Goedert et al., 1991b, Perry et al., 1991).

Pharmacological Treatment of Alzheimer's Disease: Molecular and Neurobiological Foundations,
Edited by Brioni and Decker
ISBN 0-471-16758-4   © 1997 Wiley-Liss, Inc.

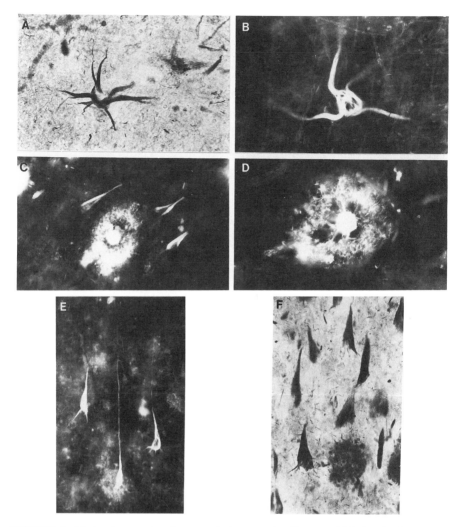

FIGURE 1. Photomicrographs of neuropathology used to diagnose Alzheimer's disease. (A and B) Neurofibrillary tangles, (D) neuritic plaque with a clear core of amyloid protein, (C, E and F) NFTs and NPs in close apposition. Note in (A) and (B) the coiled shape of the neurofibrils forming the NFTs and in (A) and (F) the dystrophic neurites in the extracellular space.

2. *Neuritic plaques (NPs)*

The second form of neuropathology in AD is the presence of neuritic plaques, which are accumulations of β-amyloid protein in the extracellular space containing dystrophic neurites with abnormally phosphorylated tau. These are frequently studded and surround a dense core of amyloid [for review see Selkoe (1994)]. Abundant diffuse β-amyloid containing masses are typically part of the microscopic picture as well, but these are also seen to some degree in elderly, nondemented individuals. A third type, but less understood neuropathological change in AD is neuronal loss, and this can occur in nontangle-containing neurons (Clinton et al., 1994). Neuronal loss is difficult to assess even with gliosis. Its assessment is not required for the diagnose of AD.

This review will focus mainly on the neuroanatomical distribution of NFTs in the central nervous system of AD cases because their density and distribution are correlated best with clinical symptoms of dementia (Samuel et al., 1991; Berg et al., 1993; Arriagada et al., 1992) whereas NPs are not. A brief example of neuronal loss, without development of NFTs, will be mentioned in the "modularity" section, to highlight the complexity of the progression of this devastating illness. We start with the most general observations, the gross appearance of the AD brain at autopsy (Figure 2).

GROSS ANATOMICAL CHANGES IN ALZHEIMER'S DISEASE

Even though the exact neuroanatomy of the human brain varies between individuals, all AD brains show gyral atrophy as manifested by the widening of sulci and the flattening of the gyri. Discoloration of the atrophic areas is not uncommon. In cases where atrophy is substantial, especially after a long duration of illness, the pre- and postcentral gyri appear conspicuously as islands of normal cortex since neighboring association areas of the frontal, parietal, and temporal lobes are atrophic.

Frontal Lobe

Changes in the frontal lobe are very common especially in the anterior parts of the superior frontal lobule, posterior and medial orbitofrontal cortex, and the subgenual areas located along the rostrum of the corpus callosum. Involvement of the inferior frontal lobule, including Broca's area, are not uncommon. Least common in our experience is heavy damage to the middle frontal lobule.

Parietal Lobe

Parietal lobe atrophy is common in AD and typically includes the inferior parietal lobule, ventral to the intraparietal sulcus (including the supramarginal and angular gyri to variable degrees), and the superior parietal lobule. The medial component of the parietal lobe, the precuneus, located between the marginal branch of the cingulate sulcus and the parieto-occipital sulcus, is typically very atrophic and shrunken. In contrast, the primary somatosensory cortex of the postcentral gyrus (Brodmann's areas 3, 1, and 2) is spared.

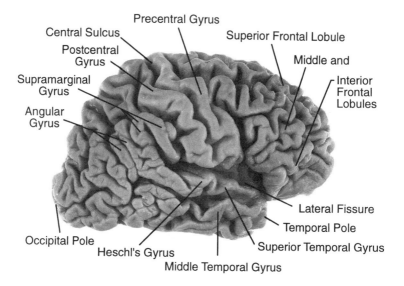

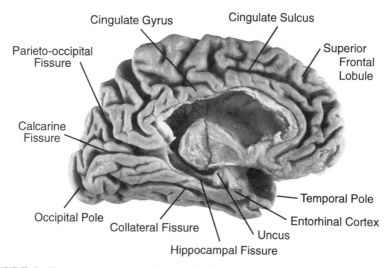

FIGURE 2. Gross specimen at end-stage AD depicting the variety of areas that develop atrophy and discoloration as a result of the illness. In contrast, note the normal appearance of primary areas such as the pre- and postcentral gyri and the occipital pole [From Van Hoesen GW and Solodkin A (1994). With permission of Ann. NY Acad Sci.]

Occipital Lobe

At the gross macroscopic level, the occipital cortex shows a knoblike appearance due in part to the relative sparing of primary visual cortex (Brodmann's area 17), mild atrophy of visual association areas, and substantial atrophy of inferior and medial parietal cortex. If atrophy is extensive in posterior temporal association areas, the occipital pole is literally surrounded by a belt of atrophic association cortex.

Temporal Lobe

This lobe is invariantly affected by AD (Arnold et al., 1991; Hooper and Vogel, 1976; Mann, 1985). The area that shows the greatest atrophy is the temporal pole (Brodmann's area 38), which in the worst cases has a bladelike appearance with a "pitted" surface (Arnold et al., 1994). In addition, superior, medial, and inferior temporal gyri (Brodmann's areas 20, 21, and 22) at end stages are typically atrophic too. However, the posterior part of the superior temporal gyrus including Heschl's gyrus, the primary auditory cortex (Brodmann's areas 41 and 42), may be spared as well as the adjacent temporal part of Wernicke's area.

Limbic Lobe

The term "limbic lobe" was coined by Broca (1878) to denote the cortex forming the "limbus" or border of the hemisphere around the upper parts of the brainstem, thalamus, and basal ganglia. Included are the cingulate cortex dorsally, the parahippocampal gyrus ventrally, and the many bridging areas that link them together. The limbic lobe is the first and most affected area in AD cases (Arnold et al., 1991; Hooper and Vogel, 1976; Braak and Braak, 1991; Corsellis, 1970). Most affected are the anterior portion of the parahippocampal gyrus, the entorhinal cortex (Brodmann's area 28), followed by temporal pole, and posterior parahippocampal gyrus. Entorhinal changes can range from a slight flattening to a gross atrophy (Van Hoesen, 1985; Van Hoesen and Damasio, 1987; Van Hoesen et al., 1991). With the atrophy of the entorhinal cortex, the uncus of the hippocampus becomes prominent (Figures 7A and B). The posterior cingulate cortex appears uncommonly narrow and atrophic, but its anterior part (Brodmann's area 24) is often spared. Pathology in other parts of the limbic lobe have not been studied systematically.

DISTRIBUTION OF PATHOLOGICAL CHANGES OF AD IN RELATION TO CORTICAL TYPES

All types of cortex are affected in AD, but changes among them are not uniform. An account of the changes taking place in different types of cortex follows (Figure 3).

Allocortical Areas

This is the least elaborate cortex and is comprised of only two or three layers with at least one being acellular. The main cellular types are modified pyramidal cells

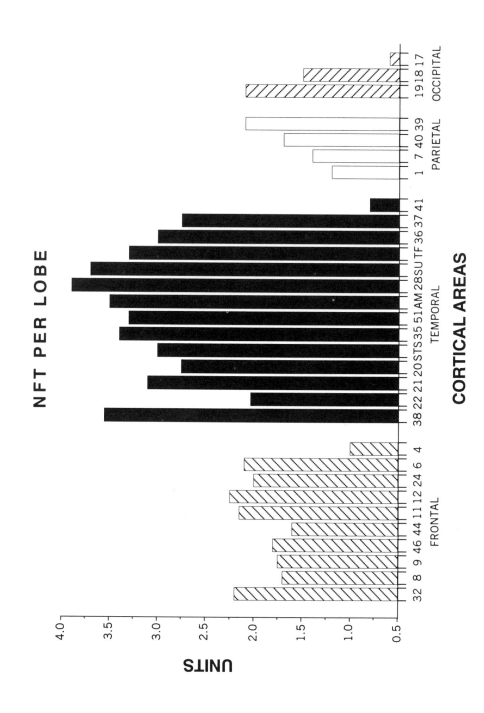

NFT PER LOBE

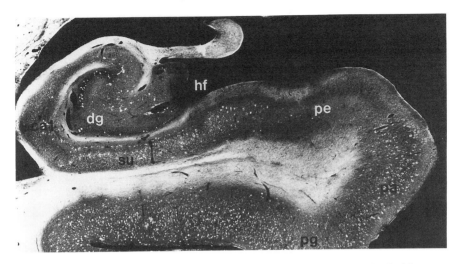

FIGURE 4. Photomicrograph depicting the distribution of NFTs and NPs in the hippocampal formation in AD. Not all areas are affected equally. Some are deeply affected (subiculum, parasubiculum, and CA1) whereas their immediate neighbors (dentate gyrus and presubiculum) are spared. Abbreviations: pg, parahippocampal gyrus; pa, parasubiculum; pe, presubiculum; su, subiculum; dg, dentate gyrus; hf, hippocampal fissure.

whose apical dendrites form a wide molecular layer. Examples of allocortical areas include the hippocampus, subiculum, periamygdaloid cortex, and the olfactory cortices. All of these are affected heavily in AD, but not uniformly. For example, in the hippocampal formation, many of the pyramidal cells of the subiculum and CA1 sector are invested with NFTs. Other parts of the hippocampal formation like the dentate gyrus and the CA3 sector seldom contain pathology (Figure 4). Cortical amygdaloid nuclei, the periamygdaloid area, and the olfactory cortices are also heavily affected (Herzog and Kemper, 1980; Esiri and Wilcock, 1984; Brashear et al., 1988; Brady and Mufson, 1990; Kromer-Vogt et al., 1990; Unger et al., 1991).

Periallocortical Areas

This unusual type of cortex is multilaminated but resembles a hybrid whose deeper layers are similar to the adjacent allocortical areas and whose superficial layers remind one more those of the isocortex.

Examples of this type of cortex are the entorhinal, parasubicular, presubicular, and retrosplenial cortices. As with the allocortices, however, the involvement of

---

FIGURE 3. Graphical representation of the mean density of NFTs ("units") in the different areas within each cortical lobe. Note that the largest density of NFTs is found in the temporal lobe, and also note the large contrast between limbic and primary sensory and motor areas [From Van Hoesen GW and Solodkin A (1994). With permission of Ann. NY Acad Sci.]

these areas is not uniform. The entorhinal cortex, for example, is one of the first and most affected areas showing both types of lesions (Hyman et al., 1984; Arnold et al., 1991; Braak and Braak, 1991). The adjacent parasubicular cortex is equally heavily affected as well, but its immediate neighbor, the presubicular cortex, is spared in AD and contains largely unaggregated β-amyloid deposits (Kalus et al., 1989). Alternatively, its neighbor, the subicular cortices, are damaged heavily (Hyman et al., 1985).

Proisocortical Areas

The third type of cortex found in the limbic lobe along with the allo and periallo-cortices is the proisocortex. The most prominent examples of this type of cortex are the posterior parts of the orbitofrontal cortex, cingulate, retrocalcarine, posterior-parahippocampal, perirhinal, temporal polar, and anterior insular cortices. In cytoarchitectural terms, they resemble the isocortical layers, but some of their layers are atypical. Some, for example, are incipient, and nearly always, layers V and VI are difficult to segregate.

In end-stage AD, these areas are uniformly and heavily affected even though individual changes appear to happen at different intervals of the disease. For example, the perirhinal cortex (Brodmann's area 35), which shows a large density of both NFTs and NPs, is according to Kemper (1978) and Braak and Braak (1991) the area that shows the first signs of pathology. The neighboring areas, posterior parahippocampal gyrus (Brodmann's area 36) and the temporal pole (Brodmann's area 38) anteriorly, are also heavily affected during the course of the illness (Kemper, 1978; Braak and Braak, 1985; Arnold et al., 1994).

The posterior orbitofrontal, agranular insula, the subgenual part of the cingulate cortex (Brodmann's area 25), as well as the posterior cingulate cortex (Brodmann's area 23) may all be affected at end-stage AD (Brun and Gustafson, 1976; Minoshima et al., 1994), but it is not unusual to see evidence of sparing in one or more of these if the duration of illness is abbreviated.

The anterior cingulate cortex (Brodmann's area 24) is frequently an exception since it is not uniformly affected. In some cases a heavy density of NFTs and NPs are present, but not in others (Brun and Gustafson, 1976; Brun and Englund, 1981).

Isocortical Areas

As evident from gross inspection, there is not a uniform involvement of the isocortical areas in AD, and the association areas of the temporal, parietal, and frontal cortices bear the brunt of isocortical pathology. In contrast, the primary sensory and motor cortices are not affected greatly. The relative sparing of these is consistent with the paucity of motor and sensory impairment in AD.

The association cortices affected in AD are also called homotypical cortices. In the frontal lobe they are formed by Brodmann's areas 9, 10, 11, 12, 13, 14, and 46. In the parietal lobe they form Brodmann's areas 7, 39, and 40. In the temporal cortex, the best examples are Brodmann's areas 20, 21, 22, and 37. These areas have the classical six-layered pattern of isocortex and represent the largest part of the cerebral cortex in human and nonhuman primate. Layer II is well developed and is formed largely by small pyramidal cells. Layer III is wide and formed by medium-sized pyramidal cells. Layer IV is composed of small pyramidal or stellate-shaped cells. Layer V is formed mainly by large pyramidal cells with long freely branching apical dendrites, and it can be separated from layer VI because the latter is formed by cells with a variety of shapes and sizes. The homotypical cortices give rise to the long corticocortical association projections that interconnect the lobes and project to limbic cortical areas (Pandya and Kuypers, 1969; Jones and Powell, 1970).

In summary, the degree of involvement of the isocortical association areas in AD is not uniform, ranging from a paucity of lesions to very extensive damage. More consistent, however, are the changes in the proisocortices, the anterior parahippocampal gyrus, and the allocortex of the hippocampal formation. It is not clear, however, if this represents early involvement or a different degree of involvement of these areas or both. Among isocortical association areas the parietotemporal and occipitotemporal regions seem to be the most affected in AD (Brun and Englund, 1981).

FUNCTIONAL CORRELATES OF CORTICAL AREAS AFFECTED IN AD

Limbic Area Involvement

Evidence clearly indicates that all the cortical types found in the limbic lobe (allocortex, periallocortex, and proisocortex) are affected heavily in AD (Figure 5). Hence, it should not be surprising to find functional deficits in this disorder that reflect the location of these lesions. Memory impairments are one of the behavioral hallmarks of AD. Anterograde memory deficits have been associated with the ventromedial temporal lobe, including the hippocampal formation since the middle of this century. This area always shows a large density of pathology in AD. In particular, the involvement of the entorhinal and perirhinal cortices is relevant since they provide the main cortical input to the hippocampal formation and are the recipients of hippocampal efferents. Neurons receiving the latter project widely to limbic and association cortices. The integrity of the entorhinal and perirhinal cortices is essential for the assimilation of new learning and its more long-term registration elsewhere in the cortex.

Other functional sequelae relating to the damage of the limbic lobe are not so easily characterized, but some predictions seem appropriate. For example, the pathology present in orbitofrontal and temporal pole areas may produce alterations in social behavior, decision making, and affect. In Brodmann's area 25 may produce alterations in autonomic control since this area has powerful connections to subcortical autonomic centers. Some have shown autonomic dysregulation in AD (Aharon-Peretz et al., 1992; Borson et al., 1992). Pathology in the posterior cingulate cortex may produce alterations in spatial awareness of both personal and extrapersonal spaces because the heavy interactions of this cortex with the frontal, parietal, and temporal association cortices.

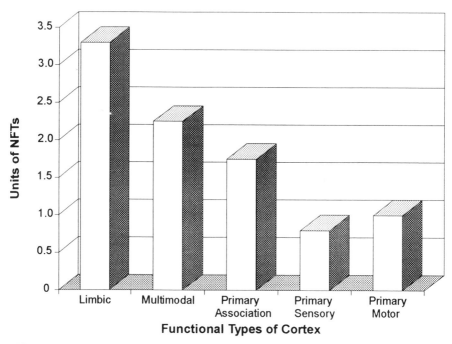

FIGURE 5. Graphic representation of the density of NFTs in relation to the functional type of cortex in which they are located. Note that the distribution of these lesions is not homogeneous through these cortices. Their distribution is skewed toward limbic cortices whereas motor and primary sensory cortices are largely spared.

Multimodal Area Involvement

Multimodal or polysensory areas are defined by virtue of the fact that they receive input from three or more association areas that themselves receive primary sensory input (Pandya and Seltzer, 1982; Pandya and Yeterian, 1985). Notable examples are the upper bank of the superior temporal sulcus, parts of the prefrontal association cortex, the occipitotemporal cortices (Brodmann's areas 36 and 37), and parts of the inferior parietal lobule. All of these areas are affected heavily in AD, and we suspect that their integrity may be essential for several cognitive functions. For example, they may be involved in the integration of perceptions involving multiple ongoing environmental stimuli. These same areas are also thought to evoke combinations of precepts stored in other parts of the association cortices so that mental images of complex sensations can be retroactivated (Damasio, 1989; Damasio et al., 1990). Whatever the case, at end-stage AD, there is a profound cognitive impairment with a minimal ability to deal meaningfully with the past or present. Pathology in multimodal association areas may be at the core of these behavioral changes.

Primary Association Area Involvement

The primary association cortices lie adjacent to primary sensory cortices and are dedicated to the respective sensory modality. These areas are only mildly affected in AD; hence, behavioral changes produced by their alterations may be minimal or difficult to discern. However, we suspect that the range of the sensory experiences, their meaning, and richness may be compromised in AD even though the blueprint of such experiences may remain intact.

Primary Sensory and Motor Area Involvement

Even at the gross anatomical level, it is evident that in the vast majority of AD cases, primary sensory and motor areas contain few pathological changes. In functional terms, this is consistent with the preservation of motility until very late in the disease process and the general central registry of sensory information with exception of olfaction (Warner et al., 1986).

LAMINAR SPECIFICITY OF CORTICAL PATHOLOGY IN ALZHEIMER'S DISEASE

The topographical specificity of AD pathology in terms of cortical types is paralleled by a cellular and laminar specificity within affected areas. This is clearly the case for NFTs. For example, neurons that form predominantly layers III and V contain this cytoskeletal alteration whereas their immediate neighbors in adjacent layers may be unaltered (Hyman et al., 1984; Van Hoesen et al., 1986; Pearson et al., 1985; Braak and Braak, 1985; Lewis et al., 1987). The same applies to some extent to the NP distribution (Rogers and Morrison, 1985; Duyckaerts et al., 1986). Although this pathological marker may have a broader distribution in terms of laminar location (Pearson et al., 1985), there are many examples in the cerebral cortex where plaques are found largely in selective cortical layers. It is less clear whether cell loss, in addition to that attributable to NFTs, follows a laminar-specific pattern (Mann et al., 1985; Terry, 1983; Terry et al., 1981), but it appears that larger cortical neurons are lost to a greater degree than small neurons in both AD and normal aging (Hof et al., 1990; Hof and Morrison, 1990; Morrison et al., 1987b). On the basis of studies of cortical connectivity in nonhuman primates, it is plausible to argue that the pathological targets of AD especially affect the long association systems that are responsible for linking the various association areas of the hemisphere among themselves and with the cortex of the limbic lobe as well as with subcortical structures. Both the feedforward systems of connections that disseminate cortical information throughout the cortex and the feedback systems that reciprocate them are implicated. Indeed, the laminar origins and some of the terminal fields of these systems correspond remarkably with the patterns of pathology observed in the cortex in AD (Hyman et al., 1984; Lewis et al., 1987; Pearson et al., 1985; Rogers and Morrison, 1985).

CONNECTIONAL SPECIFICITY OF PATHOLOGY IN ALZHEIMER'S DISEASE

It is apparent that pathological changes in AD are skewed toward the multimodal association and limbic cortices. As reported by Van Hoesen (1982), association areas are a major input to the limbic system and are a major recipient of limbic system output (Van Hoesen, 1982; Porrino et al., 1981; Kosel et al., 1982; Amaral and Price, 1984). Also, they are the major source of long corticocortical projections that link together the various parts of the cerebral cortex. Their destruction of the magnitude noted in AD would suggest that devastating cognitive changes should ensue.

The critical nature of these changes can be appreciated if one considers the connectional relation between the hippocampal formation and the cerebral cortex (Figure 6). The hippocampal formation receives few direct inputs from cortical association areas. Instead, its major cortical input arises from the entorhinal cortex. The entorhinal cortex through the perforant pathway carries the strongest source of input to the hippocampal formation and forms its main link to the remainder of the cortex. The input to the entorhinal cortex thus becomes a critical issue (Van Hoesen, 1982; Van Hoesen and Pandya, 1975; Van Hoesen et al., 1975; Amaral, 1987; Amaral and Insausti, 1990). Most afferents arise from neighboring cortical areas

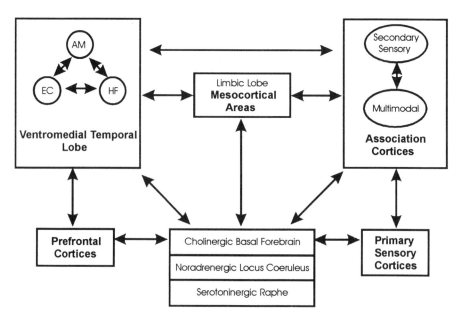

FIGURE 6. Diagram summarizing the bi-directional connections between several brain areas, cortical and subcortical. In AD, even though the pathology is in specific systems, practically all feedforward and feedback projections will be disrupted if the disease is of long duration.

such as the subicular complex, periamygdaloid and prepiriform cortices, and proisocortical areas of the temporal lobe. The latter includes the perirhinal cortex, posterior parahippocampal cortex, occipitotemporal cortex, and the temporal pole (Amaral, 1987; Van Hoesen, 1982). All of these areas are the recipients of powerful corticocortical association input from sensory association and multimodal association areas and in turn project powerfully to the superficial layers of the entorhinal cortex. The critical relay neurons in areas 35, 36, 37, and 38 are the pyramids in layers III and V. Briefly, it is probably accurate to state that a large component of the feedforward system of cortical sensory connections converges onto the entorhinal cortex, where it is relayed to the hippocampal formation by the perforant pathway.

Nearly all the key components of these neural systems are affected in AD. For example, in areas 35, 36, 37, and 38, the most common distribution of NFTs is in cortical layers III and V. NPs are abundant in their terminal zone in the entorhinal cortex layers I and III, and particularly, layer III. Moreover, the cells of origin for the perforant pathway, the large layer II stellate neurons, and more superficial layer III pyramids are laden with NFTs and often destroyed totally in AD (Hyman et al., 1986; Figures 7C and D). There is a strong likelihood that the specific cortical neurons that form neural systems conveying cortical association input to the hippocampal formation are destroyed in AD. The reciprocal of this relationship also seems compromised greatly (Hyman et al., 1984). This feedback system arises primarily from the subiculum and CA1 part of the hippocampus and from the entorhinal layer IV, which itself receives a large subicular projection. Both the subiculum and the entorhinal layer IV typically contain NFTs in AD. Such observations lead to the prediction that the pathological distribution of NFTs and NPs in AD dissects neural systems of the temporal lobe with a cellular precision that effectively isolates the hippocampal formation from the remainder of the cerebral cortex (Hyman et al., 1984; Van Hoesen and Damasio, 1987; Van Hoesen et al., 1986).

MODULAR SPECIFICITY OF ALZHEIMER'S DISEASE PATHOLOGY

The term "modular" has been used in a generic sense to characterize many different types of discrete neural organization and especially to periodicity in the grouping of neurons, their axons, their transmitters, their enzymes, and their functional properties (Mountcastle, 1957; Goldman-Rakic, 1984; DeFelipe et al., 1990; Purves and LaMantia, 1990; Purves et al., 1992; Hevner and Wong-Riley, 1992). Many different forms of modularity have been described in the cerebral cortex, mainly in primary sensory cortices (Hubel and Wiesel, 1977; Jones et al., 1975).

Interestingly, several reports have suggested that the distribution of pathology in AD (both NFTs and NPs) may be modular (Van Hoesen and Solodkin, 1993; Akiyama et al., 1993; Armstrong, 1993), and some have suggested that the modular distribution parallels the patterns of corticocortical connections (Hiorns et al., 1991; Morrison et al., 1987a; Saper et al., 1987; Armstrong, 1993). This would be of great

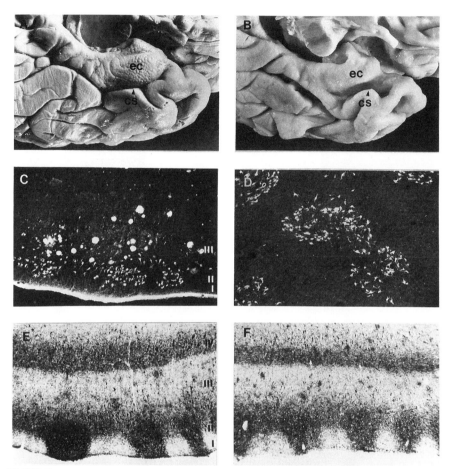

FIGURE 7. The distribution of NFTs in the entorhinal cortex (EC) will affect elements comprising its modules. At the gross microscopic level, modularity is clear by the elevations or *verrucae* on the EC surface of controls (A) which disappear in AD cases (B). Examples of modular distribution of pathology in the EC layer II. Thioflavine-S NFTs as seen in the coronal (C) and tangential (D) planes. (E and F) NFTs highlighted with the Alz-50 antibody. Note the repetitive pattern in the distribution of these lesions.

interest if proven. We are favorably disposed to the disconnection model but believe as well that AD also destroys elements of modular organization, perhaps stripping the cortex of key morphological units that support and underlie the functional operations of the cortex. An excellent example of such changes can be found in the temporal cortex where the pathology of AD targets specifically elements forming modules in several types of this cortex.

A clear case can be found in the entorhinal cortex (Figure 7) where modularity is suggested even at the gross macroscopic level of control cases because its surface is characterized by a mosaic of small elevations known as *verrucae*. These correspond to the patches of layer II multipolar cells and their associated interneurons. In AD the multipolar neurons of the entorhinal layer II suffer extensive damage since virtually all develop NFTs if the patients survive the illness for a long period of time. Layer II neurons of the entorhinal cortex (Van Hoesen and Solodkin, 1993, 1994; Solodkin and Van Hoesen, 1996) are the key elements of a modular organization, and they are destroyed or heavily damaged in all cases of AD (Hyman et al., 1984; Braak and Braak, 1991). Ancillary information reinforcing the idea of a destruction of temporal cortex modularity in AD is the difference in the fate of interneurons associated or not associated with the entorhinal cortex modules. One of the more common strategies to understand the alterations taking place in AD has been the detection of vulnerable neurons by means of changes in particular neurochemical systems. A notable example is the proposed role of cholinergic changes in the development and etiology of this illness (Davies and Maloney, 1976; Whitehouse et al., 1981; Hansen et al., 1988; Geula and Mesulam, 1989; Giacobini, 1990). However, at the present time, it is not clear if the alteration is in a specific neurochemical system or rather the combination of several processes acting simultaneously. Even though this question is difficult to solve, an alternative approach has been the evaluation of chemically specific cells less vulnerable. It has been reported for instance, that local circuit neurons containing some calcium-binding proteins [and hence, gamma amino butyric acid (GABA)], are resistant to the toxic effects of β-amyloid in AD (Ferrer et al., 1991, Hof et al., 1991, 1993; Mufson and Brandabur, 1994). In a recent study (Solodkin and Van Hoesen, 1996, Figure 8), we have found that the density of parvalbumin neurons does not decrease when associated with NPs. However, neurons containing this calcium-binding protein that are in close association with the modules of layer II are depleted in direct proportion to the density of NFTs present in that layer. In the cases where AD pathology is severe, these cells are completely depleted. These observations suggest that neuronal death may not be a direct consequence of the etiological variables of the disease process (since they do not develop NFTs themselves), but rather, an indirect effect related to the reduction in the availability of their postsynaptic targets or NFT-containing projection neurons.

A somewhat different pattern of modular change occurs in the perirhinal cortex (area 35; Figure 9). Here, NFTs form distinct columns, usually four to five cell diameters in width, that can be seen in layers II and III. Pathology-free interspaces occur between the columns of NFTs.

In summary, a growing body of evidence suggests that AD pathology affects at least some aspects of the modular organization of the cortex. If these are linked to its functional organization, even a small change in terms of pathology could be devastating in terms of behavior.

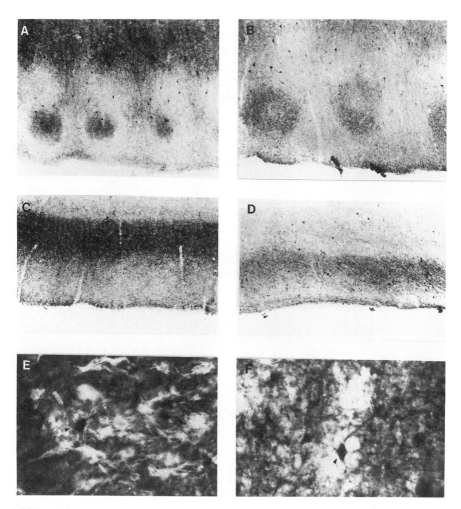

FIGURE 8. Interneurons lost during the development of AD are associated with the NFTs of layer II but not with the NPs of layer III where their density is maintained. GABAergic interneurons in the EC of controls, are highlighted in (A) by parvalbumin immunostaining and in (B) with glutamic acid decarboxylase (GAD) immunostaining. (C and D): Two examples showing the decrease and even disappearance of the parvalbumin immunostaining in layer II. (E) Arrowhead points to a parvalbumin neuron in coexistence with the NFTs developing in layer II at the beginning of the illness. Later, however, such staining disappears. (F) Coexistence of parvalbumin neuron (arrowhead) with the NPs of layer III. This cell may survive.

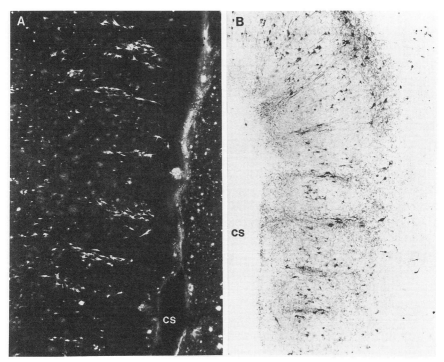

FIGURE 9. Different type of modularity emerges in the perirhinal cortex of AD cases. Here, at the beginning of the illness, NFTs are distributed in columns. Examples seen with Thioflavine-S and Alz-50 stainings are shown in (A) and (B) respectively. Abbreviations: cs, collateral sulcus.

ANATOMICAL ALTERATIONS IN SUBCORTICAL STRUCTURES IN ALZHEIMER'S DISEASE

Even though the majority of the lesions in AD are in the cerebral cortex, subcortical changes should not be overlooked (Hertz, 1989; Brun et al., 1990). Well-studied cognitive abnormalities have been reported with purely subcortical lesions, and they can affect processes such as memory (Damasio, 1984; von Cramon et al., 1985). In addition, many subcortical structures implicated in AD provide sources of input and/or output to and from the cortex.

Telencephalic Structures

The structures that form the basal forebrain are clearly implicated in AD. For example, the septum, the nuclei of the horizontal, and vertical limbs of the diagonal bands of Broca, the substantia innominata and its associated nucleus basalis of Meynert, and the amygdala are major parts. Anatomically these are characterized by reciprocal connections with at least one part of the preoptic/hypothalamic area and reciprocal connections with at least one part of the cerebral cortex. They serve as intermediaries between those parts of the brain that largely subserve and interact with the internal environment and those that more prominently interact with the external environment.

Nucleus Basalis of Meynert. The nucleus basalis of Meynert has attracted attention for two major reasons: One, it sends axons to much of the cerebral cortex (Divac, 1975; Jones et al., 1976; Kievet and Kuypers, 1975; Mesulam and Van Hoesen, 1976; Pearson et al., 1983), and two, it is the major source of cholinergic input to the cortex (Mesulam and Van Hoesen, 1976; Mesulam et al., 1983, Mesulam and Geula, 1994). Thus, it was of interest to find that basal forebrain neurons are greatly reduced in AD (Arendt et al., 1983; Candy et al., 1983; Whitehouse et al., 1981; Wilcock et al., 1983). This pathology would seem parsimonious with the memory impairments of AD (Samuel et al., 1994; Coyle et al., 1983). There is little doubt that the loss of neurons in the nucleus basalis of Meynert is a notable feature in some cases of AD. Nevertheless, the extent of pathology in this region can be as variable as in other vulnerable brain areas (Arendt et al., 1983; Mann et al., 1984), and many cases show minimal change. NFTs may be present or absent and NPs can vary widely.

Amygdala. The amygdala is the largest basal forebrain structure, and its various nuclei receive powerful cortical projections from all types of cortex. In nearly all instances, these consist of reciprocal connections that send feedback to parts of the cortex that originally projected to individual amygdaloid nuclei (Amaral and Price, 1984; Porrino et al., 1981). Prominent subcortical input arises from the hypothalamus, periaqueductal gray, peripeduncular nucleus, ventral tegmental area, suprammamillary nucleus, and various midline thalamic nuclei. The involvement of the amygdala in AD is well known (Kromer-Vogt et al., 1990; Tsuchiya and Kosaka, 1990; Kemper, 1983). NPs can be found in at least some parts of the structure, as can NFTs. Major cell loss has been noted in the superficial amygdaloid nuclei. The role that amygdaloid pathology plays in the cognitive defects of AD is not known, but this structure is unquestionably involved in many types of motivated and emotional behavior.

Basal Ganglia. Other subcortical components of the telencephalon do not escape the pathological processes of AD (Selden et al., 1994; Rudelli et al., 1984). For example, the claustrum contains both types of pathology, NFTs and NPs. Also, the caudate nucleus and the putamen are not exempted of NFTs. Interestingly, these occur in a mosaiclike pattern reminiscent of the modular pattern of certain afferents to these structures as well as the distribution of some receptors.

Diencephalic Structures

Surprisingly, diencephalic areas seem to be largely spared in AD. However, even though the pathological changes are not as dense as in other places, several hypothalamic areas have been implicated in AD. Among them, the tuberal, anterior, paraventricular, dorsal, and lateral nuclei (de Lacalle et al., 1993). Also the mammillary complex and the lateral preoptic area have been implicated (Mann et al., 1985; Nakamura et al., 1993). In the thalamus, the nuclei affected in AD are ventral anterior, reticular, ventro-lateral, dorsomedial, lateral posterior, lateral dorsal, centromedian, parafascicular, paracentral, and central lateral (Rudelli et al., 1984). Interestingly, the nuclei affected have reciprocal connections with the limbic cortices, whereas the major relay lemniscal nuclei are spared.

Mesencephalic and Myelencephalic Structures

Raphe Nuclei. There are several reports of abnormalities in the raphe complex in AD (Aletrino et al., 1992; Yamamoto and Hirano, 1985). This is of particular interest because the raphe nuclei are the main source of serotoninergic afferents to the cerebral cortex, which is significantly decreased in AD (Tejani-Butt et al., 1995).

Periaqueductal Gray (PAG). This area located around the central canal at the level of the midbrain has been implicated in the coordination of a variety of behavior including threat, stress, pain, and sexual behavior (Bandler and Shipley, 1994). So far, little is known about alterations of this area in AD, even though it has powerful connections with limbic areas such as the amygdala and prefrontal cortex, which are heavily affected. The lack of emphasis is due perhaps, to the fact that Alzheimer's pathological changes are not seen here in mild cases. However, in more severe cases, the presence of NFTs and NPs is clear. Moreover, both types of lesions show a distinct segregation within the PAG; NPs have a preferential location in dorso-lateral areas and NFTs in lateral and ventro-lateral areas. This may have special significance since each one of these areas has been implicated in different functions [for review see Depaulis and Bandler (1991)].

Locus Coeruleus. This nucleus is the major source of noradrenergic neurons projecting to the cortex, and it is also damaged in AD (Bondareff et al., 1982; Forno, 1978; Mann et al., 1984; Tomlinson et al., 1981; Hoogendijk et al., 1995). The cortical projections of this nucleus are especially widespread, and the loss of adrenergic neurons in this nucleus, as the presence of NFTs has suggested, produces a concomitant reduction in noradrenergic innervation in the cerebral cortex (Perry and Perry, 1986). The locus coeruleus is not uniformly affected in AD, but interestingly, in the cases where the cell loss in this nucleus is more pronounced, there are associated clinical symptoms of depression (Chan-Palay and Asan, 1989).

SUMMARY AND CONCLUSIONS

From a neuroanatomical perspective, the topography of AD pathology is highly selective, affecting some types of cortex and sparing others. There is no foothold in current research for understanding this. AD pathology is also highly selective within affected areas, destroying some cortical layers and sparing their neighbors. Again, there is no foothold to understand this either. Larger cortical neurons acquire NFTs more so than smaller ones. Hence, NFT-targeted neurons have long axons of the corticocortical and corticofugal variety that connect various parts of the cortex together with subcortical structures. However, it is not appropriate to consider AD as a disconnection syndrome since there are many corticocortical and corticofugal axons spared.

From a neural systems point of view, it is tempting to believe that multisynaptic pathways are targeted by pathology in AD. But this leaves serious gaps. For example, why are the primary sensory areas spared when they are the first cortical link in the multisynaptic neural systems? Or, why are the granule cells of the dentate gyrus spared since they receive a massive entorhinal input?

Neuroanatomical observations of the distribution of AD pathology have increased our appreciation of the selectivity of the lesion and in some instances this has been correlated with behavioral changes. For example, it is clear that the hippocampal formation is nearly isolated from the remainder of the cortex and can be correlated with memory impairments. Unfortunately, the same analysis cannot be applied to other neural systems.

As mentioned previously, a useful new direction may be emerging where the vertical/modular organization and spatial patterns of pathological changes in AD are appreciated. These could be highly selective and disruptive from a functional point of view and not conspicuous from a neuropathological point of view. From a cognitive point of view it could bring the system down in a brain that otherwise appears relatively unaffected.

REFERENCES

Aharon-Peretz J, Harek T, Revach M, Ben Haim SA (1992): Increased sympathetic and decreased parasympathetic cardiac innervation in patients with Alzheimer's disease. Arch Neurol 49:919–922.

Akiyama H, Yamada T, McGeer PL, Kawawata T, Tooyama I, Ishii T (1993): Columnar arrangement of β-amyloid protein deposits in the cerebral cortex of patients with Alzheimer's disease. Acta Neuropathol 85:400–403.

Aletrino MA, Vogels OJM, Van Domburg PHMF, Ten Donkelaar, HJ (1992): Cell loss in the nucleus raphe dorsalis in Alzheimer's disease. Neurobiol Aging 13:461–468.

Alzheimer A (1907):Über eine eigenartige Erkrankung der Hirnrinde. Allgemeine Z Psychiatr 64:146–148.

Amaral DG (1987): Memory: anatomical organization of candidate brain regions. In Plum F (ed): "Handbook of Physiology: Sec. 1. The Nervous System." Bethesda, MD: American Physiological Society, pp 211–294.

Amaral DG, Insausti R (1990): Hippocampal formation. In Paxinos G (ed): "The Human Nervous System." New York, Academic Press, pp 711–755.

Amaral DG, Price JL (1984): Amygdalo-cortical projections in the monkey (*Macaca fascicularis*). J Comp Neurol 230:465–496.

Arendt T, Bigl V, Arendt A, Tennstedt A (1983): Loss of neurons in the nucleus basalis of Meynert in Alzheimer's disease, paralysis agitants and Korsakoff's disease. Acta Neuropath 61:101–108.

Armstrong RA (1993): Is the clustering of neurofibrillary tangles in Alzheimer's patients related to the cell of origin of specific cortico-cortical projections? Neurosci Lett 160: 57–60.

Arnold SE, Hyman BT, Van Hoesen GW (1994): Neuropathologic changes of the temporal pole in Alzheimer's disease and Pick's disease. Arch Neurol 51:145–150.

Arnold SE, Hyman BT, Flory J, Damasio AR, Van Hoesen GW (1991): The topographical and neuroanatomical distribution of neurofibrillary tangles and neuritic plaques in the cerebral cortex of patients with Alzheimer's disease. Cereb Cortex 1:103–116.

Arriagada PV, Growdon JH, Hedley-Whyte T, Hyman BT (1992): Neurofibrillary tangles but not senile plaques parallel duration and severity of Alzheimer's disease. Neurology 42:631–639.

Bandler R, Shipley MT (1994): Columnar organization on the midbrain periaqueductal gray: Modules for emotional expression? TINS 17:379–389.

Berg L, McKeel DW, Miller P, Baty J, Morris JC (1993): Neuropathological indexes in Alzheimer's disease in demented and nondemented persons aged 80 years and older. Arch Neurol 50:349–358.

Bondareff W, Mountjoy CQ, Roth M (1982): Loss of neurons of adrenergic projection to cerebral cortex (nucleus locus coeruleus) in senile dementia. Neurology 32:164–169.

Borson S, Lampe T, Raskind MA, Veith RC (1992): Autonomic nervous system dysfunction in Alzheimer's disease: Implications for pathophysiology and treatment. In Morely JE, Coe RM, Strong RJ, Grossberg (eds): "Memory Function and Aging and Age-related Disorders." New York: Springer, pp 175–189.

Braak H, Braak E (1991): Neuropathological staging of Alzheimer's-related changes. Acta Neuropathol (Berl) 82:239–259.

Braak H, Braak E (1985): On areas of transition between entorhinal allocortex and temporary isocortex in the human brain. Normal morphology and lamina-specific pathology in Alzheimer's disease. Acta Neuropath 68:325–332.

Brady DR, Mufson EJ (1990): Amygdaloid pathology in Alzheimer's disease: Qualitative and quantitative analysis. Dementia 1:5–17.

Brashear HR, Godec MS, Carlson J (1988): The distribution of neuritic plaques and acetylcholinesterase staining in the amygdala in Alzheimer's disease. Neurology 38:1694–1699.

Broca P (1878): Anatomie comparée des circonvolutions cérébrales. Le grand lobe limbique et la scissure limbique dans la série des mammiféres. Revue d'anthropologie Ille serie tl. 385–498.

Brun A, Englund E (1981): Regional pattern of degeneration of Alzheimer's disease: Neuronal loss and histopathological grading. Histopathology 5:549–564.

Brun A, Gustafson L (1976): Distribution of cerebral degeneration in Alzheimer's disease. Arch Psychiatry 223:15–33.

Brun A, Gustafson L, Englund E (1990): Subcortical pathology of Alzheimer's disease. Adv Neurol 51:73–77.

Candy JM, Perry RH, Perry EK, Irving D, Blessed G., Fairbairn AF, Tomlinson BE (1983): Pathological changes in the nucleus of Meynert in Alzheimer's and Parkinson's diseases. J Neurol Sci 59:277–289.

Chan-Palay V, Asan E (1989): Alterations in chatecholamine neurons of the locus coeruleus in senile dementia of the Alzheimer's type and in Parkinson's disease with and without dementia and depression. J Comp Neurol 287:373–392.

Clinton J, Blackman SEA, Royston MC, Roberts GW (1994): Differential synaptic loss on the cortex in Alzheimer's disease: A study using archival material. Neuroreport 5: 497–500.

Corsellis JAN (1970): The limbic areas in Alzheimer's disease and in other conditions associated with dementia. In Wolstenhome GEW, O'Connor M (eds): "Alzheimer's Disease and Related Conditions." London: Churchill, pp 37–45.

Coyle JT, Price DL, DeLong MR (1983): Alzheimer's disease: A disorder of cortical cholinergic innervation. Science 29:1184–1190.

Damasio AR (1989): Multiregional retroactivation: A systems level model for some neural substrates of cognition. Cognition 33:25–62.

Damasio AR (1984): The anatomic basis of memory disorders. Semin Neurol 4:223–225.

Damasio AR, Damasio H, Tranel D, Brandt JP (1990): The neural regionalization of knowledge access devices: Preliminary evidence. In "Symposia on Quantitative Biology, Vol. 55." Cold Spring Harbor, NY: Cold Spring Harbor Laboratory.

Davies P, Malone AJF (1976): Selective loss of central cholinergic neurons in Alzheimer's disease. Lancet 2:1403.

de Lacalle S, Iraizoz I, Gonzalo LM (1993): Cell loss in supraoptic and paraventricular nucleus in Alzheimer's disease. Brain Res 609:154–158.

de Felipe J, Hendry SHC, Hashikawa T, Molinari M, Jones EG (1990): A microcolumnar structure of monkey cerebral cortex revealed by immunocytochemical studies of double bouquet cell axons. Neuroscience 37:655–673.

Depaulis A, Bandler R (1991): "The Midbrain Periaqueductal Gray Matter. Functional, Anatomical and Neurochemical Organization." New York: Plenum.

Divac I (1975): Magnocellular nuclei of the basal forebrain project to neocortex, brain stem and olfactory bulb: Review of some functional correlates. Brain Res 93:385–398.

Duyckaerts C, Hauw J-J, Bastenaire F, Piette F, Poulain C, Rainsard V, Javoy-Agid F, Berthaux P (1986): Laminar distribution of neocortical senile plaques in senile dementia of the Alzheimer type. Acta Neuropathol (Berl) 70:249–256.

Esiri MM, Wilcock GK (1984): The olfactory bulbs in Alzheimer's disease. J Neurol Neurosurg Psychiatry 47:56–60.

Ferrer I, Soriano E, Tuñon T, Fonseca M, Guionnet N (1991): Parvalbumin immunoreactive neurons on normal human temporal cortex and in patients with Alzheimer's disease. J Neurol Sci 106:135–141.

Forno LS (1978): The locus coeruleus in Alzheimer's disease. J Neuropathol Exp Neurol 37:614.

Geula C, Mesulam MM (1989): Cortical cholinergic fibers in aging and Alzheimer's disease: A morphometric study. Neuroscience 33:469–481.

Giacobini E (1990): Cholinergic receptors in human brain: Effects of aging and Alzheimer's disease. J Neurosci Res 27:548–560.

Goedert M, Sisodia SS, Price DL (1991a): Neurofibrillary tangles and β-amyloid deposits in Alzheimer's disease. Curr Opin Neurobiol 1:441–447.

Goedert M, Spillantini MG, Crowther RA (1991b): Tau proteins and neurofibrillary degeneration. Brain Pathol 1:279–286.

Goldman-Rakic PS (1984): Modular organization of pre-frontal cortex. TINS 7:419.

Hansen LA, DeTeresa R, Davies P, Terry RD (1988): Neocortical morphometry, lesion counts and cholin acetyltransferase levels in the age spectrum of Alzheimer's disease. Neurology 38:48–54.

Hertz L (1989): Is Alzheimer's disease an anterograde degeneration, originating in the brainstem, and disrupting metabolic and functional interactions between neurons and glial cells? Brain Res Rev 14: 335–353.

Herzog T, Kemper AS (1980): Amygdaloid changes in aging and dementia. Arch Neurol 37:625–629.

Hevner RF, Wong-Riley MTT (1992): Entorhinal cortex of the human, monkey and rat: Metabolic map as revealed by cytochrome oxidase. J Comp Neurol 326:451–459.

Hiorns RW, Neal JW, Pearson RCA, Powell TPS (1991): Clustering of ipsilateral cortico-cortical projection neurons to area 7 in the rhesus monkey. Proc R Soc Lond [Biol] 246:1–9.

Hof PR, Morrison JH (1990): Quantitative analysis of a vulnerable subset of pyramidal neurons in Alzheimer's disease. II. Primary and secondary visual cortices. J Comp Neurol 301:55–64.

Hof PR, Nimchinsky EA, Celio MR. Bouras C, Morrison JH (1993): Calretinin-immunoreactive neocortical interneurons are unaffected in Alzheimer's disease. Neurosci Lett 152: 145–149.

Hof PR, Cox K, Young WG, Celio MR, Rogers J, Morrison JH (1991): Parvalbumin-immunoreactive neurons in the neocortex are resistant to degeneration in Alzheimer's disease. J Neuropathol Exp Neurol 50:451–462.

Hof PR, Cox K, Morrison JH (1990): Quantitative analysis of a vulnerable subset of pyramidal neurons in Alzheimer's disease: I. Superior frontal and inferior temporal cortex. J Comp Neurol 301:44–54.

Hoogendijk WJG, Pool CW, Troost D, van Zwieten E, Swaab DF (1995): Image analyzer-assisted morphometry of the locus coeruleus in Alzheimer's disease, Parkinson's disease and amyotrophic lateral sclerosis. Brain 118:131–143.

Hooper MW, Vogel FS (1976): The limbic system in Alzheimer's disease. Am J Pathol 85:1–13.

Hubel DH, Wiesel TN (1977): Functional architecture of macaque monkey visual cortex. Proc R Soc Lond [Biol] 198:1–59.

Hyman BT, Van Hoesen GW, Kromer LJ, Damasio AR (1986): Perforant pathway changes and the memory impairment of Alzheimer's disease. Ann Neurol 20:472–481.

Hyman BT, Van Hoesen GW, Kromer LJ, Damasio AR (1985): The subicular cortices in Alzheimer's disease: Neuroanatomical relationships and the memory impairment. Soc Neurosci Abstr 11:458.

Hyman BT, Damasio AR, Van Hoesen GW, and Barnes CL (1984): Alzheimer's disease: Cell specific pathology isolates the hippocampal formation. Science 225:1168–1170.

Jones EG, Powell TPS (1970): An anatomical study of converging sensory pathways within the cerebral cortex of the monkey. Brain 93:793–820.

Jones EG, Burton H, Saper CB, Swanson LW (1976): Midbrain, diencephalic and cortical relationships of the basal nucleus of Meynert and associated structures in primates. J Comp Neurol 167:385–420.

Jones EG, Burton H, Porter R (1975): Commissural and cortico-cortical columns in the somatic sensory cortex of primates. Science 190:572–574.

Kalus P, Braak H, Braak E, Bohl J (1989): The presubicular region in Alzheimer's disease: topography of amyloid deposits and neurofibrillary changes. Brain Res 494:198–203.

Katzman R, Kawas CH (1994): The epidemiology of dementia and Alzheimer disease. In Terry RD, Katzman R, Bick KL (eds): "Alzheimer's Disease." New York: Raven, pp 105–122.

Kemper TL (1983): Organization of the neuropathology of the amygdala in Alzheimer's disease. In Katzman R (ed): Banbury Report, Vol. 15. "Biological Aspects of Alzheimer's Disease." Cold Spring Harbor, NY: Cold Spring Harbor Laboratory, pp 31–35.

Kemper T (1978): Senile dementia: A focal disease in the temporal lobe. In Nandy K (ed): "Senile dementia: A Biomedical Approach." New York: Elsevier, pp 105–113.

Kievet J, Kuypers HGJM (1975): Basal forebrain and hypothalamic connections to the frontal and parietal cortex in the rhesus monkey. Science, 187:660–662.

Kosel KC, Van Hoesen GW, Rosene DL (1982): Nonhippocampal cortical projections from the entorhinal cortex in the rat and rhesus monkey. Brain Res 244:201–213.

Kromer-Vogt LJ, Hyman BT, Van Hoesen GW, Damasio AR (1990): Pathological alterations in the amygdala in Alzheimer's disease. Neuroscience 37(2):377–385.

Lee VM-Y, Trojanowski JQ (1992): The disordered neuronal cytoskeleton in Alzheimer's disease. Curr Opin Neurobiol 2:653–656.

Lewis DA, Campbell MJ, Terry RD, Morrison JH (1987): Laminar and regional distributions of neurofibrillary tangles and neuritic plaques in Alzheimer's disease. A quantitative study of visual and auditory cortices. J Neurosci 7:1799–1808.

Mann DMA (1985): The neuropathology of Alzheimer's disease: A review with pathogenetic, aetiological and therapeutic considerations. Mech Aging Dev 31:213–255.

Mann DMA, Yates PO, Marcyniuk B (1985): Some morphometric observations on the cerebral cortex and hippocampus in presenile Alzheimer's disease, senile dementia of Alzheimer type and Down's syndrome in middle age. J Neurol Sci 69:139–159.

Mann DMA, Yates PO, Marcyniuk B (1984): A comparison of changes on the nucleus basalis and nucleus coeruleus in Alzheimer's disease. J Neurol Neurosurg Psychiatry 47:201–203.

Mesulam MM, Geula C (1994): Chemoarchitectonics of axonal and perikaryal acetylcholinesterase along information processing systems of the human cerebral cortex. Brain Res Bull 33:137–153.

Mesulam MM, Van Hoesen GW (1976): Acetylcholinesterase-rich projections from the basal forebrain of the rhesus monkey to neocortex. Brain Res 109:152–157.

Mesulam MM, Mufson EJ, Levey AL, Wainer BH (1983): Cholinergic innervation of cortex by the basal forebrain: Cytochemistry and cortical connections of the septal area, diagonal band nucleus basalis (substantia innominata), and hypothalamus in the rhesus monkey. J Comp Neurol 214:170–197.

Minoshima S, Foster NL, Kuhl D (1994): Posterior cingulate cortex in Alzheimer's disease. Lancet 344:895.

Morrison JH, Lewis DA, Campbell MJ (1987a): Distribution of neurofibrillary tangles and nonphosphorylated neurofilament protein-immunoreactive neurons in cerebral cortex: Implications for loss of corticocortical circuits in Alzheimer's disease. In Davies P, Finch CE (eds): Banbury Report, Vol. 27, "Molecular Neuropathology of Aging." Cold Spring Harbor, NY: Cold Spring Harbor Laboratory, pp 109–124.

Morrison JH, Lewis DA, Campbell MJ, Huntley GW, Benson DL, Bouras CA (1987b): A monoclonal antibody to non-phosphorylated neurofilament protein marks the vulnerable cortical neurons in Alzheimer's disease. Brain Res 416:331–336.

Mountcastle VB (1957): Modality and topographic properties of single neurons of cat's somatic sensory cortex. J Neurophysiol 20:408–434.

Mufson EJ, Brandabur MM (1994): Sparing NADPH-diaphorase striatal neurons in Parkinson's and Alzheimer's diseases. Neuroreport 5:705–708.

Nakamura S, Takemura M, Ohnishi K, Suenaga T, Nishimura M, Akiguchi I, Kimura J, Kimura T (1993): Loss of large neurons and occurrence of neurofibrillary tangles in the tuberomammillary nucleus of patients with Alzheimer's disease. Neurosci Lett 151: 196–199.

Olshansky SJ, Carnes BA, Cassel CK (1993): The aging of the human species. Sci Am 268: 46–52.

Pandya DN, Kuypers HGJM (1969): Cortico-cortical connections on the rhesus monkey. Brain Res 13:16–36.

Pandya DN, Seltzer B (1982): Association areas of the cerebral cortex. TINS 5:386–390.

Pandya DN, Yeterian EH (1985): Architecture and connections of cortical association areas. In Peters A, Jones EG (eds): "Cerebral Cortex, Vol. 4, Association and Auditory Cortices." New York: Plenum, pp. 3–61.

Pearson RCA, Esiri MM, Hiorns RW, Wilcock GK, Powell TPS (1985): Anatomical correlates of the distribution of the pathological changes in the neocortex in Alzheimer disease. Proc Natl Acad Sci U S A 82:4531–4534.

Pearson RCA, Gatter KC, Brodal P, Powell TPS (1983): The projection of the basal nucleus of Meynert upon the neocortex on the monkey. Brain Res 259:132–136.

Perry EK, Perry RH (1986): A review of neuropathological and neurochemical correlates of the Alzheimer's disease. Danish Med Bull 32:27–34.

Perry G, Kawai M, Tabaton M, Onorato M, Mulvihill P, Richey P, Morandi A, Connolly JA, Gambetti P (1991): Neuropil threads of Alzheimer's disease show a marked alteration of the normal cytoskeleton. J Neurosci 11:1748–1755.

Porrino LJ, Crane AM, Goldman-Rakic PS (1981): Direct and indirect pathways form the amygdala to the frontal lobe in rhesus monkeys. J Comp Neurol 198:121–136.

Purves D, LaMantia AS (1990): Construction of modular circuits in the mammalian brain. Cold Spring Harbor Symp Quant Biol 55:362–368.

Purves D, Riddle DR, LaMantia AS (1992): Iterated patterns of brain circuitry (or how the cortex gets its spots). TINS 15:362–368.

Rogers J, Morrison JH (1985): Quantitative morphology and regional and laminar distributions of senile plaques in Alzheimer's disease. J Neurosci 5:2801–2808.

Rudelli RD, Ambler MW, Wisniewski HM (1984): Morphology and distribution of Alzheimer neuritic (senile) and amyloid plaques in striatum and diencephalon. Acta Neuropathol 64: 273–286.

Samuel W, Terry RD, DeTeresa R, Butters N, Masliah E (1994): Clinical correlates of cortical and nucleus basalis pathology in Alzheimer dementia. Arch Neurol 51:772–778.

Samuel WA, Henderson VW, Miller CA (1991): Severity of dementia in Alzheimer disease and neurofibrillary tangles in multiple brain regions. In Matsuyama SS and Jarvik LS (eds) "Alzheimer Disease and Associated Disorders, Vol. 5." New York: Raven, pp 1–11.

Saper CB, Wainer BH, German DC (1987): Axonal and transneuronal transport in the transmission of neurological disease: Potential role in system degeneration, including Alzheimer's disease. Neuroscience 23:389–398.

Selden N, Mesulam M-M, Geula C (1994): Human striatum: The distribution of neurofibrillary tangles in Alzheimer's disease. Brain Res 648:327–331.

Selkoe DJ (1994): Cell biology of the amyloid β-protein precursor and the mechanism of Alzheimer's disease. Ann Rev Cell Biol 10:373–403.

Solodkin A, Van Hoesen GW (1996): The entorhinal cortex modules of the human brain. J Comp Neurol 365:1–18.

Solodkin A, Van Hoesen GW (1996): Contingent vulnerability of entorhinal parvalbumin-containing neurons in Alzheimer's disease. J Neurosci 16:3311–3321.

Tejani-Butt SM, Yang J, Pawlyk AC (1995): Altered serotonin transporter sites in Alzheimer's disease raphe and hippocampus. Neuroreport 6:1207–1210.

Terry RD (1983): Cortical morphometry in Alzheimer's disease. In Katzman R (ed): Banbury report. "Biological Aspects of Alzheimer's Disease, Vol. 15." Cold Spring Harbor, NY: Cold Spring Harbor Laboratory, pp 95–103.

Terry RD, Peck A, DeTeresa R, Schechter T, Horoupian DS (1981): Some morphometric aspects of the brain in senile dementia of the Alzheimer type. Ann Neurol 10:184–192.

Tomlinson BE, Irving D, Blessed G (1981): Cell loss in the locus coeruleus on senile dementia of Alzheimer type. J Neurol Sci 49:419–428.

Tsuchiya K, Kosaka K (1990): Neuropathological study of the amygdala in presenile Alzheimer's disease. J Neurol Sci 100:165–173.

Unger JW, Lapham LW, McNeil TH, Eskin TA, Hamill RW (1991): The amygdala in Alzheimer's disease: Neuropathology and Alz-50 immunoreactivity. Neurobiol Aging 12:389–399.

Van Hoesen GW (1985): Neural systems of the non-human primate forebrain implicated in memory. In Corkin S, Gramzu E, Olton D (eds): "Memory Dysfunctions, Vol. 444," New York: Academy Sciences, pp 97–112.

Van Hoesen GW (1982): The parahippocampal gyrus: New observations regarding its cortical connections in the monkey. TINS 5:345–350.

Van Hoesen GW, Damasio AR (1987): Neural correlates of cognitive impairment in Alzheimer's disease. In Mountcastle VB, Plum F, Geiger SR (eds): "Handbook of Physiology—The Nervous System. Vol. V, Higher Functions of the Brain," Pt 1. Bethesda, MD: American Physiological Society, pp 871–898.

Van Hoesen GW, Pandya DN (1975): Some connections of the entorhinal (area 28) and perirhinal (area 35) cortices of the rhesus monkey. I: Temporal lobe afferents. Brain Res 91:1–24.

Van Hoesen GW, Solodkin A (1994): Cellular and systems neuroanatomical changes in Alzheimer's disease. In Disterhoft JF, Khachaturian ZS (eds): "Calcium Hypothesis of Aging and Dementia, Vol. 747." New York: Ann NY Acad Sci USA, pp 12–35.

Van Hoesen GW, Solodkin A (1993): Some modular features of temporal cortex in humans as revealed by pathological changes in Alzheimer's disease. Cereb Cortex 3:465–475.

Van Hoesen GW, Hyman BT, Damasio AR (1991): Entorhinal cortex pathology in Alzheimer's disease. Hippocampus 1:1–18.

Van Hoesen GW, Hyman BT, and Damasio AR (1986): Cell-specific pathology in neural systems of the temporal lobe in Alzheimer's disease. In Swaab D (ed): "Progress in Brain Research, Vol. 70." Amsterdam: Elsevier, pp 361–375.

Van Hoesen GW, Pandya DN, Butters N (1975): Some connections of the entorhinal (area 28) and perirhinal (area 35) cortices of the rhesus monkey. II. Frontal lobe afferents. Brain Res 95:25–38.

von Cramon DY, Hebel N, Schuri U (1985): A contribution to the anatomic basis of thalamic amnesia. Brain 108:993–1008.

Warner MD, Peabody OA, Flattery JJ, Tinklenberg JR (1986): Olfactory deficits and Alzheimer's disease. Biol Psychiatry 21:116–118.

Whitehouse PJ, Price DL, Clark AW, Coyle JT, DeLong MR (1981): Alzheimer disease: Evidence for selective loss of cholinergic neurons in the nucleus basalis. Ann Neurol 10:122–126.

Wilcock GK, Esiri MM, Bowen T, Smith CCT (1983): The nucleus basalis in Alzheimer's disease—Cell counts and cortical biochemistry. Neuropathol Appl Neurobiol 9:175–179.

Yamamoto T, Hirano A (1985): Nucleus raphe dorsalis in Alzheimer's disease. Neurofibrillary tangles and the loss of large neurons. Ann Neurol 17:573–577.

CHAPTER 8

Normal Brain Aging and Alzheimer's Disease Pathology

RAJI P. GREWAL and CALEB E. FINCH

Department of Neurology, School of Medicine, and Division of Neurogerontology, Andrus Gerontology Center, University of Southern California, Los Angeles, California 90089-0191

Aging is the most significant risk factor for the development of Alzheimer's disease (AD). The prevalence of AD appears to accelerate exponentially after 60 years, with a doubling time of about 5 years in all human populations examined (Katzman and Klawas, 1994). Prevalence rates of up to 57% are reported in those 95 years of age or older (Ebly et al., 1994; Wernicke and Reischies, 1994). Even in those cases of familial AD where single gene defects have been defined, increased age is a risk factor since there are no apparent manifestations of the disease at birth or early in life. The doubling time for AD prevalence with increasing age is faster than that of the general acceleration of mortality in adult human populations, which doubles each 7–8 years up through life expectancy (Finch et al., 1990). This discrepancy may be attributed to the uncertainty in the onset or risk of detecting AD, since preclinical phases may be quite lengthy (Katzman and Klawas, 1994).

The close association between aging and AD has led some to speculate that Alzheimer's disease is an inevitable part of aging, or is a segmental acceleration of aging (Martin, 1982), and that if we live long enough, we will all become demented (Ebly et al., 1994; Von Dras and Blumenthal, 1992). Nonetheless, the oldest person alive, Jeanne Calment (Robine et al., 1994), does not give indications of AD at 121.5 years (informal impressions communicated to CEF). Moreover, the epidemiological literature regarding the incidence or prevalence of AD in the oldest old contains conflicting data, and the question of the inevitability of AD remains open (Drachman, 1994). However, the issue of the relationship of the neuropathological changes observed in AD and those related to aging becomes relevant to this question.

Pharmacological Treatment of Alzheimer's Disease: Molecular and Neurobiological Foundations,
Edited by Brioni and Decker
ISBN 0-471-16758-4   © 1997 Wiley-Liss, Inc.

By gross pathological measures, there is a general trend for brain atrophy that may reach a loss in wet weight of up to 100 g in nondemented elderly. In AD, there is typically a much greater loss of weight, with shrinkage of both gray and white matter with widening of the sulci and ventricles (Tomlinson and Corsellis, 1984). This loss of tissue in aging is more attributed to atrophy of neurons than to neuron death, as discussed below. Metabolic imaging studies also show major differences between normal aging and AD, for example, in resting glucose utilization, which is sharply reduced in temporoparietal regions of AD brains, but not in the brains of the clinically normal elderly (Foster, 1994).

Microscopically, AD even at early clinical stages is marked by the presence of neurofibrillary tangles (NFT) and senile plaques (SP), particularly in neocortical regions (Braak and Braak, 1991). The relevance of these lesions in pathophysiology of AD remains controversial (Roush, 1995). The current neuropathologic diagnostic criteria involve the quantitation or semiquantitation of senile plaques because abundant SPs are present in most if not all cases of AD (Khachaturian, 1985; Mirra et al., 1991). However, there have been cases of clinically diagnosed AD with postmortem examinations demonstrating many SPs and few NFTs (Terry et al., 1987b). Although cases of NFT-predominant AD have also been reported, they are rare (Bancher and Jellinger, 1994).

The role of SP in AD is supported by abundant genetic and molecular neurobiologic associations with Aβ, the 39–43 amino acid peptide formed from the ubiquitous precursor, APP, that is a major constituent of SP (Selkoe, 1994; Schubert, 1994). Experimental studies are now in general agreement that highly aggregated Aβ can be toxic to rodent and human neurons in cell culture and when infused into rodent brain (e.g., Pike et al., 1993; Oka et al., 1995). Furthermore, overexpression in transgenic mice of a human amyloid mutant associated with a rare form of familial AD can also cause neurodegeneration (e.g., Games et al., 1995).

The argument against the role of SP as the critical event in AD is supported by their presence to varying degrees in the cerebral cortex of older nondemented individuals (Katzman et al., 1988). The following question is then raised: to what extent are these histopathologic lesions related to aging? The presence in cerebral cortex of diffuse SP (amorphous or fibrillar deposits of Aβ without neuritic pathology) has been reported to be an age-related phenomenon and unrelated to AD (Delaere et al., 1990; Dickson et al., 1991; Tagliavini et al., 1988, Crystal et al., 1993). Furthermore, some studies report a lack of correlation between the quantitative distribution of SPs and the degree of cognitive deterioration (Bouras et al., 1994; Arriagada et al., 1992a,b). Another issue is that the number of SP does not show much change between the onset of clinical symptoms and the further course of the disease (e.g., Arriagada et al., 1992a). Some have proposed that the differences in plaque density between aging and AD may be merely quantitative rather than qualitative and an aging-disease continuum may exist (Von Dras and Blumenthal, 1992).

In part, these divergent findings may have been due to technical problems in estimating the amyloid load. A recent study by image analysis with immunocytochemistry for Aβ showed a very strong correlation ($r = -0.93$) between Aβ load in the entorhinal cortex and cognition (Cummings and Cotman, 1995). Alternatively, it has been suggested that older individuals with significant numbers of SP may represent "pathological" aging or presymptomatic AD (Dickson et al., 1991; Berg et al., 1993). Each of these proposals assumes that some of the individuals in whom SP are found were truly nondemented (Crystal et al., 1988; Katzman et al., 1988). We note that recent publication of an analysis from longitudinal cognitive and behavioral observations of normal elderly and quantitative postmortem analysis from the Washington University (St. Louis) Alzheimer Center (Morris et al., 1996). These careful studies on "nondemented" (ND) individuals showed subtle, even cryptic, cognitive changes in correlation with the presence of abundant diffuse SP in the hippocampus, but without formation of neuritic plaques. More studies will be needed to determine if, as this report suggests, a high density of cortical senile plaques of the diffuse type represents individuals at the threshold of detectable dementia. Tronsco et al., (1996) drew similar conclusions from individuals in the Baltimore Longitudinal Study. Together, both reports show that some individuals reach advanced ages without the neuropathologic signs of AD.

In contrast to younger demented cases, a postmortem study of the brains of nonagenarians and centenarians reveals a correlation between neocortical plaque numbers in the superficial layers of the inferior temporal and superior frontal cortices with the severity of dementia (Giannakopoulos et al., 1995), which suggests that AD pathology may be distinctive in very old individuals. These studies, often with conflicting conclusions, demonstrate the difficulties in addressing the role of SP in AD. Comparisons between studies are difficult to make since different brain regions are studied with a lack of uniform staining protocols or quantification criteria.

Aβ may accumulate in some individuals after 50 and in the brains of future AD patients prior to the development of neuritic plaques and tangles (Morris et al., 1996; Declaere et al., 1990). Cerebral amyloid is deposited in ND brains as documented by a variety of techniques including Congo red staining, immunostaining, and extraction of amyloid from brain tissue (Ogomori et al., 1988; Delaere et al., 1993). These techniques vary in sensitivity and show that, even when cerebral amyloid was not detectable by Congo red staining, quantitation of extracted amyloid showed an age-related increase. Vascular Aβ is increased in other species of mammals that live at least 10 years (Selkoe, 1994; Schubert, 1994), suggesting that a certain amount of time is needed for deposition to occur. In view of the recent report that Aβ can cause vascular endothelial contraction and production of superoxide radicals (Thomas et al., 1996), the presence of cerebrovascular Aβ may not be benign as once thought.

Another approach exploring the relationship between amyloid and aging is to the processing of amyloid precursor molecules (Nordstedt et al., 1991). The ratio of Aβ peptides of slightly different length (Aβ_{1-40} to Aβ_{1-42}) varies by 10-fold between brains from nondemented controls and those with sporadic AD (Naslund et al., 1994).

The presence of NFTs in AD has been correlated with the duration and severity of dementia (Arriagada et al., 1992b; Mckee et al., 1991). NFT accumulate slowly during aging in humans in the hippocampus, entorhinal cortex, and inferior temporal cortex but increased density in particular brain regions may characterize the presence of full-blown AD (Morris et al., 1996; Tronsco et al., 1996). In postmortem analysis of the brains of the nonagenarians and centenarians, differences in the NFT distribution and density exist when compared to younger individuals (Giannakopoulos et al., 1995). In AD, there is a hierarchical pattern of progression of NFT distribution from initial involvement of limbic structures to subsequent involvement of neocortex (Braak and Braak, 1991). Involvement of the neocortex appears to be crucial for the development of overt clinical signs of dementia.

The relationship of the hallmark pathologic lesions of SP and NFTs and aging depends on the relationship of these lesions to AD. The role or significance of these lesions to the pathophysiology of AD has not been unequivocally determined. The development of techniques which have increased sensitivity and specificity are being evaluated including paired helical filament (PHF) immunoreactivity synaptophysin immunoreactivity, and synapse number. These techniques may well provide insights into the relationship of the classic lesions of SP and NFTs to AD and the significance of their presence in normal aging.

Neuropathological changes associated with aging and AD are not restricted to SPs and NFTs. Traditionally, it was believed that extensive neuronal loss occurs with aging, even without neurological disease (reviewed in Finch and Morgan, 1990). More recent studies challenge this concept and suggest that in the absence of disease, cortical neuron numbers may be stable in both aged human and rodent brains (Haug, 1984; Terry et al., 1987a; West, 1993). The interpretation of age-related neuronal loss may be related to which brain region is studied (Finch and Morgan, 1990).

As a first example in this perplexing topic, no neuron loss is observed in the inferior olive or the oculomotor nuclei, even into the 90s in humans (Brody and Vijayashankar, 1977). The inferior olive is particularly striking, since these neurons also accumulate particularly large depots of aging pigments (lipofuscin) in their perikarya, frequently displacing the nucleus from its normal position. A corresponding example in mice is the absence of cholinergic forebrain neuron loss up to 53 months (Hornberger et al., 1985), which is in the 1% survivorship.

Recent technical advances may help resolve the extent of neuron loss in other brain regions. West's benchmark studies of human (West, 1993) and rat (Rasmussen et al., 1996) use the technique of "optical dissection" to minimize double counting of neurons. Figure 1 presents three regions from these studies of aging in the hippocampus of human and rat brains, granule neuron layer, CA1 pyramidal neuron layer, and the anatomically contiguous subiculum. In brains from cognitively nor-

---

FIGURE 1. General stability of neuron number during normal aging is observed in two regions of the hippocampal formation of human and rat brain. The brains of humans were selected to eliminate individuals with stroke or Alzheimer's disease. The anatomically contiguous subiculum shows a significant trend for loss in human but not rat brain. The 24-month-old rats are functionally divided into two groups: O-N, which were indistinguishable from 3-month-old young rats (Y-N) in a spatial memory test using the Morris water maze, and O-IMP, which showed impairments on this test. [Figure redrawn from West (1993) and Rasmussen et al. (1996).]

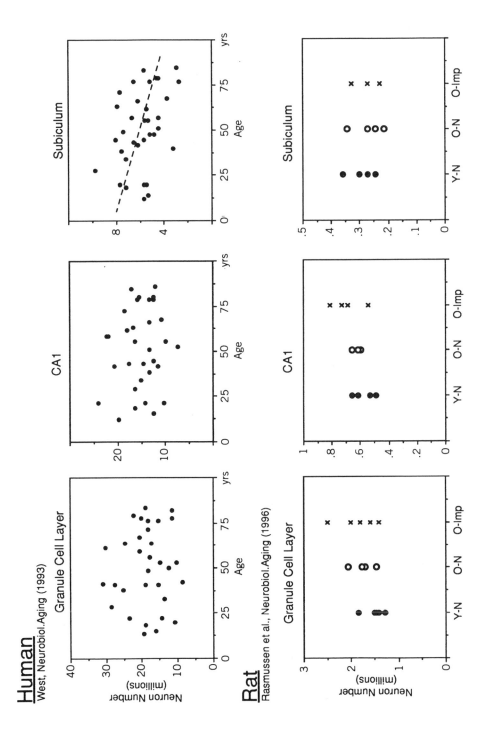

Human
West, Neurobiol.Aging (1993)

Rat
Rasmussen et al., Neurobiol.Aging (1996)

183

mal individuals aged 13–85 years, a regionally specific loss of neurons was observed in the aging human hippocampus, such that neuron loss declined progressively during aging in the hilus and subiculum, but not in the CA1 or CA2-CA3 pyramidal neuron layers (West, 1993). Note that this pattern is distinct from that of AD, in which there is typically massive loss of CA1 neurons (Braak and Braak, 1991). The changes observed are similar to those that occur in epilepsy and ischemia suggesting distinct etiological factors from those of AD (West, 1993). The rat hippocampus was examined by this technique and did not show any neuron loss in these same regions during aging (Figure 1; Rasmussen et al., 1996). The study included 24-month-old rats that were tested for spatial memory and showed no difference from the young controls (O-N) or showed impairments (O-IMP). Neither subcategory showed any neuron loss with aging.

Despite the statistically significant loss of hilar and subicular neurons in humans, which are well described by a linear regression, the scatter plots provided in Figure 1 clearly show that some human individuals at later ages have numbers of subicular and hilar neurons that are above the average for young ages (<50 years). The broad scatter in the numbers of neurons found at all ages suggests that there are substantial individual variations in the numbers of neurons present at maturity in most brain regions. If this is true, then it will be difficult to ascertain more precisely if those individuals with normal neuron numbers at later ages started life with a higher neuronal endowment, such that subsequent putative neuron loss placed them in an average range.

Alternatively, there could be individuals whose genotype protects against any neuron loss. In the near future the distribution of apoE alleles will further resolve these key questions of brain aging, particularly the apoE4 allele, which is associated with high incidence of AD, vascular disease, and shortened life expectancy (Roses et al., 1994; Poirier et al., 1993; Schächter et al, 1994). We also note reports of progressive age-related loss of motor neurons in lumbosacral segments of the spinal cord (Tomlinson and Corsellis, 1984).

Due to the wide variation displayed by aging neurons, it is important to establish which changes are canonical, that is, those that occur during aging in all individuals of related species (Finch, 1993). No example of canonical loss of brain cells is established during the aging of neurologically normal mammals. However, even if neuron numbers remain intact, a variety of studies suggest that age-related neuronal changes do occur. Shrinkage of certain types of neurons may develop as an age-related phenomenon (Finch, 1993). The pyramidal neurons of cortical layer III and the forebrain cholinergic projections are among several distinct types of neurons that exhibit these changes (Finch, 1993; Hornberger et al., 1985). The decreased neuronal size may relate in part to changes in various cellular compartments including the perikaryon, nuclei, or nucleoli. In different neuronal cell types, different compartments may be selectively affected. The relationship between neuron atrophy and cellular dysfunction or cell death is unclear. In some cells, there is no apparent cellular dysfunction noted associated with atrophy, e.g., hepatocytes. Changes in dendrites may also occur as an age-related phenomenon. Golgi studies of dendritic trees show that they are less extensive in pyramidal neurons in aged nondemented brain (Scheibel et al., 1975). Similar studies of the six types of striatal neurons show that dendritic atrophy and regression occur in selected neuronal types in aged animals (Rafols et al., 1989).

Although neuronal atrophy and dendritic extent have not been studied as extensively as SP and NFTs in AD, reports suggest that changes do occur in AD. Atrophy of large neurons may be intensified in AD when compared to age-matched nondemented controls (Coleman and Flood, 1987). The dendritic extent of several regions in AD show decreases when compared to age-matched controls including those of the hippocampus, cerebellum, and nucleus basalis. This has led some to suggest that AD represents, in part, a failure to mount a successful compensatory dendritic response to changes in the neuronal environment (Coleman and Flood, 1987).

A variety of other neuropathological changes have been observed in aged brains, but the relationship to AD is unclear. Intraneuronal accumulation of lipofuscin and melanin are strongly correlated with age (Brody and Vijayashankar, 1977), but there is no compelling evidence to suggest that these substances are involved in the pathophysiology of AD. Similarly, the significance of age-related changes of granulovacuolar degeneration and Hirano bodies is unknown, although both lesions are more common in AD. Corpora amylacea, which are intracytoplasmic bodies found in astrocytes, are frequently found in the gray matter close to the pia or around blood vessels in the white matter in the brains of the aged. A recent study shows that corpora amylacea contain a number of inflammatory mediators, including complement proteins (Singhrao et al., 1995).

The presence of complement proteins in the brain in the absence of autoimmune reactions such as found in multiple sclerosis is a new and controversial subject. Senile plaques of AD brains also contain complement proteins, which might be made by endogenous brain cells as inferred by the presence of mRNAs for several complement factors including C1q, C4, and apoJ ($=$ clusterin, which is also an inhibitor of the membrane attack complex of complement) (Johnson et al., 1992; Oda et al., 1994; Pasinetti et al., 1992; Finch and Marchalonis, 1996). Table 1 summarizes findings from the literature that are discussed in detail in Finch and Marchalonis (1996) and other accompanying articles in a special issue of the *Neurobiology of Aging*. In view of the findings of some of these components in corpora amylacea of normal aging brains, particularly epitopes to C1, C5, and apoJ suggest the presence of shared inflammatory processes during normal aging as well as in AD. Among other indexes of age-related inflammatory processes is the activation of microglia (Perry et al., 1993; Gordon et al., 1994) and astrocytes (Landfield et al., 1981; Nichols et al., 1993), which seems to be a general outcome of aging. The relationships between activation of microglia and astrocytes during aging and in AD are poorly understood.

Neurochemical studies show alterations associated with aging in cholinergic, serotonergic, dopaminergic systems, and noradrenaline metabolism, which are regionally and pathway-specific (Morgan and May, 1990; Finch, 1994). Age-related declines in the key enzyme of acetyl choline synthesis, choline acetyl transferase, occur in brains of rodents and humans (Gottfries, 1990). Neurochemical studies in association with histological analysis of the cholinergic neurons in the nucleus basalis of Meynert

TABLE 1. Inflammatory Components of Senile Plaques in AD

Inflammatory Protein	Cell Types
Amyloid β-peptides (Aβ)	Astrocytes
Amyloid precursor protein (APP)	Microglia
α_1-Antichymotrypsin (ACT)	Abnormal neurites
α_2-Macroglobulin	
apoE	
apoJ	
CRP	
BChE	
Collagen IV	
Complement factors: C1q, C3, C4a, C9	
Complement regulators: C1-Inh, apoJ, CD59, vitronectin	
Cytokines: IL-1, IL-6, TGF-β1, TNF-γ, GAP43	
Heparin sulfate glycoproteins (HSPG), including perlecan	
Integrin receptors: α_3, α_6, β_6	
Lactoferrin	
Laminin	
NACP	
S100-β	
SAP	
Not detected in senile plaques	
Albumin	B cells
Complement components	T cells
Classical path: C1r, C1s, C5, C7;	
Alternte path: B, P, D	
Complement system regulators	
Properdin	
Protease nexin-1 (PN-1)	
Fibronectin	
IgG, IgM	
c-prion protein	

For details, including cell-type localization of many of the mRNAs corresponding to the above list, see Johnson et al. (1992), Pasinetti et al. (1992), Finch and Marchalonis (1996), and Veerhuis et al. (1996).

have led to the suggestion that loss of these cholinergic neurons plays a pathogenic role in AD. Forebrain cholinergic neurons have been studied intensively for changes during aging, particularly the basal nucleus of Meynert, the diagonal band of Broca and the medial septum. Studies of these systems in aged brains suggest that with aging, neuronal atrophy occurs in a number of species of rodents and mammals (Mesulum et al., 1987; Finch, 1993). In contrast to most aging rodents, humans and rhesus monkeys show hypertrophy of these neurons in middle age followed by atrophy in the later stages of life. In the nucleus basalis of normal humans, neuron hypertrophy was progressive up to the age of 60 years throughout this structure, irrespective of neuron loss. After age 60 years, cell size declined slowly. In a smaller sample of humans, there was nucleolar shrinkage with age that may represent a later atrophic phase. However, the delayed atrophy may be confounded by two issues; the first is tissue fixation postmortem, and cross-sectional data do not indicate whether those subjects who survived to later ages had smaller cells throughout life.

Analysis of postmortem human brains in age groups above 65 have shown age-related reductions in the concentrations of 5-hydroxytryptamine (5-HT), the neurochemical marker of serotonergic cells. The presence of a disturbed 5-HT metabolism in AD is supported by the findings of NFT and neuronal loss in the dorsal raphe nucleus of AD patients (Gottfries, 1990; Morgan and May, 1990). The concentration of noradrenaline is also significantly reduced with age, and reduced concentrations have been reported from AD patients (Gottfries, 1990). Neuron atrophy also is observed in the locus coeruleus during normal aging in humans and is accentuated in AD (Zweig et al., 1988).

Is AD disease inevitable if we live long enough? Similar to the epidemiological data, the neuropathological data does not provide a definitive answer to the question. Perhaps more answers may emerge as the nature of the relationship of the neurochemical and neuropathological lesions to AD become understood.

REFERENCES

Arriagada PV, Marzloff K, Hyman BT (1992a): Distribution of Alzheimer-type pathologic changes in non-demented elderly individuals matches the pattern in Alzheimer's disease. Neurology 42:1681–1688.

Arriagada PV, Growdon JH, Hedley-Whyte T, Hyman BT (1992b): Neurofibrillary tangles but not senile plaques parallel duration and severity of Alzheimer's disease. Neurology 42:631–639.

Bancher C, Jellinger KA (1994): Neurofibrillary tangle predominant form of senile dementia of Alzheimer type: A rare subtype in very old subjects. Acta Neuropathol 88:565–570.

Berg L, McKeel DW, Jr, Miller JP, Baty J, Morris JC (1993): Neuropathological indexes of Alzheimer's disease in demented and nondemented persons aged 80 years and older. Arch Neurol 50:349–358.

Bouras C, Hof PR, Giannakopoulos P, Michel JP, Morrison JH (1994): Regional distribution of neurofibrillary tangles and senile plaques in the cerebral cortex of elderly patients: A quantitative evaluation of a 1-year autopsy population. Cereb Cortex 4:138–150.

Braak H, Braak E (1991): Neuropathological stageing of Alzheimer-related changes. Acta Neuropathol 82:239–259.

Brody H, Vijayashankar N, (1977): Anatomical changes in the nervous system. In Finch C, Hayflick L, (eds): "Handbook of the Biology of Aging," 1st ed., New York: Van Nostrand Reinhold, pp 241–261.

Coleman PD, Flood DG (1987): Neuron numbers and dendritic extent in normal aging and Alzheimer's Disease. Neurobiol Aging 8:521–545.

Crystal HA, Dickson DW, Sliwinski MJ, Lipton RB, Grober E, Marks-Nelson H, Antis P (1993): Pathological markers associated with normal aging and dementia in the elderly. Ann Neurol 34:566–573.

Crystal H, Dickson D, Fuld P, Masur D, Scott R, Mehler M, Masdeu J, Kawas C, Aronson M, Wolfson L. (1988): Clinico-pathologic studies in dementia: Nondemented subjects with pathologically confirmed Alzheimer's disease. Neurology 38:1682–1687.

Cummings BJ, Cotman CW (1995) Image analysis of β-amyloid load in Alzheimer's disease and relation to severity. Lancet 346:1524–1528.

Delaere P, Fayet G, Duyckaerts C, Hauw JJ (1993): B A4 deposits are constant in the brain of the oldest old: An immunocytochemical study of 20 French centenarians. Neurobiol Aging 14:191–194.

Delaere P, Duyckaerts C, Masters C, Beyreuther K, Piette F, Hauw JJ (1990): Large amounts of neocortical BA4 deposits without neuritic plaques nor tangles in a psychometrically assessed, non-demented person. Neurosci Lett 116:87–93.

Dickson D, Crystal HA, Mattiace LA, Masur DM, Blau AD, Davies P, Yen S, Aronson MK (1991): Identification of normal and pathological aging in prospectively studied nondemented elderly humans. Neurobiol Aging 13:179–189.

Drachman D (1994): If we live long enough, will we all be demented? Neurology 44:1563–1565.

Ebly EM, Parhad IM, Hogan DB, Fung TS (1994): Prevalence and types of dementia in the very old: Results from the Canadian Study of Health and Aging. Neurology 44: 1593–1600.

Finch CE (1994): Biochemistry of aging in the mammalian brain. In "Basic Neurochemistry," 5th ed. Siegel GJ, Agranoff BW, Albers RW, Molinoff PW (eds): pp 627–644.

Finch CE (1993): Neuron atrophy during aging: Programmed or sporadic? TINS 16:104–110.

Finch CE, Marchalonis J (1996): An evolutionary perspective on amyloid and inflammatory features of Alzheimer disease. Neurobiol Aging, 17:809–815.

Finch CE, Morgan DG (1990): RNA and protein metabolism in the aging brain. Annu Rev Neurosci 13:75–88.

Finch CE, Pike MC, Witten M (1990): Slow mortality rate accelerations during aging in animals approximate that of humans. Science 249:902–905.

Finch CE, Pike MC (1996): Maximum lifespan predictions from the Gompertz mortality model. J Gerontol 51:B183–194.

Foster NL (1994) PET imaging. In Terry RD, Katzman R, Bick KL (eds): "Alzheimer Disease," New York: Raven, pp 87–103.

Games D, Adams D, Alessandrini R, Barbour R, Bethelette P, Blackwell C, Carr T, Clemens J, Donaldson T, Gillespie F, Guido T, Hagopian S, Johnson-Wood K, Khan K, Lee M, Leibowitz P, Lieberburg I, Little S, Masliah E, McConlogue L, Montoya-Zavala M, Mucke L, Paganini L, Penniman E, Power M, Schenk D, Seubert P, Snyder B, Soriano F, Tan H, Vitale J, Wadsworth S, Wolozin B and Zhao J (1995): Alzheimer-type neuropathology in transgenic mice overexpressing V717F β-amyloyd precursor protein. Nature 373:523–527.

Gordon MN, Holcomb LA, Schreier WA, Morgan DG (1994) MHC class II antigen expression by microglial after deafferentation in aged rats. Soc Neurosci Abstr 20:1033.

Gottfries CG (1990): Neurochemical aspects on aging and diseases with cognitive impairment. J Neurosci Res 27:541–547.

Giannakopoulos P, Hof PR, Giannakopoulos AS, Herrmann FR, Michel JP, Bouras C (1995): Regional distribution of neurofibrillary tangles and senile plaques in the cerebral cortex of very old patients. Arch Neurol 52:1150–1159.

Haug H (1984): Macroscopic and microscopic morphometry of the human brain and cortex. A survey in the light of new results. In "Brain Pathol, Vol. I, 123–149.

Hornberger JC, Buell SJ, Flood DG, McNeill TH and Coleman PD (1985): Stability of numbers but not size of mouse forebrain cholinergic neurons to 53 months. Neurobiol Aging 6:269–275.

Johnson SA, Lampert-Etchells M, Rozovsky I, Pasinetti G, Finch C (1992): Complement mRNA in the mammalian brain: Responses to Alzheimer's disease and experimental lesions. Neurobiol Aging 13:641–648.

Katzman R, Klawas C (1994): The epidemiology of dementia and Alzheimer disease. In Terry RD, Katzman R, Bick KL (eds): "Alzheimer Disease," New York: Raven, pp 105–122.

Katzman R, Terry R, DeTeresa R, Brown T, Davies P, Fuld P, Reubing X, Peck A (1988): Clinical, pathological, and neurochemical changes in dementia: A subgroup with preserved mental status and numerous neocortical plaques. Ann Neurol 23:138–144.

Khachaturian ZS (1985): Diagnosis of Alzheimer's disease. Arch Neurol 42:1097–1105.

Landfield PW, Braun LD, Pitler TA, Lindsey JD, Lynch G (1981) Hippocampal aging in rats: A morphometric study of multiple variables in semithin sections. Neurobiol Aging 2:265–275.

Martin GM (1982) Syndromes of accelerated aging. Natl Canc Inst Monogr 60:241–247.

McKee AC, Kosik KS, Kowall NW (1991): Neuritic pathology and dementia in Alzheimer's disease. Ann Neurol 30:156–165.

Mesulam MM, Mufson EJ, Rogers J (1987): Age-related shrinkage of cortically projecting cholinergic neurons: A selective effect. Ann Neurol 22:31–36.

Mirra SS, Heyman A, McKeel DW, et al. (1991): The Consortium to Establish a Registry for Alzheimer's Disease (CERAD). Part II. Standardization of the neuropathologic assessment of Alzheimer's disease. Neurology 41:479–486.

Morgan DG, May PC (1990): Age-related changes in synaptic neurochemistry. In Schneider EL, Rowe JW (eds): "Handbook of the Biology of Aging," 3rd ed. San Diego: Academic, pp 219–254.

Morris JC, Storandt M, McKeel DW, Rubin EH, Price JL, Grant EA, Berg L, (1996): Cerebral amyloid deposition and diffuse plaque in "normal" aging: Evidence for presymptomatic and very mild Alzheimer's disease. Neurology, 46:707–719.

Naslund J, Schierhorn A, Hellman U, Lannfelt L, Roses AD, Tjernberg LO, Silberring J, Gandy SE, Winblad B, Greengard P, Nordstedt C, Terenius L (1994): Relative abundance of Alzheimer amyloid beta peptide variants in Alzheimer disease and normal aging. Proc Natl Acad Sci U S A 91:8378–8382.

Nichols NR, Day JR, Laping NJ, Johnson SA, Finch CE (1993): GFAP mRNA increases with age in rat and human brain. Neurobiol Aging 14:421–429.

Nordstedt C, Gandy SE, Alafuzoff I, Caporaso GL, Iverfeldt K, Grebb JA, Winblad B, Greengard P (1991): Alzheimer beta/A4 amyloid precursor protein in human brain: Aging-associated increases in holoprotein and in a proteolytic fragment. Proc Natl Acad Sci U S A 88:8910–8914.

Oda T, Wals P, Osterburg HH, Johnson SA, Pasinetti GM, Morgan TE, Rozovsky I, Stine WB, Snyder SW, Holzman TF, Krafft GA, Finch CE (1995): Clusterin (apoJ) alters the aggregation of amyloidβ-peptide ($A\beta_{1-42}$) and forms slowly sedimenting Aβ complexes that cause oxidative stress. Exp Neurol 136:22–31.

Oda T, Pasinetti GM, Osterburg HH, Anderson C, Johnson SA, Finch CE (1994): Purification and characterization of brain clusterin. Biochem Biophys Res Comm 204: 1131–1136.

Ogomori K, Kitamoto T, Tateishi J, Sato Y, Tashima T (1988): Aging and cerebral amyloid: Early detection of amyloid in the human brain using biochemical extraction and immunostain. J Gerontol Bio Sci 43:B157–162.

Pasinetti GM, Johnson SA, Rozovsky I, Lampert-Etchells M, Morgan DG, Gordon MN, Morgan TE, Willoughby DA, Finch CE (1992): Complement mRNA responses to lesioning in rat brain. Exp Neurol 118:117–125.

Perry VH, Matyszak MK, Fearn S (1993): Altered antigen expression of microglia in the aged rodent CNS. GLIA 7:60–67.

Pike CJ, Burdick D, Walencewicz AJ, Glabe CG, Cotman CW (1993): Neurodegeneration induced by beta-amyloid peptides in vitro: The role of peptide assembly state. J Neurosci 13:1676–1687.

Poirier J, Davignon J, Bouthillier S, Kogan P, Bertrand S, Gauthier (1993): Apolipoprotein E polymorphisms and Alzheimer's disease. Lancet 342:697–699.

Rasmussen T, Schliemann T, Sorensen JC, Zimmer J, West MJ (1996): Memory impaired aged rats: No loss of principal hippocampal and subicular neurons. Neurobiol Aging 17:143–147.

Rafols JA, Cheng HW, McNeill TH (1989): Golgi study of the mouse striatum: Age-related dendritic changes in different neuronal populations. J Comp Neurol 279:212–222.

Robine JM, Andrieux M, Allard M (1994): Is 120 years the real theoretical maximum life span in humans? About the J.C.D. case. Gerontologist 34 (Special Issue 1): 12 (abstract).

Roush W (1995): Protein studies try to puzzle out Alzheimer's tangles. Science 267: 793–794.

Roses A, Strittmatter WJ, Pericak-Vance MA, Corder EH, Saunders AM, Schmechel DE (1994): Clinical application of apolipoprotein E genotyping to Alzheimer's disease. Lancet 343:1564–1565.

Schächter F, Faure-Delanef L, Guénot F, Rouger H, Froguel P, Lesueur-Ginot L, Cohen D (1994): Genetic associations with human longevity at the APOE and ACE loci. Nat Genet 6:29–33.

Scheibel ME, Lindsay RD, Tomiyasu U, Scheibel AB (1975): Progressive dendritic changes in aging human cortex. Exp Neurol 47:392–403.

Schubert D (1994): "The Structure and Function of Alzheimer's Amyloid Beta Proteins." Austin: RG Landes.

Selkoe DJ (1994): Normal and abnormal biology of the β-amyloid precursor protein. Ann Rev Neurosci 17:489–517.

Singhrao SK, Morgan BP, Neal JW, Newman GR (1995): A functional role for corpora amylacea based on evidence from complement studies. Neurodegeneration 4:335–345.

Tagliavini F, Giaccone G, Frangione B, Bugiani O (1988): Preamyloid deposits in the cerebral cortex of patients with Alzheimer's disease and nondemented individuals. Neurosci Lett 93:191–196.

Terry RD, DeTeresa R, Hansen LA (1987a): Neocortical cell counts in normal human adult aging. Ann Neurol 21:530–539.

Terry RD, Hansen LA, DeTeresa R, Davies P, Tobias H, Katzmann R (1987b): Senile dementia of the Alzheimer's type without neocortical neurofibrillary tangles. J Neuropathol Exp Neurol 46:262–268.

Thomas T, Thomas G, McLendon C, Sutton T, Mullan M (1996) β-amyloid-mediated vasoactivity and vascular endothelial damage. Nature 380:168–171.

Tomlinson BE, Corsellis JAN (1984): Ageing and Dementias. In Adams JH, Corsellis JAN, Duchen LW (eds): "Greenfield's Neuropathology." New York: Wiley-Medical, pp 1026–1097.

Tronsco JC, Martin LJ, Dal Forno G, Klawas CH (1996): Neuropathology in controls and demented subjects from the Baltimore Longitudinal Study of Aging. Neurobiol Aging 17:365–371.

Veerhuis R, Janssen I, Hack CE, Eikelenboom P (1996): Early complement components in Alzheimer's disease brains. Acta Neuropath 91:53–60.

Von Dras DD, Blumenthal HT (1992): Dementia of the aged: Disease or atypical-accelerated aging? Biopathological and psychological perspectives. J A Geriatr Soc 40:285–294.

Wernicke TF, Reischies FM (1994): Prevalence of dementia in old age: Clinical diagnoses in subjects aged 95 years and older. Neurology 44:250–253.

West MJ (1993): Regionally specific loss of neurons in the aging human hippocampus. Neurobiol Aging 14:287–293.

Zweig RM, Ross CA, Hedreen JC, Steele C, Cardillo JE, Whitehouse PJ, Folstein MF, Price DL (1988): The neuropathology of aminergic nuclei in Alzheimer's disease. Ann Neurol 24:233–242.

CHAPTER 9

Recent Developments in the Genetics of Alzheimer's Disease

ROBERT F. CLARK and ALISON M. GOATE

Department of Psychiatry, Washington University School of Medicine,
St. Louis, Missouri 63110

GENETIC EPIDEMIOLOGY OF ALZHEIMER'S DISEASE

Alzheimer's disease (AD) was first described in 1907 by Alois Alzheimer in a demented 51-year-old woman (Alzheimer, 1907). It was reported in 1925 that AD ran in families (Meggendorfer, 1925). Twin studies have shown increased (but not complete) concordance in monozygotic compared to dizygotic twins (Nee et al., 1987; St. George-Hyslop et al., 1989). Monozygotic twin pairs concordant for AD have a significantly higher frequency of positive family history than do discordant monozygotic twin pairs, suggesting that concordant monozygotic twin pairs with AD have a heritable form of disease (Rapoport et al., 1991; Raiha et al., 1996).

Many epidemiological surveys have been carried out to identify risk factors for AD. However, apart from advanced age and Down syndrome, the only variable consistently found to have an effect is the presence of a positive family history of the disease (Brody 1982; Heyman et al., 1984; van Duijn et al., 1991b). Other risk factors that have been investigated are head trauma, thyroid disease, education level, and aluminum intake. Of these the only one to show any significant correlation with AD is head trauma (van Duijn et al., 1991c). The most striking evidence suggesting the importance of genetic factors in the etiology of AD is the existence of pedigrees in which the disease segregates in a manner consistent with fully penetrant autosomal-dominant transmission (Schottky 1932; Nee et al., 1983; Foncin et al., 1986). The disease in these families is often referred to as familial Alzheimer's disease (FAD). However, most cases of AD do not appear to be familial and are

Pharmacological Treatment of Alzheimer's Disease: Molecular and Neurobiological Foundations,
Edited by Brioni and Decker
ISBN 0-471-16758-4   © 1997 Wiley-Liss, Inc.

classified as sporadic, though sporadic AD does not necessarily imply a nongenetic etiology. Two subsets of FAD have been recognized on the basis of age of onset: late-onset AD (LOAD) with age of onset over 65 years and early-onset AD (EOAD) with age of onset under 65 years. No consistent phenotypic differences have been observed between the two groups, although the disease in the EOAD cases generally progresses more rapidly with more pronounced clinical and pathological features, and the disease is clearly inherited as an autosomal-dominant disorder in some cases of EOAD. First-degree relatives of AD patients have an increased risk of AD, though there is wide disagreement on the extent of the risk from 5% (Appel 1981) to nearly 100% (if the relative lives long enough) (Breitner et al., 1988). This variability in risk could be attributed to several factors. First, the disease is common in the elderly with prevalence estimates reaching as high as 18.7% in the 75–84 year age group (Evans et al., 1989). Thus, clustering of cases in a given family does not necessarily indicate inheritance of a common genetic factor. Multiple cases in a kindred could be the result of chance or of a mixed etiology, including both familial and sporadic forms of AD. Second, other causes of death may remove individuals from the study population before maximum risk for AD occurs, resulting in age censoring. This not only confounds analysis but also makes evaluation of large pedigrees difficult. Third, accurate diagnosis of AD in the elderly population is confounded by other causes of dementia, including multi-infarct disease, depression, and overmedication.

GENETIC LINKAGE STUDIES: CHROMOSOME 21

The observation of AD neuropathology in all Down syndrome individuals, who have an extra copy of chromosome 21, over the age of 30 years (Heston and Mastri, 1977) led researchers to test for genetic linkage between AD and markers on the long arm of chromosome 21, especially around the Down's obligate region 21q22, in four large pedigrees multiply affected by early-onset AD (St. George-Hyslop et al., 1987). Linkage was detected between the disease and several markers (D21S1/S11 and D21S16) in the proximal region of the long arm of the chromosome, outside the Down syndrome critical region (Figure 1). The majority of the positive linkage data came from a single French–Italian family FAD4. At about the same time, the gene encoding the β-amyloid precursor protein (APP) gene was cloned and localized to the same chromosomal region (Goldgaber et al., 1987; Kang et al., 1987; Robakis et al., 1987; Tanzi et al., 1987a). However, the discovery of multiple examples of recombinants between APP and AD (Tanzi et al., 1987b; van Broeckhoven et al., 1987) soon led to the dismissal of a mutation in the APP gene being the cause of AD. In following years, both positive (Goate et al., 1989) and negative (Schellenberg et al., 1988; Pericak-Vance et al., 1988) linkage results were reported, and it was suggested that the original chromosome 21 linkage was either a false positive or that AD showed nonallelic heterogeneity. Collaborative efforts by a number of labs supported the heterogeneity hypothesis (St. George-Hyslop et al., 1990; Schellenberg et al., 1991). No evidence has linked late-onset AD to chromosome 21. In addition, multipoint linkage data from many early-onset families also suggested the possibility that early-onset AD was genetically heterogeneous with only a small proportion of the families being linked to chromosome 21 markers.

It was this possibility that led Goate et al. (1991) to examine the segregation of chromosome 21 markers in a single family in which there was evidence for linkage. The disease locus in this family was localized to the central portion of the long arm with no recombination between AD and the APP gene in this family. Sequencing of the APP gene led to the identification of a single point mutation at bp2149 that causes a valine-to-isoleucine substitution in codon 717 of APP770 (Figure 2). Subsequent analyses of hundreds of AD cases has identified a total of 14 families in which this mutation segregates with the disease, strongly supporting the hypothesis that this mutation is pathogenic (Naruse et al., 1991; Yoshioka et al., 1991; Karlinsky et al., 1992; Fidani et al., 1992; Sorbi et al., 1993; Campion et al., 1996). The mean age of onset in families with this mutation ranges from 48 to 58 years (Hardy et al., 1991). The APP mutation in codon 717 has not been discovered in several hundred families that do not have a history of moderately early-onset AD (Chartier-

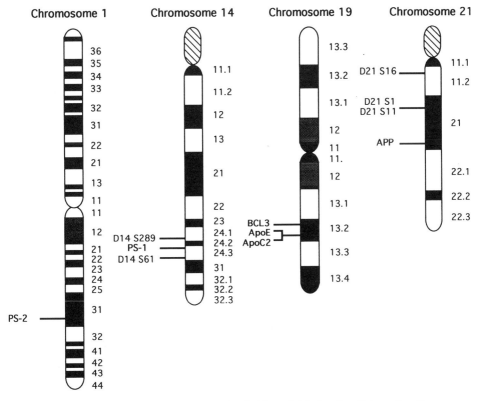

FIGURE 1. Ideograms of chromosomes 1, 14, 19, and 21 showing Geimsa banding patterns and locations of markers and genes that have been linked to AD.

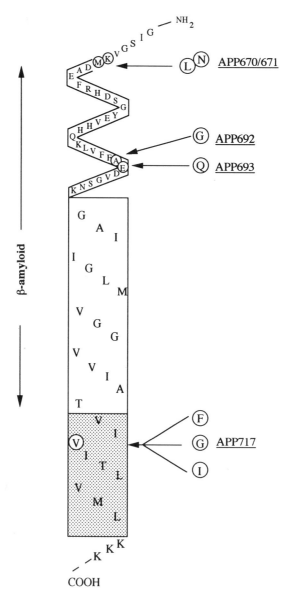

FIGURE 2. Schematic representation of part of APP showing amino acid substitutions in exons 16 and 17, which are associated with AD and HCHWA-D. The codon numbers are those of the APP770 transcript. The transmembrane domain of APP is represented by the thick boxed region, and the Aβ is represented by the unshaded boxed region.

Harlin et al., 1991b; Goate et al., 1991; Schellenberg et al., 1991; van Duijn et al., 1991a).

The description of six other mutations, all in exons 16 and 17, support the hypothesis that these mutations are pathogenic (Figure 2). Two of the mutations are at the same codon as the first mutation, APP717, but change the valine to glycine or phenylalanine, respectively (Chartier-Harlin et al., 1991a; Murrell et al., 1991). A double-point mutation in exon 16 leads to the substitution of two consecutive amino acids, at codons 670 and 671 (Mullan et al., 1992b); the mutation at 670 seems to be the mutation of secondary importance since in vitro studies suggest that the 671 mutation alone produces the same change in APP processing (Citron et al., 1992; Cai et al., 1993). All the families found with the 717 and 670/671 mutations show the classic pathology of AD and have an early age of onset of disease, with family age-of-onset means for APP717 ranging from 39 to 55 years and for APP670/671 ranging from 45 to 61 years. Inheritance is dominant with complete penetrance by the early 60s. Sequencing and single stranded conformation analysis of the other 16 exons and promoter of the APP gene has failed to detect any additional mutations in any of the British families in which APP mutations have been detected (Crawford et al., 1991; Fidani et al., 1992).

The first mutation to be reported in the APP gene was a point mutation at APP693 that leads to a glutamine for glutamic acid substitution (Figure 2). This mutation was reported in a family with a rare autosomal-dominant disorder, hereditary cerebral hemorrhage with amyloidosis–Dutch type (HCHWA-D) (Levy et al., 1990). Patients with this disease die as a result of multiple cerebral hemorrhages in their forties and fifties. Neuropathological examination has revealed the presence of large numbers of β-amyloid (Aβ) deposits in the cerebral blood vessels and diffuse plaques within the parenchyma. This disease could therefore be described as a vascular form of AD. A second family highlighting the link between these disorders was described by Hendriks et al. (1992). Four individuals have the symptoms of cerebral hemorrhage onsetting at around 40 years of age while seven others present with presenile dementia at about 49 years old. All affected individuals have an amino acid substitution at codon 692. The factors that determine which symptoms an individual gets remain to be elucidated but could be any combination of environmental and/or genetic factors. The observation that the HCHWA-D mutation and the AD mutations within the APP gene lead to quite different phenotypes is interesting and may lead to a reclassification of the term "Alzheimer's disease."

A number of other point mutations have been described that have no clear association with a disease phenotype: either they were reported in normal individuals or they have been reported in a single affected individual with no evidence for segregation with disease (Jones et al., 1992; Carter et al., 1992) (Figure 2). No mutations in the other 17 exons, promoter, or introns of the APP gene have been identified as pathogenic, but several base-pair changes have been found (Balbin et al., 1992; Kamino et al., 1992; Zubenko et al., 1992). Mutations in the APP gene account for, at most, 15% of the FAD families.

It has been suggested that Aβ deposition is central to the disease process and that, in these cases, mutations in the APP gene lead to premature deposition of Aβ, while in Down syndrome overexpression of APP due to an extra copy of the normal gene leads to the same pathology. Further evidence in support of the hypothesis has recently come from the introduction of an APPV717F transgene into mice (Games et al., 1995). These mice develop an age-related neurodegeneration and deposit large amounts of Aβ peptide in their brains. The hypothesis also predicts that other mutations that lead to AD will be in genes involved in the regulation or processing of APP.

APP MUTATIONS AND THEIR EFFECTS

Aβ deposition in Down syndrome may be a consequence of overexpression of APP, due to the 50% increase in gene dosage. Evidence has been presented that APP is expressed in Down syndrome brains at levels fivefold above those seen in normal individuals (Rumble et al., 1989). This increase in expression is postulated to lead to an increase in the amount of the protein that is processed via pathways that lead to Aβ production. This observation is the basis of the hypothesis that the APP mutations modify APP processing in a way that results in increased Aβ products and deposition.

Two normal proteolytic pathways for APP have been identified. A constitutive secretory pathway involves cleavage at Aβ amino acid 16 (Sisodia et al., 1990; Esch et al., 1990), an event that results in the release of a large soluble APP derivative and retention of a 8.7-kD membrane-bound peptide. This endoproteolytic cleavage destroys the Aβ peptide and thus cannot contribute to amyloid generation. The protease that performs this cleavage, called α-secretase, has not been identified. Initially, the α-secretase pathway was thought to represent normal processing, and the production of Aβ was thought to be a disease process. Subsequent work has now shown that normal cells produce Aβ (Shoji et al., 1992; Seubert et al., 1992; Haass et al.,1992). Moreover, the detection of Aβ in normal cerebrospinal fluid (Shoji et al., 1992; Seubert et al., 1992) demonstrates that Aβ is produced in the absence of disease. The proteolytic activities responsible for Aβ production are called β-secretase and γ-secretase, neither of which have been identified.

The AD-causing mutations appear to flank the Aβ sequence, suggesting that they may interfere with the degradation of APP by modulating the β- and γ-secretase pathways, thus causing an increase in the concentration of amyloidogenic fragments. In vitro transfection experiments have shown that cells transfected with APP constructs with the APP670/671 mutation secrete five- eight-fold more Aβ compared to cells transfected with wild-type APP cDNA (Citron et al., 1992; Cai et al., 1993). Fibroblast cultures from patients with the APP670/671 mutation secrete three-fold more Aβ than control fibroblasts; this increase in secretion was seen in cultures from both affected and presymptomatic carriers (Citron et al., 1994). In cells transfected with the APP717 mutation, the ratio of Aβ1-42 to Aβ1-40 is increased (Suzuki et al., 1994; Tamaoka et al., 1994). Aβ1-42 forms amyloid fibrils more readily than Aβ1-40 and is thus postulated to be more pathogenic (Hilbich et al., 1991).

GENETIC LINKAGE STUDIES: CHROMOSOME 14

The APP gene has been excluded as the disease locus in most early-onset AD families either by genetic linkage analysis or mutation screening. This led several groups to initiate a genome search for other genetic loci predisposing to AD. In 1992, genetic linkage was reported between early-onset AD and markers on the long arm of chromosome 14 (Schellenberg et al., 1992). This first report was quickly followed by three others confirming this observation (van Broeckhoven et al., 1992; St. George-Hyslop et al., 1992; Mullan et al., 1992a). Linkage was first reported to D14S43 and localized to a region of about 23 cM between D14S52 and D14S53 (Figure 1). Of the 48 families tested in these papers, all with family mean onset ages of less than 53 years, nine showed significant linkage (i.e., gave individual lod scores above 3) with at least one marker; only the seven Volga Germans and one other family gave negative lod scores with all markers tested. The vast majority of families gave results that were consistent with linkage to chromosome 14. The isolation of additional genetic markers led to the candidate region being narrowed to a distance of 6.4 cM between D14S89 and D14S61 (Cruts et al., 1995a). Complete yeast artificial chromosome (YAC) contigs were developed between these flanking markers (Clark et al., 1995a; Cruts et al., 1995a).

A positional cloning strategy led to the identification of five missense mutations in a novel gene from this region in seven families multiply affected by early-onset AD (Sherrington et al., 1995). The gene S182 or presenilin 1 (PS-1) appears to code for an integral membrane protein with 6–9 transmembrane (Tm) domains. The PS-1 gene is localized within a 75 kb region, and the coding region of PS-1 is made up of 10 exons (Clark et al., 1995b). Twenty-four different mutations have been found in 42 families, including families of Caucasian, Japanese, Ashkenazi-Jewish, and Hispanic origins (Figure 3) Sherrington et al., 1995; Clark 1995b; Campion et al., 1995; Cruts et al., 1995b; Rogaev et al., 1995; Wasco et al., 1995; Hutton et al., 1996; Boteva et al., 1996; Rossor et al., 1996). The distribution of the mutations suggest clustering at Tm2 and the large hydrophilic loop encoded by exons 8 and 9 (Hutton et al., 1996). There can be a difference of up to 20 years in the familial mean age of onset among different PS-1 families, ranging from 35 to 55 years depending on the site of the mutation. When the same mutation is present in several families, the mean age of onset is very similar.

As yet, PS-1 mutations have only been identified in families with early-onset FAD. However, since some mutations result in a later age of onset, perhaps due to a milder effect on PS-1 function, it cannot be excluded that PS-1 mutations may also result in late-onset AD. Initially, no significant linkage was found between chromosome 14 markers in close proximity to PS-1 and late-onset FAD (Schellenberg et al., 1993). Also, no mutations were found in a region accounting for about one-third of the open reading frame of PS-1 in a series of LOAD cases (Tsuda et al., 1995). Recently, however, using a biallelic polymorphism in intron 8 of the PS-1 gene, an association has been found between PS-1 and late-onset AD (Wragg et al., 1996). A statistically significant difference in both allele frequency and genotype distribution was observed between late-onset AD cases and controls in a Caucasian population.

```
                                                                                                                                              90
1 Human PS-2  MLTFMASDSEEEVCD ERTSLMSAESPTPRS CQEGRQEPEGENTA QWRSQENEEDGEEDP DRYVCSGVPGRPPGL EEELTLKYGAKHVIM   90
4 Mouse PS-1  -----MTEIPAPLSY FQNAQMSEDSHSSSA IRSQNDSQERQQQHD RQRLDNPEPISNGRP QS-NSRQVVEQDEEE DEELTLKYGAKHVIM   84
5 Rat PS-1    -----MTEIPAPLSY FQNAQMSEDSHSSS- VRSQNDNQERQQHHD RQRLDNPESISNGRP QSNFTRQVIEQDEEE DEELTLKYGAKHVIM   84
6 Human PS-1  -----MTELPAPLSY FQNAQMSEDNHLSNT VRSQNDNRERQEHND RRSLGHPEPLSNGRP QG-NSRQVVEQDEEE DEELTLKYGAKHVIM   84
7 SEL-12      ------------MPST RRQQBGGGADAETHT VYGTNLLTNRNSQ-- ED----------ENV VEEAELKYGASHVIH   52

1 Human PS-2  LFVPVTLCMIVVVAT IKSVRFYTEKNG-QL IYTTFTEDTPSVSQR LLNSVLNTLIMISVI VVMTIFLVVLYKYRC YKFIHGWLIMSSLML  179
4 Mouse PS-1  LFVPVTLCMVVVVAT IKSVSFYTRKDG-QL IYTPFTEDTETVSQR ALHSILNAAIMISVI VIMTILLVVLYKYRC YKVIHAWLIISSLLL  173
5 Rat PS-1    LFVPVTLCMVVVVAT IKSVSFYTRKDG-QL IYTPFTEDTETVSQR ALHSILNAAIMISVI VVMTILLVVLYKYRC YKVIHAWLIVSSLLL  173
6 Human PS-1  LFVPVTLCMVVVAT  IKSVSFYTRKDG-QL IYTPFTEDTETVSQR ALHSILNAAIMISVI VVMTILLVVLYKYRC YKVIHAWLIISSLLL  173
7 SEL-12      LFVPVSLCMALIVFT MNTITFVSQNNGRHL LYTPFVRETDSIVEK GLMSLGNALVMLCVV VLMTVLLIVFVKYKF YKLIHGWLIVSSFLL  142

1 Human PS-2  LFLFTYIYLGEVLKT YNVAMDYPTLLLTVW NFGAVGMVCIHWKGP LVLQQAYLIMISALM ALVFIKYLPEWSAWV ILGAISVDLVAVLC   269
4 Mouse PS-1  LFFFSFIYLGEVFKT YNVAVDYVTVALLIW NFGVVGMIAIHWKGP LRLQQAYLIMISALM ALVFIKYLPEWTAWL ILAVISVDLVAVLC   263
5 Rat PS-1    LFFFSFIYLGEVFKT YNVAVDYITVALLIW NFGVVGMIAIHWKGP LRLQQAYLIMISALM ALVFIKYLPEWTAWL ILAVISVDLVAVLC   263
6 Human PS-1  LFFFSFIYLGEVFKT YNVAVDYITVALLIW NFGVVGMISIHWKGP LRLQQAYLIMISALM ALVFIKYLPEWTAWL ILAVISVDLVAVLC   263
7 SEL-12      LFLFTTIYVQEVLKS FDVSPSALLVLFGLG NYGVLGMMCIHWKGP LRLQQFYLITMSALM ALVFIKYLPEWTVWF VLFVISWDLVAVLT   232

1 Human PS-2  PKGPLRMLVETAQER NEPIFPALIYSSAMV WTVGMAKLDPSSQGA LQLP------YDPEM EED--SYDSFGEP-- -SYPEVFEPPLTGYP  348
2 Rat PS-2    -------------- -------------- -------------- -------------- ------DSFGEP-- -SYPEAFEAPQGYP   20
3 Mouse PS-2  -------------- -------------- -------------- -------------- --------------GYP    3
4 Mouse PS-1  PKGPLRMLVETAQER NETLFPALIYSSTMV WLVNMAEGDPEAQRR VPKNPK-----YNTQR AER-ETQDSGSGNDD GGFSEEWEAQRDSHL  348
5 Rat PS-1    PKGPLRMLVETAQER NETLFPALIYSSTMV WLVNMAEGDPEAQRR VPKNPK-----YSTQG TEREETQDTGTGSDD GGFSEEWEAQRDSHL  349
6 Human PS-1  PKGPLRMLVETAQER NETLFPALIYSSTMV WLVNMAEGDPEAQRR VSKNSK-----YNAES TER-ESQDTVAENDD GGFSEEWEAQRDSHL  348
7 SEL-12      PKGPLRYLVETAQER NEPIFPALIYSSGVI YPYVLVTAVENTTDP REPISSDSNTSTAFP GEASCSSETPKRPKV KRIPQKVQIESNTTA  322

1 Human PS-2  G---------EE EEERGVKLGLGDFIF YSVLVGKAAATGSGD WNTTIACFVAILIGL CLTLLLLAVFKKALP  414
2 Rat PS-2    G---------EE EEERGVKLGLGDFIF YSVLVGKAAATGNGD WSTTLACFIAILIGL CLTLLLLAVFKKALP   86
3 Mouse PS-2  G---------EE EEERGVKLGLGDFIF YSVLVGKAAATGNGD WSTTLACFIAILIGL CLTLLLLAVFKKALP   69
4 Mouse PS-1  GPH------RSTPESR AAVQELSGSILTSED PEERGVKLGLGDFIF YSVLVGKASATASGD WNTTIACFVAILIGL CLTLLLAIFKKALP  433
5 Rat PS-1    GPH------RSTPESR AAVQELSGSILTSED PEERGVKLGLGDFIF YSVLVGKASATASGD WNTTIACFVAILIGL CLTLLLAIFKKALP  434
6 Human PS-1  GPH------RSTPESR AAVQELSSSILAGED PEERGVKLGLGDFIF YSVLVGKASATASGD WNTTIACFVAILIGL CLTLLLLAIFKKALP  433
7 SEL-12      STTQNSGVRVERELA AERPTVQDANFHRHE EEERGVKLGLGDFIF YSVLLGKASSY--FD WNTTIACYVAILIGL CFTLVLLAVFKKRALP  410

1 Human PS-2  ALPISITFGLIFYFS TDNLVRPFMDTLASH QLYI  448
2 Rat PS-2    A---------- ----- QLYI   87
3 Mouse PS-2  ALPISITFGLIFYFS TDNLVRPFMDTLASH QLYI  103
4 Mouse PS-1  ALPISITFGLVFYFA TDYLVQPFMDQLAFH QFYI  467
5 Rat PS-1    ALPISITFGLIFYFA TDYLVQPFMDQLAFH QFYI  468
6 Human PS-1  ALPISITFGLVFYFA TDYLVQPFMDQLAFH QFYI  467
7 SEL-12      ALPISIFSGLIFYFC TRWLITPFVTQVSQK CLLY  444
```

Homozygosity of allele 1 in the PS-1 gene was associated with a doubling of risk for late-onset AD compared with 12 and 22 genotypes. The proportion of AD cases in the sample that could be attributed to homozygosity of this locus is estimated by attributable fraction as 0.22. There was no evidence that PS-1 genotype altered age of onset in the sample. This initial study will need to be replicated in other populations to verify the association of PS-1 with late-onset AD.

Studies of the clinical and neuropathological features of PS-1 families show that AD in these families is severe. Onset can occur as early as 30 years of age, and disease duration is shorter than observed in late-onset AD. The clinical features characteristic of AD in these families include prominent seizures, myoclonus, and paratonia, all features that usually occur later in the course of the disease in other forms of AD. For the most part, though, the clinical and neuropathological phenotypes of PS-1 families overlap those observed on other forms of AD. Inheritance is autosomal dominant, and fully penetrant by the age of 50 in many families and by the late 50s in others. Except for the presence of one splice acceptor PS-1 mutant family, which exhibits an inframe deletion of exon 9 (Perez-Tur et al., 1995), only missense mutations have been reported for PS-1, suggesting that mutations in the PS-1 gene lead to a dysfunction, rather than loss of function, of the PS-1 protein. The PS-1 mutation families account for roughly 60% of the FAD families, making it the major gene for familial presenile dementia.

GENETIC LINKAGE STUDIES: CHROMOSOME 1

The presenilin 1 gene shows substantial homology to three expressed sequence tags (ESTs) in the public databases that were subsequently mapped to chromosome 1. At about the same time, genetic linkage was established in Volga German FAD kindreds between AD and markers on the distal long arm of chromosome 1 (Levy-Lahad et al., 1995a). These families have been extensively studied, and no linkage had previously been established for chromosomes 21, 19, or 14 (Schellenberg et al., 1988; 1992; Yu et al., 1994). The disease was localized to a 14-cM region between D1S225 and D1S217. As would be expected for a founder effect, the same rare allele of D1S479 [112 base pairs (bp)] segregated with the disease in most of the Volga German kindreds. Mapping of the ESTs showed that they mapped to the same YACs as D1S479, suggesting that it could be the site of mutation in the Volga

---

FIGURE 3. Alignment of the putative peptide sequences for the presenilin genes and *sel*-12. Protein sequences (Sherrington et al., 1995; Levy-Lahad et al., 1995b; Levitan and Greenwald, 1995; Vito et al., 1996; Takahashi et al., 1996) were aligned to maximum homology with BLAST. The *sel*-12 sequence was amended using Genbank sequence U41540. The rat PS-2 sequence was derived from the rat EST 110123 (Genbank sequence H33787) (Lee et al., 1995). All known FAD mutations are to underlined amino acids (Sherrington et al., 1995; Clark et al., 1995b; Campion et al., 1995; Cruts et al., 1995b; Rogaev et al., 1995; Wasco et al., 1995; Hutton et al., 1996; Boteva et al., 1996; Levy-Lahad et al., 1995b; J. Collinge, et al., 1996).

German families. Sequencing of the presenilin 2 (PS-2) cDNA from AD cases from these families led to the identification of a single-point mutation that causes a substitution of N141I (Levy-Lahad et al., 1995b) (Figure 3). Moreover, mutations in PS-2 are not restricted to Volga German families as a second missense mutation M239V has been found in an Italian FAD family (Rogaev et al., 1995).

Both presenilin proteins have roughly 450 amino acids and share an overall homology of 67%. The homology between PS-1 and PS-2 is particularly high over regions encoding the putative Tm domains. Indeed, all of the amino acids that cause AD when mutated in PS-1 or PS-2 are conserved (Figure 3). The PS-2 gene may therefore encode a subunit isoform of PS-1, a different subunit of a protein complex, or a closely related protein.

Both presenilin genes are ubiquitously expressed with alternative splice forms identified in different tissues. The PS-2 gene, which is encoded by 11 exons, shows splice forms that include an in-frame deletion of exon 8, a simultaneous omission of exons 3 and 4, and a deletion of exon 12 (Prihar et al., 1996). The alternative splicing of exon 8 in PS-2 is more prominent in leukocytes than in brain (Rogaev et al., 1995). Since many of the PS-1 mutations are clustered at exon 8, and there is an association between an intronic polymorphism on intron 8 and LOAD, this domain may be of particular significance to the function or pathogenicity of the presenilins. A splice form of exon 3 of PS-1, which uses an alternate splice donor site, deletes the four amino acids valine-arginine-serine-glutamine (VRSQ) (Clark et al., 1995b). At present, the functional significance of this is undetermined, although similar alternate splicing with VRXQ motif also occurs in both human tyrosine hydroxylase (Grima et al., 1987) and chicken gamma-aminobutyric acid (GABA) receptor $\beta 4$ subunit (Bateson et al., 1991) without any physiological consequences. Recently, another splice form of PS-1 was reported in liver, spleen, and kidney, where insertion of an additional 92 bp exon between exons 10 and 11 of the major brain transcripts results in a frameshift to produce a truncated PS-1 of 374 amino acids (Sahara et al., 1996).

FUNCTION OF THE PRESENILINS

It is, at this stage, premature to be definite about the role of the presenilins, PS-1 and PS-2 and their relationship, if any, to the amyloidogenesis of AD. However, Younkin and colleagues (Scheuner et al., 1996) have reported an increase in the ratio of $A\beta 1$-$42 : A\beta 1$-40 in the culture medium of fibroblasts and in plasma from chromosome 14 and chromosome 1 FAD cases. Such an observation is very similar to the effect of the APP717 mutations and may suggest an abnormality in the γ-secretase processing pathway. Such an abnormality could be either direct (i.e., PS-1 and/or PS-2 may be γ-secretase) or indirect.

Recently, the rat homologue of PS-1 has been cloned and sequenced (Takahashi et al., 1996). The predicted amino acid sequence shows high homology to the other known presenilin genes (Figure 3). During brain development, the expression and the number of transcripts of the rat PS-1 gene are increased between embryonic day 12 and day 15, suggesting a role in neurogenesis (Takahashi et al., 1996). In situ hybridization and Northern blot analyses have shown that human and rat PS-1's show a similar localization pattern, with predominant neuronal and low glial expression levels in the brain (Suzuki et al., 1996). In rat brain, the highest levels of expression are observed in the hippocampus, choroid plexus, cortex, and cerebellum (Kovacs et al., 1996).

The PS-1 protein (or a carboxyl fragment) has been immunologically localized to the amyloid plaques in patients with Aβ-related amyloidoses, including sporadic AD and PS-1-linked AD patients (Wisniewski et al., 1995). Recently, the presenilin proteins have been localized in the endoplasmic reticulum and Golgi complex in cells transfected in vitro with tagged presenilin constructs (Kovacs et al., 1996). FAD-associated mutations did not significantly alter their subcellular localization pattern. Confirmation of this immunolocalization study will have to be attained with antibodies to the native proteins, which were not able to be localized.

The structural similarity of the presenilins to ion channel subunits is striking, particularly in view of the clustering of mutations in Tm2 (Figure 3). Within a transmembrane domain α-helix, a series of mutations every 3–4 residues will align along one face of the helix. The possibility that the presenilins are ion channel subunits is further strengthened by the observation that most mutations are located in predicted hydrophobic domains or at the interfaces of hydrophilic and hydrophobic domains. Thus an attractive model is one where PS-1/PS-2 acts as an ion channel, with mutations that disrupt the pore internally or interfere with the interaction of subunits, or that cluster at the surface of the pore opening. In the glutamate receptor, for example, mutations in Tm2 alter the regulation of ion flow (Verdoon et al., 1991).

Recently, yet another function has been proposed for the presenilin protein using *Caenorhabditis elegans* as the model organism. In *C. elegans, lin*-12 and *glp*-1 genes are members of the Notch family of receptors. The Notch family of proteins mediates the specification of numerous cell fates during development and has been studied extensively in *Drosophila* and *C. elegans*. When Levitan and Greenwald screened for mutations in *C. elegans* that would suppress *lin*-12 gain of function mutations, a new gene was identified (*sel*-12), which appears to function by facilitating the signaling mediated by *lin*-12 and *glp*-1 (Levitan and Greenwald, 1995). This *sel*-12 gene is remarkably homologous to PS-1 and PS-2 in humans, mice, and rats (Figure 3) (50% amino acid identity between human PS-1 and *sel*-12 over the length of the sequence). Furthermore, of the 24 known mutations in PS-1 or PS-2 that lead to early-onset AD, 20 alter amino acids that are identical in *sel*-12 and human and mouse PS-1 and PS-2. This high degree of conservation suggests that the function of the *sel*-12 and presenilin proteins may also be conserved.

In a recent study, using a "death-trap" assay to identify genes that protect against T-cell receptor-induced apoptosis in a T-cell hybridoma, a mouse clone showing 98% homology to the C-terminal 103 amino acids of human PS-2 was identified (Vito et al., 1996). Since it was not demonstrated that protein was actually expressed from this partial cNDA, it was not clear whether the protective effect was due to protein or RNA. Therefore, one can only speculate on what that function of the presenilin might be, with functions as a receptor, ligand channel, or membrane structural protein as good initial candidates.

GENETIC LINKAGE STUDIES: CHROMOSOME 19

Although disease transmission studies in AD families had shown that in some LOAD families the disease was also inherited as an autosomal-dominant trait, it was recognized that in the majority of the LOAD families other factors, both genetic and environmental, contributed to the transmission pattern (Farrer et al., 1990). To more clearly define the mode of inheritance of AD, complex segregation studies were performed in a large series of AD families with a mean age of 67.5 years (Farrer et al., 1991). The genetic model that best fit the observed clustering of AD in families was of a major autosomal-dominant gene acting with a multifactorial component. Only 24% of the total variance in the AD transmission could be explained by a major gene effect, with the possession of other genes or environmental risk factors that modulate in expression.

A genome search was started using genetic markers on different chromosomes and positive evidence for a gene causing or predisposing to late-onset AD was reported with a cluster of markers (BCL3, D19S13, and ATP1A3) at chromosome 19q13.2 (Pericak-Vance et al., 1991) (Figure 1) using both parametric and nonparametric methods of analysis. Positive genetic association results had also been reported for an allele of a restriction fragment length polymorphism locus at apoCII (Schellenberg et al., 1987).

Strittmatter et al. (1993) reported that apolipoprotein E (apoE) was an Aβ binding factor in cerebrospinal fluid. The apoE gene is part of an apolipoprotein gene cluster at chromosome 19q13.2 that spans ~40 kb and contains apoE, apoCII, apoCI, and an apoCI pseudogene. In the same study, the relevance of apoE to late-onset AD was examined by genotyping patients from LOAD kindreds for apoE protein polymorphisms. These polymorphisms result from single-base changes at codons 112 and 158, which encode C112 and C158 for the ϵ2 allele, C112 and R158 for the ϵ3 allele, and R112 and R158 for the ϵ4 allele. In Caucasion controls, the allele frequencies for the ϵ2, ϵ3, and ϵ4 alleles are 0.08, 0.78, and 0.14, respectively. A strong allelic association between AD and the ϵ4 allele of apoE was reported in late-onset AD families with an increase in the ϵ4 allele to 0.52 (Strittmatter et al., 1993).

The apoE e4 association with AD has been confirmed in multitudinous studies of late-onset AD including familial samples (Payami et al., 1993; Saunders et al., 1993a; Yu et al., 1994), autopsy series (Rebeck et al., 1993; Saunders et al., 1993b), clinic-based cases (Poirier et al., 1993; Brousseau et al., 1994), and population-based studies (Mayeux et al., 1993; Tsai et al., 1994). The highest ϵ4 frequencies reported have been in late-onset FAD pedigrees (0.51–0.52) (Strittmatter et al., 1993; Yu et al., 1994). The ϵ4 frequencies for sporadic cases range from 0.24 in a French clinic population (Brousseau et al., 1994) to 0.40 in an autopsy series derived from a clinic population (Poirier et al., 1993). The association has also been reported in a number of different ethnic groups including Japanese (Noguchi et al., 1993), African Americans (Hendrie et al., 1995; Maestre et al., 1995), and Hispanics (Maestre et al., 1995). The fact that the allelic association is observed in different ethnic groups indicates that the observed relationship between AD and the $\epsilon 4$ allele is not an artifact of population stratification.

The $\epsilon 4$ allele also appears to act as a dose-dependent age-of-onset modifier (Corder et al., 1993). The highest risk is associated with the $\epsilon 4/\epsilon 4$ genotype, with intermediate risk associated with the $\epsilon 3/\epsilon 4$ genotype. In a late-onset FAD sample, each copy of the e4 allele reduces the age of onset by $7-9$ years, with onset mean ages of 68.4 y, 75.5 y, and 84.3 years reported for two $\epsilon 4$ alleles, one $\epsilon 4$ allele, and no $\epsilon 4$ alleles, respectively. This dose-dependent age-of-onset effect has also been seen in other FAD groups (Payami et al., 1994; Houlden et al., 1994), in late-onset sporadics (Lucotte et al., 1994), and in a population-based study (Tsai et al., 1994).

In many studies, the $\epsilon 2$ allele frequency in AD patients is lower than controls, suggesting that $\epsilon 2$ may be protective against AD (Chartier-Harlin et al., 1994; Brousseau et al., 1994; Corder et al., 1994; Talbot et al., 1994; Tsai et al., 1994; Yoshizawa et al., 1994; Yu et al., 1994). Most of the evidence for a protective effect of $\epsilon 2$ comes from the decreased risk associated with the $\epsilon 2/\epsilon 3$ genotype over the $\epsilon 3/\epsilon 3$, since the $\epsilon 2/\epsilon 2$ genotype is very rare. There is still disagreement about the protective effect of the $\epsilon 2$ allele (Sorbi et al., 1994; van Duijn et al., 1995).

The effects of the apoE genotypes have been investigated in families in which APP mutations cause disease. For the APP 670/671 mutation, apoE $\epsilon 2/\epsilon 3$ cases had onset ages of $57-60$ years, $\epsilon 3/\epsilon 3$ had onset ages of $51-54$ years, and a single case of $\epsilon 4/\epsilon 4$ had the earliest onset at 44 years (Alzheimer Disease Collaborative Group, 1993). Similarly in a different family with the V7171 mutation with a mean onset age of 47.6 years, the affected subjects are $\epsilon 3/\epsilon 4$, while one mutation carrier who is $\epsilon 2/\epsilon 3$ remains unaffected at an age two standard deviations past the onset mean of the family (St. George-Hyslop et al., 1994). Though sample sizes are small in both studies, data is consistent with apoE genotypes modifying the age of onset in APP mutation families. However, no such interaction was seen in HCHWA-D and APP692 mutation families in a much larger study (Haan et al., 1994; 1995). Furthermore, apoE genotypes do not influence the expression of AD in chromosome 14 FAD pedigrees (van Broeckhoven et al., 1994; Locke et al., 1995).

The genetic evidence for a strong allelic association between apoE and AD indicates that either the $\epsilon 4$ allele is the gene product involved in AD pathogenesis or that the actual disease gene is a closely linked locus in linkage disequilibrium with apoE $\epsilon 4$. The findings that $\epsilon 4$ increases risk in a dose-dependent manner and that $\epsilon 2$ is protective supports but does not prove the hypothesis that apoE is the pathogenic locus. Indeed, in an African American population the elevated AD risk population includes all $\epsilon 4$-containing genotypes, as well as the $\epsilon 2/\epsilon 3$ genotype (Maestre et al., 1995). Though this elevated $\epsilon 2/\epsilon 3$ risk was not seen in another study of African Americans (Hendrie et al., 1995), it is possible that the true disease locus has a different disequilibrium pattern with apoE in Caucasians versus African Americans. Genetic analysis may not be able to definitively demonstrate that apoE is the disease locus. Biochemical or transgenic animal studies are needed to unambiguously establish the role of apoE in AD pathogenesis. Such studies are underway (see Chapter 12).

CONCLUSIONS

Approximately 75% of AD patients have an onset of the disease after the age of 60 years, and 60% of AD patients have no family history of the disease. In some cases of EOAD, the disease is clearly inherited in an autosomal-dominant manner. The APP gene on chromosome 21, the PS-1 gene on chromosome 14, and the PS-2 gene on chromosome 1 have all been characterized as genes whose mutations lead to familial EOAD. For late-onset AD, the work on apoE indicates that the ϵ4 allele is a risk factor for developing AD. However, 35–50% of all AD patients do not have an ϵ4 allele. Other loci contributing to late-onset AD remain to be mapped and characterized. As in other complex disorders, these additional loci may involve genetic interactions with the known AD loci. Identification of all susceptibility loci for AD is a major goal in resolving the pathogenesis of AD

REFERENCES

Alzheimer A (1907): A peculiar disease of the cerebral cortex. Alg Z Psychiatr 64:146–148.

Alzheimer's Disease Collaborative Group (1993): Apolipoprotein E genotype and Alzheimer's disease. Lancet 342:737–738.

Appel S (1981): A unifying hypothesis for the cause of amyotrophic lateral sclerosis, Parkinsonism, and Alzheimer's disease. Ann Neurol 20:499–505.

Balbin M, Abrahamson M, Gustafson L, Nilsson K, Brun A, Grubb A (1992): A novel mutation in the beta-protein coding region of the amyloid beta-protein precursor (APP) gene. Hum Genet 89:580–582.

Bateson A, Lasham A, Darlison M (1991): Gamma-aminobutyric acid A receptor heterogeneity is increased by alternative splicing of a novel beta-subunit gene transcript. J Neurochem 56:1437–1440.

Boteva K, Vitek M, Mitsuda H, de Silva H, Xu P-T, Small G, Gilbert JR (1996): Mutation analysis of presenilin 1 gene in Alzheimer's disease. Lancet 347:130–131.

Brody J (1982): An epidemiologists view of senile dementia—facts and fragments. Am J Epidemiol 115:155–162.

Breitner JC, Murphy EA, Silverman JM, Mohs RC, Davis KL (1988): Age-dependent expression of familial risk in Alzheimer's disease. Am J Epidemiol 128:536–548.

Brousseau T, Legrain S, Berr C, Gourlet V, Vidal O, Amouyel P (1994): Confirmation of the epsilon 4 allele of the apolipoprotein E gene as a risk factor for late-onset Alzheimer's disease. Neurology 44:342–344.

Cai X-D, Golde TE, Younkin SG (1993): Release of excess amyloid β protein from a mutant amyloid β protein precursor. Science 259:514–516.

Campion D, Flaman J-M, Brice A, Hannequin D, Dubois B, Martin C, Moreau V, Charbonnier F, Didierjean O, Tadieu S, Penet C, Puel M, Pasquier F, Le Doze F, Bellis G, Calenda A, Heilig R, Martinez M, Mallet J, Bellis M, Clerget-Darpoux F, Agid Y, Frebourg T (1995): Mutations of the presenilin 1 gene in families with early-onset Alzheimer's disease. Hum Mol Genet 4:2373–2377.

Campion D, Brice A Hannequin D, Charbonnier F, Dubois B, Martin C, Michon A, Penet C, Bellis M, Calenda A, Martinez M, Agid Y, Clerget-Darpoux F, Frebourg T, French

Alzheimer Disease Study Group (1996): No founder effect in three novel Alzheimer's disease families with APP717 Val→Ile mutation. J Med Genet 33:661–664.

Carter DA, Desmarais E, Bellis M, Campion D, Clerget-Darpoux F, Brice A, Agid Y, Jaillard-Serradt A, Mallet J (1992): More missense in amyloid gene. Nat Genet 2:255–256.

Chartier-Harlin MC, Parfitt M, Legrain S, Perez-Tur J, Brousseau T, Evans A, Berr C, Vidal O, Roques P, Gourlet V, Fruchart J-C, Delacourte A, Rossor M, Amouyel P (1994): Apolipoprotein E, Epsilon 4 allele as a major risk factor for sporadic early and late-onset forms of Alzheimer's disease: Analysis of the 19q13.2 chromosomal region. Hum Mol Genet 3:569–574.

Chartier-Harlin MC, Crawford F, Houlden H, Warren A, Hughes D, Fidani L, Goate A, Rossor M, Roques P, Hardy J, Mullan M (1991a): Early onset Alzheimer's disease caused by mutations at codon 717 of the β-amyloid precursor protein gene. Nature 353:844–846.

Chartier-Harlin MC, Crawford F, Hamandi K, Mullan M, Goate A, Backhovens H, Martin JJ, Van Broeckhoven C (1991b): Screening for the β-amyloid precursor protein mutation (APP:Val→Ile) in extended pedigrees with early onset Alzheimer's disease. Neurosci Lett 129:134–135.

Citron M, Vigo-Pelfrey C, Teplow DB, Miller C, Schenk D, Johnston J, Winblad B, Venizelos N, Lannfelt L, Selkoe DJ (1994): Excessive production of amyloid beta-protein by peripheral cells of symptomatic and presymptomatic patients carrying the Swedish familial Alzheimer disease mutation. Proc Natl Acad Sci U S A 91:11993–11997.

Citron M, Oltersdorf T, Haass C, McConlogue L, Hung AY, Seubert P, Vigo-Pelfry C, Lieberburg I, Selkoe DJ (1992): Mutation of the β-amyloid precursor protein in familial Alzheimer's disease increases β-protein production. Nature 360:672–674.

Clark RF, Cruts M, Korenblat K, He C, Talbot C, Van Broeckhoven C, Goate AM (1995a): A yeast artificial chromosome contig from human chromosome 14q24 spanning the Alzheimer's disease locus, AD3. Hum Mol Genet 4:1347–1354.

Clark RF, Hutton M, Fuldner RA, Froelich S, Karran E, Talbot C, Crook R, Lendon C, Prihar G, He C, Korenblat K, Martinez A, Wragg M, Busfield F, Behrens MI, Myers A, Norton J, Morris J, Mehta N, Pearson C, Lincoln S, Baker M, Duff K, Zehr C, Perez-Tur J, Houlden H, Ruiz A, Ossa J, Lopera F, Arcos M, Madrigal L, Collinge J, Humphreys C, Asworth T, Sarner S, Fox N, Harvey R, Kennedy A, Roques P, Cline RT, Philips CA, Venter JC, Forsell L, Axelman K, Lilius L, Johnston J, Cowburn R, Viitanen M, Winblad B, Kosik K, Haltia M, Poyhonen M, Dickson D, Mann D, Neary D, Snowden J, Lantos P, Lannfelt L, Rossor M, Roberts GW, Adams MD, Hardy J, Goate A (1995b): The structure of the presenilin 1 (S182) gene and identification of six novel mutations in early onset AD families. Nat Genet 11:219–222.

Corder EH, Saunders AM, Risch NJ, Strittmatter WJ, Schmechel DE, Gaskell PC Jr, Rimmler JB, Locke PA, Conneally PM, Schmader KE, Small GW, Roses AD, Haines JL, Pericak-Vance MA (1994): Protective effect of apolipoprotein E type 2 allele for late onset Alzheimer disease. Nat Genet 7:180–184.

Corder EH, Saunders AM, Strittmatter WJ, Schmechel DE, Gaskel PC, Small GW, Roses AD, Haines JL, Pericak-Vance MA (1993): Gene dose of apolipoprotein E type 4 allele and the risk of Alzheimer's disease in late onset families. Science 261:921–923.

Crawford F, Hardy J, Mullan M, Goate A, Hughes D, Fidani L, Roques P, Rossor M, Chartier-Harlin MC (1991): Sequencing of exons 16 and 17 of the β-amyloid precursor protein gene in families with early onset Alzheimer's disease fails to reveal mutations in the β-amyloid sequence. Neurosci Lett 133:1–2.

Cruts M, Backhovens H, Theuns J, Clark RF, Le Paslier D, Weissenbach J, Goate AM, Martin J-J, Van Broeckhoven C (1995a): Genetic and physical characterization of the early-onset Alzheimer's disease AD3 locus on chromosome 14q24.3. Hum Mol Genet 4:1355–1364.

Cruts M, Backhovens H, Wang S-Y, Van Gassen G, Theuns J, De Jonghe C, Wehnert A, De Voecht J, De Winter G, Cras P, Bruyland M, Datson N, Weissenbach J, den Dunnen JT, Martin J-J, Hendriks L, Van Broeckhoven C (1995b): Molecular genetic analysis of familial early-onset Alzheimer's disease linked to chromosome 14q24.3. Hum Mol Genet 4:2363–2371.

Esch FS, Keim PS, Beattie EC, Blacher RW, Culwell A, Oltersdorf T, McClure D, Ward PJ (1990): Cleavage of amyloid beta peptide during constitutive processing of its precursor. Science 248:1122–1124.

Evans DA, Funkenstein HH, Albert MS, Schrerr PA, Cook NR, Chown MJ, Hebert LE, Hennekens CH, Taylor JO (1989): Prevalence of Alzheimer's disease in a community population of older persons. Higher than previously reported. JAMA 262:2551–2556.

Farrer LA, Myers RH, Connor L, Cupples A, Growdon JH (1991): Segregation analysis reveals evidence of a major gene for Alzheimer disease. Am J Hum Genet 48:1026–1033.

Farrer LA, Myers RH, Cupples LA, St. George-Hyslop PH, Bird TD, Rossor MN, Mullan MJ, Polinsky R, Lee L, Heston L, Van Broeckhoven C, Martin J, Crapper-McLachlan D, Growdon JH (1990): Transmission and age-of-onset patterns in familial Alzheimer's disease. Neurology 40:395–403.

Fidani L, Rooke K, Chartier-Harlan MC, Hughes D, Tanzi R, Mullan M, Roques P, Rossor M, Hardy J, Goate AM (1992): Screening for mutations in the open reading frame and promoter of the β-amyloid precursor protein gene in familial Alzheimer's disease: Identification of a further family with APP717 Val→Ile. Hum Mol Genet 1:165–168.

Foncin JF, Salmon D, Bruni AC (1986): Genetics of Alzheimer's disease: A large kindred with apparent Mendelian transmission; possible implications for a linkage study. In Brilley M, Kato A, Weber M (eds): "New Concepts in Alzheimer's Disease." London: Macmillan, pp 242–256.

Games D, Adams D, Alessandrini R, Barbour R, Berthelette P, Blackwell C, Carr T, Clemens J, Donaldson T, Gillespie F, Guido T, Hagopian S, Johnson-Wood K, Khan K, Lee M, Leibowitz P, Liberburg I, Little S, Masliah E, Montoya-Zavala M, Mucke L, Paganini L, Penniman E, Power M, Schenk D, Seubert P, Snyder B, Soriano F, Tan H, Vitale J, Wadsworth S, Wolozin B, Zhao J (1995): Alzheimer-type neuropathology in transgenic mice overexpressing V717F β-amyloid precursor protein. Nature 373:523–527.

Goate A, Chartier Harlin MC, Mullan M, Brown J, Crawford F, Fidani L, Giuffra L, Haynes A, Irving N, James L, Mant R, Newton P, Rooke K, Roques P, Talbot C, Pericak-Vance M, Roses A, Williamson R, Rossor M, Owen M, Hardy J (1991): Segregation of a missense mutation in the amyloid precursor protein gene with familial Alzheimer's disease. Nature 349:704–706.

Goate AM, Haynes AR, Owen MJ, Farrall M, James LA, Lai LY, Mullan MJ, Roques P, Rossor MN, Williamson R, Hardy J (1989): Predisposing locus for Alzheimer's disease on chromosome 21. Lancet 1:352–355.

Goldgaber D, Lerman MI, McBride OW, Saffiotti U, Gajdusek DC (1987): Characterization and chromosomal localization of a cDNA encoding brain amyloid of Alzheimer's disease. Science 235:877–880.

Grima B, Lamouroux A, Boni C, Julien JF, Javoy-Agig F, Mallet J (1987): A single human gene encoding multiple tyrosine hydroxylases with different predicted functional characteristics. Nature 326:707–711.

Haan J, Roos RA, Bakker E (1995): No protective effect of apolipoprotein E epsilon 2 allele in Dutch hereditary cerebral amyloid angiopathy. Ann Neurol 37:282.

Haan J, van Broeckhoven C, van Duijn CM, Voorhoeve E, van Harskamp F, van Swieten JC, Maat-Schieman ML, Roos RA, Bakker E (1994): The apolipoprotein E epsilon 4 allele does not influence the clinical expression of the amyloid precursor protein gene codon 693 or 692 mutations. Ann Neurol 36:434–437.

Haass C, Schlossmacher M, Hung A, Vigo-Pelfrey C, Mellon A, Ostaszewski B, Lieberburg I, Koo E, Schenk D, Teplow D, Selkow D (1992): Amyloid β-peptide is produced by cultured cells during normal metabolism. Nature 359:322–325.

Hardy J, Mullan M, Chartier Harlin MC, Brown J, Goate A, Rossor M, Collinge J, Roberts G, Luthert P, Lantos P, Naruse S, Kaneko K, Tsuji S, Miyatake T, Shimizu T, Kojima T, Nakano I, Yoshioka K, Sakaki Y, Katsuya T, Ogihara T, Roses A, Pericak-Vance M, Haan J, Roos R, Lucotte G, Favid F (1991): Molecular classification of Alzheimer's disease. Lancet 337;1342–1343.

Hendrie HC, Hall KS, Hui S, Unverzagt FW, Yu CE, Lahiri DK, Sahota A, Farlow M, Musick B, Class CA, Brashear A, Burdine VE, Osuntokun BO, Ogunniyi AO, Gureje O, Baiyewu O, Schellenberg GD (1995): Apolipoprotein E genotypes and Alzheimer's disease in a community study of elderly African Americans. Ann Neurol 37:118–120.

Hendriks L, van Duijn C, Cras P, Cruts M, van Hul W, van Harskamp F, Warren A, McGinnis M, Antonorakis S, van Broeckhoven C (1992); Presenile dementia and cerebral haemorrhage linked to a mutation at codon 692 of the β-amyloid precursor protein gene. Nat Genet 1:218–221.

Heston L, Mastri A (1977): The genetics of Alzheimer's disease: Associations with hematologic malignancy and Down syndrome. Arch Gen Psychiatry 34:976–981.

Heyman A, Wilkinson WE, Stafford JA, Helms MJ, Sigmon AH, Weinberg T (1984): Alzheimer's disease: A study of epidemiological aspects. Ann Neurol 15:335–341.

Hilbich C, Kisters Woike B, Reed J, Masters CL, Beyreuther K (1991): Aggregation and secondary structure of synthetic amyloid beta A4 peptides of Alzheimer's disease. J Mol Biol 218:149–163.

Houlden H, Crook R, Hardy J, Roques P, Collinge J, Rossor M (1994): Confirmation that familial clustering and age of onset in late onset Alzheimer's disease are determined at the apolipoprotein E locus. Neurosci Lett 174:222–224.

Hutton M, Busfield F, Wragg M, Crook R, Perez-Tur J, Clark RF, Prihar G, Talbot C, Phillips H, Wright K, Baker M, Lendon C, Duff K, Martinez A, Houlden H, Nichols A, Karran E, Roberts G, Roques P, Rossor M, Venter JC, Adams MO, Cline RT, Philips CA, Fuldner RA, Hardy J, Goate A (1996): Complete analysis of the presenilin 1 gene in early onset Alzheimer's disease. Neuroreport 7:801–805.

Jones C, Morris S, Yates C, Moffoot A, Sharpe C, Brock D, St. Clair D (1992): Mutation in codon 713 of beta-amyloid precursor protein gene presenting with schizophrenia. Nat Genet 1:306–309.

Kamino K, Orr HT, Payami H, Wijsman EM, Alonso E, Pulst SM, Anderson L, O'dahl S, Nemens E, White JA, Sadovnick AD, Ball MJ, Kaye J, Warren A, McInnis M, Antonarakis SE, Korenberg JR, Sharma V, Kukull W, Larson E, Heston LL, Martin GM,

Bird TD, Schellenberg GD (1992): Linkage and mutational analysis of familial Alzheimer's disease kindreds for the APP gene region. Am J Hum Genet 51:998–1014.

Kang J, Lemaire HG, Unterbeck A, Salbaum JM, Masters CL, Grzeschik KH, Multhaup G, Beyreuther K, Muller Hill B, (1987): The precursor of Alzheimer's disease amyloid A4 protein resembles a cell-surface receptor. Nature 325:733–736.

Karlinsky H, Vaula G, Haines JL, Ridgley J, Bergeron C, Mortilla M, Tupler RG, Percy ME, Robitaille Y, Noldy NE, Yip TCK, Tanzi RE, Gusella JF, Becker R, Berg JM, Crapper-McLachlan DR, St. George-Hyslop PH (1992): Molecular and prospective phenotypic characterization of a pedigree with familial Alzheimer's disease and a missense mutation in codon 717 of the β-amyloid precursor protein gene. Neurology 42:1445–1453.

Kovacs DM, Fausett HJ, Page KJ, Kim T-W, Moir RD, Merriam DE, Hollister RD, Hallmark OG, Mancini R, Felsenstein KM, Hyman BT, Tanzi RE, Wasco W (1996): Alzheimer-associated presenilins 1 and 2: Neuronal expression in brain and localization to intracellular membranes in mammalian cells. Nat Med 2:224–229.

Lee NH, Weinstock KG, Kirkness EF, Earle-Hughes JA, Fuldner RA, Marmaras S, Glodek A, Gocayne JD, Adams MD, Kerlavage AR, Fraser CM, Venter JC (1995): Comparative expressed sequence tag analysis of differential gene expression profiles in PC-12 cells before and after nerve growth factor treatment. Proc Natl Acad Sci U S A 92:8303–8307.

Levitan D, Greenwald I (1995): Facilitation of lin-12-mediated signalling by sel-12, a Caenorhabditis elegans S182 Alzheimer disease gene. Nature 377:351–354.

Levy E, Carman MD, Fernandez Madrid IJ, Power MD, Lieberburg I, van Duinen SG, Bots GT, Luyendijk W, Frangione B (1990): Mutation of the Alzheimer's disease amyloid gene in hereditary cerebral hemorrhage. Dutch type. Science 248:1124–1126.

Levy-Lahad E, Wijsman EM, Nemens E, Anderson L, Goddard KAB, Weber JL, Bird TD, Schellenberg GD (1995a): A familial Alzheimer's disease locus on chromosome 1. Science 269:970–973.

Levy-Lahad E, Wasco W, Poorkaj P, Romano DM, Oshima J, Pettingell WH, Yu C, Jondro PD, Schmidt SD, Wang K, Crowley AC, Fu Y-H, Guenette SY, Galas D, Nemens E, Wijsman EM, Bird TD, Schellenberg GD, Tanzi RE (1995b): Candidate gene for the chromosome 1 familial Alzheimer's disease locus. Science 269:973–977.

Locke PA, Conneally PM, Tanzi RE, Gusella JF, Haines JL (1995): Apoplipoprotein E4 allele and Alzheimer's disease: Examination of allelic association and effect on age of onset in both early- and late-onset cases. Genet Epidemiol 12:83–92.

Lucotte G, Turpin J-C, Landais P (1994): Apolipoprotein E-epsilon 4 allele doses in late-onset Alzheimer's disease. Ann Neurol 36:681–682.

Maestre G, Ottmann R, Stern Y, Gurland B, Chun M, Tang M-X, Shelanski M, Tycko B, Mayeux R (1995): Apolipoprotein E and Alzheimer's disease: Ethnic variation in genotypic risk. Ann Neurol 37:254–259.

Mayeux R, Stern Y, Ottmann R, Tatemichi TK, Tang M, Maestre G, Nagai C, Tycko B, Ginsberg H (1993): The apolipoprotein epsilon 4 allele in patients with Alzheimer's disease. Ann Neurol 34:752–754.

Meggendorfer F (1925): Uber familiengeschichtliche Untersuchungen bei arteriosklerotischer und seniler Demenz. Zentralbl Neurol Psychiatr 40:359.

Mullan M, Houlden H, Windelspecht M, Fidani L, Lombardi C, Diaz P, Rossor M, Crook R, Hardy J, Duff K, Crawford F (1992a): A locus for familial early-onset Alzheimer's disease on the long arm of chromosome 14, proximal to the α1-antichymotrypsin gene. Nat Genet 2:340–342.

Mullan M, Crawford F, Axelman K, Houlden H, Lilius L, Winblad B, Lannfelt L (1992b): A pathogenic mutation for probable Alzheimer's disease in the APP gene at the N-terminus of β-amyloid. Nat Genet 1:345–347.

Murrell J, Farlow M, Ghetti B, Benson M (1991): A mutation in the amyloid precursor protein associated with hereditary Alzheimer's disease. Science 254:97–99.

Naruse S, Igarashi S, Kobayashi H, Aoki K, Inuzuka T, Kaneko K, Shimizu T, Iihara K, Kojima T, Miyatake T, Tsuji S (1991): Mis-sense mutation Val→Ile in exon 17 of amyloid precursor protein gene in Japanese familial Alzheimer's disease. Lancet 337:978–979.

Nee LE, Eldridge R, Sunderland T, Thomas CB, Katz D, Thompson KE, Weingartner H, Weiss H, Julian C, Cohen R (1987): Dementia of the Alzheimer type: Clincial and family study of 22 twin pairs. Neurology 37:359–363.

Nee LE, Polinsky RJ, Eldridge R, Weingartner H, Smallberg S, Ebert M (1983): A family with histologically confirmed Alzheimer's disease. Arch Neurol 40:203–208.

Noguchi S, Murakami K, Yamada N (1993): Apolipoprotein E genotype and Alzheimer's disease. Lancet 342:737.

Payami H, Montee KR, Kaye JA, Bird TD, Yu CE, Wijsman EM, Schellenberg GD (1994): Alzheimer's disease, apolipoprotein E4, and gender. JAMA 271:1316–1317.

Payami H, Kaye J, Heston LL, Bird TD, Schellenberg GD (1993): Apolipoprotein E genotype and Alzheimer's disease. Lancet 342:738.

Perez-Tur J, Froelich S, Prihar G, Crook R, Baker M, Duff K, Wragg M, Busfield F, Lendon C, Clark RF, Roques P, Fuldner RA, Johnston J, Cowburn R, Forsell C, Axelman K, Lilius L, Houlden H, Karran E, Roberts GW, Rossor M, Adams MD, Hardy J, Goate A, Lannfelt L, Hutton M (1995): A mutation in Alzheimer's disease destroying a splice acceptor site in the presenilin-1 gene. Neuroreport 7:297–301.

Pericak-Vance MA, Bebout JL, Gaskell PC Jr, Yamaoka LH, Hung WY, Alberts MJ, Walker AP, Bartlett RJ, Haynes CA, Welsh KA, Earl NL, Heyman A, Clark CM, Roses AD (1991): Linkage studies in familial Alzheimer disease: Evidence for chromosome 19 linkage. Am J Hum Genet 48:1034–1050.

Pericak-Vance MA, Yamaoka LH, Haynes CS, Speer MC, Haines JL, Gaskell PC, Hung WY, Clark CM, Heyman AL, Trofatter JA, Eisenmenger JP, Gilbert JR, Lee JE, Alberts MJ, Dawson DV, Bartlett RJ, Earl NL, Siddique T, Vance JM, Conneally PM, Roses AD (1988): Genetic linkage studies in familial Alzheimer's disease. Exp Neurol 102:271–279.

Poirier J, Davignon J, Bouthilier D, Kogan S, Bertrand P, Gauthier S (1993): Apolipoprotein E polymorphism and Alzheimer's disease. Lancet 342:697–699.

Prihar G, Fuldner RA, Perez-Tur J, Lincoln S, Duff K, Crook R, hardy J, Philips CA, Venter JC, Talbot C, Clark RF, Goate A, Li J, Potter H, Karran E, Roberts GW, Hutton M, Adams MD (1996): Structure and alternate splicing of the presenilin-2 gene. Neuroreport in press.

Raiha I, Kaprio J, Koskenvuo M, Rajala T, Sourander L (1996): Alzheimer's disease in Finnish twins. Lancet 347:573–578.

Rapoport S, Pettigrew K, Schapiro M (1991): Discordance and concordance of dementia of the Alzheimer type (DAT) in monozygotic twins indicate heritable and sporadic forms of Alzheimer's disease. Neurology 41:1549–1553.

Rebeck GW, Reiter JS, Stickland DK, Hyman BT (1993): Apolipoprotein E in sporadic Alzheimer's disease: Allelic variation and receptor interactions. Neuron 11:575–580.

Robakis NK, Wisniewski HM, Jenkins EC, Devine Gage EA, Houck GE, Yao XL, Ramakrishna N, Wolfe G, Silverman WP, Brown WT (1987): Chromosome 21q21 sublocalisation of gene encoding beta-amyloid peptide in cerebral vessels and neuritic (senile) plaques of people with Alzheimer disease and Down syndrome. Lancet 1:384–385.

Rogaev EI, Sherrington R, Rogaeva EA, Levesque G, Ikeda m, Liang Y, Chi H, Lin C, Holman K, Tsuda T, Mar L, Sorbi S, Nacmias B, Placentini S, Amaducci L, Chumakov I, Cohen D, Lannfelt L, Fraser PE, Rommens JM, St. George-Hyslop PH (1995): Familial Alzheimer's disease in kindreds with missense mutations in a gene on chromosome 1 related to the Alzheimer's disease type 3 gene. Nature 376:775–778.

Rossor MN, Fox NC, Beck J, Campbell TC, Collinge J (1996): Incomplete penetrance of familial Alzheimer's disease in a pedigree with a novel presenilin-1 gene mutation. Lancet 347:1560.

Rumble B, Retallack R, Hilbich C, Simms G, Multhaup G, Martins R, Hockey A, Montgomery P, Beureuther K, Masters CL (1989): Amyloid A4 protein and its precursor in Down's syndrome and Alzheimer's disease. N Engl J Med 320:1446–1452.

Sahara N, Yahagi Y, Takagi H, Kondo T, Okochi M, Usami M, Shirasawa T, Mori H (1996): Identification and characterization of presenilin I-467, I-463, and I-374. FEBS Lett 381:7–11.

St. George-Hyslop P, Crapper-McLachlan D, Tsuda T, Rogaev E, Karlinsky H, Lippa CF, Pollen D (1994): Alzheimer's disease and possible gene interaction. Science 263:537.

St. George-Hyslop P, Haines J, Rogaev E, Mortilla M, Vaula G, Pericak-Vance M, Foncin J-F, Montesi M, Bruni A, Sorbi S, Rainero I, Pinessi L, Pollen D, Polinsky R, Nee L, Kennedy J, Macciardi F, Rogaeva E, Liang Y, Alexandrova N, Lukiw W, Schlumpf K, Tanzi R, Tsuda T, Farrer L, Cantu J-M, Duara R, Amaducci L, Bergamini L, Gusella J, Roses A, Crapper-McLachlan D (1992): Genetic evidence for a novel familial Alzheimer's disease locus on chromosome 14. Nat Genet 2:330–334.

St. George-Hyslop PH, Haines JL, Farrer LA, Polinsky R, van Broeckhoven C, Goate A, McLachlan DR, Orr H, Bruni AC, Sorbi S, Rainero I, Foncin J-F, Pollen D, Cantu J-M, Tupler R, Voskresenskaya N, Mayeux R, Growdon J, Fried VA, Myers RH, Nee L, Black hovens H, Martin J-J, Rossor M, Owen MJ, Mullan M, Percy ME, Karlinsky K, Rich S, Heston L, Montesi M, Mortilla M, Nacmias N, Gusella JF, Hardy J (1990): Genetic linkage studies suggest that Alzheimer's disease is not a single homogeneous disorder. FAD Collaborative Study Group. Nature 347:194–197.

St. George-Hyslop PH, Tanzi RE, Haines JL, Polinsky RJ, Farrer L, Myers RH, Gusella JF (1989): Molecular genetics of familial Alzheimer's disease. Eur Neurol 29(Suppl 3):25–27.

St. George-Hyslop PH, Tanzi RE, Polinsky RJ, Haines JL, Nee L, Watkins PC, Myers RH, Feldman RG, Pollen D, Drachman D, Growdon J, Bruni A, Foncin J-F, Salmon D, Frommelt P, Amaducci L, Sorbi S, Piacantini S, Stewart GD, Hobbes WJ, Conneally PM, Gusella JF (1987): The genetic defect causing familial Alzheimer's disease maps on chromosome 21. Science 235:885–890.

Saunders AM, Schmader K, Breitner JCS, Benson MD, Brown WT, Goldfarb L, Goldgaber D, Manwaring MG, Szymanski MH, McCown N, Dole KC, Schmechel DE, Strittmatter WJ, Pericak-Vance MA, Roses AD (1993a): Apolipoprotein E epsilon 4 allele distributions in late-onset Alzheimer's disease and in other amyloid-forming diseases. Lancet 342:710–711.

Saunders AM, Strittmatter WJ, Schmechel D, St. George-Hyslop PH, Pericak-Vance MA, Joo SH, Rosi BL, Gusella JF, Crapper-MacLachlan DR, Alberts MJ, Hulette C, Crain B, Goldgaber D, Roses AD (1993b): Association of apolipoprotein E allele E4 with late-onset familial and sporadic Alzheimer's disease. Neurology 43:1467–1472.

Schellenberg GD, Payami H, Wijsman EM, Orr HT, Goddard KAB, Anderson L, Nemens E, White JA, Alonso ME, Ball MJ, Kaye J, Morris JC, Chui H, Sadovnick AD, Heston LL, Martin GM, Bird TD (1993): Chromosome 14 and late-onset familial Alzheimer's disease (FAD). Am J Hum Genet 53:619–628.

Schellenberg GD, Bird TD Wijsman EM, Orr HY, Anderson L, Nemens E, White JA, Bonny-castle L, Weber JL, Alonso ME, Potter H, Heston LL, Martin GM (1992): Genetic link-age evidence for a familial Alzheimer's disease locus on chromosome 14. Science 258:668–671.

Schellenberg GD, Pericak-Vance MA, Wijsman EM, Moore DK, Gaskell PCJ, Yamaoka LA, Bebout JL, Anderson L, Welsh KA, Clark CM, Martin GM, Roses AD, Bird TD (1991): Linkage analysis of familial Alzheimer disease, using chromosome 21 markers. Am J Hum Genet 48:563–583.

Schellenberg GD, Bird TD, Wijsman EM, Moore DK, Boehnke M, Bryant EM, Lampe TH, Nochlin D, Sumi SM, Deeb SS, Beyreuther K, Martin GM (1988): Absence of linkage of chromosome 21q21 markers to familial Alzheimer's disease. Science 241:1507–1510.

Schellenberg GD, Deeb SS, Boehnke M, Bryant EM, Martin GM, Lampe TH, Bird TD (1987): Association of an apolipoprotein CII allele with familial dementia of the Alzheimer type. J Neurogenet 4:97–108.

Scheuner D, Eckman C, Jensen M, Song X, Citron M, Suzuki N, Bird TD, Hardy J, Hutton M, Kukull W, Larson E, Levy-Lahad E, Viitanen M, Poskind E, Poorkaj P, Schellenberg G, Tanzi R, Wasco W, Lannfelt L, Selkoe D, Younkin S (1996): Secreted amyloid β-pro-tein similar to that in the senile plaques of Alzheimer's disease is increased in vivo by the presenilin 1 and 2 and APP multations linked to familial Alzheimer's disease. Nature Medicine 2:864–870.

Schottky J (1932): Uber Prasenile Verblodungen. Z Neurol Psychol 140:333–397.

Seubert P, Vigo-Pelfrey C, Esch F, Lee M, Dovey H, Davis D, Sinha S, Schlossmacher M, Whaley J, Swindlehurst C, McCormack R, Wolfert R, Selkoe D, Lieberburg I, Schenk D (1992): Isolation and quantification of soluble Alzheimer's β-peptide from biological flu-ids. Nature 359:325–327.

Sherrington R, Rogaev E, Liang Y, Rogaeva E, Levesque G, Ikeda M, Chi H, Lin C, Holman K, Tsuda T, Mar L, Foncin J-F, Bruni A, Montsei M, Sorbi S, Rainero I, Pinessi L, Nee L, Chumakov I, Pollen D, Brookes A, Sanseau P, Polinsky R, Wasco W, da Silva H, Haines J, Pericak-Vance M, Tanzi R, Roses A, Fraser P, Rommens J, St. George-Hyslop P (1995): Cloning of a gene bearing mis-sense mutations in early-onset familial Alzheimer's disease. Nature 375:754–760.

Shoji M, Golde T, Ghiso J, Cheung TT, Estus S, Shaffer LM, Cai X-D, McKay DM, Tintner R, Frangione B, Younkin SG (1992): Production of the Alzheimer amyloid beta-protein by normal proteolytic processing. Science 258:126–129.

Sisodia S, Koo E, Beyreuther K, Unterbeck A, Price D (1990): Evidence that beta-amy-loid protein in Alzheimer's disease is not derived by normal processing. Science 248:492–494.

Sorbi S, Nacmias B, Forleo P, Latorraca S, Gobbini I, Bracco L, Piacentini S, Amaducci L (1994): ApoE allele frequencies in Italian sporadic and familial Alzheimer's disease. Neu-rosci Lett 177:100–102.

Sorbi S, Nacmias B, Forleo P, Piacentini S, Amaducci L (1993): APP717 and Alzheimer's disease in Italy. Nat Genet 4:10.

Strittmatter WJ, Saunders AM, Schmechel D, Pericak-Vance M, Enghild J, Salvesen GS, Roses AD (1993): High-avidity binding to β-amyloid and increased frequency of type 4 allele in late-onset familial Alzheimer disease. Proc Natl Acad Sci U S A 90:1977–1981.

Suzuki T, Nishiyama K, Murayama S, Yamamoto A, Sato S, Kanazawa I, Sakaki Y (1996): Regional and cellular presenilin 1 gene expression in human and rat tissues. Biochem Biophys Res Commun 218:708–713.

Suzuki N, Cheung T, Cai X-D, Odaka A, Otvos L, Eckman C, Golde T, Younkin S (1994): An increased percentage of long amyloid β protein secreted by familial amyloid β protein precursor (βAPP717) mutants. Science 264:1336–1340.

Takahashi H, Murayama M, Takashima A, Mercken M, Nakazato Y, Noguchi K, Imahori K (1996): Molecular cloning and expression of the rat homologue of presenilin-1. Neurosci Lett 206:113–116.

Talbot C, Lendon C, Craddock N, Shears S, Morris JC, Goate A (1994): Protection against Alzheimer's disease with apoE epsilon 2. Lancet 343:1432–1433.

Tamaoka A, Odaka A, Ishibashi Y, Usami M, Sahara N, Suzuki N, Nukina N, Mizusawa H, Shoji S, Kanazawa I, Mari H (1994): APP717 missense mutation affects the ratio of amyloid beta protein species (A beta 1-42/43 and a beta 1-40) in familial Alzheimer's disease brain. J Biol Chem 269:32721–32724.

Tanzi RE, Gusella JF, Watkins PC, Bruns GA, St. George-Hyslop P, Van Keuren ML, Patterson D, Pagan S, Kurnit DM, Neve RL (1987a): Amyloid beta protein gene: cDNA, mRNA distribution, and genetic linkage near the Alzheimer locus. Science 235:880–884.

Tanzi RE, St. George-Hyslop PH, Haines JL, Polinsky RJ, Nee L, Foncin JF, Neve RL, McClatchey AI, Conneally PM, Gusella JF (1987b): The genetic defect in familial Alzheimer's disease is not tightly linked to the amyloid beta-protein gene. Nature 329:156–157.

Tsai M-S, Tangalos EG, Peterson RC, Smith GE, Schaid DJ, Kokmen E, Ivnik RJ, Thibodeau SN (1994): Apolipoprotein E: Risk factor for Alzheimer disease. Am J Hum Genet 54:643–649.

Tsuda T, Chi H, Liang Y, Rogaeva EA, Sherrington R, Levesque G, Ikeda M, Rogaev EI, Pollen D, Freedman M, Duara R, St. George-Hyslop PH (1995): Failure to detect missense mutations in the S182 gene in a series of late-onset Alzheimer's disease cases. Neurosci Lett 201:188–190.

van Broeckhoven C, Backhovens H, Cruts M, Martin JJ, Crook R, Houlden H, Hardy J (1994): APOE genotype does not modulate age of onset in families with chromsome 14 encoded Alzheimer's disease. Neurosci Lett 169:179–180.

van Broeckhoven C, Backhovens H, Cruts M, De Winter G, Bruyland M, Cras P, Martin J-J (1992): Mapping of a gene predisposing to early-onset Alzheimer's disease to chromosome 14q24.3. Nat Genet 2:335–339.

van Broeckhoven C, Genthe AM, Vandenberghe A, Horsthemke B, Backhovens H, Raeymaekers P, van Hul W, Wehnert A, Gheuens J, Cras P, Bruyland M, Martin J-J, Salbaum M, Multhaup G, Masters CL, Beyreuther K, Gurling HMD, Mullan MJ, Holland A, Barton A, Irving N, Williamson R, Richards SJ, Hardy JA (1987): Failure of familial Alzheimer's disease to segregate with the A4-amyloid gene in several European families. Nature 329:153–155.

van Duijn CM, de Knijff P, Wehnert A, De Voecht J, Bronzova JB, Havekes LM, Hofman A, van Broeckhoven C (1995): The apolipoprotein E epsilon 2 allele is associated with an increased risk of early-onset Alzheimer's disease and a reduced survival. Ann Neurol 37:605–610.

van Duijn CM, Henriks L, Cruts M, Hardy JA, Hofman A, van Broeckhoven CM (1991a): Amyloid precursor protein gene mutation in early-onset Alzheimer's disease. Lancet 337:978.

van Duijn CM, Clayton D, Chandra V, Fratiglioni L, Graves AB, Heyman A, Jorm AF, Kokmen E, Kondo K, Mortimer JA, Rocca WA, Shalat SL, Soininen H, Hofman A (1991b): Familial aggregation of Alzheimer's disease and related disorders: A collaborative re-analysis of case-control studies. Int J Epidemiol 20 (Suppl 2):S13–S20.

van Duijn CM, Stijnen T, Hofman A (1991c): Risk factors of Alzheimer's disease: Overview of the EURODEM collaborative re-analysis of case-control studies. Int J Epidemiol 20(Suppl 2):S4–S12.

Verdoon T, Burnashev N, Monyer H, Seeburg P, Sakmann B (1991): Structural determinants of ion flow through recombinant glutamate receptor channels. Science 252:1715–1718.

Vito P, Lacana E, D'Adamio L (1996): Interfering with apoptosis: $Ca2^+$-binding protein ALG-2 and Alzheimer's disease gene ALG-3. Science 271:521–525.

Wasco W, Pettingell WP, Jondro PD, Schmidt SD, Gurubhagavatula S, Rodes L, DiBlasi T, Romano DM, Guenette SY, Kovacs DM, Growdon JH, Tanzi RE (1995): Familial Alzheimer's chromosome 14 mutations. Nat Med 1:848.

Wisniewski T, Palha JA, Ghiso J, Frangione B (1995): S182 protein in Alzheimer's disease neuritic plaques. Lancet 346:1366.

Wragg M, Hutton M, Talbot C, Busfield F, Han SW, Lendon C, Clark RF, Morris JC, Edwards D, Goate A, Pfeiffer E, Crook R, Prihar G, Phillips H, Baker M, Hardy J, Rossor M, Houlden H, Karran E, Roberts G, Craddock N (1996): Genetic association between intronic polymorphism in presenilin-1 gene and late-onset Alzheimer's disease. Lancet 347:509–512.

Yoshioka K, Miki T, Katsuya T, Ogihara T, Sakaki Y (1991): The 717Val→Ile substitution in amyloid precursor protein is associated with familial Alzheimer's disease regardless of ethnic groups. Biochem Biophys Res Commun 178:1141–1146.

Yoshizawa T, Yamakawa-Kobayashi K, Komatsuzaki Y,Arinami T, Oguni E, Mizusawa H, Shoji S, Hamaguchi H (1994): Dose-dependent association of apolipoprotein E allele epsilon 4 with late-onset, sporadic Alzheimer's disease. Ann Neurol 36:656–659.

Yu C, Payami H, Olson JM, Boehnke M, Wijsman EM, Orr HT, Kukull WA, Goddard KA, Nemens E, White JA, Alonso ME, Taylor TD, Ball MJ, Kaye J, Morris J, Chui H, Sadovnick AD, Martin GM, Larson EB, Heston LL, Bird TD, Schellenberg GD (1994): The apolipoprotein E/CI/CII gene cluster and late-onset Alzheimer disease. Am J Hum Genet 54:631–642.

Zubenko GS, Farr J, Stiffler JS, Hughes HB, Kaplan BB (1992): Clinically silent mutation in the putative iron-responsive element in exon 17 of the β-amyloid precursor protein gene. J Neuropathol Exp Neurol 51:459–463.

CHAPTER 10

Neurofibrillary Tangles in Alzheimer's Disease: Clinical and Pathological Implications

CHRISTOPHER M. CLARK, JOHN Q. TROJANOWSKI, and
VIRGINIA M.-Y. LEE

Departments Neurology (C.M.C.) and Pathology and Laboratory Medicine (J.Q.T. and V.M.-Y.L.), University of Pennsylvania, School of Medicine, Philadelphia, Pennsylvania 19104

INTRODUCTION

Alzheimer's disease (AD) is a heterogeneous adult-onset neurodegenerative dementia characterized by a common set of clinical and pathological features. The diagnosis is defined clinically by impairments in memory, language, judgment, and praxis with confused thinking and often coexisting behavioral changes. The common pathological features include massive neuron loss, neuritic plaques, and neurofibrillary tangles (NFT) in the brain (Cotman et al., 1994; Su et al., 1994a; Johnson, 1994; Cotman and Anderson, 1995; Smale et al., 1995). The heterogeneous nature of the clinical picture is evident by variations in the age of onset, degree of language involvement, presence of extrapyramidal signs (parkinsonism), and expression of psychotic symptoms. The pathological heterogeneity includes variations in the anatomic distribution, frequency, and relative predominance of the two hallmark lesions of neuritic amyloid plaques, and NFTs (Arnold et al., 1991). In some cases the pathologic spectrum broadens to include intraneuronal deposits of neurofilaments (Lewy bodies) (Hulette et al., 1995).

From an etiologic standpoint, the heterogeneous nature of AD is evident by the identification of specific genetic mutations on chromosomes 21 (Mullan et al., 1992; Crawford and Goate, 1992; Liepnieks et al., 1993; Zeldenrust et al., 1993;

Pharmacological Treatment of Alzheimer's Disease: Molecular and Neurobiological Foundations,
Edited by Brioni and Decker
ISBN 0-471-16758-4   © 1997 Wiley-Liss, Inc.

Levy-Lahad et al., 1995b), 14 (Sherrington et al., 1995), and 1 (Levy-Lahad et al., 1995a,b) that are independently associated with the phenotypic expression of AD. The functional nature of the gene products have yet to be fully characterized, but all are membrane-spanning proteins.

Neurofibrillary tangles represent the pathological component that correlates best with the dementia severity, but both plaques and tangles are required to establish a diagnosis of definite AD. Yet it remains unclear if their presence is the result of the convergence of a variety of etiologically unique pathological cascades or if there may also be a process uniquely responsible for the production of plaques and tangles that are sufficient to produce the clinical and pathological expression of AD. Thus there may be a spectrum of pathological processes capable of producing plaques, tangles, and neuronal loss, some of which will be dependent on specific etiologic mechanisms.

Importance of Tau in AD

A common feature of AD and several other late-life neurodegenerative diseases associated with neuronal loss is the disruption of the neuronal cytoskeleton. Neurofilaments, which play a major role in maintaining the structure of neurons, and microtubules (MT), which are required to transport products between the cell body and the distal portions of the axons and dendrites, are two key cytoskeletal organelles responsible for maintaining the structural and functional integrity of the neuron.

Understanding the role played by the microtubule-associated protein tau in the assembly and stabilization of the microtubular system, its disruption, and the subsequent formation of NFTs composed of hyperphosphorylated tau is important for the following reasons:

1. The formation of NFTs may be a key step leading to the death of the neuron and the clinical expression of AD.
2. The identification of specific isoforms of tau in the cerebral spinal fluid (CSF) may serve as a sensitive marker of neuronal death and a specific diagnostic marker for AD.
3. Changes in the CSF levels of specific tau isoforms may serve as an in vivo marker of the progression of AD pathology, and thus provide an early objective measure of response to treatment.

Role of Tau in the Normal Brain

Tau consists of six alternatively spliced protein isoforms in the brain that are encoded by the same gene (Figure 1).

Each tau isoform contains either 3 or 4 consecutive MT binding motifs that are imperfect repeats of 31 or 32 amino acids [see Goedert (1993) for a review]. These isoforms also differ with respect to the presence or absence of 29 or 58 amino acids length polypeptides in the amino-terminal third of the protein. In contrast to the MT binding motifs, the function of these amino-terminal inserts is unknown. As a result of the alternative splicing of these different inserts, central nervous system (CNS) tau pro-

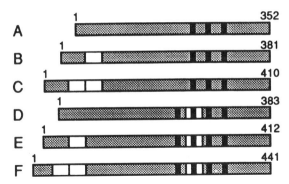

FIGURE 1. Schematic of the six isoforms of human adult tau. The number of amino acids for each isoform is noted at the carboxy end. The stippled areas indicate the regions that are common to all six isoforms. The white areas mark the location of the amino acid inserts that are used to distinguish among the isoforms. The black areas represent the tandem MT-binding repeats. Fetal brain contains only the 352 amino acid isoform (labeled A). Adult brain contains all six isoforms (labeled A through F). (Modified from The Neurofibrillary Pathology of Alzheimer's Disease in The Molecular and Genetic Basis of Neurological Disease, Second Ed., Rosenberg, RN, Prusiner SB, DiMauro S, Banchi RL, eds. [In Press] Newton MA: Butterworth Heinemann).

teins range in size from 441 amino acids in length containing 4 repeated MT binding motifs and a 58-amino-acid-long amino-terminal insert to 352 amino acids containing 3 consecutive MT binding repeats and no amino-terminal inserts. The shortest tau isoform, referred to as the "fetal" isoform, is the first to be expressed in the developing human nervous system. The other 5 alternatively spliced tau isoforms appear at a later point in development. Thus, the adult brain contains 5 "adult" and one fetal isoform.

As part of the neuronal cytoskeleton, tau proteins bind to MTs in a dynamic process to facilitate the polymerization of tubulin subunits into MTs and stabilize the newly formed MTs (Goedert, 1993; Goode and Feinstein, 1994; Matus, 1994; Trojanowski and Lee, 1994b). In the CNS they are present in neurons (Lee et al., 1991; Lee and Trojanowski, 1992) and to a lesser extent in astrocytes and oligodendrocytes (LoPresti et al., 1995). The major role of MTs is to facilitate transport of material from the cell body to the distal portions of the cell processes. Failure to maintain this transport system could lead to cell dysfunction and the eventual death of neurons. There is mounting evidence that disruption of transport in neurons could lead to their demise and thus play a major role in the pathology of AD (Trojanowski et al., 1993; Goedert et al., 1993; Trojanowski and Lee, 1994; Cotman and Anderson, 1995; Smale et al., 1995).

In the healthy neuron, the assembled MTs are most prominent in the axons and dendrites of neurons. The details of how this multistepped assembly occurs and the methods by which it is controlled remain unclear. The expression of tau and its role in the assembly and stabilization of MTs has been the subject of a number of comprehensive reviews (Mandelkow et al., 1993; Kosik, 1993; Behar et al., 1995). In addition to its role in facilitating intraneuronal transport, tau plays a part in supporting the outgrowth of neuronal processes (Shea et al., 1992).

Excessively Phosphorylated Tau as the Major Component of the NFT of AD

The role of tau in the formation of NFTs has been the subject of several reviews (Mandelkow and Mandelkow 1993; Goedert, 1993; Trojanowski et al. 1993; Trojanowski and Lee, 1994a; Mandelkow and Mandelkow, 1994, Goedert et al., 1995). Evidence that altered forms of tau comprise the core component of the paired helical filaments (PHFs) in AD NFTs comes from a number of observations. Electron micrographs (Figure 2) demonstrate that NFTs in AD are primarily composed of PHFs formed from aggregates of excessively phosphorylated tau.

These aggregates accumulate in the cell body and processes (axons and dendrites) of selectively vulnerable neuronal populations in the brain, especially in the amygdala, hippocampal formation, and neocortex (Bondareff et al., 1994). All six isoforms of tau are found in the PHFs or NFTs (Goedert et al., 1992).

The pathological cascade responsible for converting normally phosphorylated MT-associated tau to the hyperphosphorylated aggregates that make up the PHFs is not well understood. However, there is a growing line of evidence that supports the fact that hyperphosphorylated tau (also known as PHF-tau) is the primary component of the PHFs (Lee et al., 1991; Lee and Trojanowski, 1992; Trojanowski et al., 1993; Trojanowski and Lee, 1994b; Trojanowski and Lee, 1995).

Ion spray mass spectrometry studies of tau followed by sequencing of ethanethiol modified peptides have identified 19 of the 21 known phosphorylation sites (Figure 3). This schematic also indicates the approximate location of selected monoclonal and polyclonal antibody epitope sites on tau.

Table 1 compares the phosphorylation sites identified on normal biopsy-derived tau, PHF-tau, and fetal tau. All but serine-262 are located in the amino- and carboxyl-terminal flanking regions of the MT binding domain (Morishima-Kawashima et al., 1995). Eleven of the sites are known to be normally phosphorylated in the fetal tau isofom. Eleven sites are adjacent to a proline residue and are felt to be phosphorylated by proline-dependent protein kinases (PDPKs) (Singh et al., 1995b). Thus in the hyperphosphorylated state PHF-tau has an excessive number of its potential phosphate accepting sites occupied.

The mechanism responsible for the accumulation of this excessive phosphate load in PHF-tau is unclear. Since the addition and removal of phosphates from tau is a dynamic process in the life of a healthy neuron, inquiry has focused on enzymes and signaling processes involved in these two events. Protein phosphatase 2A and 2B are capable of removing phosphates in a site-specific manner from PHF-tau (Gong et al., 1994), raising the possibility that deficiencies in the activity of one or both could result in hyperphosphorylation of tau (Mawal-Dewan et al., 1994; Gong et al., 1994).

On the other side of the coin, in vitro studies demonstrate that both PDPKs such as mitogen-activated protein (MAP) kinases, glycogen synthase kinase 3 (Hanger et al., 1992; Mandelkow et al., 1992; Ishiguro et al., 1993), and cyclin-dependent kinase 5 (CDK5) (Baumann et al., 1993; Lew and Wang, 1995) as well as non-proline-dependent protein kinases (non-PDPKs) such as cyclic adenosine

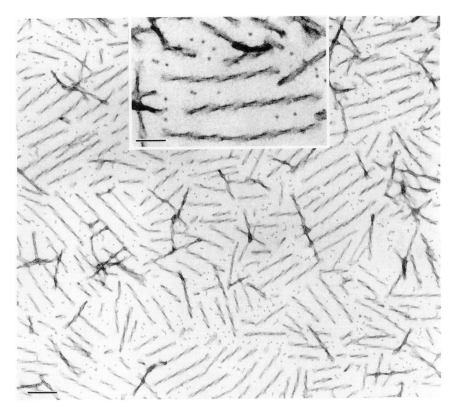

FIGURE 2. Electron micrograph of a preparation of human brain PHF-tau. The 12-mm scale bar in the lower left of the micrograph = 200 nm. The 12-mm scale bar in the lower left of the enlargement insert = 100 nm.

monophosphate (AMP)-dependent phosphokinase A, calcium/phospholipid-dependent phosphokinase C, casein kinase-1, casein kinase-2, and calcium/calmodulin-dependent protein kinase II, and a newly identified kinase known as p110[mark] (Drewes et al., 1995) are capable of adding excessive phosphate residues to tau (Singh et al., 1995a). Further, there may be a site-specific hierarchy with respect to the abnormal accumulation of phosphates at sites in PHF-tau (Su et al., 1994b). Table 2 contains a list of enzymes thought to play a role in the addition and removal of phosphate residues.

Strong evidence for a role for PHF-tau in producing the clinical features of AD comes from the relationship between the neuroanatomic distribution of the tangles and the clinical symptoms of dementia. The earliest pathological changes are found in the entorhinal cortex and hippocampus. This correlates with the observation that mild memory loss is the most common clinical feature in the earliest stage of AD. However, there is no evidence that NFTs in the entorhinal cortex and hippocampus

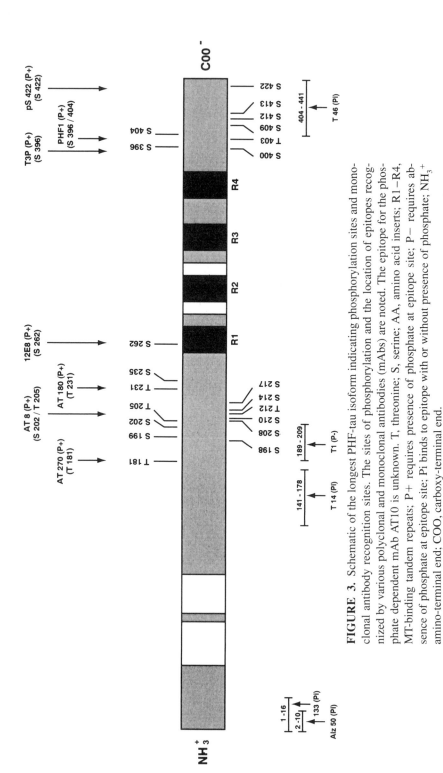

FIGURE 3. Schematic of the longest PHF-tau isoform indicating phosphorylation sites and monoclonal antibody recognition sites. The sites of phosphorylation and the location of epitopes recognized by various polyclonal and monoclonal antibodies (mAbs) are noted. The epitope for the phosphate dependent mAb AT10 is unknown. T, threonine; S, serine; AA, amino acid inserts; R1–R4, MT-binding tandem repeats; P+ requires presence of phosphate at epitope site; P– requires absence of phosphate at epitope site; Pi binds to epitope with or without presence of phosphate; NH_3^+ amino-terminal end; COO, carboxy-terminal end.

TABLE 1. Phosphorylation Sites Identified on PHF-Tau, Fetal Tau, and Biopsy Tau

Site	PHF-Tau[b]	Fetal Tau[b]	PHF-Tau[c]	Fetal Tau[c]	Biopsy Tau[c]
SP 46					
TP 181		P	P	P	P
S 198	P	P			
SP 199	P	P			
SP 202	P	P	P	P	P
TP 205			P	P	P
S 208	P				
S 210	P				
TP 212	P				
S 214	P				
TP 217	P	P			
TP 231	P	P	P	P	P
SP 235	P	P	P	P	P
S 262	P		P	P	P
S 324					
S 356					
SP 396	P	P	P	P	P
S 400	P	P			
T 403	P				
SP 404	P	P	P	P	P
S 409	P	P			
S 412	P				
S 413	P	P	P	P	P
S 416					
SP 422	P		P	P	P

[a]S, serine; SP, serine-proline; T, threonine; TP, threonine-proline.

[b]Phosphorylation sites on tau identified by chemical analysis.

[c]Phosphorylation sites identified by phosphorylation-dependent, site-specific monoclonal antibody.

are sufficient to produce symptoms of dementia since it is well known that a small number of tangles occurs in these same regions in healthy elderly individuals. Their presence may serve as a partial explanation for the clinical symptom of age-associated memory impairment (AAMI) (Crook et al., 1990). There are no unique molecular or structural characteristics that distinguish tangles associated with this "normal" age-related change from those associated with dementia. Only the number and extent of brain involvement separates individuals with AAMI from patients who have clinical symptoms of dementia. The extension of NFTs to the association neocortex appears to be one critical threshold in that even patients with mild dementia almost invariably have tangles in the association neocortex.

Further, the accumulation of abnormally phosphorylated PHF-tau is associated with a reduction in the amount of normal tau (Bramblett et al., 1992). Cortical areas that have the highest amount of normal tau seem to be most vulnerable to pathological conversion to the hyperphosphorylated state (Holzer et al., 1994).

**TABLE 2. Candidate Enzymes Involved in the
Addition and Removal of Phosphate from Tau**

Kinases
    Mitogen-activated protein (MAP) kinases
    Glycogen synthase 3 (GSK3)
    Cdk5
    Cdc2 kinase
    Proline-directed kinase and cdc2-like kinase
    110 kD protein kinase
Phosphatases
    Protein phosphatase 2A (PP2A)
    Protein phosphatase 2B (PP2B) or calcineurin

Studies demonstrating the difference between tau from patients with AD and nondemented elderly subjects have almost exclusively relied upon postmortem evaluations. This raised the possibility that some (or all) of the differences between normal tau and PHF-tau could be due to their differential sensitivity to dephosphorylation after death. To evaluate this possibility, the phosphorylation state of tau in cortical samples of normal brain tau isolated from surgical specimens from adult patients undergoing temporal lobe resection for treatment of epilepsy was compared to postmortem PHF-tau from patients with AD (Matsuo et al., 1994). Quite unexpectedly these studies showed that tau isolated from the surgical specimens was phosphorylated at many of the same sites as the PHF-tau isolated from postmortem AD brains. The implication of this finding was that autopsy-derived adult human tau from cognitively normal subjects must undergo more rapid in situ postmortem dephosphorylation than PHF-tau in the AD brain. In the surgical specimens protein phosphatases 2A (PP2A) and 2B (PP2B) dephosphorylated tau in a site-specific manner. Thus, one possible explanation for the formation of PHFs is that the normal removal of phosphates from tau is due to a down-regulation of phosphatases (i.e., PP2A and PP2B) in the brains of patients with AD thereby leading to the production of maximally phosphorylated tau accompanied by the loss of the ability of tau to bind MTs and the subsequent aggregation of PHF-tau into the abnormal filaments found in NFTs and dystrophic neurites.

Aluminum, Zinc, and Other Factors that May Influence Tau Hyperphosphorylation

In addition to specific kinases and phosphatases, cellular components that colocalize with tangles may alter the microenvironment in a manner that promotes excessive phosphorylation. Initial studies demonstrated not only that aluminum is a component of neuritic plaques (Candy et al., 1986), but it also colocalizes with NFTs (Perl and Brody, 1980; Perl, 1985; Perl and Good, 1991, 1992; Good et al., 1992). The ability to induce tanglelike lesions in the brains of rabbits or rodents exposed to aluminum (Pendlebury et al., 1988; Kowall et al., 1989; Shin et al., 1994; Savory et al., 1995) and the report of a higher than expected incidence of dementia in subjects exposed to aluminum in drinking water (Martyn et al., 1989) provided intriguing support for the notion that aluminum may somehow facilitate the neurofibrillary cascade.

Further support came from in vitro experiements that demonstrated that aluminum chloride concentrations ranging from $10nM$ to $10\mu M$ could activate the phosphorylation of tau in the presence of P334, protein kinase P (PKP), and protein kinase C (PKC) (el-Sebae et al., 1993; Abdel-Ghany et al., 1993).

However, when exposed to higher concentrations of aluminum ($\geq 400\mu M$) tau aggregated but failed to form typical fibrillar structures characteristic of NFTs (Scott et al., 1993). This finding, as well as a microprobe analysis of autopsy tissue from patients with AD reporting accumulations of aluminum in both NFT-free and NFT-bearing neurons (Lovell et al., 1993), raises questions about the pathological significance of this metal in the formation of NFTs (Candy et al., 1992; Edwardson et al., 1992; Xu et al., 1992; Lovell et al., 1993, Tokutake et al., 1995). The argument that aluminum plays a direct role in the formation of NFTs was further weakened with the finding that in a cultured rat neuron model, aluminum-induced tangles were composed primarily of neurofilaments other than tau (Langui et al., 1990).

Thus, while it remains possible that aluminum serves as a cofactor in the abnormal phosphorylation of PHF-tau and/or the accumulation of PHFs in neurons of the AD brain, its precise role remains controversial.

The role of zinc in the assembly and stabilization of MTs remains equally unclear. There is a small amount of in vitro evidence documenting the ability of zinc to increase the rate of MT polymerization when it is added to a brain preparation from animals fed a zinc-deficient diet (Hesketh, 1984; Oteiza et al., 199a,b). However, the relevance of this to AD remains to be seen.

There are a number of other factors that may influence the degree to which tau is phosphorylated, including the redox potential in the neuron, which in turn may alter the oxidation state and presence of disulfide bridges on the protein (Schweers et al., 1995). Nonetheless, the potential significance of this finding remains to be determined.

NEUROFIBRILLARY TANGLES IN OTHER DISEASES

Although it has been well established that NFTs are not unique to AD, recent studies have shown that intraneuronal NFTs and tanglelike inclusions in glial cells can be found in a number of seemingly unrelated neurologic diseases and that the abnormal tau in these disorders is similar to PHF-tau in AD (Iwatsubo et al., 1994) (see Table 3).

The regional distribution of NFTs differs for each of these conditions. It matches the areas involved in the neuropathology and is consistent with what would be expected based on the clinical presentation of the illnesses.

Further, extensive neuron loss is a common element in each condition. In every

TABLE 3. Pathologic Conditions Associated with the Presence of Neurofibrillary Tangles

Alzheimer's disease
Down syndrome
Pick's disease
Progressive supranuclear palsy
Multisystem atrophy
Dementia pugilistica
Inclusion body myositis
Gerstmann–Straussler–Scheinker
Argyrophilic grain dementia
Amyotrophic lateral sclerosis/parkinsonism-dementia
     complex of Guam
Corticobasal degeneration
Progressive supranuclear palsy
Multiple system atrophy
Niemann–Pick's disease type C
Hallervorden–Spatz disease
Subacute sclerosing panencephalitis

instance the tangles represent aggregates of hyperphosphorylated tau, and the tau proteins in these disorders are abnormally phosphorylated at the same sites as PHF-tau in AD. However, the electrophoretic mobility of these abnormal tau proteins may differ from PHF-tau in AD as exemplified by progressive supranuclear palsy (Bancher et al., 1987; Schmidt et al., 1996).

Included in this group of diseases with prominent NFTs or tau-rich inclusions are Down syndrome (DS) (Giaccone et al., 1989; Flament et al., 1990), dementia pugilistica (Roberts et al., 1990; Allsop et al., 1990), inclusion body myositis (Askanas et al., 1994), Gerstmann–Straussler–Scheinker (GSS) (Ghetti et al., 1989; Giaccone et al., 1990; Tagliavini et al., 1993), argyrophilic grain dementia (Braak and Braak, 1987; Itagaki et al., 1989), amyotrophic lateral sclerosis/parkinsonism-dementia complex of Guam (ALS/PDC) (Hof et al., 1994; Buee-Scherrer et al., 1995), Pick's disease (Perry et al., 1987; Murayama et al., 1990), corticobasal degeneration (Mori et al., 1994; Wakabayashi et al., 1994; Ksiezak-Reding et al., 1994; Feany and Dickson, 1995), progressive supranuclear palsy, (Bancher et al., 1987; Giaccone et al., 1988; Flament et al., 1991), multiple system atrophy (Papp et al., 1989), Niemann–Pick disease type C (Suzuki et al., 1995; Love et al., 1995), Hallervorden–Spatz disease (Eidelberg et al., 1987), and subacute sclerosing panencephalitis (Mandybur et al., 1977; McQuaid et al., 1994).

In some of these diseases (i.e., DS, GSS, and ALS/PDC) the abnormal tau proteins have similar isoelectric and molecular weight characteristics as that found in AD PHF-tau (Flament et al., 1990; Tagliavini et al., 1993; Buee-Scherrer et al., 1995). In some of the others [progressive supranuclear palsy (PSP), corticobasal degeneration (CBD)], the abnormal tau isoforms appear different on Western blot analysis. (Flament et al., 1991, Ksiezak-Reding et al., 1994). Thus, while the hyperphosphorylation of tau in these other diseases resembles PHF-tau in AD, both the manner in which this occurs and the resulting end product may differ in a disease-specific manner.

Patients with DS are of particular interest as all who live beyond age 40 develop both NFTs and plaques. It is difficult to establish how often these changes are associated with the progressive loss of cognitive function characteristic of dementia because of the confounding conditions of mental retardation and coexisting neurological problems such as epilepsy. Tau mRNA may be up-regulated, although it is not clear how this effects its phosphorylation (Oyama et al., 1994).

CLINICAL RELEVANCE OF TAU IN AD

Relationship between NFTs and Dementia

In elderly subjects the number of NFTs found in the hippocampus and entorhinal cortex is age related, increasing with each year beyond the sixth decade. This may represent the subclinical expression of a universal age-related pathological process or simply reflect age-related changes without the potential for dementia (Vermersch et al., 1992). It is not known if these changes bear any relationship to the clinical entity of AAMI (Crook et al., 1990). Extension of NFTs to the neocortex may represent the threshold for dementia as preliminary studies indicate that the presence of more than a "rare" or "isolated" NFT in the neocortex is almost always associated with clinical signs of an Alzheimer-like dementia (Morris et al., 1991; Weisshaar and Matus, 1993).

The correlation between the number of NFTs and the severity of the dementia provides a strong argument that the presence of PHF-tau is detrimental to normal neuronal function and by implication, that it bears at least some responsibility for the decline in cognitive function. At the cellular level this is most likely related to a disruption in the MT-based transport system since hyperphosphorylated PHF-tau does not bind to MTs. The exact mechanism by which this results in the death of neurons remains to be elucidated, but it probably involves the loss of intracellular axonal transport of critical nutrients and trophic factors. This, in turn, could lead to a "dying back" of the axon with the loss of synaptic intercellular connections and the ultimate clinical expression of the cognitive disconnection syndrome of AD.

Additional evidence supporting the hypothesis that NFTs composed of PHF-tau can disrupt neuronal function comes from biochemical and neuropathological studies of the Guamanian Chamorro population with amyotrophic lateral sclerosis/parkinson dementia complex (ALS/PDC). The PHFs in the brains of these patients are structurally and immunologically similar to those seen in patients with AD (Hof et al., 1994; Buee-Scherrer et al., 1995). Since amyloid plaques, Lewy bodies, and other lesions associated with neurodegenerative diseases are rare to absent, this suggests that neuron death may be due to NFTs or some as yet unrecognized lesion. Additional support for the "cognitive toxicity" of NFTs comes from the recognition of patients with "tangle-only" AD-like dementia (Sumi et al., 1992; Hof et al., 1994; Bancher and Jellinger, 1994; Buee-Scherrer et al., 1995).

Thus, it seems reasonable that the progressive conversion of normal CNS tau into PHF-tau in the AD brain could lead to the degeneration or loss of corticocortical connections and incremental impairments of synaptic transmission followed by the emergence of the type of cognitive impairments seen in AD. Ultimately, the accumulation of PHFs in the neuron may disrupt critical cellular functions, including the entrapment of cellular organelles and blockage of both orthograde and retrograde intraneuronal transport, followed by the death of neurons.

As a final step in this scenario, cellular debris, including normal tau, Aβ, and fragments of amyloid precursor proteins (APPs) could be released into the extracellular space and contribute to amyloid plaque formation by serving as "pathological chaperones" or as a nidus for the aggregation and fibrillogenesis of constitutively secreted, extracellular Aβ.

As attractive as this hypothetical scenario may be, it remains just that. Simply a speculative model of one possible pathological cascade in what is undoubtedly a etiologically and pathologically multifaceted phenomenon.

Use of CSF Tau Levels as Diagnostic Marker for AD

Once it was established that NFTs were composed of aggregates of hyperphosphorylated tau (Lee et al., 1991), the next clinically relevant step was to see if the presence of abnormal amounts of tau in the CSF could serve as a diagnostic marker for PHF-related pathology (Mandelkow and Mandelkow, 1993). The results of such studies are encouraging but have fallen short of the ideal for a definitive diagnostic tool. Nevertheless, the studies are of major clinical importance. If a therapy is developed to either stop the pathological process or slow its rate of progression, it will be critical to make an accurate diagnosis as early in the course of the disease as possible. Indeed, the ideal time would be either just before the pathological lesions develop (at the earliest) or as soon as the first symptoms appear (at the latest).

There have been a number of studies reporting elevated CSF tau levels in patients with a clinical diagnosis of AD (Wang et al., 1991; Vandermeeren et al., 1993; Delacourte, 1994; Motter et al., 1995; Arai et al., 1995; Hock et al., 1995; Vigo-Pelfrey et al., 1995; Mori et al., 1995; Jensen et al., 1995; Munroe et al., 1995; Tato et al., 1995; Blennow et al., 1995) (see Table 4).

These studies used a variety of phosphate-dependent and phosphate-independent monoclonal antibodies capable of detecting tau levels as low as 5 pg/ml in unconcentrated CSF. There was no apparent difference in tau levels when antibodies that recognized specific phosphorylated epitopes were compared to those that recognized tau independent of its phosphorylation state. While there were statistically significant differences when the average tau level of patients with a clinical diagnosis of AD was compared to both normal subjects and those with other neurological conditions, there was some overlap between the three groups. Of the 401 AD patients evaluated, 62% had total tau levels that were above the cutoff for normal used in each study. The average value was 4.3 times the average level for the group of

TABLE 4. Studies Reporting CSF Levels of Tau in AD

	AD	
Study	N	% abn.
Vandermeeren et al. (1993)	27	81.5
Wang et al. (1991)	44	77.3
Blennow et al. (1995)	44	84.1
Munroe et al. (1995)	24	37.5
Jensen et al. (1995)	15	93.3
Mori et al. (1995)	14	100.0
Vigo-Pelfrey et al. (1995)	71	39.4
Arai et al. (1995)	70	94.3
Motter et al. (1995)	50	52.0
Totals	**401**	**62.3**

298 subjects in the combined normal cohort. However, almost 4% of these "neurologically normal" subjects had tau values that exceeded the cutoff. For some the elevated level may indicate the existence of a presymptomatic condition reflecting unrecognized neuropathology.

CSF tau levels were also measured in patients with a variety of other neurologic conditions. The lack of standardized diagnostic criteria across studies makes it difficult to evaluate the correlation between CSF tau levels and specific diseases. However, elevated levels were found in some (but not all) patients who had a clinical diagnosis of other neurologic conditions associated with inflammation, ischemia, hypoxia, or neurodegenerative conditions. Included in this list acquired immunodeficiency syndrome (AIDS), encephalitis, stroke, carbon monoxide poisoning, epilepsy, ALS, frontal lobe dementia, GSS, and Parkinson dementia (Table 5).

Undoubtedly the list will grow as investigators gain more experience using the assay in other neurological diseases.

Thus there are a number of factors that limit the diagnostic utility of a finding of elevated CSF tau levels. Among them is the pragmatic observation that the correlation between CSF tau levels and the underlying pathology is based on a premortem clinical diagnosis. In only a few subjects has the clinical diagnosis been confirmed by a postmortem evaluation. In expert hands, the clinical diagnosis of AD is confirmed at postmortem about 90% of the time. This gives an expected error rate of

TABLE 5. CSF Tau Results in Subjects Who Do Not Have a Clinical Diagnosis of AD

Clinical Diagnostic Category	Number	% > Upper Limit of Normal
Normal	155	3.9%
Neurodegenerative	89	22.5%
Vascular	39	69.2%
Inflammatory	64	43.8%

about 10% for these clinical studies. At best this could account for only a fraction of the clinically diagnosed AD patients who had normal tau levels. An additional fraction may represent variations of AD with low tangle counts, such as the Lewy body variant of AD. However, the true explanation will have to await autopsy analysis of the neuropathology found in those AD subjects who had low levels of CSF tau.

A somewhat surprising finding is the lack of a correlation between the CSF tau levels and the severity of the disease. This observation is based on cross-sectional analysis of the study cohorts rather than serial values in prospectively followed patients and thus must be interpreted with caution. There have been only a few anecdotal reports where repeated CSF tau measurements separated by intervals greater than 12 months were done in the same patient. However, the few that have been done failed to find an increase in CSF tau levels as the patient's disease progressed. One possible explanation for this finding would be the presence of a steady-state dynamic between the rate of neuronal death and progression of the disease.

When considered as a group, patients with AD tend to have the highest CSF tau levels. Nevertheless, they are also elevated in some patients with AIDS, carbon monoxide poisoning, ALS, encephalitis, and stroke, suggesting that CSF tau may simply be a marker for any lesion capable of producing significant neuronal cell death. Many of these conditions do not represent a differential diagnostic conundrum for experienced clinicians evaluating a patient with symptoms of dementia. However, distinguishing between various neurodegenerative causes of dementia, such as frontal lobe dementia, diffuse Lewy body disease, GSS syndrome, Creutzfeldt–Jakob disease, and ischemic vascular dementia can be clinically quite challenging. It is in sorting out of these disorders where a definitive diagnostic test would be most useful. So far the existing studies of CSF tau are not adequate to establish the diagnostic specificity of elevated tau levels in eliminating any of these conditions from consideration in the evaluation of an individual patient.

Ultimately the most useful CSF tau test will come with the identification of a specific PHF-tau epitope that is uniquely linked to AD. This could be on the basis of specific phosphorylation site on tau that only occurs in AD or the finding of a level of phosphorylation on a subset of the CSF tau proteins that occur only in the presence of NFTs. However, it may be that both normal and abnormal tau is modified by phosphatases after it is secreted into the CSF, thereby eliminating unique isoforms related to the presence of NFTs.

Implications for Treatment

Rational and effective treatments for AD will only come with a better understanding of conditions responsible for the key pathological processes responsible for the functional disruption of the neuron and ultimate neuronal death. Within the NFT cascade, efficacious treatment could come from agents that enhance the stability of the MT system, block the addition of excessive phosphate molecules to tau, remove phosphate residues from hyperphosphorylated tau, prevent the formation of NFTs, or enhance neuronal function in the face of accumulating PHFs.

CONCLUSION

AD is an etiologically heterogeneous neurodegenerative disorder of the elderly that produces a common set of hallmark pathological lesions (i.e., extracellular deposits of Aβ-rich amyloid plaques, intraneuronal neurofibrillary lesions) and a protean, yet recognizable, dementing syndrome characterized by memory loss, language impairment, apraxia, mental confusion, and behavioral changes.

This chapter has focused on the role of tau in the pathobiology of this disorder. We have discussed the physiologic role of normal tau in promoting MT formation and stability and how the conversion of tau to a hyperphosphorylated state could result in the disruption of the MT system and the formation of intracellular PHFs and NFTs with the eventual death of affected neurons. We have speculated on the possible mechanisms responsible for this pathological cascade and reviewed the supporting data.

We have also reviewed the implications that the expanding knowledge of tau has on the development of a diagnostic test for AD, which will be specific and sensitive in the course of the illness.

Lastly we have briefly reviewed points in the pathological cascade that may be appropriate therapeutic targets.

REFERENCES

Abdel-Ghany M, el-Sebae AK, Shalloway D (1993): Aluminum-induced nonenzymatic phospho-incorporation into human tau and other proteins. J Biol Chem 268: 11976–11981.

Allsop D, Haga S, Bruton C, Ishii T, Roberts GW (1990): Neurofibrillary tangles in some cases of dementia pugilistica share antigens with amyloid beta-protein of Alzheimer's disease. Am J Pathol 136:255–260.

Arai H, Terajima M, Miura M, Higuchi S, Muramatsu T, Machida NX, Seiki H, Takase S, Clark CM, Lee VM, Trojanowski JQ, Sasaki H (1995): Tau in cerebrospinal fluid: a potential diagnostic marker in Alzheimer's disease. Ann Neurol 38:649–652.

Arnold SE, Hyman BT, Flory J, Damasio AR, Van Hoesen GW (1991): The topographical and neuroanatomical distribution of neurofibrillary tangles and neuritic plaques in the cerebral cortex of patients with Alzheimer's disease. Cerebral Cortex 1:103–116.

Askanas V, Engel WK, Bilak M, Alvarez RB, Selkoe DJ (1994): Twisted tubulofilaments of inclusion body myositis muscle resemble paired helical filaments of Alzheimer brain and contain hyperphosphorylated tau. Am J pathol 144:177–187.

Bancher C, Jellinger KA (1994): Neurofibrillary tangle predominant form of senile dementia of Alzheimer type: A rare subtype in very old subjects. Acta Neuropathol 88:565–570.

Bancher C, Lassmann H, Budka H, Grundke-Iqbal I, Iqbal K, Wiche GX, Seitelberger F, Wisniewski HM (1978): Neurofibrillary tangles in Alzheimer's disease and progressive supranuclear palsy: antigenic similarities and differences. Microtubule-associated protein tau antigenicity is prominent in all types of tangles. Acta Neuropathol 74:39–46.

Baumann K, Mandelkow EM, Biernat J, Piwnica-Worms H, Mandelkow E (1993): Abnormal Alzheimer-like phosphorylation of tau-protein by cyclin-dependent kinases cdk2 and cdk5. FEBS Lett 336:417–424.

Behar L, Marx R, Sadot E, Barg J, Ginzburg I (1995): Cis-acting signals and trans-acting proteins are involved in tau mRNA targeting into neurites of differentiating neuronal cells. Int J Dev Neurosci 13:113–127.

Blennow K, Wallin K, Agren H, Spenger C, Siegfried J, Vanmechelen E (1995): Tau protein in cerebrospinal fluid. A biochemical marker for axonal degeneration in Alzheimer disease. Mol Chem Neuropathol 26:231–245.

Bondareff W, Harrington CR, McDaniel SW, Wischik CM, Roth M (1994): Presence of axonal paired helical filament-tau in Alzheimer's disease: Submicroscopic localization. J Neurosci Res 38:664–669.

Braak H, Braak E (1987): Argyrophilic grains: Characteristic pathology of cerebral cortex in cases of adult onset dementia without Alzheimer changes. Neurosci Lett 76:124–127.

Bramblett GT, Tronjanowski JQ, Lee VM (1992): Regions with abundant neurofibrillary pathology in human brain exhibit a selective reduction in levels of binding-competent tau and accumulation of abnormal tau-isoforms (A68 proteins). Lab Invest 66:212–222.

Buee-Scherrer V, Buee L, Hof PR, Leveugle B, Gilles C, Loerzel AJ, Perl DP, Delacourte A (1995): Neurofibrillary degeneration in amyotrophic lateral sclerosis/parkinsonism-dementia complex of Guam. Immunochemical characterization of tau proteins. Am J Pathol 146:924–932.

Candy JM, McArthur FK, Oakley AE, Taylor GA, Chen CPL-H, Mountfort SA, Thompson JE, Chalker PR, Bishop HE, Beyreuther K, Perry G, Ward MK, Martyn CN, Edwardson JA (1992): Aluminum accumulation in relation to senile plaque and neurofibrillary tangle formation in the brains of patients with renal failure. J Neurol Sci 107:210–218.

Candy JM, Oakley AE, Klinowski J, Carpenter TA, Perry RH, Atack JRX, Perry EK, Blessed G, Fairbairn A, Edwardson JA (1986): Aluminosilicates and senile plaque formation in Alzheimer's disease. Lancet 1:354–357.

Cotman CW, Anderson AJ (1995): A potential role for apoptosis in neurodegeneration and Alzheimer's disease. [Review]. Mol Neurobiol 10:19–45.

Cotman CW, Whittemore ER, Watt JA, Anderson AJ, Loo DT (1994): Possible role of apoptosis in Alzheimer's disease. [Review]. Ann N Y Acad Sci 747:36–49.

Crawford F, Goate A (1992): Alzheimer's disease untangled. [Review]. Bioessays 14:727–734.

Crook TH, Larrabee GJ, Youngjohn JR (1990): Diagnosis and assessment of age-associated memory impairment. [Review]. Clin Neuropharmacol 13(Suppl 3):S81–91.

Delacourte A (1994): Pathological tau proteins of Alzheimer's disease as a biochemical marker of neurofibrillary degeneration. [Review]. Biomed Pharmacother 48:287–295.

Drewes G, Trinczek B, Illenberger S, Biernat J, Schmitt-Ulms G, Meyer HE, Mandelkow EM, Mandelkow E (1995): Microtubule-associated protein/microtubule affinity-regulating kinase (p110mark). A novel protein kinase that regulates tau-microtubule interactions and dynamic instability by phosphorylation at the Alzheimer-specific site serine 262. J Biol Chem 270:7679–7688.

Edwardson JA, Candy JM, Ince PG, McArthur FK, Morris CM, Oakley AEX, Taylor GA, Bjertness E (1992): Aluminum accumulation, beta-amyloid deposition and neurofibrillary changes in the central nervous system. [Review]. Ciba Found Symp 169:165–179.

Eidelberg D, Sotrel A, Joachim C, Selkoe D, Forman A, Pendlebury WWX, Perl DP (1987): Adult onset Hallervorden-Spatz disease with neurofibrillary pathology. A discrete clinico-pathological entity. Brain 110:993–1013.

el-Sebae AH, Abdel-Ghany ME, Shalloway D, Abou Zeid MM, Blancato J, Saleh MA (1993): Aluminum interaction with human brain tau protein phosphorylation by various kinases. J Environ Sci Health [B] 28:763–777.

Feany MB, Dickson DW (1995): Widespread cytoskeletal pathology characterizes corticobasal degeneration. Am J Pathol 146:1388–1396.

Flament S, Delacourte A, Verny M, Hauw JJ, Javoy-Agid F (1991): Abnormal Tau proteins in progressive supranuclear palsy. Similarities and differences with the neurofibrillary degeneration of the Alzheimer type. Acta Neuropathol 81:591–596.

Flament S, Delacourte A, Mann DM (1990): Phosphorylation of Tau proteins: A major event during the process of neurofibrillary degeneration. A comparative study between Alzheimer's disease and Down's syndrome. Brain Res 516:15–19.

Ghetti B, Tagliavini F, Masters CL, Beyreuther K, Giaccone G, Verga L, Farlow MR, Conneally PM, Dlouhy SR, Azzarelli B, Bugiani O (1989): Gerstmann-Straussler-Scheinker disease. II. Neurofibrillary tangles and plaques with PrP-amyloid coexist in an affected family. Neurology 39:1453–1461.

Giaccone G, Tagliavini F, Linoli G, Bouras C, Frigerio L, Frangione B, Bugiani O (1989): Down patients: extracellular preamyloid deposits precede neuritic degeneration and senile plaques. Neurosci Lett 97:232–238.

Giaccone G, Tagliavini F, Street JS, Ghetti B, Bugiani O (1988): Progressive supranuclear palsy with hypertrophy of the olives. An immunocytochemical study of the cytoskeleton of argyrophilic neurons. Acta Neuropathol 77:14–20.

Giaccone G, Tagliavini F, Verga L, Frangione B, Farlow MR, Bugiani O, Ghetti B (1990): Neurofibrillary tangles of the Indiana kindred of Gerstmann-Straussler-Scheinker disease share antigenic determinants with those of Alzheimer disease. Brain Res 530:325–329.

Goedert M (1993): Tau protein and the neurofibrillary pathology of Alzheimer's disease. [Review]. Trends Neurosci 16:460–465.

Goedert M, Jakes R, Crowther RA, Six J, Lubke U, Vandermeeren M, Cras P, Trojanowski JQ, Lee VM (1993): The abnormal phosphorylation of tau protein at Ser-202 in Alzheimer disease recapitulates phosphorylation during development. Proc Nat Aca Sci U S A 90:5066–5070.

Goedert M, Jakes R, Vanmechelen E (1995): Monoclonal antibody AT8 recognises tau protein phosphorylated at both serine 202 and threonine 205. Neurosci Lett 189:167–169.

Goedert M, Spillantini MG, Cairns NJ, Crowther RA (1992): Tau proteins of Alzheimer paired helical filaments: Abnormal phosphorylation of all six brain isoforms. Neuron 8:159–168.

Gong CX, Grundke-Iqbal I, Iqbal K (1994): Dephosphorylation of Alzheimer's disease abnormally phosphorylated tau by protein phosphatase-2A. Neuroscience 61:765–772.

Good PF, Perl DP, Bierer LM, Schmeidler J (1992): Selective accumulation of aluminum and iron in the neurofibrillary tangles of Alzheimer's disease: a laser microprobe (LAMMA) study. Ann Neurol 31:286–292.

Goode BL, Feinstein SC (1994): Identification of a novel microtubule binding and assembly domain in the developmentally regulated inter-repeat region of tau. J Cell Biol 124:769–782.

Hanger DP, Hughes K, Woodgett JR, Brion JP, Anderton BH (1992): Glycogen synthase kinase-3 induces Alzheimer's disease-like phosphorylation of tau: Generation of paired helical filament epitopes and neuronal localisation of the kinase. Neurosc Lett 147:58–62.

Hesketh JE (1984): Microtubule assembly in rat brain extracts. Further characterization of the effects of zinc on assembly and cold stability. Int J Biochem 16:1331–1339.

Hock C, Golombowski S, Naser W, Muller-Spahn F (1995): Increased levels of tau protein in cerebrospinal fluid of patients with Alzheimer's disease—correlation with degree of cognitive impairment [letter]. Ann Neurol 37:414–415.

Hof PR, Nimchinsky EA, Buee-Scherrer V, Buee L, Nasrallah JX, Hottinger AF, Purohit DP, Loerzel AJ, Steele JC, Delacourte A (1994): Amyotrophic lateral sclerosis/parkinsonism-dementia complex of Guam: quantitative neuropathology, immunohistochemical analysis of neuronal vulnerability, and comparison with related neurodegenerative disorders. Acta Neuropathol 88:397–404.

Holzer M, Holzapfel HP, Zedlick D, Bruckner MK, Arendt T (1994): Abnormally phosphorylated tau protein in Alzheimer's disease: Heterogeneity of individual regional distribution and relationship to clinical severity. Neuroscience 63:499–516.

Hulette C, Mirra S, Wilkinson W, Heyman A, Fillenbaum G, Clark C (1995): The Consortium to Establish a Registry for Alzheimer's Disease (CERAD). Part IX. A prospective cliniconeuropathologic study of Parkinson's features in Alzheimer's disease. Neurology 45:1991–1995.

Ishiguro K, Shiratsuchi A, Sato S, Omori A, Arioka M, Kobayashi SX, Uchida T, Imahori K (1993): Glycogen synthase kinase 3 beta is identical to tau protein kinase I generating several epitopes of paired helical filaments. FEBS Lett 325:167–172.

Itagaki S, McGeer PL, Akiyama H, Beattie BL, Walker DG, Moore GRX, McGeer EG. (1989): A case of adult-onset dementia with argyrophilic grains. Ann Neurol 26:685–689.

Iwatsubo T, Hasegawa M, Ihara Y (1994): Neuronal and glial tau-positive inclusions in diverse neurologic diseases share common phosphorylation characteristics. Acta Neuropathol 88:129–136.

Jensen M, Basun H, Lannfelt L (1995): Increased cerebrospinal fluid tau in patients with Alzheimer's disease. Neurosci Lett 186:189–191.

Johnson EM, Jr (1994): Possible role of neuronal apoptosis in Alzheimer's disease. [Review]. Neurobiol Aging 15(Suppl 2): S187–189.

Kosik KS (1993): The molecular and cellular biology of tau. [Review]. Brain Pathol 3:39–43.

Kowall NW, Pendlebury WW, Kessler JB, Perl DP, Beal MF (1989): Aluminum-induced neurofibrillary degeneration affects a subset of neurons in rabbit cerebral cortex, basal forebrain and upper brainstem. Neuroscience 29:329–337.

Ksiezak-Reding H, Morgan K, Mattiace LA, Davies P, Liu WK, Yen SHX, Weidenheim K, et al. (1994): Ultrastructure and biochemical composition of paired helical filaments in corticobasal degeneration. Am J Pathol 145:1496–1508.

Langui D, Probst A, Anderton B, Brion JP, Ulrich J (1990): Aluminum-induced tangles in cultured rat neurones. Enhanced effect of aluminum by addition of maltol. Acta Neuropathol 80:649–655.

Lee VM, Trojanowski JQ (1992): The disordered neuronal cytoskeleton in Alzheimer's disease. [Review]. Curr Opin Neurobiol 2:653–656.

Lee VM, Balin BJ, Otvos L, Jr, Trojanowski JQ (1991): A68: A major subunit of paired helical filaments and derivatized forms of normal Tau. Science 251:675–678.

Levy-Lahad E, Wasco W, Poorkaj P, Romano DM, Oshima J, Pettingell WH, Yu C, Jondo PD, Schmidt SD, Wang K, Crowley AC, Fu YH, Guenette SY, Galas D, Nemens E, Wijsman EM, Bird TD, Schellenberg GD, Tanzi RE (1995): Candidate gene for the chromosome 1 familial Alzheimer's disease locus. Science 269:973–977.

Levy-Lahad E, Wijsman EM, Nemens E, Anderson L, Goddard KAB, Weber JL, Bird TD, Schellenberg GD (1995): A familial Alzheimer's disease locus on chromosome 1. Science 269:970–973.

Lew J, Wang JH (1995): Neuronal cdc2-like kinase. [Review]. Trends Biochem Sci 20:33–37.

Liepnieks JJ, Ghetti B, Farlow M, Roses AD, Benson MD (1993): Characterization of amyloid fibril beta-peptide in familial Alzheimer's disease with APP717 mutations. Biochem Biophys Res Commun 197:386–392.

LoPresti P, Szuchet S, Papasozomenos SC, Zinkowski RP, Binder LI (1995): Functional implications for the microtubule-associated protein tau: Localization in oligodendrocytes. Proc Nat Acad Sci U S A 92:10369–10373.

Love S, Bridges LR, Case CP (1995): Neurofibrillary tangles in Niemann-Pick disease type C. Brain 118:119–129.

Lovell MA, Ehmann WD, Markesbery WR (1993): Laser microprobe analysis of brain aluminum in Alzheimer's disease Ann Neurol 33:36–42.

Mandelkow EM, Mandelkow E (1994): Tau protein and Alzheimer's disease. [Review]. Neurobiol Aging 15(Suppl 2): S85–86.

Mandelkow EM, Mandelkow E (1993): Tau as a marker for Alzheimer's disease. [Review]. Trends Biochem Sci 18:480–483.

Mandelkow EM, Biernat J, Drewes G, Steiner B, Lichtenberg-Kraag B, Wille H, Gustke N, Mandelkow E (1993): Microtubule-associated protein tau, paired helical filaments, and phosphorylation. [Review]. Ann N Y Acad Sci 695:209–216.

Mandelkow EM, Drewes G, Biernat J, Gustke N, Van Lint J, Vandenheede JR, Mandelkow E (1992): Glycogen synthase kinase-3 and the Alzheimer-like state of microtubule-associated protein tau. FEBS Lett 314:315–321.

Mandybur TI, Nagpaul AS, Pappas Z, Niklowitz WJ (1977): Alzheimer neurofibrillary change in subacute sclerosing panencephalitis. Ann Neurol 1:103–107.

Martyn CN, Barker DJ, Osmond C, Harris EC, Edwardson JA, Lacey RF (1989): Geographical relation between Alzheimer's disease and aluminum in drinking water [see comments]. Lancet 1:59–62.

Matsuo ES, Shin RW, Billingsley ML, Van deVoorde A, O'Connor M, Trojanowski JQ, Lee VM (1994): Biopsy-derived adult human brain tau is phosphorylated at many of the same sites as Alzheimer's disease paired helical filament tau. Neuron 13:989–1002.

Matus A (1994): Stiff microtubules and neuronal morphology. [Review]. Trends Neurosci 17:19–22.

Mawal-Dewan M, Henley J, Van de Voorde A, Trojanowski JQ, Lee VM (1994): The phosphorylation state of tau in the developing rat brain is regulated by phosphoprotein phosphatases. J Biol Chem 269:30981–30987.

McQuaid S, Allen IV, McMahon J, Kirk J (1994): Association of measles virus with neurofibrillary tangles in subacute sclerosing panencephalitis: A combined in situ hybridization and immunocytochemical investigation. Neuropathol Appl Neurobiol 20:103–110.

Mori H, Hosoda K, Matsubara E, Nakamoto T, Furiya Y, Endoh R, Usami M, Shoji M, Maruyama S, Hirai S (1995): Tau in cerebrospinal fluids: establishment of the sandwich ELISA with antibody specific to the repeat sequence in tau. Neurosci Lett 186:181–183.

Mori H, Nishimura M, Namba Y, Oda M (1994): Corticobasal degeneration: A disease with widespread appearance of abnormal tau and neurofibrillary tangles, and its relation to progressive supranuclear palsy. Acta Neuropathol 88:113–121.

Morishima-Kawashima M, Hasegawa M, Takio K, Suzuki M, Yoshida H, Titani K, Ihara Y (1995): Proline-directed and non-proline-directed phosphorylation of PHF-tau. J Biol Chem 270:823–829.

Morris JC, McKeel DW, Jr, Storandt M, Rubin EH, Price JL, Grant EA, Ball MJ, Berg L (1991): Very mild Alzheimer's disease: informant-based clinical, psychometric, and pathologic distinction from normal aging [see comments]. Neurology 41:469–478.

Motter R, Vigo-Pelfrey C, Kholodenko D, Barbour R, Johnson-Wood KX, Galasko D, Chang L, Miller B, Clark C, Green R, Olson D, Southwick P, Wolfert R, Munroe B, Lieberburg I, Seubert P, Schenk D (1995): Reduction of beta-amyloid peptide42 in the cerebrospinal fluid of patients with Alzheimer's disease. Ann Neurol 38:643–648.

Mullan M, Crawford F, Axelman K, Houlden H, Lilius L, Winblad BX, Lannfelt L. (1992): A pathogenic mutation for probable Alzheimer's disease in the APP gene at the N-terminus of beta-amyloid. Nature Genet 1:345–347.

Munroe WA, Southwick PC, Chang L, Scharre DW, Echols CL, Jr, Fu PC, Whaley JM, Wolfert RL (1995): Tau protein in cerebrospinal fluid as an aid in the diagnosis of Alzheimer's disease. Ann Clin Lab Sci 25:207–217.

Murayama S, Mori H, Ihara Y, Tomonaga M (1990): Immunocytochemical and ultrastructural studies of Pick's disease. Ann Neurol 27:394–405.

Oteiza PI, Cuellar S, Lonnerdal B, Hurley LS, Keen CL (1990a): Influence of maternal dietary zinc intake on in vitro tubulin polymerization in fetal rat brain. Teratology 41:97–104.

Oteiza PI, Hurley LS, Lonnerdal B, Keen CL (1990b): Effects of marginal zinc deficiency on microtubule polymerization in the developing rat brain. Biol Trace Elem Res 24:13–23.

Oyama F, Cairns NJ, Shimada H, Oyama R, Titani K, Ihara Y (1994): Down's syndrome: Up-regulation of beta-amyloid protein precursor and tau mRNAs and their defective coordination. J Neurochem 62:1062–1066.

Papp MI, Kahn JE, Lantos PL (1989): Glial cytoplasmic inclusions in the CNS of patients with multiple system atrophy (striatonigral degeneration, olivopontocerebellar atrophy and Shy-Drager syndrome). J Neurol Sci 94:79–100.

Pendlebury WW, Beal MF, Kowall NW, Solomon PR (1988): Neuropathologic, neurochemical and immunocytochemical characteristics of aluminum-induced neurofilamentous degeneration. Neurotoxicology 9:503–510.

Perl DP (1985): Relationship of aluminum to Alzheimer's disease. Environ Health Perspect 63:149–153.

Perl DP, Good PF (1992): Aluminum and the neurofibrillary tangle: Results of tissue microprobe studies. [Review]. Ciba Found Symp 169:217–227.

Perl DP, Good PF (1991): Aluminum, Alzheimer's disease, and the olfactory system. [Review]. Ann N Y Acad Sci 640:8–13.

Perl DP, Brody AR (1980): Alzheimer's disease: X-ray spectrometric evidence of aluminum accumulation in neurofibrillary tangle-bearing neurons. Science 208:297–299.

Perry G, Stewart D, Friedman R, Manetto V, Autilio-Gambetti LX, Gambetti P (1987): Filaments of Pick's bodies contain altered cytoskeletal elements. Am J Pathol 127:559–568.

Roberts GW, Allsop D, Bruton C (1990): The occult aftermath of boxing. J Neurol Neurosurg Psychiatry 53:373–378.

Savory J, Huang Y, Herman MM, Reyes MR, Wills MR (1995): Tau immunoreactivity associated with aluminum maltolate-induced neurofibrillary degeneration in rabbits. Brain Res 669:325–329.

Schmidt ML, Huang R, Martin JA, Henley J, Mawal-Dewan M, Hurtig HI, Lee VM-Y, Trojanowski JQ (1996): Neurofibrillary tangles in progressive supranuclear palsy contain the same epitopes identified in Alzheimer's disease PHF-tau. J Neuropathol Exper Neurol 55:534–539.

Schweers O, Mandelkow EM, Biernat J, Mandelkow E (1995): Oxidation of cysteine-322 in the repeat domain of microtubule-associated protein tau controls the in vitro assembly of paired helical filaments. Proc Nat Acad Sci U S A 92:8463–8467.

Scott CW, Fieles A, Sygowski LA, Caputo CB (1993): Aggregation of tau protein by aluminum. Brain Res 628:77–84.

Shea TB, Beermann ML, Nixon RA, Fischer I (1992): Microtubule-associated protein tau is required for axonal neurite elaboration by neuroblastoma cells. J Neurosci Res 32: 363–374.

Sherrington R, Rogaev EI, Liang Y, Rogaeva EA, Levesque G, Ikeda M, Chi H, Lin C, Li G, Holman K, Tsuda R, Mar L, Foncin F-F, Bruni AC, Montesi MP, Sorbi S, Rainero I, Pinessi L, Nee L, Chumakov I, Pollen D, Brookes A, Sanseau P, Polinsky RJ, Wasco W, Da Sliva HAR, Haines JL, Pericak-Vance MA, Tanzi RE, Roses AD, Fraser PE, Rommens JM, St George-Hyslop PH (1995): Cloning of a gene bearing missense mutations in early-onset familial Alzheimer's disease. Nature 375:754–760.

Shin RW, Lee VM, Trojanowski JQ (1994): Aluminum modifies the properties of Alzheimer's disease PHF tau proteins in vivo and in vitro. J Neurosci 14:7221–7233.

Singh TJ, Grundke-Iqbal I, Iqbal K (1995a): Phosphorylation of tau protein by casein kinase-1 converts it to an abnormal Alzheimer-like state. J Neurochem 64:1420–1423.

Singh TJ, Haque N, Grundke-Iqbal I, Iqbal K (1995b): Rapid Alzheimer-like phosphorylation of tau by the synergistic actions of non-proline-dependent protein kinases and GSK-3. FEBS Lett 358:267–272.

Smale G, Nichols NR, Brady DR, Finch CE, Horton WE, Jr (1995): Evidence for apoptotic cell death in Alzheimer's disease. Exp Neurol 133:225–230.

Su JH, Anderson AJ, Cummings BJ, Cotman CW (1994a): Immunohistochemical evidence for apoptosis in Alzheimer's disease. Neuroreport 5:2529–2533.

Su JH, Cummings BJ, Cotman CW (1994b): Early phosphorylation of tau in Alzheimer's disease occurs at Ser-202 and is preferentially located within neurites. Neuroreport 5: 2358–2362.

Sumi SM, Bird TD, Nochlin D, Raskind MA (1992): Familial presenile dementia with psychosis associated with cortical neurofibrillary tangles and degeneration of the amygdala. Neurology 42:120–127.

Suzuki K, Parker CC, Pentchev PG, Katz D, Ghetti B, D'Agostino ANX, Carstea ED. (1995): Neurofibrillary tangles in Niemann-Pick disease type C. Acta Neuropathol 89: 227–238.

Tagliavini F, Giaccone G, Prelli F, Verga L, Porro M, Trojanowski JQ, Farlow MR, Frangione B, Ghetti B, Bugiani O (1993): A68 is a component of paired helical filaments of Gerstmann-Straussler-Scheinker disease, Indiana kindred. Brain Res 616:325–329.

Tato RE, Frank A, Hernanz A (1995): Tau protein concentrations in cerebrospinal fluid of patients with dementia of the Alzheimer type. J Neurol Neurosurg Psychiatry 59:280–283.

Tokutake S, Nagase H, Morisaki S, Oyanagi S (1995): Aluminum detected in senile plaques and neurofibrillary tangles is contained in lipofuscin granules with silicon, probably as aluminosilicate. Neurosci Lett 185:99–102.

Trojanowski JQ, Lee M-Y (1995): Phosphorylation of Neuronal Cytoskeletal Proteins in Alzheimer's Disease and Lewy Body Dementias. Ann N Y Acad Sci 747:92–109.

Trojanowski JQ, Lee VM (1994a): Paired helical filament tau in Alzheimer's disease. The kinase connection. [Review]. Am J Pathol 144:449–453.

Trojanowski JQ, Lee VM (1994b): Phosphorylation of neuronal cytoskeletal proteins in Alzheimer's disease and Lewy body dementias. [Review]. Ann N Y Acad Sci 747:92–109.

Trojanowski JQ, Schmidt ML, Shin RW, Bramblett GT, Rao D, Lee VM (1993): Altered tau and neurofilament proteins in neurodgenerative diseases: Diagnostic implications for Alzheimer's disease and Lewy body dementias. [Review]. Brain Pathol 3:45–54.

Vandermeeren M, Mercken M, Vanmechelen E, Six J, Van de Voorde A, Martin JJ, Cras P (1993): Detection of tau proteins in normal and Alzheimer's disease cerebrospinal fluid with a sensitive sandwich enzyme-linked immunosorbent assay. J Neurochem 61: 1828–1834.

Vermersch P, Frigard B, David JP, Fallet-Bianco C, Delacourte A (1992): Presence of abnormally phosphorylated Tau proteins in the entorhinal cortex of aged non-demented subjects. Neurosci Lett 144:143–146.

Vigo-Pelfrey C, Seubert P, Barbour R, Blomquist C, Lee M, Lee D, Coria F, Chang L, Miller B, Lieberburg I (1995): Elevation of microtubule-associated protein tau in the cerebrospinal fluid of patients with Alzheimer's disease. Neurology 45:788–793.

Wakabayashi K, Oyanagi K, Makifuchi T, Ikuta F, Homma A, Homma YX, Horikawa Y, Tokiguchi S (1994): Corticobasal degeneration: etiopathological significance of the cytoskeletal alterations. Acta Neuropathol 87:545–553.

Wang GP, Iqbal K, Bucht G, Winblad B, Wisniewski HM, Grundke-Iqbal I (1991): Alzheimer's disease: Paired helical filament immunoreactivity in cerebrospinal fluid. Acta Neuropathol 82:6–12.

Xu N, Majidi V, Markesbery WR, Ehmann WD (1992): Brain aluminum in Alzheimer's disease using an improved GFAAS method. Neurotoxicology 13:735–743.

Zeldenrust SR, Murrell J, Farlow M, Ghetti B, Roses AD, Benson MD (1993): RFLP analysis for APP 717 mutations associated with Alzheimer's disease. J Med Genet 30:476–478.

CHAPTER 11

Amyloid Cytotoxicity and Alzheimer's Disease: Roles of Membrane Oxidation and Perturbed Ion Homeostasis

MARK P. MATTSON, KATSUTOSHI FURUKAWA, ANNADORA J. BRUCE, ROBERT J. MARK, and EMMANUELLE M. BLANC

Sanders-Brown Research Center on Aging and Department of Anatomy & Neurobiology, University of Kentucky, Lexington, Kentucky 40536

INTRODUCTION: OXIDATIVE STRESS, ALTERED ION HOMEOSTASIS, AND NEURONAL INJURY IN ALZHEIMER'S DISEASE

Age is the major risk factor for Alzheimer's disease (AD) suggesting that an understanding of the cellular and molecular mechanisms of normal aging will contribute to an understanding of the pathogenesis of AD. The "free-radical" hypothesis of aging, which was forwarded many years ago [see Sohal (1993) and Harman (1994) for review], posits that age-related accumulation of reactive oxygen species (ROS) in tissues results in damage to major molecular components of cells including proteins, nucleic acids and lipids. Evidence supporting this hypothesis continues to accumulate and includes: data showing age- and disease-associated accumulation of various ROS and ROS-modified proteins, lipids, and DNA; alterations in cellular systems involved in ROS metabolism (e.g., antioxidant enzymes and mitochondrial electron transport proteins); and intervention studies in which manipulations that suppress ROS accumulation extend lifespan or allay age-related decline in function of specific organ systems [see Sohal (1993) and Benzi and Moretti (1995) for review]. Compelling evidence supporting the free-radical theory is that dietary restriction in rodents and primates significantly reduces oxidative stress in multiple organ systems and extends maximum life span (e.g., Youngman et al., 1992). In addition, antioxidants can increase the life span

Pharmacological Treatment of Alzheimer's Disease: Molecular and Neurobiological Foundations,
Edited by Brioni and Decker
ISBN 0-471-16758-4 © 1997 Wiley-Liss, Inc.

of diverse species ranging from *Drosophila* to rodents (Orr and Sohal, 1992; Edamatsu et al., 1995). As the brain ages, levels of protein oxidation (Smith et al., 1991) and lipid peroxidation (Zhang et al., 1994) increase. Alterations in levels of antioxidant enzymes have also been reported to occur in the aging rodent brain (Carrillo et al., 1992). Antioxidants, including the spin-trapping agent phenyl-butylnitrone, delayed age-associated decline in memory function in rodents (Carney et al., 1991).

The age-related increases in oxidative stress and perturbation of antioxidant enzyme systems appear to be enhanced in AD [see Benzi and Moretti (1995) for review]. For example, protein oxidation and lipid peroxidation were reported to be increased in brain tissue from AD patients compared to brain tissue from age-matched controls (Subbarao et al., 1990; Smith et al., 1991; Lovell et al., 1995). In addition, Lovell et al. (1995) and Bruce et al. (1997) reported that activity levels of several different antioxidant enzymes were altered, to varying extents, in vulnerable regions (e.g., hippocampus) compared to less vulnerable brain regions of AD brain and to all regions of age-matched control brains.

Alterations in systems that regulate cellular ion homeostasis that occur during the aging process may be particularly pronounced in age-related neurodegenerative disorders including AD [see Landfield et al. (1992) and Mattson (1992) for review]. While calcium plays key roles as a second messenger mediating a variety of neuronal functions, it is increasingly appreciated that dysregulation of calcium homeostasis is a pivotal step in the neurodegenerative process in both acute and chronic neurodegenerative conditions. Intimately tied to dysregulation of calcium homeostasis are receptors for the excitatory neurotransmitter glutamate, which, when excessively activated (particularly under conditions of metabolic or oxidative compromise), can promote massive calcium influx and consequent cell degeneration. Free radicals and calcium appear to be final common messengers of cell death, and their actions are intimately related such that free radicals promote destabilization of calcium homeostasis and, conversely, elevation of intracellular free calcium levels ($[Ca^{2+}]_i$) induces free-radical production (Lafon-Cazal et al., 1993; Mark et al., 1995a; Mattson et al., 1995b). Increasing evidence for mechanistic links between alterations in metabolism of the β-amyloid precursor protein (βAPP) and dysregulation of free-radical metabolism and calcium homeostasis are the main topic of this chapter and would appear to strongly support central roles of free radicals and calcium in the nerve cell death that occurs in AD.

MECHANISMS OF CYTOTOXICITY OF AMYLOID β-PEPTIDE AND THE FREE-RADICAL THEORY OF ALZHEIMER'S DISEASE

Cellular Metabolism of βAPP

The amyloid β-peptide (Aβ) is a relatively small peptide fragment (40–42 amino acids) of a much larger βAPP [see Yankner and Mesulam (1991) and Selkoe (1993) for review]. βAPP is an axonally transported glycoprotein that localizes to membranes where it exists in a transmembrane configuration with a single membrane-spanning domain, a small cytoplasmic C-terminus, and a large extracellular N-terminus (Figures 1 and 2A). Alternative splicing of βAPP transcripts results in

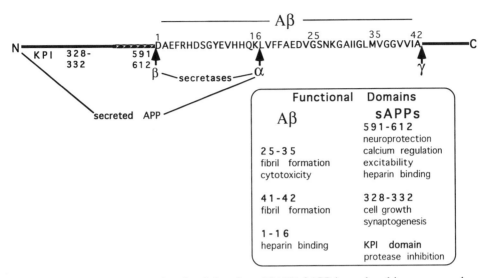

FIGURE 1. Structure and functional domains of βAPP. βAPP is produced in neurons and axonally transported to presynaptic terminals (or axonal growth cones during brain development). βAPP is inserted into plasma membrane such that a large N-terminal domain protrudes outside the cell. Aβ is situated partially outside the cell and partially within the membrane. An enzymatic cleavage toward the middle of the Aβ sequence, effected by an enzyme called α-secretase, results in release of secreted forms of βAPP (sAPPαs). An alternative cleaves at the N-terminus of Aβ releases sAPPβs and leaves intact Aβ as part of a C-terminal fragment of βAPP. Internalization and further enzymatic cleavage of the C-terminal βAPP fragment results in the release of soluble Aβ from cells. The α-secretase cleavage can be induced by electrical activity in neurons, and protein kinase C may serve as a second messenger in activity-dependent release of sAPPα. Several domains of βAPP have been identified as having important physiological and pathophysiological activities. In sAPPα, a region that extends from amino acids 591–612 of βAPP695 (overlaps the β-secretase cleavage site) has been shown to activate a signal transduction pathway in neurons, which involves generation of cGMP and opening of K^+ channels with resultant membrane hyperpolarization. Because of sAPPαs are released from presynaptic terminals in an activity-dependent manner, activation of the sAPPα signaling pathway in postsynaptic neurons modulates synaptic plasticity. Moreover, signaling via the 591–612 sAPPα domain suppresses calcium influx and protects the neurons against excitotoxicity and Aβ toxicity. Two other domains of sAPPs have been shown to have biological activities. A five-amino-acid segment of sAPP (amino acids 328–332) induces proliferation of nonneuronal cells and promotes neurite outgrowth and synaptogenesis. Some forms of βAPP contain a kunitz-type protease inhibitor (KPI) domain near the N-terminus, which is likely to play important roles in cell adhesion and other processes involving protease activities. Two different regions of Aβ appear to play important roles in fibril formation and neurotoxicity of the peptide. Amino acids 25–35 of Aβ exhibit aggregation and neurotoxicity activities similar, if not identical, to those of full-length of Aβ (Aβ1–42). Amino acids 41 and 42 of Aβ may promote Aβ fibril formation by specific interactions with amino acids in the 25–35 region.

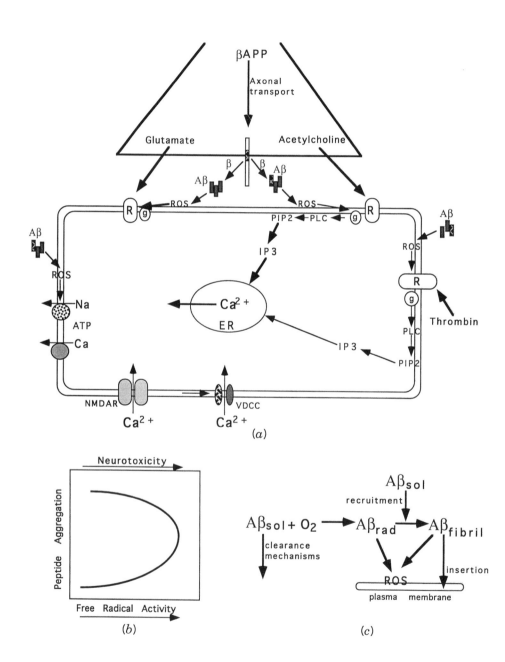

(a)

(b)

(c)

several forms of βAPP that differ only by the presence or absence of a kunitz protease inhibitor domain in their N-terminal region. Aβ is liberated from βAPP as the result of the enzymatic activity of two proteases; β-secretase cleaves at the N-terminus of the Aβ sequence and γ-secretase cleaves at the C-terminus of Aβ (Figure 1). Although the latter processing pathway normally occurs and Aβ circulates at low levels in cerebrospinal fluid (CSF) and blood, the physiological importance of the processing pathway that releases intact Aβ is unclear. From the perspective of AD, however, the significance of the β-secretase pathway seems clear; it allows release of intact Aβ, which then has the potential to form the insoluble fibrillar aggregates that comprise amyloid plaques. Together with neurofibrillary tangles, amyloid plaques are a defining feature of AD. An alternative processing pathway involves cleavage of βAPP within the Aβ sequence (between amino acids 16 and 17) by α-secretase. The latter processing pathway, which is regulated by physiological stimuli (e.g., excitatory transmitters and membrane depolarization), results in release of secreted forms of βAPP (sAPPαs), which have been shown to have neurotrophic activities, and to play important roles in developmental and synaptic plasticity (see below). It should be noted that none of the three secretase enzymes have yet been isolated.

βAPP clearly plays a central role in at least some inherited forms of AD, although the extent of its involvement in the more common sporadic forms of AD appears to be variable. Several different mutations in βAPP are causally linked to AD in affected individuals in those pedigrees [see Mullan and Crawford (1993) for review]. Each of the mutations lies close to the Aβ sequence, and studies in which the mutations were

---

FIGURE 2. Mechanisms of Aβ neurotoxicity. (*a*) β-secretase (β) cleavage of βAPP releases soluble Aβ, which, under certain environmental conditions (e.g., oxidative environment), forms fibrillar aggregates. Interaction of Aβ with the plasma membrane results in generation of reactive oxygen species (ROS) and lipid peroxidation. Free radicals may then directly or indirectly (via alteration of the lipid environment) impair the function of many different membrane-associated enzymes and signal transduction components. For example, Aβ impairs function of the Na^+/K^+-and Ca^{2+}-ATPases by a free-radical-mediated mechanism. Impairment of these key ion pumps results in membrane depolarization, calcium influx, increased vulnerability to excitotoxicity, and eventual cell death. Aβ also disrupts coupling of muscarinic cholinergic receptors to their GTP-binding protein (Gq11); this action occurs with subtoxic levels of Aβ and may impair cholinergic transmission well prior to neuronal degeneration. Aβ was also shown to alter thrombin receptor transduction resulting in aberrant calcium signaling. Other membrane systems appear less vulnerable to Aβ and free-radical-mediated damage. For example, Na^+/Ca^{2+} exchange is relatively unaltered by Aβ. (*b*) Biphasic relationship between the extent of Aβ aggregation and its free-radical-generating and neurotoxic activities suggest that chemical reactions occuring during the aggregation process, rather than the state of aggregation per se, are central to the mechanism of its neurotoxic actions. (*c*) Role of ROS in Aβ fibril formation and neurotoxicity. Oxidation promotes formation of Aβ with free-radical moieties (probably associated with methionine 35); the free-radical peptides then covalently crosslink to form fibrils.

expressed in cultured cells showed that the mutations affect enzymatic processing of βAPP in ways that result in increased production of Aβ and/or an increase in the amount of the Aβ1–42 form (Cai et al., 1993; Citron et al., 1994; Suzuki et al., 1994). Importantly, mutations that increase β-secretase cleavage result in a decrease in the amount of sAPPα, the neuroprotective form of sAPP (see below). Both the increased levels of Aβ and the decreased levels of sAPP are likely to contribute to the neurodegenerative process in AD, as will be considered in detail later.

Aggregation and Neurotoxicity of Aβ

In AD brain two different types of Aβ deposits are distinguishable: (a) Diffuse plaques contain Aβ that is largely nonfibrillar and therefore is not reactive with thioflavin or Congo Red, two dyes that recognize β-sheet structure; and (b) senile (compact neuritic) plaques are comprised of fibrillar Aβ and are associated with degenerated neurites. Two important predictions as to the role of Aβ in the pathophysiology of AD can be deduced from this fundamental histopathological information, the first being that Aβ is neurotoxic and the second being that the neurotoxicity of the peptide is related to its fibrillar structure. Experimental data have confirmed each of these predictions (Table 1). Synethetic Aβ was neurotoxic in primary rat hippocampal cell cultures (Yankner et al., 1990), and the toxicity of the peptide was shown to be directly related to the propensity of the peptide to form fibrillar aggregates (Pike et al., 1993; Lorenzo and Yankner, 1994). For reasons not yet clear, different batches of synthetic Aβ have different propensities to aggregate (May et al., 1992; Pike et al., 1993), a fact that often makes it difficult to obtain reproducible results when studying mechanisms of Aβ toxicity. Nevertheless, it is now generally agreed that Aβ can be neurotoxic and that the toxicity is correlated with transitions from soluble to fibrillar Aβ. Studies of different fragments of Aβ have revealed key structural requirements for peptide fibril formation and neurotoxicity. Aβ1–42 more readily forms fibrils than Aβ1–40 and can "seed" fibril formation of Aβ1–40 (Jarrett and Lansbury, 1993). Full-length Aβ is not required for fibril formation or neurotoxicity; Aβ25–35 readily aggregates and is highly neurotoxic in cell cultures (Yankner et al., 1990; Pike et al., 1993; Mattson et al., 1993a). Pike et al. (1995) have shown that, within the 25–35 sequence, methionine 35 plays a pivitol role in peptide aggregation and neurotoxicity.

Several environmental factors have been identified that greatly affect Aβ fibril formation and neurotoxicity. For example, the peptide aggregates much more readily at acidic pH than at physiological pH (Fraser et al., 1991; Barrow et al., 1992), and an oxidizing environment promotes Aβ aggregation (Dyrks et al., 1992). The presence of molecular oxygen appears to be required for Aβ aggregation and toxicity (Hensley et al., 1994). Different metal cations, including zinc and aluminum, can also promote aggregation of Aβ (Mantyh et al., 1993; Bush et al., 1994). Iron (Goodman and Mattson, 1994a; Schubert and Chevion, 1995) and aluminum (Kuroda and Kawahara, 1994) were also reported to enhance the toxicity of Aβ in cultured neurons. Each of these metals have been implicated in the pathogenesis of AD (Wisniewski and Wen, 1992; Bush et al., 1994; Gerlach et al., 1994).

TABLE 1. Actions of Aβ on Neuronal and Nonneuronal Cells that May Contribute to the Pathogenesis of Neuronal Degeneration in Alzheimer's Disease

Cell Type	Effects of Amyloid β-peptide	References
Rat hippocampal neurons	Neurotoxicity, exacerbation of excitotoxicity	Yankner et al (1990), Mattson et al. (1993a)
Rat cortical neurons	Neurotoxicity, exacerbation of excitotoxicity	Koh et al. (1990), Pike et al. (1993)
Human cortical neurons	Neurotoxicity, exacerbation of excitotoxicity	Mattson et al. (1992)
Rat cortical neurons	Apoptotic death	Loo et al. (1993)
Rat hippocampal neurons	Impairment of ion-motive ATPases	Mark et al. (1995)
Rat cortical neurons	Disruption of muscarinic signal transduction	Kelly et al. (1996)
Human neuroblastoma	Disruption of thrombin signal transduction	Mattson and Begley (1996)
Rat cortical astrocytes	Impairment of glutamate transport	Harris et al. (1995)
Rat cortical astrocytes	Induction of reactive phenotype	Pike et al. (1994)
Rat cortical microglia	Induction of reactive phenotype, production of neurotoxins, production of cytokines	Meda et al. (1995)
Vascular endothelial cells	Disruption of barrier function	Blanc et al. (submitted)
Vascular endothelial cells	Impairment of glucose transport	Blanc et al. (submitted)
Vascular endothelial cells	Apoptotic death	Blanc et al. (submitted)
Vascular smooth muscle	Increased Aβ production, cell degeneration	Davis-Salinas et al. (1995)
Human lymphocytes	Disruption of calcium signaling	Eckert et al. (1993)
Human red blood cells	Impairment of ion-motive ATPases, reduction of glucose uptake, cell lysis	Mark et al. (in preparation)

245

Concerning the role of peptide fibril formation in neurotoxicity of Aβ, the major emphasis has been placed on understanding secondary structure and how it might be involved in the neurotoxic mechanism (e.g., Simmons et al., 1994). In this regard, Lansbury et al. (1995) recently described an antiparallel β-sheet structural model of β-amyloid fibrils in which amino acids 41 and 42 play an important role in stabilizing the fibrils and promoting their growth. This type of structural information is very valuable and may reveal whether or not specific structural details of Aβ fibrils are mechanistically linked to toxic activity of the peptide. On the other hand, it should also be considered that it is not the secondary structure of the peptide that determines whether or not it is toxic, but rather it is the chemical process(es) leading to fibril formation that is neurotoxic. The observation that Aβ25–35 is as toxic or more toxic than Aβ1–40 or Aβ1–42 (Yankner et al., 1990; Mattson et al., 1993a) itself suggests a dissociation between fibril formation and toxic potency. In addition, cell culture data indicate that as peptide aggregation increases, neurotoxic activity first increases and then decreases. We and others have observed that Aβ can be "overaggregated" such that its toxicity is reduced (Simmons et al., 1994; Figure 2B). This suggests that, rather than being directly related to the amount of aggregated peptide, the toxicity of Aβ is greatest during the time period of maximum rate of aggregation. We have proposed that, in the presence of molecular oxygen, Aβ generates free-radical moieties that are causally involved in peptide crosslinking and fibril formation (Hensley et al., 1994; Mattson, 1995a). As considered in more detail below, the free radicals can propagate to cellular membranes and damage key regulatory systems therein; this radical-generating action of Aβ appears to play a central role in the cytotoxicity of the peptide (Figure 2C). This same mechanism may also account for the cytotoxic activities of other types of amyloidogenic peptides including human pancreatic amylin and β2-microglobulin (May et al., 1993; Mattson and Goodman, 1995).

Mechanism of Amyloid β-Peptide Toxicity Involves Generation of Reactive Oxygen Species and Disruption of Cellular Calcium Homeostasis

Studies in neuroblastoma cells and rat hippocampal and cortical neurons showed that Aβ (25–35 and 1–40) can induce accumulation of hydrogen peroxide in neurons (Behl et al., 1994a; Goodman and Mattson, 1994a). Behl et al. (1994a) and Goodman and co-workers (Goodman and Mattson, 1994a; Goodman et al., 1994) also showed that antioxidants [e.g., vitamin E, propyl gallate, and *n*-tert-butyl phenylnitrone (PBN) can protect neurons against Aβ toxicity. Additional studies have confirmed and extended the initial findings. Sagara et al. (1996) showed that neuroblastoma cell lines resistant to Aβ toxicity possessed greater antioxidant enzyme levels than did cell lines vulnerable to Aβ toxicity, suggesting a role for antioxidant enzymes in neuronal vulnerability in AD. The antioxidant U-78517F protected cultured hippocampal neurons against Aβ toxicity (Kumar et al., 1994), and Aβ induced lipid peroxidation in neocortical synaptosomes (Butterfield et al., 1994) and cultured rat hippocampal neurons (Goodman and Mattson, 1996a). In a very intriguing recent report Busciglio and Yankner (1995) showed that cultured cortical neurons from Down's syndrome fetuses spontaneously undergo apoptosis and exhibit clear increases in measures of oxidative stress. Although it is not clear whether Aβ mediates the apoptotic death of Down's syndrome neurons, it is evident that there is something intrinsically different about Down's syndrome neurons that renders them vulnerable to environment stressors.

Impairment of mitochondrial enzyme function by Aβ (Shearman et al., 1995) would be expected to increase superoxide anion radical production, which is a likely mechanism whereby Aβ causes an increase in hydrogen peroxide levels. Mitochondria are a major source of superoxide anion, and superoxide metabolism can lead to formation of several damaging free-radical species including hydroxyl radical and peroxynitrite (Figure 3). Superoxide anion is converted to hydrogen perox-

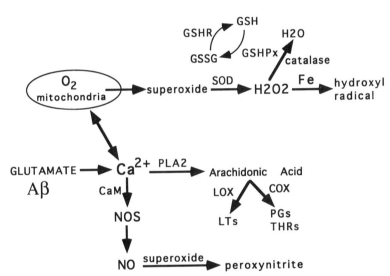

FIGURE 3. Some cellular sources of reactive oxygen species (ROS) and cellular mechanisms to prevent accumulation of the ROS. As a consequence of mitochondrial respiration, superoxide anion radical is produced. Superoxide dismutases (SOD) convert superoxide to hydrogen peroxide (H_2O_2). In the presence of ferrous iron (Fe) H_2O_2 is converted to hydroxyl radical. Hydroxyl radical formation can be avoided when catalase and glutathione peroxidase (GSHPx) are present; these enzymes detoxify H_2O_2 by converting it to H_2O. Another important enzyme that prevents oxyradical formation is glutathione reductase (GSHR), which converts oxidized glutathione (GSSG) to reduced glutathione (GSH). Stimuli that elevate intracellular calcium levels (e.g., glutamate and Aβ) can promote ROS formation via several mechanisms including: calcium disrupts mitochondrial transmembrane potential and promotes superoxide formation; calcium binds calmodulin (CaM), which then activates the enzyme nitric oxide synthase (NOS), which results in generation of nitric oxide (NO)—interaction of NO with superoxide results in the formation of peroxynitrite, a highly destructive ROS; calcium promotes activity of phospholipase A2 (PLA2), an enzyme that liberates arachidonic acid from membrane phospholipids—ROS are generated as the result of activity of lipoxygenases (LOX) and cyclooxygenases (COX) on arachidonic acid. Abbreviations: LTs, leukotrienes; PGs, prostaglandins; THRs, thromboxanes.

ide by superoxide dismutases [SOD (Cu/Zn-SOD and Mn-SOD)]. While hydrogen peroxide itself is relatively innocuous, in the presence of Fe^{2+}, hydrogen peroxide is rapidly converted to the highly destructive hydroxyl radical. The antioxidant enzymes glutathione peroxidase and catalase convert hydrogen peroxide to water and thereby prevent hydroxyl radical formation. In addition to being a precursor to hydrogen peroxide and hydroxyl radical, superoxide can interact with nitric oxide to form peroxynitrite, another damaging ROS (Beckman, 1994; Lipton et al., 1994).

Cell culture data and studies of synaptosomes indicate that the plasma membrane is the major site at which Aβ induces generation of ROS. When added to primary neuronal cultures, Aβ (1–38, 1–40, or 1–42) accumulates on the plasma membrane; very little or no Aβ enters these cells (Mattson et al., 1993a,b). Electron paramagnetic resonance spectroscopy studies using nitroxylstearate spin labels that report lipid peroxidative events have shown that Aβ induces lipid peroxidation in synaptosomes (Butterfield et al., 1994). Similar results were obtained in membranes isolated from PC12 cells; when membranes were exposed to Aβ, there was a highly significant reduction in 12-nitroxylstearate paramagnetic signal intensity indicating the presence of free radicals within the membrane phospholipid bilayer (Figure 4). Interestingly, the signal from a spin label (5-nitroxylstearate) that reports free-radical signals from the outer edge of the membrane bilayer was also affected by Aβ,

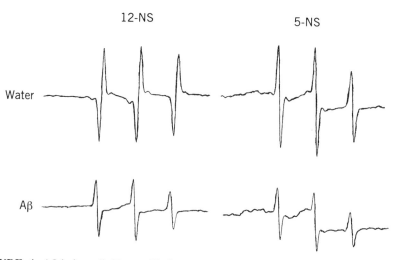

FIGURE 4. Aβ induces lipid peroxidation and oxidation of cell surface molecules in membranes from cultured PC12 cells. Cell membranes (crude membrane preparation) were isolated from PC12 cells and were exposed for 30 min to either vehicle (water) or 380 μM Aβ25–35 in the presence of either 12-NS (12-nitroxylstearate) or 5-NS (5 nitroxylstearate) spin probes. Shown are representative electron paramagnetic resonance spectroscopic (EPR) traces. The 12-NS probe reports a signal from deep within the membrane phospholipid bilayer, while the 5-NS probe localizes to the lipid–water interface. Aβ caused a reduction in the amplitude of EPR signals from both the 12-NS and 5-NS probes suggesting oxidative damage to membrane lipids and cell surface molecules, respectively.

suggesting that Aβ may damage molecules at the cell surface (Figure 4). Consistent with Aβ inducing free radicals within the plasma membrane are reports showing that Aβ can impair the function of plasma membrane systems involved in the regulation of ion homeostasis. Mark et al. (1995a) reported that exposure of cultured rat hippocampal neurons, and synaptosomes from adult human hippocampus, to Aβ results in selective impairment of Na^+/K^+-ATPase and Ca^{2+}-ATPase activities; activities of other Mg^{2+}-dependent ion-motive ATPases and the Na^+/Ca^{2+} exchanger were unaffected by Aβ. Free radicals mediated the impairment of ion-motive ATPases because antioxidants (e.g., propyl gallate and vitamin E) prevented impairment of the ion-motive ATPases. Impairment of ion-motive ATPases appears to be an early event in the mechanism of Aβ cytotoxicity. As with Aβ, ouabain (a specific inhibitor of the plasma membrane Na^+/K^+-ATPase) caused membrane depolarization and increased neuronal vulnerability to excitotoxicity (Brines et al., 1995). Inhibition of the Na^+/K^+-ATPase may play a role in the elevation of intracellular free calcium levels ($[Ca^{2+}]_i$) and increased neuronal sensitivity to excitotoxicity previously reported in studies of cultured human cortical and rat hippocampal neurons exposed to Aβ (Mattson et al., 1992, 1993a; Hartmann et al., 1993). Aβ may have similar calcium-amplifying effects in nonneuronal cells including lymphocytes (Eckert et al., 1993). Impairment of Na^+/K^+-ATPase in neurons exposed to Aβ preceded elevation of $[Ca^{2+}]_i$, and calcium influx induced by Aβ was causally involved in the neurotoxic mechanism of the peptide because removal of extracellular calcium (Mattson et al., 1993a) and calcium channel blockers (Weiss et al., 1994) protected neurons against Aβ toxocity. Moreover, neurons expressing calbindin (Mattson and Furukawa, 1996) and calretinin (Pike et al., 1995) were resistant to Aβ toxicity; such calcium-binding proteins are known to protect neurons against calcium-mediated death, further suggesting a role for calcium in the cell death process.

Further studies have provided evidence for additional interactions of Aβ with membranes that may account for its ability to disrupt ion homeostasis. Arispe et al. (1993) reported that synthetic Aβ can insert into membranes and form pores that conduct cations. Electrophysiological data also indicate that Aβ can induce nonselective ion conductances (Simmons and Schneider, 1993; Furukawa et al., 1994) and calcium conductances (Davidson et al., 1994) in cultured neurons (Figure 5). Additional intriguing findings come from the work of Etcheberrigaray et al. (1994) who reported that Aβ, at quite low (nM) concentrations, caused the virtual disappearance of a particular type of potassium channel conductance in cultured human fibroblasts. They showed that this same alteration in potassium channel properties occurred in fibroblasts from patients with inherited forms of AD (Etcheberrigaray et al., 1993). If such an alteration also occurs in neurons, it would be expected to promote sustained membrane depolarizations with resultant calcium influx neuronal injury.

The importance of cellular systems that regulate calcium homeostasis in neuronal physiology and plasticity cannot be overstated. Neurons possess a myriad of proteins whose function is to control the movement of Ca^{2+} into and out of the cell and between different subcellular compartments. For example, the plasma membrane contains ligand-gated and voltage-dependent calcium channels that are

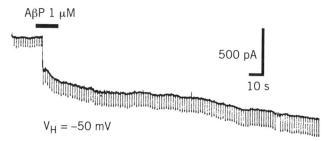

FIGURE 5. Aβ induces large inward currents in cultured neocortical neurons. A typical patch clamp current recording (voltage clamp node) prior to, during, and following focal application of Aβ25–35 (1μM). The horizontal bar indicates the time period during which Aβ was applied. The holding potential was -50 mV; 10-mV hyperpolarizing pulses were applied every 2 sec. Note that Aβ induced a large and sustained inward current. Modified from Furukawa et al. (1994).

activated by excitatory neurotransmitters, Ca^{2+}-ATPases that provide a major mechanism for removing Ca^{2+} from the cell and maintaining the calcium concentration gradient, and a Na^+/Ca^{2+} exchanger that has a high capacity to remove Ca^{2+} following a stimulus that induces calcium influx. Calcium can be concentrated in the smooth endoplasmic reticulum via activity of a specific Ca^{2+}-ATPase, and calcium is released from endoplasmic reticulum stores in response to inositol triphosphate, the latter being liberated from membrane phosphatidyl inositol bisphosphate in response to signals such as acetylcholine linked to phospholipase C. Calcium acts as a second messenger that mediates a variety of neuronal responses to environmental stimuli. For example, calcium influx is the trigger for vesicle fusion and neurotransmitter release from presynaptic terminals. By regulating cytoskeletal elements, calcium plays a prominent role in controlling behaviors of neuronal growth cones and in regulating synaptic plasticity in the adult nervous system (Mattson, 1992). The centrality of calcium in neuronal function and plasticity is underscored by the adverse consequences of dysregulation of calcium homeostasis in the nervous system. Prolonged elevations of $[Ca^{2+}]_i$ have been causally linked to neuronal degeneration and death in both acute and chronic neurodegenerative conditions. For example, disruption of cellular calcium homeostasis plays a major role in neuronal degeneration in ischemic brain injury (Choi, 1995), traumatic brain injury (Mattson, 1995b), epilepsy (Scharfmann and Schwartzkroin, 1989), amyotrophic lateral sclerosis (Smith et al., 1994), and AD (Mattson et al., 1993b).

Glutamate is the major excitatory neurotransmitter in the human brain. While glutamate therefore plays major roles in synaptic transmission and related processes such as learning and memory, it has become quite clear that glutamate can also damage and kill neurons, particularly when receptors are excessively stimulated during periods of reduced energy availability. Several different subtypes of glutamate receptor have been identified. Ionotropic glutamate receptors include the

N-methyl-D-aspartate receptor, the AMPA receptor, and the kainate receptor. The NMDA receptor itself is a calcium channel that when activated provides a conduit that allows large amounts of Ca^{2+} to enter the cell. AMPA and kainate receptors mainly flux Na^+ and thereby depolarize the membrane resulting in activation of voltage-dependent Ca^{2+} channels. Metabotropic glutamate receptors are not ion channels; rather they are linked to GTP-binding proteins and the inositol phospholipid cascade. Neurons that are particularly vulnerable in AD (e.g., hippocampal CA1 neurons and entorhinal layer II cells) express particularly high levels of ionotropic glutamate receptors.

Many neurons that degenerate in AD exhibit abnormal filamentous accumulations (straight and paired-helical filaments) of the microtubule-associated protein tau. Both oxidative stress and disruption of calcium homeostasis have been linked to neurofibrillary tangle formation. Tau fibril formation in vitro can be induced by oxidation of cysteine residues (Troncoso et al., 1993; Schweers et al., 1995), and tau is modified by advanced glycation end products (Yan et al., 1994), suggesting a contribution of oxidative stress to neurofibrillary tangle formation. Cell culture studies of human and rat cortical and hippocampal neurons have shown that prolonged elevation of $[Ca^{2+}]_i$ can induce some cytoskeletal alterations similar (although clearly not identical) to those seen in the neurofibrillary tangles in AD (Mattson, 1990; Sautierre et al., 1992). The changes include loss of microtubles, antigenic changes in tau, and accumulation of ubiquitin. Such tanglelike changes in cultured neurons were also induced by glucose deprivation (Cheng and Mattson, 1992) and, in a cooperative manner, by Aβ and excitatory amino acids (Mattson et al., 1992). In vivo studies have also shown that excitotoxic insults can induce calcium-mediated cytoskeletal alterations reminiscent of neurofibrillary tangles (Elliott et al., 1993; Stein-Behrens et al., 1994). The latter studies also showed that glucocorticoids and physiological stress can exacerbate neuronal injury and cytoskeletal alterations induced by excitotoxins. Yankner and co-workers recently showed clearly that Aβ can induce paired helical filament-(PHF)-like antigenic changes in tau and reduced microtubule binding in cultured human neurons (Busciglio et al., 1995), although in their paradigm calcium may not play a major role in the tau alterations. Collectively, these findings suggest possible roles for metabolic compromise, excitotoxicity and Aβ toxicity in the pathogenesis of neurofibrillary pathology in AD.

Apoptosis and Necrosis: Different Manifestations of Shared Mechanisms

While the evidence that free radicals and calcium play central roles in neurodegenerative processes in AD is compelling, it is unclear whether neurons dye by apoptosis or necrosis. Cells dying by apoptosis and necrosis are quite different when they are observed with either the light or electron microscope (McGahon et al., 1995). Apoptosis manifests as cell shrinkage, cell surface blebbing, and nuclear DNA condensation and fragmentation; the cell membrane remains intact until the cell is dead. Necrotic cells are swollen and vacuolated, and ultimately spill their contents into the extracellular space as they die. Evidence supporting an apoptotic mechanism of neuronal death in AD comes from data showing that Aβ can induce apoptosis in cultured brain neurons (Loo et al., 1993; Forloni et al., 1993; Gshwind and Huber, 1995). On the other hand, Schubert and co-workers provided evidence that Aβ can kill neurons by necrosis rather than apoptosis (Behl et al., 1993, 1994b). In addition to neurons, cultured vascular endothelial cells dying as the result of exposure to Aβ exhibit DNA condensation and fragmentation and are protected by inhibitors of RNA synthesis, protein synthesis, and endonucleases (Blanc et al., 1966; Figure 6). Recent studies of postmortem AD brain have provided evidence for DNA strand breakage and induction of apoptosis-related genes in neurons in vulnerable brain regions such as the hippocampus (Cotman and Anderson, 1995).

While there is general agreement that the vast majority of cases of cell death can be categorized as either apoptosis or necrosis based on morphological criteria, it is much less clear whether distinct mechanisms underlie each form of cell death and, by extension, whether knowing whether neurons in AD are dying by apoptosis or necrosis will alter therapeutic strategies to prevent the degeneration. Many

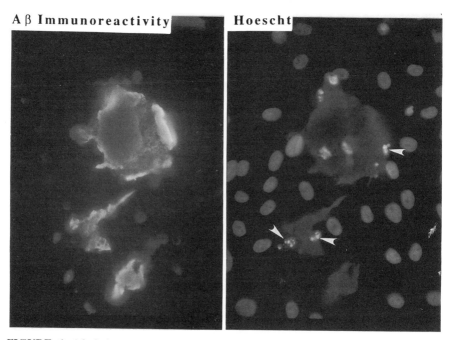

FIGURE 6. Aβ induces apoptosis in cultured vascular endothelial cells. Cultures of porcine pulmonary vascular endothelial cells were exposed to 20μM Aβ1–40 for 18 hr, and then double-stained with an antibody to Aβ (left; the "A") and Hoescht dye (right). Note the large Aβ aggregate ("A" in left panel), and that cells apposed to the Aβ aggregate exhibited condensed DNA (e.g., arrowheads) while cells not contacted by Aβ appeared undamaged.

"cell deathologists" have used the term *programmed cell death* as a synonym for apoptosis; programmed cell death being defined as an active death process requiring expression of new gene products (death genes). In invertebrates such as the nematode *Caenorhabditis elegans* there is indeed evidence that certain gene products such as the interleukin-1β converting enzyme (ICE) are causally involved in developmental apoptotic cell death (Yuan, 1995). On the other hand, increasing data indicate that many signal transduction pathways activated in injured neurons serve neuroprotective functions. For example, neurotrophic factor and cytokine signaling pathways have been shown to induce expression of antioxidant enzymes and proteins involved in stabilization of ion homeostasis [see Mattson and Furukawa (1966) for review]. One of the cornerstone pieces of evidence that neuronal death in a particular condition is programmed cell death is that the protein synthesis inhibitor cycloheximide prevents the cell death. For example, death of sympathetic neurons resulting from nerve growth factor (NGF) withdrawal can be delayed or prevented by exposing the cells to cycloheximide (Johnson and Deckwerth, 1993). Interestingly, recent findings indicate that the interpretation that cycloheximide protects neurons by preventing expression of death gene products may not be correct. It has been observed in several paradigms that maximum effectiveness of cycloheximide occurred within a certain concentration range of this compound such that higher levels were ineffective or even toxic (Figure 7). It turns out that the neuroprotective concentrations of cycloheximide do not, in fact, inhibit protein synthesis to any appreciable extent. In fact, neuroprotective concentrations of cycloheximide induced expression of c-Fos protein and antioxidant enzymes in rat hippocampal cell cultures (Furukawa et al., 1997). It therefore may be the case that cycloheximide can protect neurons by inducing the expression of cytoprotective proteins. If this is correct, then cycloheximide may substitute for NGF by activating survival-promoting genetic programs.

It has been proposed that cells constantly rely on the presence of growth factors produced by neighbors and/or themselves and that apotosis occurs when levels of such factors fall below a certain threshold level (Jacobson et al., 1994). This concept could be extended to neurodegenerative disorders, whether acute (e.g., stroke or traumatic brain injury) or chronic (AD, Parkinson's disease, amyotropic lateral sclerosis), wherein injury mobilizes several different neuroprotective signaling pathways. In order to emphasize the preeminent role of cell survival signal pathways over cell death-promoting pathways, we believe it is useful to consider the concept of *programmed cell life* (Mattson and Furukawa, 1996). In this view, pathological neuronal death (apoptosis or necrosis) occurs when neuroprotective signaling pathways are unable to overcome the injury process. Programmed cell life mechanisms are many, as indicated by hundreds of studies showing that brain injury induces the expression of neurotrophic factors and cytokines, and that activation of signal transduction pathways of these factors can protect neurons against insults (e.g., excitotoxins, metabolic insults, and Aβ) relevant to the pathogenesis of neurodegenerative disorders [see Mattson et al. (1993c) and Mattson and Furukawa (1996) for review].

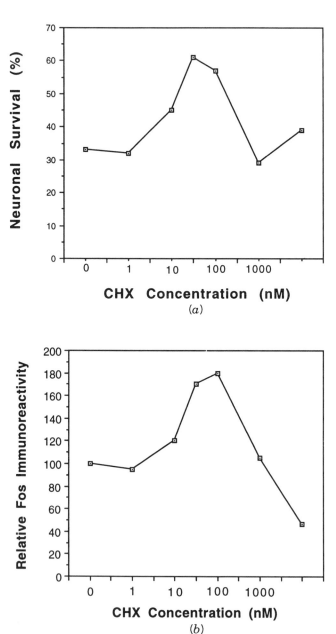

FIGURE 7. Cycloheximide protects hippocampal neurons against Aβ toxicity and induces c-Fos protein expression in a concentration-dependent manner. (*a*) Cultures were pretreated for 12 hr with the indicated concentrations of cycloheximide (CHX) and were then exposed to 5μ*M* Aβ25–35 for 24 hr. Neuronal survival was quantified by cell counts, and values are expressed as percentage of initial number of the viable neurons prior to exposure to Aβ. With CHX concentrations of 10, 50, and 100 nM neuronal survival was significantly increased. (*b*) Cultures were exposed to the indicated concentrations of CHX for 4 hr and then immunostained with a rabbit polyclonal antibody to c-Fos. Immunoreactivity was quantified and values are expressed native to control cultures (100% value). Note that levels of c-Fos immunoreactivity were increased in cultures exposed to 50 and 100 n*M* CHX.

Subtoxic Levels of Amyloid β-Peptide Can Disrupt Neuronal Membrane Signal Transduction Pathways

The strong evidence that Aβ can induce membrane oxidation and impair ion-motive ATPase activities suggested the possibility that subtoxic levels of Aβ might affect many different signal transduction pathways associated with the plasma membrane. Previous studies of membrane and synaptosome preparations from postmortem AD and control brain tissue suggested that coupling of muscarinic acetylcholine receptors to Gq11 (GTP-binding protein) was impaired in AD (Warpman et al., 1993; Cutler et al., 1994; FLynn et al., 1995). When cultured rat neocortical neurons were exposed to increasing concentrations of Aβ (1 nM to 50 μM) a concentration-dependent impairment of carbachol (muscarinic acetylcholine receptor agonist)-induced GTPase activity occurred (Kelly et al., 1996; Figure 8). Impairment of carbachol responses occurred within 20–60 min of exposure to Aβ and was observed with both subtoxic (10–100 nM) and toxic (1–50 μM) concentrations of Aβ. Pretreatment of neurons with Aβ also resulted in muting of carbachol-induced inositol phosphate release and calcium release from intracellular stores. Aβ did not interfere with ligand–receptor binding, indicating that the mode of action of Aβ involved "uncoupling" of muscarinic receptors from Gq11. Antioxidants, including propyl gallate and vitamin E, largely prevented the impairment of receptor–G protein coupling otherwise caused by Aβ, indicating the involvement of free radicals in the process (Kelly et al., 1996). Interestingly, Aβ does not affect all G-protein-linked signaling pathways in the same manner. For example, the ability of agonists of metabotropic glutamate receptors to induce inositol phosphate release from cultured rat neocortical neurons was less affected by Aβ (E.M. Blanc and M.P. Mattson, unpublished data).

Another receptor expressed by neurons and linked to a G protein that activates phospholipase C is the thrombin receptor (Weinstein et al., 1995). When calcium responses to thrombin were examined in neurons pretreated with Aβ for different time periods, an interesting phenomenon was observed. With short-term exposures to Aβ (e.g., 30 min) calcium responses to thrombin were enhanced, while longer exposures (e.g., 6 hr) resulted in attenuation of calcium responses to thrombin (Mattson and Begley, 1996). The enhancement of calcium responses to thrombin with short-term Aβ exposure is similar to the increased sensitivity of neurons to glutamate-induced elevation of $[Ca^{2+}]_i$ previously reported (Mattson et al., 1992; 1993a) and may be explained by impairment of ion-motive ATPase (Mark et al., 1995a). The abrogation of thrombin responses in cells exposed to Aβ for longer time periods is similar to the "uncoupling" effect of Aβ on muscarinic cholinergic signal transduction already described. Thrombin receptors are widely expressed in neurons throughout the brain, including those vulnerable in AD (Weinstein et al., 1995). Several findings suggest a possible role for thrombin signaling in the pathogenesis of AD [see Cunningham et al. (1993) for review]. Both thrombin and the thrombin inhibitor protease nexin-1 are localized to amyloid plaques (Akiyama et al., 1992). In addition, cell culture data showed that thrombin can be neurotoxic and that protease nexin-1 (PN-1) is neuroprotective (Smith-Swintosky et al., 1995a, b). The toxicity of Aβ was exacerbated by thrombin and reduced by PN-1 in studies

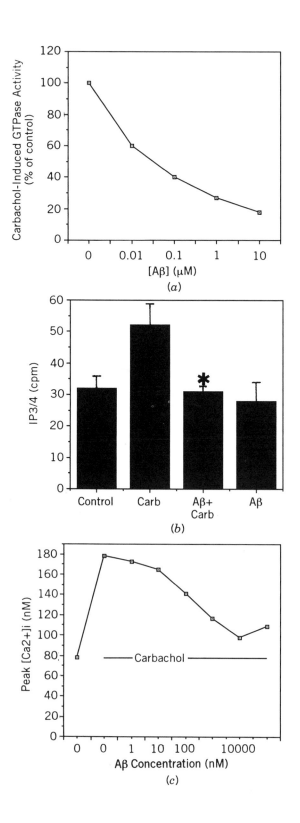

performed in rat hippocampal cell cultures (Smith-Swintosky et al., 1995b). Enhancement of Aβ toxicity by thrombin is consistent with the time course of Aβ-induced impairment of ion-motive ATPase activities (less than 30 min) while the time course of Aβ-induced impairment of thrombin receptor–G protein coupling may require more prolonged or severe oxidative damage. The data concerning effects of Aβ on various plasma membrane enzymes and signal transduction systems are summarized in Figure 2A.

Roles for Aβ in Dysfunction of, and Damage to, Glial and Vascular Cells in AD

Astrocytes subserve important neuroprotective functions in the brain (Hansson and Ronnback, 1995; Muller et al., 1995). For example, astrocytes express high levels of glutamate transporters, which are believed to be the major mechanism whereby (potentially toxic) glutamate is removed from the extracellular space. Studies have shown that the glutamate transporter is sensitive to damage by free radicals (Volterra et al., 1994). Because Aβ induces lipid peroxidation and damages membrane transport systems in several cell types, including neurons (see above) and vascular endothelial cells (see below), it is likely that Aβ also impairs glutamate transport in astrocytes and, indeed, preliminary data indicate this is the case (Harris et al., 1995). Impairment of glutamate transport would increase extracellular levels of glutamate and promote excitotoxic neuronal injury. Pike et al. (1994) reported that Aβ can induce a reactive phenotype in cultured astrocytes characterized by morphological changes and increased levels of glial fibrillary acidic protein and basic fibroblast growth factor (bFGF). The increase in bFGF levels is of interest because bFGF was previously shown to be present in plaques (Cummings et al., 1993) and to protect cultured hippocampal neurons against Aβ toxicity (Mattson et al., 1993a). Thus, some effects of Aβ on astrocytes are likely to be detrimental to neurons whereas other actions may include induction of neuroprotective substances.

Aβ can also induce multiple alterations in microglia that may impact on the neurodegenerative process in AD. Meda et al. (1995) reported that Aβ can activate cul-

---

FIGURE 8. Aβ disrupts muscarinic cholinergic signal transduction in cultured cortical neurons. (*a*) Rat cortical cell cultures were exposed for 4 hr to vehicle or the indicated concentrations of Aβ25–35. Basal and carbachol-induced GTPase activity was then quantified in membranes. Values are the mean and SEM ($n = 5$). Aβ did not affect basal (unstimulated) GTPase activity, (*b*) [^{3}H]-myoinositol was incorporated into neocortical cells, and then cultures were exposed to either vehicle (Control and Carb groups) or 20 μM Aβ25–35 (Aβ and Aβ + Carb groups) for 5 hr. Cells were then exposed to vehicle or 100 μM carbachol for 20 min in the presence of LiCl. Levels of inositol polyphosphates (IP$_{3/4}$) were then quantified. Values are the mean and SEM ($n = 3$). *$p < 0.05$, compared to carbachol-treated cultures not exposed to Aβ (Carb). (*c*) Cultures were exposed to the indicated concentrations of Aβ25–35 and then exposed to vehicle or 100 μM carbachol as indicated. Values represent the peak [Ca^{2+}]$_i$ (and SEM) following exposure to vehicle or carbachol ($n = 16–24$ neurons in three separate cultures). Modified from Kelly et al. (1996).

tured microglia resulting in their production of both neurotoxic and neurotrophic substances. Prior studies had shown that activated microglia produce several different cytokines and growth factors including tumor necrosis factor-α (TNF) and transforming growth factor-β [TGFβ; see Raivich and Kreutzberg (1994) for review]. Interestingly, both TNF (Barger et al., 1995b) and TGFβ (Galindo et al., 1994) were shown to protect cultured hippocampal neurons against Aβ toxicity, suggesting a neuroprotective role for activated microglia. On the other hand, strong evidence indicates that microglia can release cytotoxic substances, including ROS (e.g., superoxide anion) and excitotoxins (Piani and Fontana, 1994). A major unresolved question is whether injury-induced activation of microglia in vivo results in a worsening or lessening of neuronal damage. In a recent study of transgenic mice lacking TNF receptors, we found that the microglial response to excitotoxic and ischemic insults was suppressed and that damage to neurons was increased when compared to wild-type mice (Bruce et al., 1996). These data suggest that microglia do not play a major role in promoting neuronal degeneration in the injured brain.

Aβ deposits accumulate in blood vessel walls in AD (Frackowiak et al., 1994). The data described above showing profound effects of Aβ on neurons and glial cells suggested that cells of the vasculature that encounter Aβ might also be adversely affected. The major cell types in the vasculature that are likely exposed to Aβ include vascular smooth muscle cells, vascular endothelial cells, red blood cells, lymphocytes, and platelets. Several different studies of postmortem AD brain tissue have clearly documented damage to vascular smooth muscle and endothelial cells (Kawai et al., 1993; Buee et al., 1994; Perlmutter, 1994; Wisniewski et al., 1994; Davis-Salinas et al., 1995; Kalaria and Hedera, 1995). Vascular endothelial cells constitute the key cellular component of the blood–brain barrier, and some data suggest that the blood–brain barrier is disrupted in AD (Kalaria and Grahovac, 1990; Mattila et al., 1994). Thomas et al. (1996) showed that Aβ can damage vascular endothelial cells in a dramatic manner, providing evidence that Aβ could contribute to altered vascular reactivity and disruption of the blood–brain barrier in AD. Consistent with the latter study, Blanc et al. (submitted) found that Aβ can disrupt barrier and glucose transport functions of vascular endothelial cells grown in monolayer culture. Aβ induced death of vascular endothelial cells, which was characterized by DNA condensation and fragmentation (Figure 6), and was prevented with inhibitors of RNA synthesis, protein synthesis, and endonucleases. Damage to the blood–brain barrier may contribute to inflammatory processes (McGeer et al., 1994) and reduced energy availability in the brain (Hoyer, 1993; Pettegrew et al., 1994).

Circulating lymphocytes and red blood cells have also been shown to be adversely affected by Aβ. For example, Eckert et al. (1993) reported that Aβ enhanced the mitogen-induced calcium response in human lymphocytes. Altered immune functions have been reported in AD, and Aβ could conceivably play a role in these alterations by perturbing immune cell functions. We have found that Aβ can also damage red blood cells disrupting ion-motive ATPase activities and inducing cell degeneration and lysis (Figure 9). Red blood cells are the major source of oxygen for the brain and damage to these cells could contribute to the well-documented detriment in energy availability to the brain parenchyma in AD.

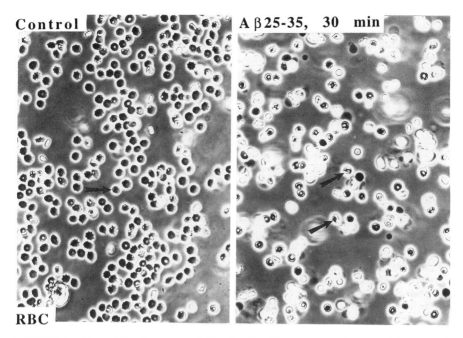

FIGURE 9. Aβ rapidly damages red blood cells. Phase-contrast images of human red blood cells that had been exposed for 30 min to vehicle (Control, left panel) or 20 μ*M* Aβ25–35 (right panel). Control cells have a smooth undamaged appearance, while many of the red blood cells exposed to Aβ appear crenated and damaged (e.g., arrows in right panel).

NORMAL FUNCTIONS OF βAPP: REGULATION OF NEURONAL EXCITABILITY, PLASTICITY, AND SURVIVAL

While Aβ is the product of βAPP that has received the bulk of attention vis-à-vis AD, data concerning the normal function of βAPP itself is rapidly accumulating. Early circumstantial evidence suggested that βAPP might be a cell surface receptor because of its predicted transmembrane configuration (Kang et al., 1987). However, as studies of βAPP functions have progressed it has become apparent that it is unlikely to function as a signal transducing receptor. Rather, it appears that the sAPP products of α-secretase cleavage of βAPP (sAPPαs) serve important intercellular signaling roles in the central nervous system (CNS). βAPP is axonally transported in the fast component (Koo et al., 1990) and immunocytochemical data indicate that βAPP accumulates in presynaptic terminals (Schubert et al., 1991) and axonal growth cones (Mattson, 1994). Release of sAPPα can be induced by excitatory neurotransmitters (Nitsch et al., 1992), electrical activity in neural circuits (Nitsch et al., 1993) and by direct activation of protein kinase C with phorbol esters (Buxbaum et al., 1990). Collectively, these data suggest the possibility that sAPPαs are released from presynaptic terminals coincident with neurotransmitters. Studies of the effects of sAPPαs on cultured hippocampal neurons have revealed roles for these βAPP derivatives in regulation of developmental and synaptic plasticity and cell survival. Calcium imaging studies showed that sAPPαs induced a rapid reduction of $[Ca^{2+}]_i$ and that calcium responses to glutamate were markedly attenuated in neurons pretreated with sAPPαs (Mattson et al., 1993d). The sAPPαs (APP695 and APP751) forms protected neurons against excitotoxicity and glucose deprivation-induced injury (Mattson et al., 1993d). Expression of βAPP in cultured neuroblastoma cells protected them against glutamate toxicity (Schubert and Behl, 1993), which, in that system, is likely mediated by oxyradical production. sAPPαs were subsequently shown to be effective in protecting cultured hippocampal neurons against Aβ toxicity by a mechanism involving suppression of free-radical accumulation (Goodman and Mattson, 1994a).

Whole-cell and single-channel patch clamp recordings showed that sAPPαs activate a high conductance, charybdotoxin-sensitive K^+ channel resulting in membrane hyperpolarization (Furukawa et al., 1996). The latter study also showed that sAPPαs suppress synaptically driven action potentials (Figure 10). The sAPPαs

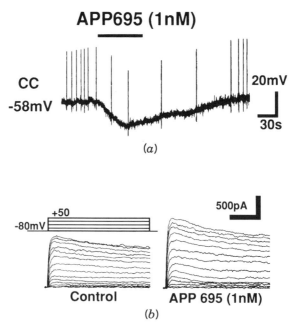

(a)

(b)

FIGURE 10. Secreted APPs reduce membrane excitability and suppress synaptic activity by activating K^+ channels in hippocampal neurons. (a) Spontaneous action potentials recorded in current clamp (CC) mode in a cultured hippocampal neuron prior to, during, and following exposure to sAPP695. The sAPP elicited a reversible hyperpolarization and greatly reduced the firing rate of synaptically driven action potentials. (b) Representative voltage-activated K^+ current recordings in a neuron prior to (Control) and 5 min following exposure to sAPP695. The pulses were applied in voltage steps from -80 to $+50$ mV. Modified from Furukawa et al. (1996).

were very potent with picomolar concentrations causing rapid activation of K^+ channels and suppression of glutamate-induced calcium influx. Using antibodies directed against different domains of sAPPα, it was shown that a region just N-terminal to the Aβ sequence mediated the actions of sAPPαs on neuronal excitability and calcium homeostasis (Mattson et al., 1993d; Furukawa et al., 1996). The receptor mediating these actions of sAPPαs has yet to be isolated, but the signal transduction pathway may involve a membrane-associated guanylate cyclase (Barger and Mattson, 1995; Barger et al., 1995a; Furukawa et al., 1996).

In addition to the roles of the functional domain of sAPPs just described, data suggest roles for a different domain of sAPPs, namely, amino acids 328–332 (RERMS), which lies just C-terminal to the kunitz protease insert site. Saitoh and co-workers reported that the RERMS domain was responsible for the mitogen actions of sAPPs, which they had previously described (Saitoh et al., 1989; Roch et al., 1993). Moreover, this peptide promoted neurite outgrowth in cultured cells (Jin et al., 1994) and synaptogenesis *in vivo* (Roch et al., 1994). Collectively, the data indicate that sAPPs may serve several fundamental roles in regulating neuronal plasticity and survival.

INTEGRATION OF AMYLOID TOXICITY MECHANISMS WITH OTHER HYPOTHESES OF THE PATHOGENESIS OF NEURONAL INJURY IN AD

As research into the pathophysiology of AD progressed, it became clear that many factors other than Aβ play important roles in determining whether AD develops in a particular individual. In this section we consider some of the factors for which considerable evidence supports roles in AD. These factors include hormones such as estrogens and glucocorticoids, cytokines such as TNF and TGFβ, neurotrophic factors such as bFGF and brain-derived neurotrophic factor (BDNF), proteases and their inhibitors (e.g., thrombin and protease nexin-1), and apolipoprotein E.

Laudable Estrogens and Deplorable Glucocorticoids

Animal studies and clinical data from postmenopausal women receiving estrogen replacement therapy have clearly shown that estrogens have a positive impact on multiple organ systems in the aging body including the nervous system. The abilities of estrogens to retard bone loss and suppress the development of atherosclerosis are well known (Schwartz et al., 1995; Prestwood et al., 1995). Estrogens may also suppress age-related neurodegenerative disorders including AD. Recent studies have shown a clear reduction in the incidence of AD in postmenopausal women receiving estrogens compared to those who did not receive estrogens (Henderson et al., 1994; Tang et al., 1996). The mechanisms whereby estrogens suppress age-related neurodegenerative processes are not well understood, although recent data suggest the involvement of antioxidant mechanisms. Earlier studies of the anti-atherosclerotic actions of estrogens showed that estrogens can suppress free-radical-mediated injury to vascular endothelial cells induced by oxidized low-density lipoprotein (Keaney et al., 1994). Studies of estrogen actions in neuroblastoma cell cultures showed that 17β-estradiol can protect cells against oxidative insults (Behl et al., 1995). Goodman et al. (1996) showed that 17β-estradiol and estriol could suppress membrane oxidation and disruption of ion homeostasis induced by Aβ in hippocampal neurons, while other steroids including testosterone, aldosterone, and vitamin D were ineffective (Figure 11). The neuroprotective actions of estrogens were not mediated by the classic steroid receptor–transcription pathway because high concentrations of estrogens were required and the estrogens were effective in the presence of RNA and protein synthesis inhibitors (Behl et al., 1995; Goodman et al., 1996). Taken together with data concerning the mechanism of Aβ cytotoxicity described above, the data indicate that the inherent antioxidant activity of estrogens may play a role in protecting neurons against oxidative insults believed to mediate the neurodegenerative process in AD. However, additional transcription-dependent actions of estrogens could also contribute to neuroprotective activities. For example, estrogens were shown to increase the expression of neurotrophic factors in the rodent brain in vivo (Singh et al., 1995). Finally, suppression of the development of atherosclerotic damage to cerebral blood vessels could play a role in the antidementia actions of estrogens.

Glucocorticoids are produced by adrenal cortical cells in response to environmental and psychological stressors that signal through the hypothalamic–pituitary–adrenal axis. While short-term activation of this neuroendocrine system mobilizes energy stores and enhances responses to the stressor, long-term activation of this system can adversely affect many different organ systems including the immune system (Wilckens, 1995) and the brain (Landfield et al., 1992; Sapolsky, 1994). In vitro and in vivo studies have shown that elevated levels of circulating glucocorticoids can exacerbate injury to hippocampal and cortical neurons induced by excitotoxic, metabolic, and oxidative insults. For example, corticosterone increased the vulnerability of hippocampal neurons to excitotoxic (Elliott et al., 1993) and ischemic (Smith-Swintosky et al., 1996a) injury (Figure 12). It was also shown that excitotoxic injury was enhanced in rats subjected to a physiological stress regimen prior to administration of kainic acid (Stein-Behrens et al., 1994). Cell culture studies have shown that glucocorticoids can impair glucose uptake (Horner et al., 1990), destabilize calcium homeostasis (Elliott and Sapolsky, 1993), and exacerbate free-radical production in neurons exposed to oxidative insults (Goodman et al., 1996). Several laboratories have reported rather pronounced abnormalities in regulation of the hypothalamic–pituitary–adrenal axis in AD patients compared to age-matched controls (Hatzinger et al., 1995; Raadsheer et al., 1995). Therapies aimed at suppressing the stress response early in the course of AD should be pursued. Animal studies indicate that inhibitors of glucocorticoid synthesis (e.g., metyrapone) can reduce ischemia- and excitotoxin-induced damage to hippocampal neurons of adult rats (Smith-Swintosky et al., 1996a), suggesting that effects of chronic administration of such compounds in animal models of AD should be explored.

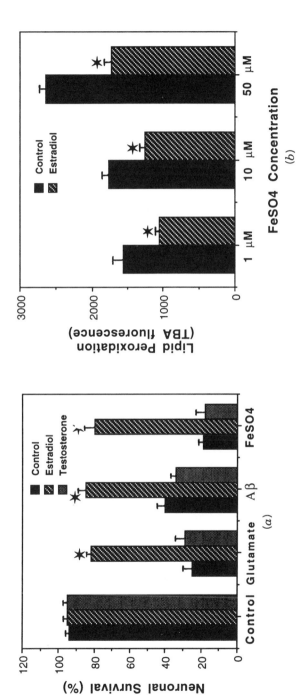

FIGURE 11. Estradiol protects cultured hippocampal neurons against excitotoxicity, Aβ toxicity, and oxidative injury and suppresses membrane lipid peroxidation. (*a*) Hippocampal cultures were pretreated with vehicle (Control), 1 μ*M* 17β-estradiol or 1 μ*M* testosterone and were then exposed to saline (24 hr, Control), glutamate (10 μ*M* for 20 hr), Aβ (2 μ*M* Aβ25–35 for 24 hr), or FeSO₄ (5 μ*M* for 6 hr). Values for neuronal survival are expressed as percentage of initial number of viable neurons and represent the mean and SEM of determinations made in four separate cultures. *$p <$ 0.01 compared to corresponding values in Control and testosterone-treated cultures. (*b*) Cultures were pretreated with vehicle (Control) or 1 μ*M* 17β-estradiol for 2 hr and were then exposed to the indicated concentrations of FeSO₄ for 1 hr. Cells were then fixed in thiobarbituric acid (TBA) fixative and cellular fluorescence was quantified from confocal laser scanning microscope images. Values represent the mean and SEM of determinations made in 18–23 neurons in three separate cultures. Modified from Goodman et al. (1996).

263

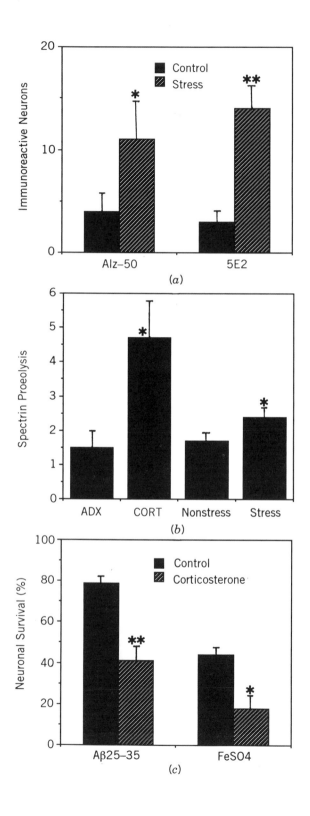

Cytokines

Inflammatory mediators have recently attracted a great deal of attention among AD researchers. Studies of AD brain have revealed the presence of a variety of immune response factors in association with amyloid plaques [see Eikelenboom et al. (1994) and McGeer et al. (1994) for review]. Complement cascade components, complement activators, amyloid P component, thrombin, and apolipoprotein E are all associated with plaques. Activated microglia, which represent a major cellular component of inflammatory processes in the brain, are a prominent feature of AD lesions. Further evidence that inflammatory processes contribute to the pathogenesis of AD comes from a study suggesting that nonsteroidal anti-inflammatory agents reduce the risk of developing AD (Breitner et al., 1994). On the other hand, some cytokines associated with the inflammatory process may be beneficial to neurons. Both TNF (Cheng et al., 1994a; Barger et al., 1995b) and TGFβ (Prehn et al., 1993; Galindo et al., 1994) were reported to protect hippocampal and cortical neurons against excitotoxicity and Aβ toxicity. Neurons pretreated with TNF were relatively resistant to glutamate toxicity, glucose deprivation-induced death, Aβ toxicity and $FeSO_4$ toxicity (Cheng et al., 1994a; Barger et al., 1995b). The elevation of $[Ca^{2+}]_i$ normally induced by glutamate and Aβ was suppressed in neurons pretreated with TNF. As well, lipid peroxidation and hydrogen peroxide accumulation induced by $FeSO_4$ and Aβ were suppressed in neurons pretreated with TNF (Barger et al., 1995b). Interestingly TNF also induced expression of calbindin in astrocytes, a cell type in which calbindin is not normally expressed (Mattson et al., 1995a).

In the case of TNF the neuroprotective signal transduction mechanism has been elucidated. Two different receptors for TNF have been isolated and cloned, p55 and

---

FIGURE 12. Glucocorticoids and physiological stressors exacerbate cytoskeletal alterations and neuronal degeneration induced by excitotoxins and Aβ. (*a*) Adult rats were subjected to stressors or a battery of physiological stressors. Kainic acid was then injected into the dorsal hippocampus of rats in each group, and 3 hr later the rats were killed and coronal brain sections immunostained with tau antibodies Alz-50 and 5E2. Immunoreactive neurons in region CA3 of the hippocampus were counted, and values represent the mean and SEM of determinations made in 8 rats/group. $*p < 0.05$, $** p < 0.01$ compared to the Control value. (*b*) Four groups of adult rats were prepared including: ADX, adrenalectomized and administered a control pellet ($n = 16$); CORT, adrenalectomized and received a 100% corticosterone pellet or corticosterone injection ($n = 16$); Nonstress, unstressed controls ($n = 5$); Stress, exposure for 24 hr to a battery of stressful conditions *(n = 5)*. Kainic acid was then injected into the dorsal hippocampus of rats in each group, and 3 hr later the rats were killed and spectrin proteolysis in the injected hippocampus quantified by densitometric analysis of immunoreactive bands corresponding to spectrin breakdown products on Western blots. $*p < 0.05$ compared to ADX value and nonstress value. (*c*) Rat hippocampal cell cultures were pretreated for 2 hr with either vehicle (Control) or 1 μ*M* corticosterone. Cultures were then exposed to either 2 μ*M* Aβ25–35 for 24 hr or 2 μ*M* $FeSO_4$ for 6 hr. Neuronal survival was quantified and values represent the mean and SEM of determination made in four separate cultures. $*p < 0.05$, $**p < 0.01$ compared to Control value. Modified from Stein-Behrens et al. (1994) and Goodman et al. (1996).

p75. Binding of TNF to the p55 receptor results in activation of a sphingomyelinase that cleaves membrane-associated sphingomyelin releasing the compound ceramide. Ceramide then appears to activate a kinase that may then activate the transcription factor NFκB (Kolesnick and Golde, 1994). NFκB is a cytosolic complex of three proteins; p50 and p65 are the transcription factor dimer and IκB is a subunit that tonically inhibits activity of the transcription factor dimer. Signals that activate NFκB do so by causing dissociation of IκB from p50–p65; the dimer then translocates to the nucleus and binds the enhancer region of DNA in NFκB responsive genes. In cultured rat hippocampal neurons TNF activated NFκB and induced the expression of the calcium-binding protein calbindin (Cheng et al., 1994a; Barget et al., 1995b) and the antioxidant enzymes MnSOD and Cu/Zn-SOD (M. P. Mattson, unpublished data). The following data indicate that NFκB is mechanistically involved in the neuroprotective actions of TNF (Figure 13). Pretreatment of hippocampal cell cultures with a membrane-permeant ceramide analog protected neurons against excitotoxicity, $FeSO_4$ toxicity and Aβ toxicity (Goodman and Mattson, 1996a). Ceramide also induced an increase in calbindin levels in cultured hippocampal cells. Exposure of cultured hippocampal neurons to IκB (MAD3) antisense oligodeoxynucleotides resulted in an increase in NFκB activity, suppressed Aβ-induced elevation of $[Ca^{2+}]_{i,}$ and protected the neurons against Aβ toxicity (Barger et al., 1995b). There has recently been a rapid increase in interest in the function of NFκB in the nervous system, and the data just described suggest this transcription factor may play important roles in neurodegenerative disorders. NFκB is of particular interest with respect to the role of oxidative processes in the injury of neurons in AD, because exposure of cells to oxidative insults results in activation of NFκB (Schreck et al., 1992). This suggests that activation of NFκB may constitute a cytoprotective signaling pathway that induces expression of protective gene products such as calbindin and antioxidant enzymes.

FIGURE 13. Activators of the transcription factor NFkB protect neurons against Aβ toxicity and oxidative insults. (*a*) Rat hippocampal cell cultures were pretreated for 20 hr with the indicated concentrations of C2-ceramide (C2) or dihydroceramide (DHC) and were then exposed to 10 μM Aβ25–35 for 24 hr. Values for neuronal and survival are expressed as percent initial number of viable neurons prior to exposure to Aβ and represent the mean and SEM of determinations made in four–six separate cultures. Neuronal survival was significantly increased in cultures pretreated with C2 concentrations of 100 nM ($p < 0.01$), 1 μM ($p < 0.001$), and 10 μM ($p < 0.01$). (*b*) Rat hippocampal cell cultures were pretreated for the indicated time periods with 1 μM C2 and were then exposed to either 10 μM glutamate for 24 hr, 10 μM $FeSO_4$ for 4 hr, or 10 μM Aβ1–40 for 24 hr. Each value is the mean and SEM ($n = 4$–6). (*c*) Mouse hippocampal cultures were pretreated for 24 hr with 20 μM MAD3 (IκB) antisense oligonucleotide, mismatch control oligonucleotide, or no oligonucleotide (Control). Cultures were then exposed to 20 μM Aβ25–35 for 24 hr and neuronal survival was quantified. Values are the mean and SEM of determinations made in three separate cultures. *$p < 0.05$ compared to corresponding values for Control and mismatch cultures. Modified from Barger et al. (1995b) and Goodman and Mattson (1996a).

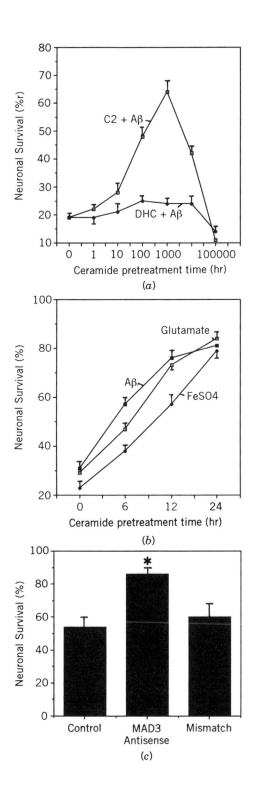

(a)

(b)

(c)

Neurotrophic Factors

Interest in roles for neurotrophic factors in the pathogenesis of AD was sparked by the observations that basal forebrain cholinergic neurons degenerate in AD and express NGF receptors, and that NGF supports the survival of basal forebrain cholinergic neurons in animal "models" of AD [see Hefti (1994) for review]. The second major impetus for studies of neurotrophic factors in AD was the finding that bFGF and NGF can protect hippocampal and cortical neurons against metabolic and excitotoxic insults (Mattson et al., 1989; Cheng and Mattson, 1991), and subsequent studies show that several different neurotrophic factors can protect neurons against insults relevant to the pathogenesis of AD including excitotoxins, metabolic insults, and Aβ [see Mattson et al. (1993c) and Mattson and Furukawa (1996) for review]. From the standpoint of oxidative processes and neuronal degeneration in AD, it was shown that bFGF, NGF, and BDNF can suppress accumulation of free radicals in neurons exposed to glutamate (Mattson et al., 1995b). The latter three neurotrophic factors induced increases in the activity of one or more antioxidant enzymes including Cu/Zn-SOD, catalase, glutathione peroxidase, and glutathione reductase. Basic FGF stabilized cellular calcium homeostasis and protected cultured rat hippocampal neurons against Aβ toxicity (Mattson et al., 1993a). Several other neurotrophic factors have been reported to protect neurons against oxidative insults, including insulinlike growth factors (Zhang et al., 1993), neurotrophins 3 and 4/5 (Cheng and Mattson, 1994; Cheng et al., 1994b), and platelet-derived growth factors (Cheng and Mattson, 1995). At this point it is quite clear that administration of neurotrophic factors can be very effective in protecting neurons against insults relevant to AD. It is much less clear whether alterations in neurotrophic factor systems contribute to the disease process. Different laboratories have reported that expression of BDNF is reduced in hippocampus from AD patients compared to age-matched controls [see Hellweg and Jockers-Scherubl (1994)]. Levels of NGF may be increased in cerebral cortex and reduced in basal forebrain (Scott et al., 1995); this alteration in NGF distribution may be the result of degeneration of basal forebrain neurons rather than an antecedent event.

Apolipoprotein E

In light of the mounting evidence that vascular alterations contribute to the pathogenesis of AD (see above), it is likely that the increased propensity to develop AD at an earlier age in individuals carrying the apolipoprotein E4 (apoE4) allele is due to the atherogenic action of this apoE allele (Kosunen et al., 1995). However, many laboratories are pursuing the general hypothesis that the apoE link to AD is the result of some action of apoE in the brain parenchyma [see Strittmatter and Roses (1995) for review]. Initial studies that focused on possible interactions between apoE and Aβ have yielded positive data; but, unfortunately, the data are often conflicting and no clear picture has emerged. For example, Castano et al. (1995) reported that apoEs promote Aβ aggregation and that apoE4 is more effective than apoE3. On the other hand seemingly opposite results were obtained by LaDu et al. (1994) who found that apoE3 bound more tightly to Aβ than did apoE4. Further complicating matters are reports apoE inhibits Aβ fibril formation (Evans et al., 1995). More recent work indicates that the presence of lipid can greatly influence binding of apoEs to Aβ (LaDu et al., 1995).

THERAPEUTIC IMPLICATIONS

Knowledge of cellular and molecular mechanisms in the following areas have revealed a wide array of potential therapeutic targets and approaches (Table 2) including: (1) regulation of βAPP processing, (2) prevention of Aβ aggregation, (3) stabilization of cellular ion homeostasis, (4) suppression of oxidative processes and free-radical metabolism, (5) blockade of excitotoxic processes, (6) activation of neurotrophic signal transduction pathways, and (7) anti-apoptotic agents. Figure 14 summarizes the various relevant therapeutic targets at which some compounds act to reduce neuronal degeneration, at least in cell culture paradigms of injury believed relevant to the pathogenesis of AD (e.g., Aβ toxicity, excitotoxicity, and oxidative injury).

Although identification and characterization of compounds that affect βAPP processing are being vigorously pursued, no data has yet been published. It is known that agents that activate protein kinase C (e.g., phorbol esters) can induce α-secretase cleavage and thereby reduce release of intact Aβ from cells (Buxbaum et al., 1990; Nitsch et al., 1993). Certain serum-derived growth factors may also promote α-secretase cleavage of βAPP (LeBlanc, 1995). Several neurotrophic factors are known to utilize receptors linked to phospholipase C and protein kinase C activation (e.g., bFGF), and therefore have the potential to protect neurons in several different ways (βAPP processing, enhancement of calcium homeostasis, and suppression of free-radical accumulation; see above).

Because aggregation of Aβ is strongly linked to its neurotoxic actions (see above), many investigators are working to identify compounds that prevent aggregation of the peptide. Such compounds exist and are effective in in vitro systems. For example, Congo Red prevents Aβ fibril formation and protects cultured neurons against Aβ toxicity (Lorenzo and Yankner, 1994). Proteins that may normally play roles in clearance of soluble Aβ are also being studied. For example, apoE can affect Aβ aggregation and toxicity (Whitson et al., 1994), and small peptide inhibitors of Aβ aggregation exist and may have therapeutic potential. Finally, oxidative stress may contribute to Aβ aggregation in the aging brain and in AD (Dyrks et al., 1992), and antioxidants have been shown to protect neurons against Aβ toxicity (see above).

The largest number of compounds with therapeutic potential in AD reported to date appear to fall into the category of agents that protect neurons against Aβ neurotoxicity. Several compounds that stabilize cellular ion homeostasis were reported to be effective in attenuating the toxic actions of Aβ in cultured neurons. For example, calcium channel blockers (Weiss et al., 1994) and sodium channel blockers (Mark et al., 1995a) protected cultured neurons against Aβ toxicity. In addition, potassium channel openers such as diazoxide and levocromakalim were very effective in protecting cultured hippocampal neurons against Aβ toxicity, as well as excitotoxicity and oxidative injury (Goodman and Mattson, 1996b). Potassium channel openers are routinely used to treat cardiovascular disorders and are therefore poised for rapid movement to clinical trials in AD. Many of these agents are also very effective in protecting neurons against excitotoxic and metabolic insults in vivo. Several different anticonvulsants, including valproic acid, phenytoin, and carbamazepine, protected cultural hippocampal neurons against excitotoxicity and Aβ toxicity (Mark et al., 1995b). Moreover, neurotrophic factors (e.g., bFGF) and cy-

TABLE 2. Neuroprotective Agents with Potential to Slow the Progression of Alzheimer's Disease

Agent	Mechanism of Action	References
Congo red	Prevents peptide aggregation	Lorenzo and Yankner (1994)
Vitamin E	Chain-breaking antioxidant	Goodman and Mattson (1994), Behl et al. (1994)
Propyl gallate	Antioxidant	Mark et al. (1995a)
Phenyl-butyl-nitrone (PBN)	Spin trap (antioxidant	Mark et al. (1995a)
Nordihydroguaiaretic acid	Antioxidant, lipoxygenase inhibitor	Goodman et al. (1994)
Nifedipine	L-type calcium channel blocker	Weiss et al. (1994)
MK-801, APV	NMDA receptor antagonists	Mattson et al. (1993a)
Phenytoin, carbamazepine	Sodium channel blockers	Mark et al. (1995b)
Valproic acid	GABA agonist, sodium channel blocker	Mark et al. (1995b)
Diazoxide, pinacidil, chromakalim	Potassium channel openers	Goodman and Mattson (1996b)
K-252a, K-252b, staurosporine	Activate neurotrophic factor signaling pathways (tyrosine kinase cascades)	Cheng et al. (1994), Goodman and Mattson (1994b)
bFGF, BDNF, NGF, NT-3 NT-4/5, IGF-1, TGFβ	Tyrosine phosphorylation, MAP kinase, and gene expression	Mattson and Scheff (1994) (review) Mattson and Furukawa (1996) (review)
TNFα and TNGβ	NFκB activation and gene expression	Barger et al. (1995b)
sAPPs	Activate potassium channels and NFkB	Furukawa et al. (1996), Barget and Mattson (1996)
Ceramide	Activate NFκB	Goodman and Mattson (1996a)
Estrogens	Antioxidant activity	Goodman et al. (1996) Behl et al., (1995)
Metyrapone	Blocks glucocorticoid production	Smith-Swintosky et al. (1996a)
Cytochalasin D	Actin depolymerization/decr. calcium influx	Furukawa et al. (1995)
		Furukawa and Mattson (1995a)
Taxol	Microtubule stabilizer/decr. calcium influx	Furukawa and Mattson (1995b)

tokines (TNF) that can protect cultured neurons against Aβ toxicity have been shown to stabilize calcium homeostasis, possibly by inducing the expression of the calcium-binding protein calbindin (Mattson et al., 1993a; Cheng et al., 1994a; Barget et al., 1995b). Finally, additional calcium-stabilizing agents are being identified that have novel and intriguing mechanisms of action. For example, cytochalasins were shown to protect cultured neurons against excitotoxicity and Aβ toxicity and also protected hippocampal neurons against excitotoxic injury in vivo (Furukawa et al., 1995; Furukawa and Mattson, 1995a). In the latter studies it was shown that the mechanism of action of cytochalasins involves depolymerization of actin and suppression of calcium influx through NMDA receptors and voltage-dependent calcium channels. Apparently, depolymerization of actin induced by prolonged elevation of $[Ca^{2+}]_i$ is not simply an adverse consequence of calcium influx but rather is functionally involved in a neuroprotective feedback pathway that limits further calcium influx (Furukawa et al., 1995). Interestingly, the microtubule-stabilizing agent taxol was also effective in protecting cultured hippocampal neurons against excitotoxicity (Furukawa and Mattson, 1995b).

Another category of neuroprotective agents with considerable therapeutic potential in AD is antioxidants. Such agents include vitamin E, the spin-trapping compound PBN, and propyl gallate (Behl et al., 1994a; Goodman and Mattson, 1994a). These compounds were effective in protecting cultured neurons against an array of insults relevant to the pathogenesis of AD, including Aβ toxicity, excitotoxicity, and direct oxidative insults such as exposure to iron sulfate. In vivo studies have shown that several antioxidants are effective in protecting brain cells against ischemic and excitotoxic injuries (Hall et al., 1992; Carney and Carney, 1994). Neurotrophic factors can also be considered as having antioxidant properties in that they can induce the expression of antioxidant enzymes in brain cells (see above). Also falling into the category of antioxidants are estrogens, which may exhibit intrinsic antioxidant activity or may act in an indirect manner by inducing the expression of neurotrophic factors (see above). Clinical trials of several antioxidants in AD patients are in progress.

Antiexcitotoxic agents have been most intensively studied from the perspective of acute neurodegenerative conditions such as stroke and traumatic brain injury (Lipton, 1993). However, as described above there is considerable evidence that neuronal degeneration in AD includes an excitotoxic component. Many different antagonists of different subtypes of glutamate receptors exist including those that block NMDA receptors and AMPA/kainate receptors. Such compounds are of potential benefit in suppressing the neurodegenerative process in AD, although adverse side effects are likely to continue to be a problem.

A rapidly growing therapeutic approach involves identifying compounds that activate neuroprotective signal transduction pathways. As described above, receptor tyrosine kinase cascades and cytokine signaling pathways involving NFκB can activate a host of cellular defense mechanisms in neurons. Administration of the ligands themselves is one approach to activating these pathways in brain cells of AD patients and, indeed, clinical trials of neurotrophic factors are in progress (Olson et al., 1994). However, such neurotrophic factors are large proteins that do not readily access the brain when administered peripherally. Therefore, two alternative approaches are being pur-

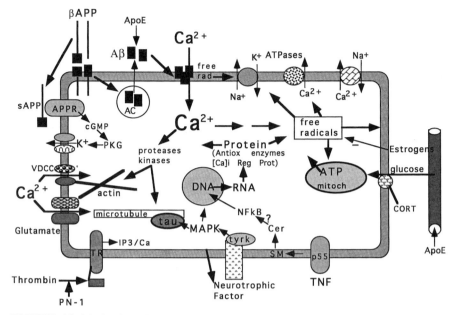

FIGURE 14. Mechanisms that promote or prevent oxidative cell injury and disruption of ion homeostasis are relevant to the pathogenesis of neuronal injury in AD. βAPP is proteolytically cleaved by either α-secretase resulting in release of secreted forms of βAPP (sAPP) from the cell surface or β-secretase resulting in release of amyloid β-peptide (Aβ). The sAPPs bind to a putative receptor (APPR) linked to elevation of cyclic GMP levels, activation of cGMP-dependent protein kinase (PKG), and activation of a high-conductance K^+ channel. The sAPPs thereby hyperpolarize the membrane and counteract the depolarizing actions of glutamate, energy failure, and Aβ. By reducing levels of α-secretase-derived sAPPs, mutations in βAPP may promote neuronal degeneration. In response to age-related factors (e.g., increased oxidative stress), Aβ forms fibrils and induces free-radical production in neurons resulting in impairment of Na^+/K^+-ATPase and Ca^{2+}-ATPase activities. Impairment of the ion pumps results in membrane depolarization, Ca^{2+} influx, and increased sensitivity to excitotoxicity. Ca^{2+} induces production of several free radicals including superoxide anion, hydroxyl radical, and nitric oxide. Estrogens act as antioxidants and thereby suppress accumulation of free radicals.

Glutamate activates NMDA and AMPA receptors resulting in Ca influx through the NMDA receptor channel and voltage-dependent calcium channels (VDCC). Calcium activates proteases, kinases, and other calcium-regulated proteins that affect cytoskeletal polymerization and ion channel function. Reduced glucose availability to neurons occurs in AD resulting in ATP depletion, compromise of Na^+/K^+-ATPase activity, and increased vulnerability to excitotoxicity; glucocorticoids may exacerbate energy depletion by impairing glucose transport into neurons. Neuroprotective signaling pathways that stabilize calcium homeostasis and suppress accumulation of ROS include neurotrophic factors that activate receptor tyrosine kinases (tyrk). Activation of the NTF receptors results in a cascade of phosphorylation reactions involving intermediate kinases, mitogen-activated protein kinases (MAPK), and transcription factors. Genes induced by NTFs include proteins involved in regulation of $[Ca^{2+}]_i$ (e.g., calcium-binding proteins) and antioxidant enzymes (e.g., superoxide dismutases, catalase, and glutathione peroxidase). Kinases activated by neurotrophic factors may also phosphorylate cytoskeletal proteins such as the microtubule-associated protein tau. Cytokines such as tumor necrosis factor (TNF) are likely to play important roles in inflammatory processes in AD. In neurons TNF binds to a receptor (p55) linked to sphingomyelin sued. One approach is to identify small lipophilic compounds that activate neuroprotective signaling pathways. Cell culture and in vivo studies of paradigms of neuronal injury relevant to AD have revealed several such molecules. The bacterial alkaloids K252a and staurosporine were shown to activate receptor tyrosine kinase signaling cascades and protected cultured rat hippocampal and cortical neurons against metabolic and excitotoxic insults (Cheng et al., 1994c). Moreover, these bacterial alkaloids protected adult rats against hippocampal damage and memory loss induced by severe seizure activity (Smith-Swintosky et al., 1996b). Another example is the compound ceramide, which is known to activate NFκB. Ceramide protected cultured hippocampal neurons against excitotoxicity and oxidative insults including Aβ toxicity (Goodman and Mattson, 1996a). In vivo trials of ceramide are in progress. A second approach is to identify compounds that induce the expression of endogenous neurotrophic factors. Nabeshima and co-workers have reported on several such compounds that look promising (Nitta et al., 1993; Nabeshima et al., 1994).

To this point, cell culture models have been instrumental in identifying potential therapeutic approaches. However, it is now critical to employ animal models of AD currently being developed in order to screen such compounds in vivo and then move on to primate studies and clinical trials in humans. Animal models such as the V717F mouse (Games et al., 1995) should be used extensively as a key bridge between basic research and clinical trials. It is expected that similar animal models based on mutations known to cause AD in humans including those in βAPP. S182 [chromosome 14 gene product; Sherrington et al. (1995)] and STM2 [chromosome 1 gene product; Levy-Lahad et al. (1995)] will be developed in the near future. The latter mutations appear to promote neuron degeneration by disrupting calcium homeostasis (Guo et al., 1996) and altering βAPP processing (Scheuner et al., 1996). It is hoped that such animals will be made available to the increasing number of AD researchers who can make major contributions and accelerate the development of effective preventative and therapeutic agents for this devastating disorder.

ACKNOWLEDGMENTS

We thank J. G. Begley, S. Bose, and R. Pelphrey for technical support and G. Sears for editing of the manuscript. Original research from the author's laboratory was supported by grants to M. P. M. from the NIH, the Alzheimer's Association (Evelyn Stone fund and Zenith Award), and the Metropolitan Life Foundation. A. J. B. is a recipient of an NIH training grant fellowship. R. J. M. was supported by a neurobiology of aging training grant from the NIA. E. M. B. is the recipient of a Fellowship from the DRET (#93811-50).

(SM) hydrolysis and release of ceramide; ceramide (via intervening kinases) activates the transcription factor NKκB resulting in induction of neuroprotective gene products. Thrombin has been shown to influence neuronal vulnerability to metabolic and oxidative insults by activating a receptor linked to inositol phospholipid hydrolysis and release of calcium from intracellular stores. Glial cells produce the thrombin inhibitor protease nexin-1 (PN-1), which can block actions of thrombin.

REFERENCES

Akiyama H, Ikeda K, Kondo H, McGeer PL (1992): Thrombin accumulation in brains of patients with Alzheimer's disease. Neurosci Lett 146:152–154.

Arispe N, Pollard HB, Rojas E (1993): Giant multilevel cation channels formed by Alzheimer disease amyloid β-protein [ABP-(1-40)] in bilayer membranes. Proc Natl Acad Sci U S A 90:10573–10577.

Barger SW, Mattson MP (1995): Secreted form of the Alzheimer's amyloid precursor protein stimulates a membrane-associated guanylate cyclase. Biochem J 311:45–47.

Barger SW, Fiscus RR, Ruth P, Hofmann F, Mattson MP (1995a): Role of cyclic GMP in the regulation of neuronal calcium and survival by secreted forms of β amyloid precursor. J Neurochem 64:2087–2096.

Barger SW, Horster D, Furukawa K, Goodman Y, Krieglstein J, Mattson MP (1995b): TNFα and TNFβ protect hippocampal neurons against amyloid β-peptide toxicity: Evidence for involvement of a κB-binding factor and attenuation of peroxide and Ca^{2+} accumulation. Proc Natl Acad Sci U S A 92:9328–9332.

Barger SW, Mattson MP (1996): Induction of neuroprotective κB-dependent transcription by secreted forms of the Alzheimer's β-amyloid precursor. Mol Brain Res 40:116–126.

Barrow CJ, Yasuda A, Kenny PT, Zagorski MG (1992): Solution conformations and aggregational properties of synthetic amyloid beta-peptides of Alzheimer's disease: Analysis of circular dichroism spectra. J Mol Biol 225:1075–1093.

Beckman JS (1994): Peroxynitrite versus hydroxyl radical: The role of nitric oxide in superoxide-dependent cerebral injury. Ann N Y Acad Sci 738:69–75.

Behl C, Davis J, Lesley R, Schubert D (1994a): Hydrogen peroxide mediates amyloid β protein toxicity. Cell 77:817–827.

Behl C, Davis JB, Klier FG, Schubert D (1994b): Amyloid beta peptide induces necrosis rather than apoptosis. Brain Res 645:253–264.

Behl C, Hovey L, Krajewski S, Schubert D, Reed JC (1993): BCL-2 prevents killing of neuronal cells by glutamate but not by amyloid beta protein. Biochem Biophys Res Commun 197:949–956.

Behl C, Widmann M, Trapp T, Holsboer F (1995): 17-β estradiol protects neurons from oxidative stress-induced cell death in vitro. Biochem Biophys Res Commun 216:473–482.

Beckman JS (1994): Peroxynitrite versus hydroxyl radical: The role of nitric oxide in superoxide-dependent cerebral injury. Ann N Y Acad Sci 738:69–75.

Benzi G, Moretti A (1995): Are reactive oxygen species involved in Alzheimer's disease? Neurobiol Aging 16:661–674.

Blanc Em, Toborek M, Mark RJ, Mattson MP (submitted): Amyloid β-peptide disrupts barrier and transport functions and induces apoptosis in vascular endothelial cells.

Breitner JCS, Gau BA, Welsh KA, Plassman BL, McDonald WM, Helms MJ, Anthony JC (1994): Inverse association of anti-inflammatory treatments and Alzheimer's disease. Neurology 44:227–232.

Brines ML, Dare AO, de Lanerolle NC (1995): The cardiac glycoside ouabain potentiates excitotoxic injury of adult neurons in rat hippocampus. Neurosci Lett 191:145–148.

Bruce AJ, Boling W, Kindy MS, Peschon J, Kraemer PJ, Carpenter MK, Holtsberg FW, Mattson MP (1996): Altered neuronal and microglial responses to brain injury in mice lacking TNF receptors. Nature Medicine 2:788–794.

Bruce AJ, Bose S, Fu W, Butt CM, Mirault ME, Taniguchi N, Mattson MP (1996): Amyloid β-peptide alters the profile of antioxidant enzymes in hippocampal cultures in a manner similar to that observed in Alzheimer's disease. Pathogenesis. In press.

Buee L, Hof PR, Bouras C, Delacourte A, Perl DP, Morrison JH, Fillit HM (1994): Pathological alterations of the cerebral microvasculature in Alzheimer's disease and dementing disorders. Acta Neuropathol 87:469–480.

Busciglio J, Yankner BA (1995): Apoptosis and increased generation of reactive oxygen species in Down's syndrome neurons in vitro. Nature 378:776–779.

Busciglio J, Lorenzo A, Yeh J, Yankner BA (1995): β-amyloid fibrils induce tau phosphorylation and loss of microtubule binding. Neuron 14:879–888.

Bush AI, Pettingell WH, Multhaup G, Paradis M, Vonsattel JP, Gusella JF, Beyreuther K, Master CL, Tanzi RE (1994): Rapid induction of Alzheimer β-amyloid formation by zinc Science 265:1464–1467.

Butterfield DA, Hensley K, Harris M, Mattson MP, Carney J (1994): β-amyloid peptide free radical fragments initiate synaptosomal lipoperoxidation in a sequence-specific fashion: Implications to Alzheimer's disease. Biochem Biophys Res Commun 200:710–715.

Buxbaum JD, Gandy SE, Cicchetti P, Ehrlich ME, Czernik AJ, Fracasso RP, Ramabhadran TV, Unterbeck AJ, Greengard P (1990): Processing of Alzheimer beta/A4 amyloid precursor protein: Modulation by agents that regulate protein phosphorylation. Proc Natl Acad Sci U S A 87:6003–6006.

Cai X, Golde T, Youkin S (1993): Release of excess amyloid β protein from a mutant amyloid B protein precursor. Science 259:514–516.

Carney JM, Carney AM (1994): Role of protein oxidation in aging and in age-associated neurodegenerative diseases. Life Sci 55:2097–2103.

Carney JM, Starke-Reed PE, Oliver CN, Landum RW, Cheng MS, Wu JF, Floyd RA (1991): Reversal of age-related increase in brain protein oxidation, decrease in enzyme activity, and loss in temporal and spatial memory by chronic administration of the spin-trapping compound N-tert-butyl-alpha-phenylnitrone. Proc Natl Acad Sci U S A 88:3633–3636.

Carillo MC, Kanai S, Sato Y, Kitani K (1992): Age-related changes in antioxidant enzyme activities are region and organ, as well as sex, selective in the rat. Mech Ageing Dev 65:187–198.

Castano EM, Prelli F, Wisniewski T, Golabek A, Kumar RA, Soto C, Frangione B (1995): Fibrillogenesis in Alzheimer's disease of amyloid beta peptides and apolipoprotein E. Biochem J 306:599–604.

Cheng B, Mattson MP (1995): PDGFs protect hippocampal neurons against energy deprivation and oxidative injury: Evidence for induction of antioxidant pathways. J Neurosci 15:7095–7104.

Cheng B, Mattson MP (1994): NT-3 and BDNF protect hippocampal, septal, and cortical neurons against metabolic compromise. Brain Res 640:56–67.

Cheng B, Mattson MP (1992): Glucose deprivation elicits neurofibrillary tangle-like antigenic changes in hippocampal neurons: Prevention by NGF and bFGF. Exp Neurol 117:114–123.

Cheng B, Mattson MP (1991): NGF and bFGF protect rat and human central neurons against hypoglycemic damage by stabilizing calcium homeostasis. Neuron 7:1031–1041.

Cheng B, Christakos S, Mattson MP (1994a): Tumor necrosis factors protect neurons against excitotoxic/metabolic insults and promote maintenance of calcium homeostasis. Neuron 12:139–153.

Cheng B, Goodman Y, Begley JG, Mattson MP (1994b): Neurotrophin 4/5 protects hippocampal and cortical neurons against energy deprivation- and excitatory amino acid-induced injury. Brain Res 650:331–335.

Cheng B, Barger SW, Mattson MP (1994c): Staurosporine, K-252a and K-252b stabilize calcium homeostasis and promote survival of CNS neurons in the absence of glucose. J Neurochem 62:1319–1329.

Choi DW (1995): Calcium: Still center-stage in hypoxic-ischemic neuronal death. Trends Neurosci 18:58–60.

Citron M, Vigo-Pelfrey C, Teplow DB, Miller C, Schenk D, Johnston J, Winblad B, Venizelos N, Lannfelt L, Selkoe DJ (1994): Excessive production of amyloid β-protein by peripheral cells of symptomatic and presymptomatic patients carrying the Swedish familial Alzheimer disease mutation. Proc Nat Acad Sci U S A 91:11993–11997.

Cotman CW, Anderson AJ (1995): A potential role for apoptosis in neurodegeneration and Alzheimer's disease. Mol Neurobiol 10:19–45.

Cummings BJ, Su JH, Cotman CW (1993): Neuritic involvement within bFGF immunopositive plaques of Alzheimer's disease. Exp Neurol 124:315–325.

Cunningham DD, Pulliam L, Vaughan PJ (1993): Protease nexin-1 and thrombin: Injury related processes in the brain. Thromb Haemost 70:168–171.

Cutler R, Joseph JA, Yamagami K, Villalobos-Molina R, Roth GS (1994): Area specific alterations in muscarinic stimulated low K_m GTPase activity in aging and Alzheimer's disease: Implications for altered signal transduction. Brain Res 664:54–60.

Davidson RM, Shajenko L, Donta TS (1994): Amyloid β-peptide (AβP) potentiate a nimodipine-sensitive L-type barium conductance in N1E-115 neuroblastoma cells. Brain Res 643:324–327.

Davis-Salina J, Saporito-Irwin SM, Cotman CW, Van Nostrand WE (1995): Amyloid beta-protein induces its own production in cultured degenerating cerebrovascular smooth muscle cells. J Neurochem 65:931–934.

Dyrks T, Dyrks E, Hartmann T, Masters C, Beyreuther KE (1992): Amyloidogenicity of beta A4 and beta A4-bearing amyloid protein precursor fragments by metal-catalyzed oxidation. J Biol Chem 267:18210–18217.

Eckert A, Hartmann H, Muller WE (1993): Beta-amyloid protein enhances the mitogen-induced calcium response in circulating human lymphocytes. FEBS Lett 330:49–52.

Edamatsu R, Mori A, Packer L (1995): The spin-trap N-tert-alpha-phenyl-butylnitrone prolongs the life span of the senescence accelerated mouse. Biochem Biophys Res Commu 211:847–849.

Eikelenboom P, Zhan SS, van Gool WA, Allsop D (1994): Inflammatory mechanisms in Alzheimer's disease. Trends Pharmacol Sci 15:447–450.

Elliott EM, Sapolsky RM (1993): Corticosterone impairs hippocampal neuronal calcium regulation—possible mediating mechanisms. Brain Res 602:84–90.

Elliott E, Mattson MP, Vanderklish P, Lynch G, Chang I, Sapolsky RM (1993): Corticosterone exacerbates kainate-induced alterations in hippocampal tau immunoreactivity and spectrin proteolysis in vivo. J Neurochem 61:57–67.

Etcheberrigaray R, Ito E, Kim CS, Alkon DL (1944): Soluble β-amyloid induction of Alzheimer's phenotype for human fibroblast K+ channels. Science 264:276–279.

Etcheberrigaray R, Ito E, Oka K, Tofel-Grehl B, Gibson GE, Alkon DL (1993): Potassium channel dysfunction in fibroblasts identifies patients with Alzheimer disease. Proc Natl Acad Sci U S A 90:8209–1823.

Evans KC, Berger EP, Cho CG, Weisgraber KH, Lansbury PT (1995): Apolipoprotein E is a kinetic but not a thermodynamic inhibitor of amyloid formation: Implications for the pathogenesis and treatment of Alzheimer disease. Proc Natl Acad Sci U S A 92:763–767.

Flynn DD, Ferrari-Dileo G, Mash DC, Levey AI (1995): Differential regulation of molecular subtypes of muscarinic receptors in Alzheimer's disease. J Neurochem 64:1888–1891.

Forloni G, Chiesa R, Smiroldo S, Verga L (1993): Apoptosis mediated neurotoxicity induced by chronic application of beta amyloid fragment 25-35. Neuroreport 4:523–526.

Frackowiak J, Zoltowska A, Wisniewski HM (1994): Non-fibrillar beta-amyloid protein is associated with smooth muscle cells of vessel walls in Alzheimer disease. J Neuropathol Exp Neurol 53:637–645.

Fraser PE, Nguyen JT, Surewicz WK, Kirschner DA (1991): pH-dependent structural transitions of Alzheimer amyloid peptides. Biophys J 60:1190–1201.

Furukawa K, Mattson MP (1995a): Cytochalasins protect hippocampal neurons against amyloid β-peptide toxicity: Evidence that actin depolymerization suppresses Ca^{2+} influx. J Neurochem 65:1061–1068.

Furukawa K, Mattson MP (1995b): Taxol stabilizes $[Ca^{2+}]_i$ and protects hippocampal neurons against excitotoxicity. Brain Res 689:141–146.

Furukawa K, Barger SW, Blalock E, Mattson MP (1996): Activation of K^+ channels and suppression of neuronal activity by secreted β-amyloid precursor protein. Nature 379:74–78.

Furukawa K, Sopher B, Rydel RE, Begley JG, Martin GM, Mattson MP (1996): Increased activity-regulating and neuroprotective efficacy of α-secretase-derived secreted APP is conferred by a C-terminal heparin-binding domain. J Neurochem 67:1882–1896.

Furukawa K, Smith-Swintosky VL, Mattson MP (1995): Evidence that actin depolymerization protects hippocampal neurons against excitotoxicity by stabilizing $[Ca^{2+}]_i$. Exp Neurol 133:153–163.

Furukawa K, Abe Y, Akaike N (1994): Amyloid β protein-induced irreversible current in rat cortical neurones. Neuroreport 5:2016–2018.

Furukawa K, Estus S, Fu W, Mattson MP (1997): Neuroprotective action of cycloheximide involves induction of Bcl-2 and antioxidant pathways. J Cell Biol, submitted.

Galindo MF, Prehn JHM, Bindokas VP, Miller RJ (1994): Potential role of TGFβ-1 in Alzheimer's disease: Regulation of APP expression and inhibition of βAP neurotoxicity. Soc Neurosci Abstr 14:1248.

Games D, Adams D, Alessandrinl R, Barbour R, Berthelette P, Blackwell C, Carr T, Clemens J, Donaldson T, Gillespie F, Guido T, Hagoplan S, Johnson-Wood K, Khan K, Lee M, Lelbowitz E, McConlogue S, Montoya-Zavala M, Mucke L, Paganini L, Penniman E, Power M, Schenk D, Seubert P, Snyder B, Soriano F, Tan H, Vitale J, Wadsworth S, Wolozin B, Zhao J (1995): Alzheimer-type neuropathology in transgenic mice overexpressing V717F β-amyloid precursor protein. Nature 373:523–527.

Gerlach M, Ben-Shachar D, Riederer P, Youdim MB (1994): Altered brain metabolism of iron as a cause of neurodegenerative diseases? J Neurochem 63:793–807.

Goodman Y, Mattson MP (1994b): Staurosporine and K-252 compounds protect hippocampal neurons against amyloid β-peptide toxicity and oxidative injury. Brain Res 650:170–174.

Goodman Y, Mattson MP (1996a): Ceramide protects hippocampal neurons against excitotoxic and oxidative insults, and amyloid β-peptide toxicity. J Neurochem 66:869–872.

Goodman Y, Mattson MP (1996b): K^+ channel openers protect hippocampal neurons against oxidative injury and amyloid β-peptide toxicity. Brain Res 706:328–332.

Goodman Y, Bruce AJ, Cheng B, Mattson MP (1996): Estrogens attenuate and corticosterone exacerbates excitotoxicity, oxidative injury, and amyloid β-peptide toxicity in hippocampal neurons. J Neurochem 66:869–872.

Goodman Y, Mattson MP (1994a): Secreted forms of β-amyloid precursor protein protect hippocampal neurons against amyloid β-peptide-induced oxidative injury. Exp Neurol 128:1–12.

Goodman Y, Steiner MR, Steiner SM, Mattson MP (1994): Nordihydroguaiaretic acid protects hippocampal neurons against amyloid β-peptide toxicity, and attenuates free radical and calcium accumulation. Brain Res 654:171–176.

Gschwind M, Huber G (1995): Apoptotic cell death induced by beta-amyloid 1–42 peptide is cell type dependent. N Neurochem 65:292–300.

Guo Q, Furukawa K, Sopher BL, Pham DG, Robinson N, Martin GM, Mattson MP (1996): Alzheimer's PS-1 mutation perturbs calcium homeostasis and sensitizes PC12 cells to death induced by amyloid β-peptide. NeuroReport 7: in press.

Hall ED, Yonkers PA, Andrus PK, Cox JW, Anderson DK (1992): Biochemistry and pharmacology of lipid antioxidants in acute brain and spinal cord injury. N Neurotrauma 9: S425–S442.

Hansson E, Ronnback L (1995): Astrocytes in glutamate neurotransmission. FASEB J 9:343–350.

Harman D (1994): Free-radical theory of aging. Increasing the functional life span. Ann N Y Acad Sci 717:1–15.

Harris ME, Wang Y, Pedigo N, Carney JM (1995): Astrocytes and L-glutamate transport: Effects of oxidation and amyloid peptides in relation to Alzheimer's disease. Soc Neurosci Abstr 21:477.

Hartmann H, Eckert A, Muller WE (1993): Beta-amyloid protein amplifies calcium signalling in central neurons from the adult mouse. Biochem Biophys Res Commun 194:1216–1220.

Hatzinger M, Z'Brun A, Hemmeter Y, Seifritz E, Baumann F, Holsboer-Trachsler E, Heuser IJ (1995): Hypothalamic-pituitary-adrenal system function in patients with Alzheimer's disease. Neurobiol Aging 16:205–209.

Hefti F (1994): Neurotrophic factor therapy for nervous system degenerative diseases. J Neurobiol 25:1418–1435.

Hellweg R, Jockers-Scherubl M (1994): Neurotrophic factors in memory disorders. Life Sci 55:2165–2169.

Henderson VW, Paganini-Hill A, Emanuel CK, Dunn ME, Buckwalter JG (1994): Estrogen replacement therapy in older women. Comparisons between Alzheimer's disease cases and nondemented control subjects. Arch Neurol 51:896–900.

Hensley K, Carney JM, Mattson MP, Aksenova M, Harris M, Wu JF, Floyd R, Butterfield DA (1994): A model for β-amyloid aggregation and neurotoxicity based on free radical generation by the peptide: Relevance to Alzheimer's disease. Proc Natl Acad Sci U S A 91:3270–3274.

Horner HC, Packan DR, Sapolsky RM (1990): Glucocorticoids inhibit glucose transport in cultured hippocampal neurons and glia. Neuroendocrinology 52:57–64.

Hoyer S (1993): Abnormalities in brain glucose utilization and its impact on cellular and molecular mechanisms in sporadic dementia of Alzheimer type. Ann N Y Acad Sci 695:77–80.

Jacobson MD, Burne JF, Raff MC (1994): Mechanisms of programmed cell death and Bcl-2 protection. Biochem Soc Trans 22:600–602.

Jarrett JT, Lansbury PT (1993): Seeding "One-dimensional crystallization" of amyloid: A pathogenic mechanism in Alzheimer's disease and scrapie? Cell 73:1055–1058.

Jin LW, Ninomiya H, Roch JM, Schubert D, Masliah E, Otero DA, Saitoh T (1994): Peptides containing the RERMS sequence of amyloid beta/A4 protein precursor bind cell surface and promote neurite extension. J Neurosci 14:5461–5470.

Johnson EM, Deckwerth TL (1993): Molecular mechanisms of developmental neuronal death. Annu Rev Neurosci 16:31–46.

Kalaria N, Grahovac I (1990): Serum amyloid P immunoreactivity in hippocampal tangles, plaques and vessels: Implications for leakage across the blood-brain barrier in Alzheimer's disease. Brain Res 516:349–353.

Kalaria RN, Hedera P (1995): Differential degeneration of the cerebral microvasculature in Alzheimer's disease. Neuroreport 6:477–480.

Kang J, Lemaire HG, Unterbeck A, Salbaum JM, Masters CL, Grzeschick KH, Multhaup G, Beyreuther K, Muller-Hill B (1987): The precursor of Alzheimer's disease amyloid A4 protein resembles a cell surface receptor. Nature 325:733–736.

Kawai M, Kalaria RN, Cras P, Siedlak SL, Velasco ME, Shelton ER, Chan HW, Greenberg BD, Perry G (1993): Degeneration of vascular muscle cells in cerebral amyloid angiopathy of Alzheimer disease. Brain Res 623:142–146.

Keaney JF Jr, Shwaery GT, Xu A, Nicolosi RJ, Loscalzo J, Foxall TL, Vita JA (1994): 17 Beta-estradiol preserves endothelial vasodilator function and limits low-density lipoprotein oxidation in hypercholesterolemic swine. Circulation 89:2251–2259.

Kelly J, Furukawa K, Barger SW, Mark RJ, Rengen MR, Blanc EM, Roth GS, Mattson MP (1996): Amyloid β-peptide disrupts carbachol-induced muscarinic cholinergic signal transduction in cortical neurons. Proc Natl Acad Sci USA 93:6753–6758.

Kolesnick R, Golde DW (1994): The sphingomyelin pathway in tumor necrosis factor and interleukin-1 signaling. Cell 77:325–328.

Koo EH, Sisodia SS, Archer DR, Martin LJ, Weidemann A, Beyreuther K, Fischer P, Masters CL, Price DL (1990): Precursor of amyloid protein in Alzheimer disease undergoes fast anterograde axonal transport. Proc Natl Acad Sci U S A 87:1561–1565.

Kosunen O, Talasniemi S, Lehtovirta M, Heinonen O, Helisalmi S, Mannermaa A, Paljarvi L, Ryynanen M, Riekkinen PJ Sr, Soininen H (1995): Relation of coronary atherosclerosis and apolipoprotein E genotypes in Alzheimer patients. Stroke 26:743–748.

Kumar U, Dunlop DM, Richardson JS (1994): The acute neurotoxic effect of beta-amyloid on mature cultures of rat hippocampal neurons is attenuated by the anti-oxidant U-78517F. Int J Neurosci 79:185–190.

Kuroda Y, Kawahara M (1994): Aggregation of amyloid beta-protein and its neurotoxicity: Enhancement by aluminum and other metals. Tohoku J Exp Med 174:263–268.

LaDu MJ, Pederson TM, Frail DE, Reardon CA, Getz GS, Falduto MT (1995): Purification of apolipoprotein E attenuates isoform-specific binding to β-amyloid. J Biol Chem 270:9039–9042.

LaDu MJ, Falduto MT, Manelli AM, Reardon CA, Getz GS, Frail DE (1994): Isoform-specific binding of apolipoprotein E to beta-amyloid. J Biol Chem 269:23403–23406.

Lafon-Cazal M. Pietri S, Cuicasi M, Bockaert J (1993): NMDA-dependent superoxide production and neurotoxicity. Lett Nat 364:535–537.

Landfield PW, Thibault O, Mazzanti ML, Porter NM, Kerr DS (1992): Mechanisms of neuronal death in brain aging and Alzheimer's disease: Role of endocrine-mediated calcium dyshomeostasis. J Neurobiol 23:1247–1260.

Lansbury PT, Costa PR, Griffiths JM, Simon EJ, Auger M, Halverson KJ, Kocisko DA,

Hendsch ZS, Ashburn TT, Spencer RGS, Tidor B, Griffin RG (1995): Structural model for the β-amyloid fibril: Interstrand alignment of an antiparallel β sheet comprising a C-terminal peptide. Nature Struct Biol 2:990–998.

LeBlanc A (1995): Increased production of 4 kDa amyloid β peptide in serum deprived human primary neuron cultures: Possible involvement of apoptosis. J Neurosci 15:7837–7846.

Levy-Lahad E, Wasco W, Poorka JP, Romano DM, Oshima J, Pettingell WH, Yu CE, Jondro PD, Schmidt SD, Wang K (1995): Candidate gene for the chromosome 1 familial Alzheimer's disease locus. Science 269:973–977.

Lipton SA (1993): Prospects for clinically tolerated NMDA antagonists: Open channel blockers and alternative redox states of nitric oxide. Trends Neurosci 16:527–532.

Lipton SA, Singel DJ, Stamler JS (1994): Nitric oxide in the central nervous system. Prog Brain Res 103:359–364.

Loo DT, Copani A, Pike CJ, Whittemore ER, Walencewicz AJ, Cotman CW (1993): Apoptosis is induced by beta-amyloid in cultured central nervous system neurons. Proc Natl Acad Sci U S A 90:7951–7955.

Lorenzo A, Yankner BA (1994): β-amyloid neurotoxicity requires fibril formation and is inhibited by Congo red. Proc Natl Acad Sci U S A 91:12243–12247.

Lovell MA, Ehmann WD, Butler SM, Markesbery W (1995): Elevated thiobarbituric acid-reactive substances and antioxidant enzyme activity in the brain in Alzheimer's disease. Neurology 45:1594–1601.

Mantyh PW, Ghilardi JR, Rogers S, DeMaster E, Allen CJ, Stimson ER, Maggio JE (1993): Aluminum, iron, and zinc ions promote aggregation of physiological concentrations of beta-amyloid peptide. J Neurochem 61:1171–1174.

Mark RJ, Hensley K, Butterfield DA, Mattson MP (1995a): Amyloid β-peptide impairs ionmotive ATPase activities: Evidence for a role in loss of neuronal Ca^{2+} homeostasis and cell death. J Neurosci 15:6239–6249.

Mark RJ, Ashford JW, Mattson MP (1995b): Anticonvulsants attenuate amyloid β-peptide neurotoxicity and promote maintenance of calcium homeostasis. Neurobiol Aging 16:187–198.

Mattila KM, Pirtilla T, Blennow K, Wallin A, Viitanen M, Frey H (1994): Altered blood-brain barrier function in Alzheimer's disease? Acta Neurol Scand 89:192–198.

Mattson MP, Murrain M, Guthrie PB, Kater SB (1989): Fibroglast growth factor and glutamate: Opposing roles in the generation and degeneration of hippocampal neuroarchitecture. J Neurosci 9:3728–3740.

Mattson MP, Begley JG (1996): Amyloid β-peptide alters thrombin-induced calcium responses in cultured human neural cells. Amyloid 3:28–40.

Mattson MP Furukawa K (1996): Programmed cell life: Anti-apoptotic signaling and therapeutic strategies in neurodegenerative disorders. Restorative Neurol Neurosci 9:191–205.

Mattson MP (1995b): Role of calcium in CNS trauma. In Ohnishi TS, Ohnishi T (eds): "Central Nervous System Trauma: Research Techniques." Boca Raton, FL: CRC Press, pp 59–73.

Mattson MP (1995a): Untangling the pathophysiochemistry of β-amyloid. Nature Struct Biol 2:926–928.

Mattson MP (1994): Secreted forms of β-amyloid precursor protein modulate dendrite outgrowth and calcium responses to glutamate in cultured embryonic hippocampal neurons. J Neurobiol 25:439–450.

Mattson MP, Scheff SW (1994): Endogenous neuroprotection factors and traumatic brain injury: mechanisms of action and implications for therapies. J Neurotroma 11:3–33.

Mattson MP (1992): Calcium as sculptor and destroyer of neural circuitry. Exp Gerontology 27:29–49.

Mattson MP (1990): Antigenic changes similar to those seen in neurofibrillary tangles are elicited by glutamate and calcium influx in cultured hippocampal neurons. Neuron 4:105–117.

Mattson MP, Goodman Y (1995): Different amyloidogenic peptides share a similar mechanism of neurotoxicity involving reactive oxygen species and calcium. Brain Res 676:219–224.

Mattson MP, Cheng B, Baldwin S, Smith-Swintosky VL, Keller J, Geddes JW, Scheff SW, Christakos S (1995a): Brain injury and tumor necrosis factors induce expression of calbindin D-28k in astrocytes: A cytoprotective response. J Neurosci Res 42:357–370.

Mattson MP, Lovell MA, Furukawa K, Markesbery WR (1995b): Neurotrophic factors attenuate glutamate-induced accumn of peroxides, elevation of $[Ca^{2+}]_i$ and neurotoxicity, and increase antioxidant enzyme activities in hippocampal neurons. J Neurochem 65: 1740–1751.

Mattson MP, Tomaselli K, Rydel (RE (1993a): Calcium-destabilizing and neurodegenerative effects of aggregated β-amyloid peptide are attenuated by basic FGF. Brain Res 621: 35–49.

Mattson MP, Barger SW, Cheng B, Lieberburg I, Smith-Swintosky VL, Rydel RE (1993b): β-amyloid precursor protein metabolites and loss of neuronal calcium homeostasis in Alzheimer's disease. Trends Neurosci 16:409–415.

Mattson MP, Cheng B, Smith-Swintosky VL (1993c): Growth factor-mediated protection from excitotoxicity and disturbances in calcium and free radical metabolism. Semin Neurosci 5:295–307.

Mattson MP, Cheng B, Culwell A, Esch F, Lieberburg I, Rydel RE (1993d): Evidence for excitoprotective and intraneuronal calcium-regulating roles for secreted forms of β-amyloid precursor protein. Neuron 10:243–254.

Mattson MP, Cheng B, Davis D, Bryant K, Lieberburg I, Rydel RE (1992): β-amyloid peptides destabilize calcium homeostasis and render human cortical neurons vulnerable to excitotoxicity J Neurosci 12:376–389.

May PC, Boggs LN, Fuson KS (1993): Neurotoxicity of human amylin in rat primary hippocampal cultures: Similarity to Alzheimer's disease amyloid-beta neurotoxicity. J Neurochem 61:2330–2333.

May PC, Gitter BD, Waters DC, Simmons LK, Becker GW, Small JS, Robison PM (1992): β-Amyloid peptide in vitro toxicity: Lot-to-lot variability. Neurobiol Aging 13:605–607.

McGahon AJ, Martin SJ, Bissonnette RP, Mahboubi A, Shi Y, Mogil RJ, Nichioka WK, Green DR (1995): The end of the (cell) line: Methods for the study of apoptosis in vitro. Methods Cell Biol 46:153–185.

McGeer PL, Klegeris A, Walker DG, Yasuhara O, McGeer EG (1994): Pathological proteins in senile plaques. Tohoku J Exp Med 174:269–277.

Meda L, Cassatella MA, Szendrei GI, Otvos L Jr, Baron P, Villalba M, Ferrari D, Rossi F (1995): Activation of microglial cells by beta-amyloid protein and interferon-gamma. Nature 374:647–650.

Mullan M, Crawford F (1993): Genetic and molecular advances in Alzheimer's disease. Trends Neurosci 16:398–403.

Muller HW, Junghans U, Kappler J (1995): Astroglial neurotrophic and neurite-promoting factors. Pharmacol Ther 65:1–18.

Nabeshima T, Nitta A, Fuji K, Kameyama T, Hasegawa T (1994): Oral administration of NGF synthesis stimulators recovers reduced brain NGF content in aged rats and cognitive dysfunction in the basal-forebrain-lesioned rats. Gerontology 2:46–56.

Nitsch RM, Farber SA, Growdon JH, Wurtman RJ (1993): Release of amyloid beta-protein precursor derivatives by electrical depolarization of rat hippocampal slices. Proc Natl Acad Sci U S A 90:5191–5193.

Nitsch RM, Slack BE, Wurtman RJ, Growdon JH (1992): Release of Alzheimer amyloid precursor derivatives stimulated by activation of muscarinic acetylcholine receptors. Science 258:304–307.

Nitta A, Hasegawa T, Nabeshima T (1993): Oral administration of idebenone, a stimulant of NGF synthesis, recovers reduced NGF content in aged rat brain. Neurosci Lett 163:219–222.

Olson L, Backman L, Ebendal T, Eriksdotter-Jonhagen M, Hoffer B, Humpel C, Freedman R, Giacobini M, Meyerson B, Nordberg A (1994): Role of growth factors in degeneration and regeneration in the central nervous system; clinical experiences with NGF in Parkinson's and Alzheimer's diseases. J Neurol 242:S12–15.

Orr WC, Sohal RS (1992): The effects of catalase gene overexpression on life span and resistance to oxidative stress in transgenic Drosophila melangoster. Arch Biochem Biophys 297:35–41.

Perlmutter LS (1994): Microvascular pathology and vascular basement membrane components in Alzheimer's disease Mol Neurobiol 9:33–40.

Pettegrew JW, Panchalingam K, Klunk WE, McClure RJ, Muenz LR (1994): Alterations of cerebral metabolism in probable Alzheimer's disease: A preliminary study. Neurobiol Aging 15:117–132.

Piani D, Fontana A (1994): Macrophage-induced glutamate-dependent cytotoxicity to neurons. J Immunol 152:3578–3585.

Pike CJ, Cotman CW (1995): Calretinin-immunoreactive neurons are resident to β-amyloid toxicity in vitro. Brain Res 671:293–298.

Pike CJ, Walencewicz-Wasserman AJ, Kosmoski J, Cribbs DH, Glabe CG, Cotman CW (1995): Structure-activity analyses of β-amyloid peptides: Contributions of the β25-35 region to aggregation and neurotoxicity. J Neurochem 64:253–265.

Pike CJ, Cummings BJ, Monzavi R, Cotman CW (1994): β-amyloid-induced changes in cultured astrocytes parallel reactive astrocytosis associated with senile plaques in Alzheimer's disease. Neurosci 63:517–531.

Pike C, Burdick D, Walencewicz A, Glabe C, Cotman C (1993): Neurodegeneration induced by β-amyloid peptides in vitro: The role of peptide assembly state. J Neurosci 13:1676–1686.

Prehn JH, Backhauss C, Krieglstein J (1993): Transforming growth factor-β1 prevents glutamate neurotoxicity in rat neocortical cultures and protects mouse neocortex from ischemic injury in vivo. J Cereb Blood Flow Metab 13:521–525.

Prestwood KM, Pilbeam CC, Raisz LG (1995): Treatment of osteoporosis. Ann Rev Med 46:249–256.

Raadsheer FC, van Heerikhuize JJ, Lucassen PJ, Hoogendijk WJ, Tilders FJ, Swaab DF (1995): Corticotrophin-releasing hormone mRNA levels in the paraventricular nucleus of patients with Alzheimer's disease and depression. Am J Psychiatry 152:1372–1376.

Raivich G, Kreutzberg GW (1994): Pathophysiology of glial growth factor receptors. Glia 11:129–146.

Roch JM, Masliah E, Roch-Levecq AC, Sundsmo MP, Otero DA, Veinbergs I, Saitoh T (1994): Increase of synaptic density and memory retention by a peptide representing the trophic domain of the amyloid beta/A4 protein precursor. Proc Natl Acad Sci U S A 91:7450–7454.

Roch JM, Jin LW, Ninomiya H, Schubert D, Saitoh T (1993): Biologically active domain of the secreted form of the amyloid beta/A4 protein precursor. Ann N Y Acad Sci 695: 149–157.

Sagara Y, Dargusch R, Klier FG, Schubert D, Behl C (1996): Increased antioxidant enzyme activity in amyloid beta protein- resistant cells. J Neurosci 16:497–505.

Saitoh T, Sundsmo M, Roch J-M, Ximura M, Cole G, Schubert D, Oltersdorf T, and Schenk DB (1989): Secreted form of amyloid β protein precursor is involved in the growth regulation of fibroblasts. Cell 58:615–622.

Sapolsky RM (1994): The physiological relevance of glucocorticoid endangerment of the hippocampus. Ann N Y Acad Sci 746:294–304.

Sautiere P-E, Sindou P, Couratier P, Hugon J, Wattez A, Delacourte A (1992): Tau antigenic changes induced by glutamate in rat primary culture model: A biochemical approach. Neurosci Lett 140:206–210.

Scharfman HE, Schwartzkroin PA (1989): Protection of dentate hilar cells from prolonged stimulation by intracellular calcium chelation. Science 246:257–260.

Scheuner D, Eckman CJM, Song X, Citron M, Suzuki N, Bird TD, Hardy J, Hutton M, Kukull W, Larson E, Levy-Lahad E, Vitanen M, Peskind E, Poorkaj P, Schellenberg G, Tanzi R, Wasco W, Lannfelt L, Selkoe D, Younkin S (1996): Secreted amyloid β-protein similar to that in the senile plaques of Alzheimer's disease is increased in vivo by the presenilin 1 and 2 and APP mutations linked to familial Alzheimer's disease. Nature Med 2:864–870.

Schreck R, Albermann K, Baeuerle PA (1992): Nuclear factor kappa B: An oxidative stress-responsive transcription factor of eukaryotic cells. Free Radic Res Comm 17:221–237.

Schubert D, Behl C (1993): The expression of amyloid beta protein precuror protects nerve cells from beta-amyloid and glutamate toxicity and alters their interaction with the extracellular matrix. Brain Res 629:275–282.

Schubert D, Chevion M (1995): The role of iron in beta amyloid toxicity. Biochem Biophys Res Commun 216:702–707.

Schubert W, Prior R, Weidemann A, Dircksen H, Multhaup G, Masters CL, Beyreuther K (1991): Localization of Alzheimer βA4 amyloid at presynaptic terminals. Brain Res 563:184–194.

Schwartz J, Freeman R, Frishman W (1995): Clinical pharmacology of estrogens: Cardiovascular actions and cardioprotective benefits of replacement therapy in postmenopausal women. J Clin Pharmacol 35:314–329.

Schweers O, Mandelkow E, Biernat J, Mandelkow E (1995): Oxidation of cysteine-322 in the repeat domain of microtubule-associated protein tau controls the in vitro assembly of paired helical filaments. Proc Natl Acad Sci U S A 92:8463–8467.

Scott SA, Mufson EJ, Weingartner JA, Skau KA, Crutcher KA (1995): Nerve growth factor in Alzheimer's disease: Increased levels throughout the brain coupled with declines in nucleus basalis. J Neurosci 15:6213–6221.

Selkoe DJ (1993): Physiological production of the β-amyloid protein and the mechanism of Alzheimer's disease. Trends Neurosci 16:403–409.

Shearman MS, Hawtin SR, Tailor VJ (1995): The intracellular component of cellular 3-(4,5-

dimethylthiazol-2-yl)-2, 5-diphenyltetrazolium bromide (MTT) reduction is specifically inhibited by β-amyloid peptides. J Neurochem 65:218–227.

Sherrington R, Rogaev EI, Liang Y, Rogaeva EA, Levesque G, Ikeoa M, Chi H, Linc C, Li G, Holman K (1995): Cloning of a gene bearing missense mutations in early-onset familial Alzheimer's disease. Nature 375:754–760.

Simmons A, Schneider CR (1993): Amyloid beta peptides act directly on single neurons. Neurosci Lett 150:133–136.

Simmons LK, May PC, Tomaselli KJ, Rydel RE, Fuson KS, Brigham EF, Wright S, Lieberburg I, Becker GW, Brems DN (1994): Secondary structure of amyloid beta peptide correlates with neurotoxic activity in vitro. Mol Pharmacol 45:373–379.

Singh M, Meyer EM, Simpkins JW (1995): The effect of ovariectomy and estradiol replacement on brain-derived neurotrophic factor messenger ribonucleic acid expression in cortical and hippocampal brain regions of female Sprague-Dawley rats. Endocrinology 136: 2320–2324.

Smith CD, Carney JM, Starke-Reed PE, Oliver CN, Stadtman ER, Floyd RA, Markesbery WR (1991): Excess brain protein oxidation and enzyme dysfunction in normal aging and in Alzheimer disease. Proc Natl Acad Sci U S A 88:10540–10543.

Smith RG, Alexianu ME, Crawford G, Nyormoi O, Stefani E, Appel SH (1994): Cytotoxicity of immunoglobulins from amyotrophic lateral sclerosis patients on a hybrid motoneuron cell line. Proc Natl Acad Sci U S A 91:3393–3397.

Smith-Swintosky VL, Pettigrew LC, Sapolsky RM, Phares C, Craddock SD, Brooke SM, Mattson MP (1996a): Metyrapone, an inhibitor of glucocorticoid production, reduces brain injury induced by focal and global ischemia and seizures. J Cerebr Blood Flow Metab 16:585–598.

Smith-Swintosky VL, Kraemer PJ, McCants N, Maki A, Brown RW, Keller J, Goodman Y, Mattson MP (1996b): Bacterial alkaloids mitigate seizure-induced hippocampal damage and memory deficits. Exp Neurol 141:287–296.

Smith-Swintosky VL, Zimmer S, Fenton JW, Mattson MP (1995a): Protease nexin-I and thrombin modulate neuronal Ca^{2+} homeostasis and sensitivity to glucose deprivation-induced injury. J Neurosci 15:5840–5850.

Smith-Swintosky VL, Zimmer S, Fenton II JW, Mattson MP (1995b) Opposing actions of thrombin and protease nexin-1 on amyloid β-peptide toxicity and on accumulation of peroxides and calcium in hippocampal neurons. J Neurochem 65:1415–1418.

Sohal RS (1993): The free radical hypothesis of aging: an appraisal of the current status. Aging 4:3–17.

Stein-Behrens B, Mattson MP, Chang I, Yeh M, Sapolsky RM (1994): Stress exacerbates neuron loss and cytoskeletal pathology in the hippocampus. J Neurosci 14:5373–5380.

Strittmatter WJ, Roses AD (1995): Apolipoprotein E and Alzheimer disease. Proc Natl Acad Sci U S A 92:4725–4747.

Subbarao KV, Richardson JS, Ang LC (1990): Autopsy samples of Alzheimer's cortex show increased peroxidation in vitro. J Neurochem 55:342–345.

Suzuki N, Cheung TT, Cai XD, Odaka A, Otvos LJ, Eckman C, Golde TE, Younkin SG (1994): An increased percentage of long amyloid β protein secreted by familial amyloid β protein precursor ($bAPP_{717}$) mutants. Science 264:1336–1340.

Tang MX, Jacobs D, Stern Y, Marder K, Schofield P, Gurland B, Andrews H, Mayeux R (1996): Effect of oestrogen during menopause on risk and age at onset of Alzheimer's disease. Lancet 348:429–432.

Thomas T, Thomas G, McLendon C, Sutton T, Mullan M (1996): β-amyloid-mediated vasoactivity and vascular endothelial damage. Nature 380:168–171.

Troncoso JC, Costello A, Watson AL, Johnson GVW (1993): In vitro polymerization of oxidized tau into filaments. Brain Res 613:313–316.

Volterra A, Trotti D, Tromba C, Floridi S, Racagni G (1994): Glutamate uptake inhibition by oxygen free radicals in rat cortical astrocytes. J Neurosci 14:2924–2932.

Warpman U, Alafuzoff I, Nordberg A (1993): Coupling of muscarinic receptors to GTP proteins in postmortem human brain—alterations in Alzheimer's disease. Neurosci Lett 150:39–43.

Weinstein JR, Gold SJ, Cunningham DD, Gall CM (1995): Cellular localization of thrombin receptor mRNA in rat brain: Expression by mesencephalic dopaminergic neurons and codistribution with prothrombin mRNA. N Neurosci 15:2906–2919.

Weiss JH, Pike CJ, Cotman CW (1994): ca^{2+} channel blockers attenuate beta-amyloid peptide toxicity to cortical neurons in culture. N Neurochem 62:372–375.

Whitson JS, Mims MP, Strittmatter WJ, Yamaki T, Morrisett JD, Appel SH (1994): Attenuation of the neurotoxic effect of Aβ amyloid peptide by apolipoprotein E. Biochem Biophys Res Commun 199:163–170.

Wilckens T (1995): Glucocorticoids and immune function: Physiological relevance and pathogenic potential of hormonal dysfunction. Trends Pharmacol Sci 16:193–197.

Wisniewski HM, Wen GY (1992): Aluminum and Alzheimer's disease. Ciba Found Symp 169:142–154.

Wisniewski HM, Frckowiak J, Zoltowska A, Kim KS (1994): Vascular β-amyloid in Alzheimer's disease angiopathy is produced by proliferating and degenerating smooth muscle cells. Int J Exp Clin Invest 1:8–16.

Yan S-D, Chen X, Schmidt A-M, Brett J, Godman G, Zou YS, Scott CW, Caputo C, Frappier T, Smith MA, Perry G, Yen, S-H, Stern D (1994): Glycated tau protein in Alzheimer's disease: A mechanism for induction of oxidant stress. Proc Natl Acad Sci U S A 91:7787–7791.

Yankner BA, Mesulam MM (1991): β-amyloid and the pathogenesis of Alzheimer's disease. N Engl J Med 325:1849–1857.

Yankner BA, Duffy LK, Kirschner DA (1990): Neurotrophic and neurotoxic effects of amyloid beta protein: Reversal by tachykinin neuropeptides. Science 250:279–282.

Youngman LD, Park JY, Ames BN (1992): Protein oxidation associated with aging is reduced by dietary restriction of protein or calories. Proc Natl Acad Sci U S A 89: 9112–9116.

Yuan J (1995): Molecular control of life and death. Curr Opin Cell Biol 7:211–214.

Zhang JR, Andrus PK, Hall ED (1994): Age-related phospholipid hydroperoxide levels in gerbil brain measured by HPLC-chemiluminescence and their relation to hydroxyl radical stress. Brain Res 639:275–282.

Zhang Y, Tatsuno T, Carney J, Mattson MP (1993): Basic FGF, NGF, and IGFs protect hippocampal neurons against iron-induced degeneration. J Cerebral Blood Flow Metab 13:378–388.

CHAPTER 12

Role of Apolipoprotein E in Neurobiology and the Pathogenesis of Alzheimer's Disease

MICHAEL T. FALDUTO and MARY JO LADU

Immunoscience Discovery, Pharmaceutical Products Division, Abbott Laboratories, Abbott Park, Illinois 60064 (M.T.F.) and Department of Pathology, University of Chicago, Chicago, Illinois 60637 (M.J.L.)

INTRODUCTION

The neuropathological processes that result in the amyloid deposits and neurofibrillary tangles (NFT) characteristic of Alzheimer's disease (AD) remain essentially unknown. Therefore, considerable interest has been generated by recent genetic, immunohistochemical, and biochemical evidence suggesting a correlation between apolipoprotein E (apoE) allelic variations and AD. ApoE, a component of several classes of lipoproteins, acts as a ligand for cell surface lipoprotein receptors, thus regulating lipid transport and clearance. Investigation into the role of apoE in the pathogenesis of AD has produced collateral interest in the general function of apoproteins and lipids in the brain. This chapter will discuss the isoform-specific actions of apoE in lipid metabolism, neurobiology, and the pathogenic processes of AD.

APOE: CENTRAL ROLE IN LIPID METABOLISM

ApoE Structure and Function in Plasma Lipid Metabolism

In the aqueous environment of the blood, neutral lipids circulate packaged as lipoproteins. Lipoproteins are composed of a phospholipid and free cholesterol shell surrounding a triglyceride (TG) and cholesteryl-ester (CE) core. Lipoproteins

Pharmacological Treatment of Alzheimer's Disease: Molecular and Neurobiological Foundations,
Edited by Brioni and Decker
ISBN 0-471-16758-4   © 1997 Wiley-Liss, Inc.

are stabilized by surface apolipoproteins. Apolipoproteins also serve as cofactors for enzymatic reactions and ligands for lipoprotein receptors. Lipoproteins can be separated by size and density into four major classes, chylomicrons, very low density lipoproteins (VLDL), low-density lipoproteins (LDL), and high-density lipoproteins (HDL), that vary in their core TG–CE content and apolipoprotein composition. The soluble apoprotein gene family encodes proteins with amphipathic α-helical structures in the C-terminus that allow the proteins to exist at the water–lipid interface (Li et al., 1988). One such apolipoprotein is apoE.

ApoE is a 35-kD glycoprotein that circulates in the plasma associated with several classes of lipoproteins including chylomicrons, VLDL, and a subset of HDL. ApoE-containing lipoproteins are bound and internalized via receptor-mediated endocytosis by a number of receptors in the LDL receptor family of proteins including LDL receptor, LDL receptor-related protein (LRP), VLDL receptor, glycoprotein 330, and the newly described apoE receptor 2 (Kim et al., 1996). While the LDL receptor binds lipoproteins containing apoB100 and/or apoE, the other receptors recognize only apoE-containing particles. Thus, apoE is a major contributor to the transport of lipid particles to and from the bloodstream, regulating plasma lipid and cholesterol metabolism by its involvement in the three primary pathways of lipid metabolism. In the exogenous pathway, dietary lipids are packaged into chylomicrons and secreted by the intestine into the lymph, passing into the circulation via the thoracic duct. Lipoprotein lipase (LPL) anchored in the capillary endothelia hydrolyzes the TG from the chylomicron core, releasing free fatty acids (FFA) that are then available for uptake by the surrounding tissue. The apoE acquired by chylomicron remnants in the plasma allows these TG-poor particles to be cleared by apoE receptors on the liver. In the similar endogenous pathway, apoE-containing VLDL are produced by the liver and secreted into the circulation where LPL again hydrolyzes their core TG. The resulting VLDL remnants are either taken up by hepatic receptors via recognition of apoE or further modified to LDL. In reverse cholesterol transport, cholesterol from peripheral tissues is transported to the liver either directly by apoE-containing HDL or via transfer of the cholesteryl esters to larger particles.

In humans, apoE has 299 amino acids and three major isoforms that differ at two residues: E2 (Cys^{112}, Cys^{158}), E3 (Cys^{112}, Arg^{158}), and E4 (Arg^{112}, Arg^{158}) (Figure 1). The allelic variations that produce these isoforms have differing distributions in the general population. The $\epsilon3$ allele is the most common, with a gene frequency of $\sim77\%$. The frequencies of $\epsilon4$ ($\sim15\%$) and $\epsilon2$ ($\sim8\%$) are much lower but still relatively common (Davignon et al., 1988). The single amino acid changes that produce the apoE phenotypes are sufficient to influence plasma lipid metabolism and clearance. Residue 158, which is adjacent to the LDL receptor-binding site (residues 136–150), affects the interaction between the basic residues of apoE and the acidic residues of the ligand-binding domain of the LDL receptor. ApoE2 is defective in LDL receptor binding and individuals with the apoE2/2 genotype are at risk for developing type III hyperlipoproteinemia, a disorder characterized by elevated plasma TG and cholesterol. While apoE4 does not exhibit a decrease in binding to the LDL receptor in vitro, it is associated with elevated plasma cholesterol and LDL, suggesting that its interaction with other aspects of the lipoprotein pathway differs

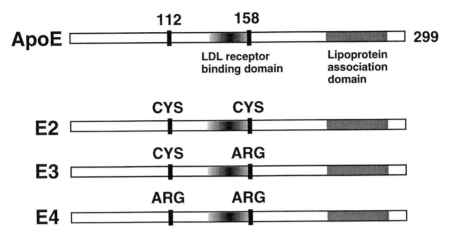

FIGURE 1. Structure of ApoE isoforms. Schematic of apoE protein including the amino acid differences between the apoE isoforms. Also indicated are the regions that comprise the LDL receptor binding domain and the domain for lipoprotein association.

from that of apoE3 (Mahley, 1988). ApoE4/4 individuals have a small but significant increased risk for coronary heart disease (Davignon et al., 1988).

In addition to the functional changes predicted by apoE phenotype, other domains of apoE have been characterized and interactions between domains observed [apoE structure–function relationships are comprehensively reviewed by Weisgraber (1994)]. A thrombin cleavage site at residue 191 divides the protein into two structural domains. The 22 kDa N-terminal fragment contains the receptor binding domain and the 10 kDa C-terminus contains several amphipathic α-helices that are important for the association of apoE with lipoproteins. In plasma, apoE2 and apoE3 preferentially bind to HDL while apoE4 binds to VLDL, though each is found in both lipoproteins. This observation illustrates that the interaction between domains is an important feature of the structure of apoE. While the C-terminus contains the lipid binding domain, the N-terminus contains the residues that confer isoform specificity. Therefore, the preferential association of the apoE isoforms with different classes of lipoproteins is the result of an interaction between the two domains.

Lipoproteins and Lipid Transport in the Brain

In the central nervous system, as in plasma, apoE may function as a lipid transport protein, redistributing lipids and participating in cholesterol homeostasis (Pitas et al., 1987b). Unlike other apoproteins, which are expressed primarily in the intestine and liver, apoE mRNA is present in most body tissues. While the major site of apoE synthesis is the liver, the brain contains the second highest abundance of apoE mRNA (Elshourbagy et al., 1985). In cerebrospinal fluid (CSF), the primary lipid-carrying particles are similar to plasma HDL in both size and density. CSF-HDL are spherical, composed of phospholipid, cholesterol, and protein, with apoE and apoA-I as the primary apolipoproteins (Pitas et al., 1987b; Borghini et al., 1995). ApoE and apoA-I appear to be present on distinct populations of particles. The source of these two sets of particles is not fully understood and they may have different origins. While the small, apoA-I containing CSF-HDL may originate from the plasma, evidence suggests that apoE is made within the blood–brain barrier. Following liver transplantation, while the plasma apoE phenotype of the recipient changes to that of the liver donor, the apoE phenotype in CSF does not change, indicating that at least the apoE component of CSF-HDL is synthesized locally (Linton et al., 1991). As an exchangeable apoprotein, apoE may displace apoA-I from plasma-derived particles or the apoE-containing particles may be synthesized within the brain.

Unlike the peripheral pathways, little is known about lipid transport and metabolism in the brain, and analysis of CSF lipoproteins provide only limited information about these processes. CSF is produced from filtered plasma by the choroid plexus. It also contains resorbed perivascular fluid, composed of interstitial fluid as well as plasma components. Thus, the synthesis, secretion, and modification of lipid particles by neural cells remains speculative. Unlike the parenchymal cells of the liver and enterocytes of the intestine, which can secrete spherical particles containing both a neutral lipid core and surface apoproteins, the cells of the brain probably secrete particles deficient in core lipids. ApoE is synthesized by glial cells (Boyles et al., 1985) and is most likely secreted associated with phospholipid as evidenced by the expression of apoE in a variety of nonhepatic cell types (Reardon et al., 1986; Basu et al., 1982). In the extracellular space, this nascent, discoidal particle may then be modified, acquiring additional surface protein components and core lipid. The redistribution of lipid to apoE-containing particles could be facilitated by lecithin : cholesterol acyltransferase (LCAT) and cholesteryl ester transfer protein (CETP). LCAT catalyzes the esterification of cholesterol in HDL, facilitating the transport of cholesterol as a component of the HDL core. LCAT mRNA is present in brain (Warden, et al., 1989), and by in situ hybridization, LCAT is synthesized by several cell types including neurons and glia (Smith et al., 1990). In plasma, CETP promotes the exchange of CE and TG between VLDL and HDL. The level of CETP activity in the CSF suggests that it is not simply present from filtration of the plasma but is synthesized within the brain (Albers et al., 1992). Whatever their origin, apoE-containing particles generated within neural tissue can redistribute their contents to the surrounding cells via uptake by apoE receptors. Further study, including in vitro co-culture models of glial cells and neurons, is needed to elucidate these pathways in the brain.

APOE AS A GENETIC RISK FACTOR FOR NEURODEGENERATIVE DISORDERS

ApoE and Alzheimer's Disease

The genetic components of Alzheimer's disease are complex. There are at least four genetic loci associated with the disease, and two of these have only very recently been defined. The β-amyloid peptide (Aβ) deposited in the senile plaques of AD patients is a proteolytic product of the amyloid precursor protein (APP) coded by a gene on chromosome 21. Mutations flanking both the amino and carboxyl terminus of Aβ within APP were discovered to be sufficient to cause early-onset AD (Goate et al., 1991; Mullan et al., 1992), strengthening the argument that Aβ deposition is an important pathogenic event in AD. In addition, Down syndrome patients, who have an extra copy of chromosome 21, display profound amyloid plaque deposition at early ages, presumably due to an APP gene dosage effect (Masters et al., 1985). In the past year, two previously unknown, yet similar, proteins whose genes are on chromosomes 1 and 14 were discovered to cause early-onset AD (Levy-Lahad et al, 1995; Sherrington et al., 1995). However, despite much speculation as well as some interesting preliminary experimental findings, neither their normal function nor the nature of their involvement in AD pathogenesis is known.

An early study demonstrated linkage of late-onset familial AD to the proximal long arm of chromosome 19, the locus of the apoE gene (Pericak-Vance et al., 1991). It was subsequently determined that individuals with late-onset familial AD, the most common form of the disease, displayed an increased frequency of the ε4 allele of apoE (Strittmatter et al., 1993a). Within the last 3 years, the genetic association of apoE with AD has been confirmed by a large number of studies that define the inheritance of the apoE ε4 allele as a major risk factor for developing both sporadic (Saunders et al., 1993b) or late-onset familial (Corder et al., 1993) AD. It appears that apoE4 lowers the age of onset of AD thereby increasing the chance of the AD phenotype presenting within a normal lifespan (Figure 2) without altering the rate of disease progression. The relative risk for AD is three- and eightfold greater in individuals with one or two copies of the ε4 gene, respectively, compared to ε3 homozygotes. Almost all individuals who are homozygous for the ε4 allele and live to be 80 years of age will develop AD (Corder et al., 1993). However, ε4 is a risk factor that, unlike the autosomal-dominant mutations at other loci, does not always result in AD. Neither is ε4 necessary for the development of AD since almost half of all AD patients have not inherited the ε4 gene. In addition to its contribution in late-onset AD, there is some evidence to suggest that ε4 gene dosage may further influence the age of disease onset in individuals with genetic mutations known to cause early-onset AD (Hardy et al., 1993). Recent genetic data has also implicated apoE2 as a protective isoform in the development of AD. Together with the increased risk of AD due to the ε4 allele, the reduced risk with ε2 indicates that over 80% of all AD cases can be attributed to genetic variance at the apoE locus (Corder et al., 1994).

It is intriguing that the VLDL receptor, an apoE receptor present in the brain, appears to have an allelic variation in the 5' untranslated region of the gene, which is present with increased frequency in patients with sporadic AD (Okuizumi et al., 1995). This small but significant risk for AD is further increased in patients homozygous for the VLDL receptor allele variant and in patients with at least one copy of the apoE ε4 allele. The significance of the VLDL receptor as a susceptibility gene for AD and any potential interactions with apoE awaits further study.

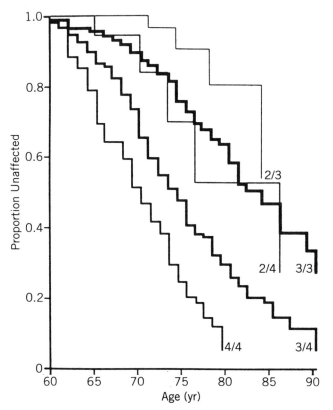

FIGURE 2. Risk of remaining unaffected by AD in relation to apoE genotype. Age of AD onset for subjects with each indicated apoE genotype. Onset curves were estimated by Kaplan–Meier product limit distributions. Data are limited to late-onset AD and should not be generalized to all populations at risk. Epidemiologically based distributions will be needed before risks can be estimated to the general population. From Roses et al. (1994): Lancet 343:1564.

APoE and Other Neurodegenerative Disorders

The influence of apoE genotype in other neurodegenerative disorders is unclear. Even in diseases where β-amyloid plaque deposition is a primary feature, the effect of the ε4 allele is unsettled. ε4 allele frequencies are increased compared to controls in Lewy body dementia (Hardy et al., 1994; Lippa et al., 1995; Pickering-Brown et al., 1994b), either the same (Nicoll et al., 1996a; Itoh et al., 1996) or increased (Greenberg et al., 1995; Kalaria et al., 1996) in cerebral amyloid angiopathy, and the same in Down syndrome (Pickering-Brown et al., 1994b; Saunders et al., 1993a). The extent of Aβ deposition after head injury correlates with the ε4 allele (Nicoll et al., 1996b). Creutzfeldt-Jakob disease is characterized by the accumulation of amyloid prion protein plaques that are apoE immunopositive (Namba et al., 1991). The role of apoE genotype in Creutzfeldt-Jakob disease is also equivocal, with the $\epsilon4$ allele either being comparable (Salvatore et al., 1995) or increased (Amouyel et al., 1994) in comparison to controls.

Parkinson's disease, Huntington's disease, and familial amyloidotic polyneuropathy appear not to be strongly linked to apoE genotype (Koller et al., 1995; Pickering-Brown et al., 1994a; Saunders et al., 1993a) though Parkinson's disease with dementia does appear to be related to the frequency of the $\epsilon4$ allele (Salvatore et al., 1995; Frisoni et al., 1994). Thus, the possibility of an apoE dependent process underlying several neurodegenerative disorders awaits further clarification.

APOE AND AD: IMMUNOLOCALIZATION OF APOE AND ITS RECEPTORS

ApoE

Investigations of apoE localization in normal human brain have been limited. Much of the information regarding apoE in normal brain tissue has come from studies in other species, including rodents (Boyles et al., 1985) and nonhuman primates (Mufson et al., 1994; Poduri et al., 1994). In these species, apoE staining is present in most major subdivisions of the CNS, primarily in the perinuclear region and processes of astrocytes. In situ hybridization confirms that astrocytes synthesize apoE (Poirier et al., 1991).

The identification of apoE as a risk factor for AD has increased interest in the immunolocalization of apoE in normal and AD brains. Recently, human cerebral cortex from all cognitively normal individuals exhibited extensive apoE staining of pyramidal neurons (Metzger et al., 1996) (Figure 3). This complements a previous observation of neuronal staining in the hippocampus from two of six control cases (Han et al., 1994b). However, it is not clear whether the apoE in human neurons is synthesized there or is the result of binding or internalization of apoE from other cellular sources. The localization of apoE to neurons appears to be altered by AD pathology, as the number of apoE-containing neurons in AD brains was significantly reduced (Metzger et al., 1996). These data suggest that apoE may have a normal function in neuronal metabolism that, when disrupted, could contribute to AD. Alternatively, apoE may be localized to neurons only in response to injury. In the nucleus basalis of Meynert and entorhinal cortex of AD brains, apoE neuronal staining mainly colocalized to neurons already immunopositive for paired helical filaments (PHF) (Benzing and Mufson, 1995). This observation also suggests that apoE may not play a pivotal role in the preliminary events that result in NFT formation.

ApoE immunostaining is also evident in association with the hallmarks of AD pathology, Aβ-containing plaques, and NFT (Namba et al., 1991; Wisniewski and Frangione, 1992) (Figure 3). The density of these deposits may be related to apoE genotype. The $\epsilon4$ allele correlates with higher plaque densities in the brains of AD patients (Rebeck et al., 1993; Schmechel et al., 1993). Specifically, apoE4 is associ-

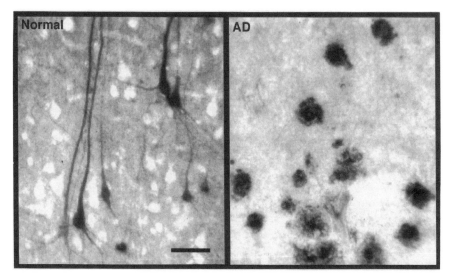

FIGURE 3. ApoE immunostaining of normal and AD cerebral cortex. Normal sections stained with ApoE antisera showing large projection neurons in cortical layer V. AD section with numerous apoE-immunoreactive senile plaques and no immunopositive neurons in cortical layer III. Magnification bar 20 μm.

ated with an increase in Aβ 1-40 positive plaques while the number of Aβ 1-42 immunoreactive plaques is similar among apoE genotypes (Gearing et al., 1996). The correlation of the ε4 allele with neuritic pathology is less clear. Though recent evidence indicates that NFT formation may be increased in ε4 carriers (Ohm et al., 1995; Nagy et al., 1995), others have observed no such difference (Schmechel et al., 1993; Gomez-Isla et al., 1996). In addition, apoE genotype does not affect the correlation between tangle density and duration of illness (Gomez-Isla et al., 1996).

In addition to apoE, other apolipoproteins have been found in senile plaques, including apoproteins A-I and J (Wisniewski et al., 1995a; McGeer et al., 1992). Apolipoprotein J (ApoJ) in plasma and CSF, as well as purified apoJ, has been shown to bind Aβ (Ghiso et al., 1993; Matsubara et al., 1995). It has been proposed that apoJ has a role in normal and pathological neural function, both for its role as a lipid and Aβ carrier, and as a complement inhibitor. However, a full review of apoJ is beyond the scope of this chapter.

ApoE has recently been observed by immunostaining in muscle fibers of patients with a common, progressive disorder known as inclusion body myositis (IBM) (Askanas et al., 1994). Like AD, the sporadic form of this disorder usually occurs later in life while an inherited form leads to disease at an earlier age. Though the pathogenesis of IBM is unknown, there are striking similarities between AD and IBM. In the muscle fibers of IBM patients, both PHF and Aβ fibrils are present and apoE colocalizes to both these structures (Askanas and Engel, 1994). Muscle atrophy resembling that seen with denervation has been observed in biopsies from both sporadic and hereditary IBM patients. Therefore, IBM may represent a testable peripheral disease model with pathogenic pathways similar to AD.

Lipoprotein Receptors

Several members of the LDL receptor family have been identified in the brain by immunostaining. The LDL receptor is found in pial cells of the arachnoid space and in the outermost layer of astrocytes in the cerebral cortex, though at levels below that seen in parenchymal cells of the liver (Pitas et al., 1987a). Deeper layers of the cortex have diffuse immunoreactivity not associated with cellular structures (Pitas et al., 1987a; Rebeck et al., 1993). The VLDL receptor is present in hippocampal neurons as well as in senile plaques of AD brains (Okuizumi et al., 1995). Neuronal VLDL receptor immunoreactivity is stronger in AD brains than control brains, indicating that this receptor may be upregulated in response to the disease.

LRP, also known as the α2-macroglobulin receptor, is involved in the clearance of a variety of ligands, including activated α2-macroglobulin, tissue and urokinase-type plasminogen activators, plasminogen activator inhibitor-1, lactoferrin, LPL, and apoE. Interestingly, a recent study has demonstrated that APP also binds and is internalized by LRP, demonstrating that a single receptor is involved in the metabolism of two proteins implicated in AD pathogenesis, suggesting a mechanism for their interaction (Kounnas et al., 1995). In normal brain, LRP is predominantly found associated with granule and pyramidal neurons of the hippocampus and pyramidal neurons of the frontal and temporal cortex (Wolf et al., 1992; Rebeck et al., 1993; Metzger et al., 1996). In AD brain, LRP is also present on senile plaques and activated, but not resting, astrocytes (Rebeck et al., 1993). The localization of LRP to plaques provides a mechanism for the accumulation of its ligands, all of which have been found associated with senile plaques (Rebeck et al., 1995). LRP binding and internalization is inhibited by receptor-associated protein (RAP). In AD hippocampus and temporal cortex, RAP colocalizes with LRP on neurons. However, RAP staining does not correspond to LRP staining in reactive astrocytes and senile plaques. This suggests that astrocytes can bind and clear LRP ligands, but neuronal clearance may be impaired by AD (Rebeck et al., 1995).

The newly described apoE receptor 2, whose preferred ligand appears to be apoE-enriched β-migrating VLDL (β-VLDL), is also highly expressed in human brain (Kim et al., 1996). By in situ hybridization in rat brain, the mRNA is localized to the cerebellar cortex, choroid plexus, ependyma, hippocampus, and cerebral cortex (Kim et al., 1996).

Other lipoprotein receptors have been localized to the CNS. The macrophage scavenger receptor, whose ligands include oxidized LDL and other glycated proteins, is expressed on microglia and particularly in association with senile plaques in AD brains (Christie et al., 1996). Similarly, the expression of the receptor for advanced glycation end products (RAGE) is increased in AD compared to control brain (Yan et al., 1996). In vitro, both these receptors appear to mediate the effects of fibrilized Aβ, causing activation and adhesion in microglia and an increase in free radical production in both microglia and neurons (El Khoury et al., 1996; Yan et al., 1996).

ROLE OF APOE IN THE PERIPHERAL AND CENTRAL NERVOUS SYSTEMS

Neuronal Growth and Development

ApoE secreted from resident macrophages and nonmyelinating glial cells in the peripheral nervous system and from astrocytes in the central nervous system may directly contribute to the growth of developing neurons. In primary dorsal root ganglia cultures, a model of peripheral nerve development, purified rabbit apoE added in the presence of β-migrating VLDL (β-VLDL), a large cholesterol-enriched lipid particle, increased neuritic growth (Handelmann et al., 1992). Using β-VLDL preenriched with human apoE isoforms, Nathan and co-workers (1994) found that apoE3 increased neuritic extension and decreased branching, while apoE4 decreased both branching and extension. Similarly, in human central nervous system derived cell lines, using either purified apoE or apoE stably expressed by the cells, apoE3 but not apoE4 increased neurite extension in the presence of exogenously added β-VLDL, CSF lipoproteins, or lipid emulsions (Holtzman et al, 1995; Bellosta et al., 1995).

In these cultures, neither purified apoE nor apoE stably expressed by the neurons has an effect on neuritic growth without the addition of exogenous lipid. This suggests that a receptor-mediated event is involved, as both LDL receptor and LRP binding requires that purified apoE be reconstituted with lipid particles. That the apoE isoform-specific effect on neurite outgrowth is mediated by receptor events has been confirmed by the demonstration that various treatments that inhibit the association of apoE with lipoprotein receptors, particularly LRP, blocked this effect (Bellosta et al., 1995; Nathan et al., 1994; Holtzman et al., 1995). While one explanation for the effect of apoE in these cultures is due to the apoE-mediated uptake of cholesterol and phospholipid for membrane remodeling, another possibility is that internalized apoE has an intracellular function. In this regard, Nathan and co-workers (1995) described a disruption in microtubule polymerization in neurons treated with β-VLDL and apoE4 but not apoE3. Even though lipid uptake by the cells was comparable for the two isoforms, more apoE3 accumulated intracellularly than apoE4. This effect may be unique to neurons as intracellular apoE was not detected in fibroblasts cultured under similar conditions.

In primary rat hippocampal cultures, both apoE3 and E4 exerted comparable neurotrophic effects on neurite development (Puttfarcken et al., 1997). In these experiments, the apoE was delivered as conditioned media from eukaryotic cells, where it is associated with small, dense particles (LaDu et al., 1995a). The uptake of these lipid poor particles is undoubtedly less than that of the apoE-enriched particles used in the experiments described above, as apoE-enriched particles are the preferred ligand for LRP (Bellosta et al., 1995). Thus, the observation that both apoE3 and E4 associated with lipid-poor particles had growth-factor-like effects may be due to a different mechanism of action from the isoform-specific effects that are dependent on receptor-mediated uptake. However, it is not clear why these growth-factor-like effects were not observed in human neuronal cell lines treated with exogenous apoE (Nathan et al., 1995) or stably expressing apoE (Bellosta et al., 1995) in the absence of exogenous lipid. Variation in developmental status of the neurons and the specific growth-promoting supplements present in the cultures may influence the reaction of neurons to apoE.

Nerve Injury and Repair

In addition to its role in neural homeostasis, apoE has been implicated in mediating the delivery of lipids to regenerating axons after peripheral nerve injury. ApoE is synthesized and secreted in large quantities by resident and monocyte-derived macrophages in degenerating peripheral nerves after acute injury (Boyles et al, 1989). This apoE is packaged with scavenged lipid, particularly cholesterol, liberated from degenerating axons (Goodrum, 1991). The high concentration of LDL receptors at axonal growth cones (Boyles et al, 1989; Ignatius et al., 1987) allows for the uptake of these apoE-containing particles in regenerating axons. Nevertheless, apoE may be sufficient, but not necessary, for peripheral nerve regeneration. Recovery from peripheral nerve injury in mice with a homozygous disruption of the apoE gene (apoE null mice) was similar to that of normal mice (Popko et al, 1993).

In the central nervous system, where the regenerative ability of neurons is limited, the deafferented hippocampus of the rat displays upregulation of apoE synthesis and secretion from astrocytes rather than macrophages (Poirier et al., 1991). This model of reactive synaptogenesis involves lesioning of the rat entorhinal cortex, which destroys over half of the synaptic input to the granule cell layer of the hippocampus. The subsequent compensatory response results in almost complete restoration of synapses within a few months. As in the peripheral nervous system, it is thought that apoE secreting astrocytes engulf and metabolize degenerating synaptic terminals, storing the lipid components for their secretion with apoE. The apoE-containing lipid particles may be internalized by neuronal apoE receptors and transported to the synaptic terminal for the synthesis of new synaptic membranes. In the hippocampus, peak levels of apoE synthesis and secretion by astrocytes after entorhinal cortex lesioning corresponded with a loss in *de novo* cholesterol synthesis and the extent of cholinergic reinnervation paralleled an increase in LDL receptor binding (Poirier et al., 1993). ApoE null mice show an accelerated loss of synapses and cytoskeletal alterations with age, as well as poor reinnervation responses when challenged by entorhinal cortex lesioning, further strengthening the argument that apoE is required for efficient reactive synaptogenesis in the brain (Masliah et al., 1994; Masliah et al., 1995). These results support the concept that cholesterol released during the breakdown of nerve terminals can be reutilized as a precursor during membrane remodeling in axonal growth and synaptogenesis.

Aβ-induced Neurotoxicity

The Aβ peptide is derived by proteolytic processing of APP, resulting in peptides that range in length from 39 to 43 amino acids. It is primarily the longer forms of the peptide that are found as insoluble aggregates in senile plaques. In vitro, Aβ (1–42,43) aggregate at a faster rate than the shorter, more soluble forms of the peptide. Aged $A\beta(1-42)$, a peptide with considerable β-sheet structure, is toxic to primary rat hippocampal cultures (Puttfarcken et al., 1996). The addition of either apoE3- or E4-containing conditioned media attenuated the Aβ-induced reduction in both neurite outgrowth and cell survival (Puttfarcken et al., 1997). The level of protection against this toxicity was proportional to the growth-promoting effect of the two apoE isoforms in these cells. In contrast, apoE did exhibit an isoform specific effect (E2 > E3 > E4) on the cytotoxicity induced by $A\beta(25-35)$ and $A\beta$ $(1-40)$, preparations that lack secondary structure (Miller et al., 1996; Miyata and Smith, 1996). These results suggest that apoE may have an isoform-specific effect at a point early in the process of Aβ aggregation, possibly due to antioxidant properties of apoE.

BIOCHEMICAL STUDIES OF APOE AND AD-ASSOCIATED PROTEINS

Aβ – ApoE Interactions

It appears certain from both the in vitro and in vivo data summarized below that apoE binds to amyloid peptides, is associated with amyloid deposits, and affects fibrillogenesis. However, the differential effects of the apoE isoforms in these functions and their relationship to the manifestation of AD remain unclear.

ApoE – Aβ Complex

The physiologic mechanism by which apoE contributes to AD pathology may be by interaction with Aβ. In separate investigations, apoE was identified as an Aβ-binding protein in CSF (Strittmatter et al., 1993a; Wisniewski et al., 1993). Subsequently, synthetic Aβ peptides were shown to form a sodium dodecyl sulfate (SDS)-stable complex with apoE from intact VLDL particles (LaDu et al., 1995b), tissue culture media (LaDu et al., 1994, 1995b; Zhou et al., 1996), and cerebrospinal fluid (Ghiso et al., 1993; Wisniewski et al., 1993), as well as purified apoE (Strittmatter et al., 1993b; Naslund et al., 1995).

The isoform-specific interaction between apoE and Aβ is dependent on the preparation of apoE used. ApoE3 and E4 purified from plasma bound $A\beta(1-40)$ with comparable avidity in SDS-resistant gel shift assays (LaDu et al., 1995b; Strittmatter et al., 1993b), though apoE4 appeared to form complex faster than apoE3 (Strittmatter et al., 1993b). When the Aβ-binding capacity of native (unpurified) apoE isoforms from both tissue culture media and intact human VLDL was examined, the level of apoE3–Aβ complex was ~20-fold greater than apoE4–Aβ complex (LaDu, et al., 1994, 1995b) (Figure 4). ApoE2 on intact VLDL bound Aβ at levels comparable to apoE3 (Pederson et al., 1995). On the other hand, apoE3 and apoE4 purified from these two sources, by a process that includes delipidation and denaturation, bound to Aβ with comparable avidity (LaDu et al., 1995b).

Whether in the extracellular fluid of cell culture or the whole animal, endogenous apoE is generally associated with lipid. In each of the native preparations described above, the apoE was lipid associated, though with different classes of particles. In tissue culture media, apoE is found in small, dense particles (LaDu et al., 1995a), while VLDL is a large buoyant particle. Thus, while native apoE from two very different sources exhibited similar isoform-specific binding to Aβ, purified apoE did not. Like the receptor-binding activity of apoE described previously, apoE–Aβ binding activity seems to be determined by its conformation. These results indicate that native preparations of apoE may be a more physiologically relevant substrate for Aβ binding with purified apoE.

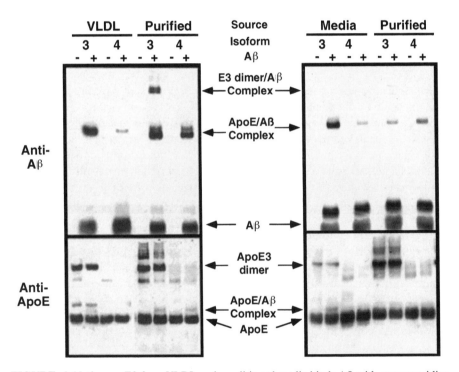

FIGURE 4. Native apoE3 from VLDL and conditioned media binds Aβ with greater avidity than apoE4. This isoform specificity is abolished when apoE is purified. Western blots of binding reactions using 25 μg/mL (~700 nM) of apoE incubated with or without 250 μM Aβ(1–40) peptide for 2 hr at room temperature. Source of apoE: (*Left*) Intact VLDL from apoE3/3 or apoE4/4 homozygotes, or purified from VLDL of apoE3/3 or apoE4/4 homozygotes; (*Right*) conditioned media of apoE3 or E4 transfected cells, or purified from conditioned media. Samples were run in nonreducing Laemmli buffer on 10–20% SDS-tricine gels, transferred to Immobilon-P membrane and probed for Aβ (*top*) or apoE (*bottom*) immunoreactivity.

Amyloidosis

Amyloidosis is characterized by the accumulation of normally soluble proteins into insoluble deposits that stain positive with Congo Red, indicating a β-pleated sheet secondary structure. In the periphery, a variety of proteins can form the fibrils that compose these deposits, including amyloid A (AA) and amyloid L (AL) in patients with Mediterranean fever and primary amyloidosis, respectively. AA and AL fibrils purified from these patients contained the C-terminal fragments of apoE, and in vitro AA formed SDS-resistant complexes with purified human apoE (Castano et al., 1995a). Amyloid deposits composed of Aβ fibrils are found in the periphery of patients with inclusion body myositis and in the brains of Lewy body and AD patients. C-terminal fragments of apoE also co-purified with Aβ extracted from the brain tissue of AD patients (Naslund et al., 1995; Wisniewski et al., 1995b). In solid phase binding assays, apoE bound to Aβ with a dissociation constant of $\sim$20nM (Golabek et al., 1996; Shuvaev and Siest, 1996). This affinity was enhanced by increased secondary structure of the peptide (Golabek et al., 1996), which explains in part the copurification of apoE with amyloid from senile plaques and systemic amyloid.

Fibrillogenesis

The influence of apoE isoforms on Aβ fibrillogenesis in vitro is equivocal. Several studies indicated that purified apoE enhances the formation of Aβ into amyloid fibrils, with apoE4 a more potent catalyst than apoE3 (Wisniewski et al., 1994; Ma et al., 1994; Castano et al., 1995b). The type of fibril formed also appeared to depend on the presence of apoE3 or E4 (Sanan et al., 1994). However, other data indicated that apoE3 and apoE4 both delay the onset of β-amyloid fibril formation (Evans et al., 1995). In addition, using native isoforms of apoE from conditioned media, apoE3 and E4 produced comparable increases in the fibrillogenesis of Aβ(1–42) (Sweeney et al., 1995). ApoE purified from plasma, primarily apoE3, also increased the fibrillogenesis of synthetic peptides of gelsolin amyloid and amyloid A (Soto et al., 1995).

Aggregation of apoE may also contribute to plaque deposition. In vitro, C-terminal peptides of apoE, like apoA-I, apoA-II, and serum amyloid A protein, can form Congo Red positive fibrils (Wisniewski et al., 1995b). This indicates that, in addition to Aβ amyloidosis, the amyloid deposits of AD may be caused by apoE amyloidosis. In addition, Aβ may influence the aggregation of apoE. Fractionation of plasma or apoE-conditioned media after preincubation with Aβ(1–40) peptide showed that apoE and Aβ coaggregate and elute as large protein complexes, much of which are SDS-sensitive (LaDu et al., 1995a). Subsequent gel-shift assays revealed that a portion of these apoE–Aβ structure are SDS-stable complexes. Isoform-specific differences in apoE aggregation have not been reported.

Aβ Association with Lipid Particles

Several mechanisms could account for an observed association of Aβ with lipoproteins, including interactions with lipid or protein components of the particles. In isolated lipoproteins, fractionated plasma, or CSF, Aβ was present in HDL particles, where a portion of it was complexed with apoE, apoJ, or apoA-I (Ghiso et al., 1993; Koudinov et al., 1996; Koudinov et el., 1994; LaDu et al., 1995a). In aqueous solutions, Aβ(1–40) and related species exist in equilibrium between random coil and β-sheet structures. Addition of negatively charged lipid vesicles induced a transition toward β-structure in the peptide at the water–lipid interface, indicating that the peptide can either aggregate at the membrane surface or intercalate into the hydrophobic part of the membrane (Terzi et al., 1995). In cortical cell homogenates, aggregated Aβ(1–40) associated with both lipid and protein components, while monomeric peptide bound only protein (Good and Murphy, 1995). When amyloid deposits from AD brains were fractionated by sucrose density gradients, Aβ copurified with lipid, specifically GM1 ganglioside (Yanagisawa et al., 1995). Thus, Aβ can probably associate with both the protein and lipid components of lipoproteins.

ApoE Interactions with Cytoskeletal Proteins

It is thought that phosphorylation of the microtubule-associated protein tau results in the formation of PHF, the primary component of NFT. Phosphorylation of tau allegedly causes it to disassociate from the microtubule and self-assemble into PHF by forming antiparallel dimers via the C-terminal microtubule binding repeat region of the protein. This process is thought to destabilize the neuron, over time leading to its degeneration. By immunostaining, apoE is present in NFT-containing neurons (Namba et al., 1991; Wisniewski and Frangione, 1992), though its association may be secondary to tangle formation (Benzing and Mufson, 1995). In vitro, purified apoE3 but not apoE4 bound full length recombinant tau, its C-terminal microtubule binding domain, and peptides of each of the four repeats in this domain (Strittmatter et al., 1994b; Huang et al., 1995). ApoE3–tau was detected by formation of an SDS-stable complex in gel shift assays. Neither apoE isoform formed complex with hyperphosphorylated tau and phosphorylation of serine 262, the residue in repeat I known to be phosphorylated in PHF-tau, abolished apoE3 binding. It has been proposed that apoE3–tau complex formation protects tau from phosphorylation and prevents self-assembly into PHF (Strittmatter et al., 1994a). Indeed, it has been demonstrated that mice lacking apoE have hyperphosphorylated tau protein (Genis et al., 1995). However, as apoE binds tau at its microtubule binding domain, it is unclear what effect the formation of apoE3–tau complex would have on normal neuronal function. ApoE3 can also form SDS-stable complex with other cytoskeletal proteins, including microtubule-associated protein MAP2C (Huang et al., 1994) and neurofilament protein (Flemming et al., 1996). In less stringent assays, both apoE3 and apoE4 bound tau and tubulin, and apoE3 also bound actin (Flemming et al., 1996). Thus, the specificity and significance of the interaction of apoE with cytoskeletal proteins, particularly in vivo, requires further clarification.

HYPOTHESES REGARDING APOE IN AD PATHOGENESIS

The isoform-specific action of apoE that affects the expression of AD pathology remains unclear. The role of apoE could be via an already established function of the protein, such as the differential association of the apoE isoforms with lipoprotein particles and its ability to transport lipid. Alternatively, the interaction between apoE and AD may be the result of a previously unidentified function of the protein, including isoform-specific interactions with either Aβ or tau. Because no definitive mechanism of apoE-related pathogenesis in AD has arisen, this section summarizes current hypotheses.

Several of these hypotheses propose a protective role for apoE3 in AD pathogenesis, a function that apoE4 lacks. Humans are the only species known to express apoE as different isoforms. With the exception of rabbits (Cys[112]), all other species have Arg at residues 112 and 158, comparable to human apoE4 at these sites. Moreover, the human apoE sequence diverges from other species at additional positions. Thus, it is possible that a protective role ascribed to apoE2 and apoE3 is unique to humans, complicating the development of transgenic animal models of AD. Whether apoE4 is pathogenic or apoE3 protects against AD clearly determines the course of development of compounds that affect apoE metabolism and prevent, delay, or reverse the onset of AD symptoms. Until these hypotheses are confirmed or rejected by experiments performed in vivo, the targeting of effective therapeutics to apoE neurobiology remains elusive.

ApoE Lipid Metabolism: Synaptogenesis, Membrane Remodeling, and Neuronal Dysfunction in AD

The development of AD is an age-related process. Over time, neuronal cell loss occurs, even in the brains of cognitively normal individuals. The mobilization and redistribution of lipid and cholesterol for membrane remodeling may be an important compensatory mechanism for maintaining normal synpatic density and neuronal function (Figure 5). ApoE plays a pivotal role in lipid transport in the brain. Anything compromising the ability of apoE to perform its normal function may result in a loss of synaptic plasticity. A gradual loss of synaptic function could lead to the cognitive decline and pathological manifestations of AD. Thus, minor differences in the ability of apoE isoforms to maintain membrane turnover could explain the expression of AD at an earlier age in carriers of the ε4 allele. Poirier (1994) has proposed that apoE4 could interfere with normal compensatory synaptogenesis and that the cholinergic systems are most vulnerable because of their reliance on intact phospholipid metabolism. In fact, choline acetyltransferase enzyme activity was reduced in brain tissue from AD patients with ε4/4 genotypes relative to controls or AD patients with no ε4 alleles (Soininen et al., 1995), indicating that ε4 carriers have a severe cholinergic defect. Evidence for apoE allelic variation in synaptogenesis is also illustrated by the loss of volume in the right hippocampus of AD patients with an ε4 allele (Lehtovirta et al., 1995). The importance of apoE in the preservation of normal neuronal function is further reflected in the data demonstrating enhanced outgrowth of neurites in the presence of apoE3 (Nathan et al., 1994; Holtzman et al., 1995; Bellosta et al., 1995), apoE immunostaining in neurons from cognitively normal brains (Metzger et al., 1996), and compromised reinnervation responses in the brains of apoE null mice (Masliah et al., 1994). This hypothesis unifies two of the primary risk factors for the development of AD, apoE genotype and age, and may help to explain why individuals without the ϵ4 gene can still develop AD, albeit with a later age of onset (Corder et al., 1993).

ApoE and Aβ: Binding, Sequestration, Uptake, and Fibrillogenesis

Several hypotheses explain the function of apoE isoforms in AD pathogenesis in terms of their interaction with the Aβ peptide. The colocalization of apoE with amyloid fibrils led Wisniewski and Frangione (1992) to classify apoE as a "pathological chaperone," targeting Aβ for amyloid deposits that can mature into senile plaques. As previously discussed, there is evidence to suggest that apoE4 can directly catalyze the formation of Aβ into insoluble fibrils (Wisniewski et al., 1994; Ma et al., 1994; Castano et al., 1995b). However, the biochemical, immunohistochemical, and genetic data are also consistent with the alternative hypothesis that apoE3 is a protective isoform in AD. Rebeck and co-workers (1993) proposed that apoE normally clears Aβ from the neuropil via uptake by LRP on neurons (Figure 5). Because apoE3 and apoE4 appear to bind LRP with equal affinity (Kowal et al., 1990), they hypothesized that apoE4 is less efficient in clearing Aβ due to either lower levels of the protein or an altered interaction with Aβ. Native apoE3 binds Aβ with higher avidity than apoE4 (LaDu et al., 1995b). Thus, apoE3 could reduce the concentration and residence time of extracellular Aβ via clearance of apoE3–Aβ by apoE receptors. Alternatively, the binding of apoE3 to Aβ could inhibit aggregation and fibril formation or otherwise affect the extracellular sequestration of this amyloidogenic species. ApoE2 on intact VLDL also binds Aβ with greater avidity than apoE4 (Pederson et al., 1995), suggesting that the protective effect of the ϵ2 allele in AD may be due to a mechanism similar to that described above for apoE3. The enhanced protection of ϵ2 compared to ϵ3 could result from variations in the concentrations of the apoE isoforms in the brain. While the plasma level of apoE in ϵ2/2 individuals may be elevated compared to other genotypes (Innerarity et al., 1986), the relative levels of apoE isoforms in the brain are not known. The relevance of SDS-stable and other types of apoE–Aβ complexes to the tissue fluid environment of the brain requires further investigation. However, the observation that apoE2 and apoE3 inhibit the neurotoxicity of soluble Aβ peptides better than apoE4 (Miller et al., 1996; Miyata and Smith, 1996) suggests that isoform-specific apoE–Aβ interactions protect neurons from extracellular Aβ.

ApoE uptake in neural tissue may exhibit an isoform specificity different than that observed in other tissues. For example, apoE ϵ2/2 and ϵ3/3 VLDL exhibit a comparable affinity for the VLDL receptor, demonstrating that the relative binding affinities of the apoE isoforms may differ for individual lipoprotein receptors (Takahashi et al., 1996). In determining the relative binding affinities of the apoE isoforms for the LDL receptor and LRP, the apoE isoforms are purified from human plasma and reconstituted with phospholipid vesicles or β-VLDL, respectively. In the context of the brain, the affinity of endogenous apoE-containing particles for apoE receptors may exhibit an isoform specificity not detected by current in vitro binding assays. Recently, in vitro binding of radioidonated apoE3 reconstituted on

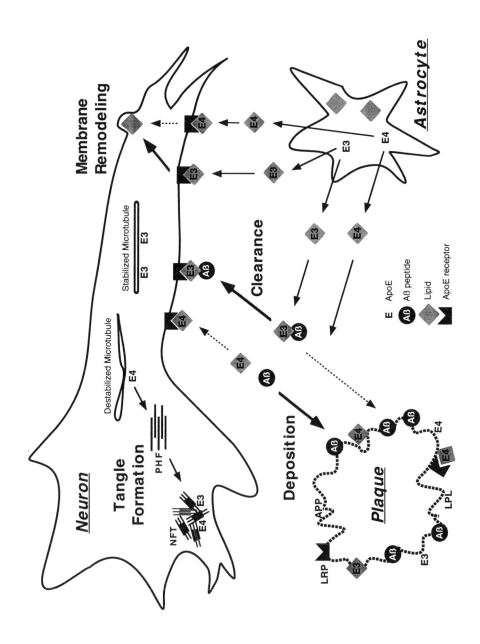

liposomes was demonstrated to preferentially bind neuronal cells while apoE4 liposomes bound astrocyte and neurons with equal affinity (Guillaume et al., 1996). ApoE2 had a significantly lower affinity than apoE3 or apoE4 in both astrocytes and neurons. In addition, the presence of another moiety, such as Aβ, may affect the binding and uptake of apoE-containing particles. Preliminary evidence suggests that in the presence of Aβ, isoform-specific uptake of apoE occurs in both primary hippocampal neurons and cortical astrocytes, an effect at least partly mediated by the LDL receptor (Beffert et al., 1995).

The preferential association of apoE3 with HDL particles may influence the pathogenic pathways of AD. Though the apoE content of CSF-HDL in ε3/3 versus ε4/4 individuals is unknown, CSF-HDL in individuals with the apoE3 phenotype could be more available for receptor-mediated clearance than apoE4 CSF-HDL due to a greater proportion of particles containing apoE3. The observation that Aβ associates with HDL-like particles in both plasma and CSF (Koudinov et al., 1994; Koudinov et al., 1996; LaDu et al., 1995a) leads to the possibility that the binding of apoE3 to Aβ and the partitioning of apoE3 and Aβ to HDL may both influence the rate of Aβ uptake from the neuropil. Over time, the cumulative effect of a reduced clearance rate by apoE4 could be increased amyloid deposition. Alternatively, Aβ interactions with lipid moieties in apoE-containing lipid particles could directly mediate Aβ aggregation. Lipid vesicles induce β-sheet structure in Aβ (Terzi et al., 1995). In addition, a variety of unsaturated FFA enhanced both Aβ aggregation and PHF extension in vitro (Wilson and Binder, 1995). The expression of LPL in the brain (Ben-Zeev et al., 1990; Vilaro et al., 1990) and its presence in the capillary endothelia is indirect evidence that FFA are readily available in the interstitial fluid via simple diffusion from the circulation. The presence of LPL in amyloid plaques (Rebeck et al., 1995) suggests that FFA may indeed participate in amyloid plaque formation. These processes may be retarded by efficient transport and clearance of lipid by apoE3-containing particles.

ApoE and Cytoskeletal Stability

Strittmatter and co-workers (1994a) have proposed that intraneuronal apoE3 binds the microtubule-associated protein tau to prevent the hyperphosphorylation that results in an accelerated rate of PHF formation and assembly into NFTs. Therefore, the ineffec-

---

FIGURE 5. Model summarizing the proposed roles for apoE3 and E4 in neuropathogenesis. *Aβ deposition and clearance:* ApoE3 avidly binds Aβ and is cleared by neuronal apoE receptors, accounting for the apoE association with neurons. The reduced efficiency of apoE4–Aβ binding allows acceleration of amyloid deposition and plaque formation. The LRP and apoE associated with plaques may also contribute to Aβ deposition. *Neurofibrillary tangle formation:* Cellular apoE4 is associated with microtubule destabilization, potentially leading to NFT formation, while apoE3 stabilizes cytoskeletal elements. *Membrane remodeling:* ApoE3 is more efficient than apoE4 in delivering lipids for membrane maintenance, eventually leading to impaired synaptogenesis.

tiveness of apoE4 in this function would be the source of the genetic correlation between ϵ4 and AD (Figure 5). The interaction of apoE with cytoskeletal proteins assumes that apoE has access to the cytoplasmic compartment. ApoE has been localized to the cytosol of neurons in vivo (Han et al., 1994a) and to the cytoplasm, endosomes, and peroxisomes of hepatocytes (Hamilton et al., 1990). In cultured neurons, apoE-enriched particles taken up from the media resulted in apoE immunoreactivity in the cells (Nathan et al., 1995). Even though a comparable amount of lipid was taken up by cells treated with apoE3- and apoE4-containing β-VLDL, more apoE3 accumulated intracellularly than apoE4, perhaps due to apoE3 binding to cytoskeletal elements (Strittmatter et al., 1994b) stabilizing both the neuronal infrastructure and the intracellular presence of apoE3. In addition, uptake of apoE4 was associated with microtubule depolymerization, suggesting that apoE4 promotes neuronal destabilization (Nathan et al., 1995).

CONCLUSION

The pathological features that define AD are the result of a gradual process. Just how gradual is illustrated by recent data from the longitudinal Nun Study (Snowdon et al., 1996). Linguistic ability measured while the participants were in their early twenties accurately predicted cognitive function late in life, correlating with the clinical manifestation of AD. Thus, a subtle difference in the function of the apoE isoforms could, over time, be sufficient to account for ϵ4 being a risk factor for AD.

In spite of an intensive research effort in the 3 years since the correlation between apoE and AD was first documented, the nature of this isoform-specific effect remains unclear. Is it the presence of apoE4 or the absence of apoE2 or apoE3 that contributes to the pathogenic process? Is the role of apoE related to its known lipid carrying and clearing function or to an activity more directly related to the development of amyloid deposits and NFT? Does apoE act extracellularly or intracellularly? The answers to these questions await additional study to further define the isoform-specific role of apoE in the development of AD.

ACKNOWLEDGMENTS

The authors wish to thank Catherine Reardon and Godfrey Getz for helpful readings of this chapter. The author's cited work was supported by Abbott Laboratories and by American Health Assistance Foundation grant 95100 and NIH grant 1F32 HL08833-01 to M.J.L.

REFERENCES

Albers JJ, Tollefson JH, Wolfbauer G, Albright RE (1992): Cholesteryl ester transfer protein in human brain. Int J Clin Lab Res 21:264–266.

Amouyel P, Vidal O, Launay JM, Laplanche JL (1994): The apolipoprotein E alleles as major susceptibility factors for Creutzfeldt–Jakob disease. Lancet 344:1315–1318.

Arai H, Muramatsu T, Higuchi S, Sasaki H, Trojanowski JQ (1994): Apolipoprotein E gene in Parkinson's disease with or without dementia. Lancet 344:889.

Askanas V, Engel WK (1994): Inclusion-body myositis: Newest advances. Brain Pathol 4:361–362.

Askanas V, Mirabella M, Engel WK, Alvarez RB, Weisgraber KH (1994): Apolipoprotein E immunoreactive deposits in inclusion-body muscle diseases. Lancet 343:364–365.

Basu SK, Ho YK, Brown MS, Bilheimer DW, Anderson RGW, Goldstein JL (1982): The biochemical and genetic studies of apoprotein E secreted by mouse macrophages and human monocytes. J Biol Chem 257:9788–9795.

Beffert U, Aumont N, Dea D, Davignon J, Poirier J (1995): Apolipoprotein E uptake is increased in the presence of β-amyloid peptide and reduced by blockade of low density lipoprotein receptor. Soc Neurosci Abst 21(1):6.

Bellosta S, Nathan BP, Orth M, Dong LM, Mahley RW, Pitas RE (1995): Stable expression and secretion of apolipoproteins E3 and E4 in mouse neuroblastoma cells produces differential effects on neurite outgrowth. J Biol Chem 270:27063–27071.

Ben-Zeev O, Doolittle MH, Singh N, Chang CH, Schotz MC (1990): Synthesis and regulation of lipoprotein lipase in the hippocampus. J Lipid Res 31:1307–1313.

Benzing WC, Mufson EJ (1995): Apolipoprotein E immunoreactivity within neurofibrillary tangles: Relationship to tau and PHF in Alzheimer's disease. Exp Neurol 132:162–171.

Borghini I, Barja F, Pometta, James RW (1995): Characterization of subpopulations of lipoprotein particles isolated from human cerebrospinal fluid. Biochem Biophys Acta 1255:192–200.

Boyles JK, Zoellner CD, Anderson LJ, Kosik LM, Pitas RE, Weisgraber KH, Hui DY, Mahley RW, Gebicke-Haerter PJ, Ignatius MJ, Shooter EM. (1989): A role for apolipoprotein E, apolipoprotein A-I, and low density lipoprotein receptors in cholesterol transport during regeneration and remyelination of the rat sciatic nerve. J Clin Invest 83:1015–1031.

Boyles JK, Pitas RE, Wilson E, Mahley RW, Taylor JM (1985): Apolipoprotein E associated with astrocytic glia of the central nervous system and with nonmyelinating glia of the peripheral nervous system. J Clin Invest 76:1501–1513.

Castano EM, Prelli F, Pras M, Frangione B (1995a): Apolipoprotein E carboxy-terminal fragments are complexed to amyloids A and L. J Biol Chem 270:17610–17615.

Castano EM, Prelli F, Wisniewski Tgolabek A, Kumar RA, Soto C, Frangione B (1995b): Fibrillogenesis in Alzheimer's disease of amyloid β peptides and apolipoprotein E. Biochem J 306:599–604.

Christie RH, Freeman M, Hyman BT (1996): Expression of the macrophage scavenger receptor, a multifunctional lipoprotein receptor, in microglia associated with senile plaques in Alzheimer's disease. Am J Pathol 148:399–403.

Corder EH, Saunders SM, Risch NJ, Strittmatter WJ, Schmechel DE, Gaskell PC, Jr, Rimmler JB, Locke PA, Conneally PM, Schmader KE, Small GW, Roses AD, Haines JL, Pericak-Vance MA (1994): Protective effect of apolipoprotein E type 2 allele for late onset Alzheimer disease. Nature Gene 7:180–184.

Corder EH, Saunders SM, Strittmatter WJ, Schmechel DE, Gaskell PC, Small GW, Roses AD, Haines JL, Pericak-Vance MA. (1993): Gene dose of apolipoprotein E type 4 allele and the risk of Alzheimer's disease in late onset families. Science 261:921–923.

Davignon J, Gregg R, Sing C (1988): Apolipoprotein E polymorphism and atherosclerosis. Arteriosclerosis 8:1–21.

El Khoury J, Hickman SE, Thomas CA, Cao L, Silverstein SC, Loike JB (1996): Scavenger receptor-mediated adhesion of microglia to β-amyloid fibrils. Nature 382:716–719.

Elshourbagy NA, Lia WS, Mahley RW, Taylor JM (1985): Apolipoprotein E mRNA is abundant in the brain and adrenals, as well as in the liver, and is present in other peripheral tissues of rats and marmosets. Proc Natl Acad Sci 82, 203–207.

Evans KC, Berger EP, Cho C, Weisgraber KH, and Lansbury PT (1995): Apolipoprotein E is a kinetic but not a thermodynamic inhibitor of amyloid formation: Implications for the pathogenesis and treatment of Alzheimer disease. Proc Natl Acad Sci U S A 92:763–767.

Fleming LM, Weisgraber KH, Strittmatter WJ, Troncoso JC, Johnson GVW (1996): Differential binding of apolipoprotein E isoforms to tau and other cytoskeletal proteins. Exp Neurol. 138:252–260.

Frisoni GB, Calabresi L, Geroldi C, Bianchetti A, D'Acquarica AL, Govoni S, Sirtori CR, Trabucchi M, Franceschini G (1994): Apolipoprotein E ε4 allele in Alzheimer's disease and vascular dementia. Dementia 5:240–242.

Gearing M, Mori H, Mirra SS (1996): Aβ-peptide length and apolipoprotein E genotype in Alzheimer's disease. Annals Neurol 39:395–399.

Genis I, Gordon I, Sehayek E, Michaelson DM (1995): Phosphorylation of tau in apolipoprotein E-deficient mice. Neurosci Lett 199:5–8.

Ghiso J, Matsubara E, Koudinov A, Choi-Miura NH, Tomita M, Wisniewski T, Frangione B (1993): The cerebral spinal-fluid soluble form of Alzheimer's amyloid beta is complexed to SP-40,40 (apolipoprotein J), an inhibitor of the complement membrane-attack complex. Biochem J 293:27–30.

Goate A, Chartier-Harlin MC, Mullan M, Brown J, Crawford F, Fidani L, Giuffra L, Haynes A, Irving N, James L, Mant R, Newton P, Rooke K, Roques P, Talbot C, Pericak-Vance M, Roses A, Williamson R, Rossor M, Owen M, Hardy JA (1991): Segregatioan of a missense in the amyloid precursor protein gene with familial Alzheimer's disease. Nature 349:704–706.

Golabek AA, Soto C, Vogel T, Wisniewski T (1996): The interaction between apolipoprotein E and Alzheimer's amyloid β-peptide is dependent on β-peptide conformation. J Biol Chem 271:10602–10606.

Gomez-Isla T, West HL, Rebeck GW, Harr SD, Growdon JH, Locascio JJ, Perls TT, Lipsitz LA, Hyman BT (1996): Clinical and pathological correlates of apolipoprotein E ε4 in Alzheimer's disease. Ann Neurol 39:62–70.

Good TA, Murphy RM (1995): Aggregation state-dependent binding of β-amyloid peptide to protein and lipid components of rat cortical lipid homogenates. Biochem Biophys Res Comm 207:209–215.

Goodrum JF (1991): Cholesterol from degenerating nerve myelin becomes associated with lipoproteins containing apolipoprotein E. J Neurochem 56:2082–2086.

Greenberg SM, Rebeck GW, Vonsattel JPG, Gomez-Isla T, Hyman BT (1995): Apolipoprotein E ε4 and cerebral hemorrhage associated with amyloid angiopathy. Ann Neurol 38:254–259.

Guillaume D, Bertrand P, Dea D, Davignon J, Poirier J (1996): Apolipoprotein E and low-density lipoprotein binding and internalization in primary cultures of rat astrocytes: Isoform-specific alterations. J Neurochem 66:2410–1418.

Hamilton RL, Wong JS, Guo LSS, Krisans S, Havel RJ (1990): Apolipoprotein E localization in rat hepatocytes by immunogold labeling of cryothin secretions. J Lipid Res 31:1589–1603.

Han S-H, Einstein G, Weisgraber KH, Strittmatter WJ, Saunders AM, Pericak-Vance M, Roses AD, Schmechel DE (1994a): Apolipoprotein E is localized to the cytoplasm of human cortical neurons: A light and electron microscopic study. J Neuropathol Exp Neurol 53:535–544.

Han S-H, Hulette C, Saunders AM, Einstein G, Pericak-Vance M, Strittmatter WJ, Roses AD, Schmechel DE. (1994b): Apolipoprotein E is present in hippocampal neurons without neurofibrillary tangles in Alzheimer's disease and in age-matched controls. Exp Neurol 128:13–26.

Handelmann GE, Boyles JK, Weisgraber KH, Mahley RW, Pitas RE (1992): Effects of a apolipoprotein E, β-very low density lipoproteins, and cholesterol on the extension of neurites by rabbit dorsal root ganglion neurons *in vitro*. J Lipid Res 33:1677–1688.

Hardy J, Crook R, Prihar G, Roberts G, Raghavan R, Perry R (1994): Senile dementia of the Lewy body type has an apolipoprotein E ε4 allele frequency intermediate between controls and Alzheimer's disease. Neurosci Lett 182:1–2.

Hardy J, Hooulden H, Collinge J (1993): Apolipoprotein-E genotype and Alzheimer's disease. Lancet 342:737–738.

Holtzman DM, Pitas RE, Kilbridge J, Nathan B, Mahley RW, Bu G, Schwartz AL (1995): Low density lipoprotein receptor-related protein mediates apolipoprotein E-dependent neurite outgrowth in a central nervous system-derived neuronal cell line. Proc Natl Acad Sci 92:9480–9484.

Huang DY, Weisgraber KH, Goedert M, Saunders AM, Roses AD, Strittmatter WJ (1995): ApoE3 binding to tau tandem repeat I is abolished by tau serine 262 phosphorylation. Neurosci Lett 192:209–212.

Huang DY, Goedert M, Jakes R, Weisgraber DH, Garner CC, Saunders AM, Pericak-Vance MA, Schmechel DE, Roses AD, Strittmatter WJ (1994); Isoform-specific interactions of apolipoprotein E with microtubule-associated protein MAP2c: Implications for Alzheimer's disease. Neurosci Lett 182:55–58.

Ignatius MJ, Shooter EM, Pitas RE, Mahley RW (1987): Lipoprotein uptake by neuronal growth cones *in vitro*. Science 236:959–962.

Innerarity TL, Hui DY, Bersot TP, Mahley RW (1986): Type III hyperlipoproteinemia: A focus on lipoprotein receptor-apolipoprotein E2 interactions. In Angel A, Frohlich J (eds): "Advances in Experimental Medicine and Biology." New York: Plenum, pp 273–288.

Itoh Y, Yamada M, Suematsu N, Matsushita M, Otomo E (1996): Influence of apolipoprotein E genotype on cerebral amyloid angiopathy in the elderly. Stroke 27:216–218.

Kalaria RN, Cohen DL, Premkumar, DRD (1996): Apolipoprotein E alleles and brain vascular pathology in Alzheimer's disease. Ann N Y Academy Sci 777:266–270.

Kim DH, Iijima H, Goto K, Sakai J, Ishii H, Kim HJ, Suzuki H, Konda H, Saeki S, Yamamoto T (1996): Human apolipoprotein E receptor 2: A novel lipoprotein receptor of the low density lipoprotein receptor family predominantly expressed in brain. J Biol Chem 271:8373–8380.

Koller WC, Glatt SL, Hubble JP, Paolo A, Troster AI, Handler MS, Horvar RT, Martin C, Schmidt K, Karst A, Wijsman EM, Yu CE, Schellenberg GD (1995): Apolipoprotein E genotype in Parkinson's disease with and without dementia. Ann Neurol 37:242–245.

Koudinov AR, Koudinova NV, Kumar A, Beavis R, Ghiso J (1996): Biochemical characterization of Alzheimer's soluble amyloid beta protein in human cerebrospinal fluid: association with high density lipoproteins. Biochem Biophys Res Commun 223:592–597.

Koudinov A, Matsubara E, Frangione B, Ghiso J (1994): The soluble form of Alzheimer's amyloid beta protein is complexed to high density lipoprotein 3 and very high density lipoprotein in normal human plasma. Biochem Biophys Res Comm 205:1164–1171.

Kounnas MZ, Moir RD, Rebeck GW, Bush A, Argraves WS, Tanzi RE, Hyman BT, Strickland DK (1995): LDL receptor-related protein, a multifunctional apoE receptor, binds secreted beta-amyloid precursor protein and mediates its degradation. Cell 82:331–340.

Kowal RC, Herz J, Weisgraber KH, Mahley RW, Brown MS, Goldstein JL (1990). Opposing effects of apolipoproteins E and C on lipoprotein binding to low density lipoprotein receptor-related protein. J Biol Chem 265:10771–10779.

LaDu MJ, Lukens JR, Pederson TM, Reardon CA, Getz GS, Falduto MT (1995a): Particle size distribution of native apolipoprotein E in the presence of β-amyloid peptide. Soc Neurosci Abst 21(1):5.

LaDu JM, Pederson TM, Frail DE, Reardon CA, Getz GS, Falduto MT (1995b): Purification of apolipoprotein E attenuates isoform-specific binding to β-amyloid. J Biol Chem 270: 9039–9042.

LaDu MJ, Falduto MT, Manelli AM, Reardon CA, Getz GS, Frail DE (1994): Isoform-specific binding of apolipoprotein E to β-amyloid. J Biol Chem 269:23403–23406.

Lehtovirta M, Laakso MP, Soininen H, Helisalmi S, Mannermaa A, Helkala E-L, Partanen K, Ryynanen M, Vainio P, Hartikainen P, Riekkinen PJ (1995): Volumes of hippocampus, amygdala and frontal lobe in Alzheimer patients with different apolipoprotein E genotypes. Neuroscience 67:65–72.

Levy-Lahad W, Wasco W, Poorkaj P, Romano DM, Ashima J, Pettengell WH, Yu C, Jondro PD, Schmidt SD, Wang K, Crowley AC, Fu YH, Guenette SY, Galas D, Nemens E, Wijsman EM, Bird TD, Schellenberg GD, Tanzi RE (1995): Candidate gene for the chromsome 1 familial Alzheimer's disease locus. Science 269:973–977.

Li W-H, Tanimura M, Luo C-C, Datta S, Chan L (1988): The apolipoprotein multigene family: Biosynthesis, structure, structure–function relationships, and evolution. J Lipid Res 29:245–271.

Linton MF, Gish R, Hubl ST, Butler E, Esquivel C, Bry WI, Boyles JK, Wardell MR, Young SG (1991): Phenotypes of apoB and apoE after liver transplantation. J Clin Invest 88: 270–281.

Lippa CF, Smith TW, Saunders AM, Crook R, Pulaski-Salo D, Davies P, Hardy J, Roses AD, Dickson D (1995): Apolipoprotein E genotype and Lewy body disease. Neurology 45:97–103.

Ma J, Yee A, Brewer HB, Jr, Das S, Potter H (1994): Amyloid-associated proteins α1-antichymotrypsin and apolipoprotein E promote assembly of Alzheimer β-protein into filaments. Nature 372:92–94.

Mahley RW (1988): Apolipoprotein E: Cholesterol transport protein with expanding role in cell biology. Science 240:622–630.

Masliah E, Mallory M, Ge N, Alford M, Veinbergs I, Roses AD (1995): Neurodegeneration in the central nervous system of apoE-deficient mice. Exper Neurol 136:107–122.

Masliah E, Mallory M, Alford M, Mucke L (1994): Abnormal synaptic regeneration in hAPP transgenic and apoE knockout mice. Neurobiol Aging 15:S11.

Masters CL, Simms G, Weinmann NA, Multhaup G, McDonald BL, Beyreuther K (1985): Amyloid plaque core protein in Alzheimer's disease and Down's syndrome. Proc Natl Acad Sci 82:4245–4249.

Matsubara E, Frangione B, Ghiso J (1995): Characterization of apolipoprotein J-Alzheimer's Aβ interaction. J Biol Chem 270:7563–7567.

McGeer PL, Kawamata T, Walker DG (1992): Distribution of clusterin in Alzheimer brain tissue. Brain Res 579:337–341.

Metzger RE, LaDu JM, Pan JB, Getz GS, Frail DE, Falduto MT (1996): Neurons of the human frontal cortex display apolipoprotein E immunoreactivity:implications for Alzheimer's disease. J Neuro Path Exp Neuro 55:372–380.

Miller RJ, Galindo MF, Jordan J, Lukens JR, LaDu MJ, Getz GS (1996): Isoform-specific effect of apolipoprotein E on β-amyloid induced toxicity in rat hippocampal pyramidal neuronal cultures. Soc Neurosci Abst 22(3):2117.

Miyata M, Smith JD (1996): Apolipoprotein E allele-specific antioxidant activity and effects on cytotoxicity by oxidative insults and β-amyloid peptides. Nature Genet 14:55–61.

Mufson EJ, Benzing WC, Cole GM, Wang H, Emerich DF, Sladek JR, Morrison JH, Kordower JH (1994): Apolipoprotein E-immunoreactivity in aged rhesus monkey cortex: Colocalization with amyloid plaques. Neurobiol Aging 15:621–627.

Mullan M, Crawford F, Axelman K, Houlden H, Lilius L, Winblad B, Lannfelt L (1992): A pathogenic mutation for probable Azheimer's disease in the APP gene at the N-terminus of β-amyloid. Nature Genet 1:345–347.

Nagy ZS, Esiri MM, Jobst KA, Johnston C, Litchfield S, Sim E, Smith AD (1995): Influence of the apolipoprotein E genotype on amyloid deposition and neurofibrillary tangle formation in Alzheimer's disease. Neuroscience 69:757–761.

Namba Y, Tomonaga M, Kawasaki H, Otomo E, Ikeda K (1991): Apolipoprotein E immunoreactivity in cerebral amyloid deposits and neurofibrillary tangles in Alzheimer's disease amd kuru plaque amyloid in Creutzfeldt-Jakob disease. Brain Res 541:163–166.

Naslund J, Thyberg J, Tjernberg LO, Wernstedt C, Karlstrom AR, Bogdanovic N, Gandy SE, Lannfelt L, Terenius L, Nordstedt C (1995): Characterization of stable complexes involving apolipoprotein E and the amyloid β peptide in Alzheimer's disease brain. Neuron 15:219–228.

Nathan BP, Chang KC, Bellosta S, Brisch E, Ge N, Mahley RW, Pitas RE (1995): The inhibitory effect of apolipoprotein E4 on neurite outgrowth is associated with microtubule depolymerization. J Biol Chem 270:19791–19799.

Nathan BP, Bellosta S, Sanan DA, Weisgraber KH, Mahley RW, Pitas RE. (1994): Differential effects of apolipoproteins E3 and E4 on neuronal growth *in vitro*. Science 264:850–852.

Nicoll JAR, Burnett C, Love S, Graham DI, Ironside JW, Vinters HV (1996a): High frequency of apolipoprotein E ε2 in patients with cerebral hemorrhage due to cerebral amyloid angiopathy. Ann Neurol 39:682.

Nicoll JAR, Roberts GW, Graham DI (1996b): Amyloid β-protein, APOE genotype and head injury. Ann N Y Acad Sci 777:271–275.

Ohm TG, Kirca M, Bohl J, Scharnagl H, Grob W, Marz W (1995): Apolipoprotein E polymorphism influences not only cerebral senile plaque load but also Alzheimer-type neurofibrillary tangle formation. Neuroscience 66:583–587.

Okuizumi K, Onodera O, Namba Y, Ikeda K, Yamamoto T, Seki K, Ueki A, Nanko S, Tanaka H, Takahashi H, Oyanagi K, Mizuasawa H, Kanazawa I, Tsuji S (1995): Genetic association of the very low density lipoprotein (VLDL) receptor gene with sporadic Alzheimer's disease. Nature Genet 11:207–209.

Pederson TM, Frail DE, Metzger RE, Manelli AM, Reardon CA, Falduto MT, Getz GS, LaDu MJ (1995): Binding of apolipoprotein E2 to β-amyloid: Comparison to apolipoprotein E3 and E4. Soc Neurosci Abst 21(3):1716.

Pericak-Vance MA, Bebout JL, Gaskell PC, Yamaoka LH, Hung WY, Alberts MJ, Walker AP, Bartlett RH, Haynes CA, Welsh KA, Earl NL, Heyman A, Clark CM, Roses AD (1991): Linkage studies in familial Alzheimer disease: Evidence for chromsome19 linkage. Am J Hum Genet 48:1034–1050.

Pickering-Brown SM, Roberts DA, Owen F (1994a): Apolipoprotein E4 alleles and non-Alzheimer's disease forms of dementia. Neurodegeneration 3:95–96.

Pickering-Brown SM, Mann DM, Bourke JP, Roberts DA, Balderson D, Burns A, Byrne J, Owen F (1994b): Apolipoprotein E4 and Alzheimer's disease pathology in Lewy body disease and in other β-amyloid-forming diseases. Lancet 343:1155.

Pitas RE, Boyles JK, Lee SH, Foss D, Mahley RW (1987a): Astrocytes synthesize apolipoprotein E and metabolize apolipoprotein E-containing lipoproteins. Biochim Biophys Acta 917:148–161.

Pitas RE, Boyles JK, Lee SH, Hui D, Weisgraber KH (1987b): Lipoproteins and their receptors in the central nervous system—Characterization of the lipoproteins in cerebrospinal fluid and identification of apolipoprotein B,E(LDL) receptors in the brain. J Biol Chem 262:14352–14360.

Poduri A, Gearing M, Rebeck GW, Mirra SS, Tigges J, Hyman BT (1994): Apolipoprotein E4 and beta amyloid in senile plaques and cerebral blood vessels of aged rhesus monkeys. Am J Pathol 144:1183–1187.

Poirier J (1994): Apolipoprotein E in animal models of CNS injury and in Alzehimer's disease. Trends Neurosci 17:525–530.

Poirier J, Baccichet A, Dea D, Gauthier S (1993): Cholesterol synthesis and lipoprotein reuptake during synaptic remodeling in hippocampus in adult rats. Neuroscience 55:81–90.

Poirier J, Hess M, May PC, Finch CE (1991): Astrocytic apolipoprotein E mRNA and GFAP mRNA in hippocampus after entorhinal cortex lesioning. Mol Brain Res 11:97–106.

Popko B, Goodrum JF, Bouldin TW, Zhang SH, Maeda N (1993): Nerve regeneration occurs in the absence of apolipoprotein E in mice. J Neurochem 60:1155–1158.

Puttfarcken PS, Manelli AM, Neilly J, Frail DE (1996): Inhibition of age-induced β-amyloid neurotoxicity in rat hippocampal cells. Exp Neurol 138:73–81.

Puttfarcken PS, Manelli AM, Falduto MT, Getz GS, LaDu MJ (1997): Effect of apolipoprotein E on neurite outgrowth and β-amyloid-induced toxicity in developing rat primary hippocampal cultures. J Neurochem (in press).

Reardon CA, Lau Y-F, Paik Y-K, Weisgraber KH, Mahley RW, Taylor JM (1986): Expression of human apolipoprotein E gene in cultured mammalian cells. J Biol Chem 261: 9858–9864.

Rebeck GW, Harr SD, Strickland DK, Hyman BT (1995): Multiple, diverse senile plaque-associated proteins are ligands of an apolipoprotein E receptor, the α2-macroglobulin receptor/low-density-lipoprotein receptor-related protein. Ann Neurol 37:211–217.

Rebeck GW, Reiter JS, Strickland DK, Hyman BT (1993): Apolipoprotein E in sporadic Alzheimer's disease: Allelic variation and receptor interactions. Neuron 11:575–580.

Salvatore M, Seeber AC, Nacmisa B, Petraroli R, D'Alessandro M, Sorbi S, Pacchiari M (1996): Apolipoprotein E in sporadic and familial Creutzfeldt-Jakob disease. Neurosci Lett 199:95–98.

Sanan DA, Weisgraber KH, Russell SJ, Mahley RW, Huang D, Saunders A, Schmechel D, Wisniewski T, Frangione B, Roses AD, Strittmatter WJ (1994): Apolipoprotein E associates with β amyloid peptide of Alzheimer's disease to form novel monofibrils. Isoform apoE4 associates more efficiently than apoE3. J Clin Invest 94:860–869.

Saunders AM, Schmader K, Breitner JC, Benson MD, Brown WT, Goldfarb L, Goldgaber D, Manwaring MG, Szymanski MH, McCown N, Dole KC, Schmechel DE, Strittmatter WJ, Pericak-Vance MA, Roses AD (1993a): Apolipoprotein E ε4 allele distribution in lateonset Alzheimer's disease and in other amyloid-forming diseases. Lancet 342:710–711.

Saunders AM, Strittmatter WJ, Schmechel D, St. George-Hyslop PH, Pericak-Vance MA, Joo SH, Rosi BL, Gusella JF, Crapper-MacLachlan DR, Alberts MJ, Hulette C, Crain B, Goldgaber D, Roses AD (1993b): Association of apolipoprotein E allele ε4 with late-onset familial and sporadic Alzheimer's disease. Neurology 43:1467–1472.

Schmechel DE, Saunders AM, Strittmtter WJ, Crain BJ, Hulette CM, Joo SH, Pericak-Vance MA, Goldgaber D, Roses AD (1993): Increased amyloid β-peptide deposition in cerebral cortex as a consequence of apolipoprotein E genotype in late-onset Alzheimer disease. Proc Natl Acad Sci 90:9649–9653.

Sherrington R, Rogaev EI, Liang Y, Rogaeva EA, Levesque G, Ikeda M, Chi H, Lin C, Li G, Holman K, Tsuda T, Mar L, Foncin J-F, Bruni AC, Montesi MP, Sorbi S, Rainero I, Pinessi L, Nee L, Chumakov I, Pollen D, Brookes A, Sanseau P, Polinsky RJ, Wasco W, Da Silva HAR, Haines JL, Pericak-Vance MA, Tanzi RE, Roses AD, Fraser PE, Rommens JM, St. George-Hyslop PH (1995): Cloning of a gene bearing missense mutations in early-onset familial Alzheimer's disease. Nature 375:754–760.

Shuvaev VV, Siest G (1996): Interaction between human amphipathic apolipoproteins and amyloid β-peptide: surface plasmon resonance studies. FEBS Letters 383:9–12.

Smith KM, Lawn RM, Wilcox JN (1990): Cellular localization of apolipoprotein D and lecithin:cholesterol acyltransferase mRNA in rhesus monkey tissues by in situ hybridization. J Lipid Res 31:995–1004.

Snowdon DA, Kemper SJ, Mortimer JA, Greiner LH, Wekstein DR, Markesbery WR (1996): Linguistic ability in early life and cognitive function and Alzheimer's disease in late life. JAMA 275:528–532.

Soininen H, Kosunen O, Helisalmi S, Mannermaa A, Paljarvi L, Talasniemi S, Ryynanen M, Riekkinen P (1995): A severe loss of choline acetyltransferase in the frontal cortex of Alzheimer patients carrying apolipoprotein ε4 allele. Neurosci Lett 187:79–82.

Soto C, Castano EM, Prelli F, Kumar RA, Baumann M (1995): Apolipoprotein E increases the fibrillogenic potential of synthetic peptides derived from Alzheimer's, gelsolin and AA amyloids. FEBS Lett 371:110–114.

Strittmatter WJ, Weisgraber KH, Goedert M, Saunders AM, Huang D, Corder EH, Dong L-M, Jakes R, Alberts MJ, Gilbert JR, Han S-H, Hulette C, Einstein G, Schmechel D, Pericak-Vance M, Roses AD (1994a): Hypothesis: Microtubule instability and paired helical filament formation in the Alzheimer disease brain are related to apolipoprotein E genotype. Exp Neurol 125:163–171.

Strittmatter WJ, Saunders AM, Goedert M, Weisgraber KH, Dong L-M, Jakes R, Huang DY, Pericak-Vance M, Schmechel D, Roses AD (1994b): Isoform-specific interactions of apolipoprotein E with microtubule-associated protein tau: Implications for Alzheimer disease. Proc Natl Acad Sci U S A 91:11183–11186.

Strittmatter WJ, Saunders AM, Schmechel D, Pericak-Vance M, Enghild J, Salvesen GS, Roses AD (1993a): Apolipoprotein E: High-avidity binding to β-amyloid and increased frequency of type 4 allele in late-onset familial Alzheimer disease. Proc Natl Acad Sci 90:1977–1981.

Strittmatter WJ, Weisgraber KH, Huang DY, Dong L-M, Salvesen GS, Pericak-Vance M, Schmechel D. Saunders AM, Goldgaber D, Roses AD (1993b): binding of human apolipoprotein E to synthetic amyloid β peptide: Isoform-specific effects and implications for late-onset Alzheimer disease. Proc Natl Acad Sci 90:8098–8102.

Sweeney D, Zhou Z, Martins R, LeVine H, Cheetham, J, Breslow J, Smith J, Greengard P, Gandy S (1995): Physiological apolipoprotein E ε3 and ε4 isoforms promote fibrillogenesis of Aβ (1–42) in a thioflavin T assay. Soc Neurosci Abst 21(3):1715.

Takahashi S, Oida K, Ookubo M, Suzuki J, Kohno M, Murase T, Yamamoto T, Nakai T (1996): Very low density lipoprotein receptor binds apolipoprotein E2/2 as well as apolipoprotein E3/3. FEBS Lett 386:197–200.

Terzi E, Holzemann G, Seelig J (1995): Self-association of β-amyloid peptide (1–40) in solution and binding to lipid membranes. J Mol Biol 252:633–642.

Vilaro S, Camps L, Reina M, Perez-Clausell J, Llobera M, Olivecrona T (1990): Localization of lipoprotein lipase to discrete areas of the guinea pig brain. Brain Res 506:249–253.

Warden CH, Langner CA, Gordon JL, Taylor BA, McLean JW, Lusis AJ (1989): Tissue-specific expression, developmental regulation, and chromosomal mapping of the lecithin:cholesterol acyltransferase gene. J Biol Chem 264:21573–21581.

Weisgraber KH (1994): Apolipoprotein E: Structure-function relationships. Adv Protein Chem 45:249–302.

Wilson DM, Binder LI (1995): In vitro polymerization of microtubule-associated protein tau and amyloid peptide A4(1–40) is stimulated by free fatty acids. Mol Biol Cell 6:37a.

Wisniewski T, Frangione B (1992): Apolipoprotein E: A pathological chaperone protein in patients with cerebral and systemic amyloid. Neurosci Lett 135:235–238.

Wisniewski T, Golabek AA, Kida E, Wisniewski KE, Frangione B (1995a): Conformational mimicry in Alzheimer's disease role of apolipoproteins in amyloidogenesis. Am J Path 147:238–244.

Wisniewski T, Lalowski M, Golabek A, Vogel T, Frangione B (1995b): Is Alzheimer's disease an apolipoprotein E amyloidosis? Lancet 345:956–958.

Wisniewski T, Castaño EM, Golabek A, Vogel T, Frangione B (1994): Acceleration of Alzheimer's fibril formation by apolipoprotein E *in vitro*. Am J Pathol 145:1030–1035.

Wisniewski T, Golabek A, Matsubara E, Ghiso J, Frangione B (1993): Apolipoprotein E: Binding to soluble Alzheimer's β-amyloid. Biochem Biophys Res Commun 192:359–365.

Wolf BB, Beatriz M, Lopes S, VandenBerg SR, Gonias SL (1992). Characterization and immunohistochemical localization of α2-macroglobulin receptor (low-density lipoprotein receptor-related protein) in human brain. Am J Pathol 141:37–42.

Yan SD, Chen X, Fu J, Chen M, Zhu H, Roher A, Slattery T, Zhao L, Nagashima M, Morser J, Migheli A, Nawroth P, Stern D, Schmidt AM (1996): RAGE and amyloid-β peptide neurotoxicity in Alzheimer's disease. Nature 382:685–691.

Yanagisawa K, Odaka A, Suzuki N, Ihara Y (1995): GM1 ganglioside-bound amyloid β-protein (Aβ): A possible form of preamyloid in Alzheimer's disease. Nature Med 1:1062–1066.

Zhou Z, Smith JD, Greengard P, Gandy S (1996): Alzheimer amyloid-β peptide forms denaturant-resistant complex with type E3 but not type E4 isoform of native apolipoprotein E. Mol Med 2:175–180.

CHAPTER 13

Animal Models Relevant to Alzheimer's Disease

DAVID R. BORCHELT, LEE J. MARTIN, KAREN K. HSIAO,
JOHN D. GEARHART, BRUCE T. LAMB, SANGRAM S. SISODIA,
and DONALD L. PRICE

Departments of Pathology (D.R.B., L.J.M., S.S.S., D.L.P.), Neuroscience (L.J.M., S.S.S.,
D.L.P.), and Neurology (D.L.P.), and Obstetrics & Gynecology (J.D.G., B.T.L.), the Division of
Reproductive & Developmental Biology (J.D.G., B.T.L.), and the Neuropathology Laboratory
(D.R.B., L.J.M., S.S.S., D.L.P.), The Johns Hopkins University School of Medicine, Baltimore,
Maryland, 21205 and the Department of Neurology (K.K.H.), University of Minnesota Medical
School, Minneapolis, Minnesota 55455

INTRODUCTION

Alzheimer's disease (AD), the most common cause of dementia in the elderly (Evans et al., 1989), is associated with dysfunction and death of populations of neurons in a variety of neural circuits in multiple brain regions. Many vulnerable neurons exhibit neurofibrillary inclusions in cell bodies [neurofibrillary tangles (NFT)] in processes (neurites, neuropil threads). Extracellular β-amyloid protein (Aβ) is abundant in diffuse deposits within the neuropil, in senile plaques, and within the walls of leptomeningeal/cerebral vessels. Synaptic inputs are reduced in the neocortex and hippocampus, and the severity of synaptic decline correlates with the clinical syndrome of dementia (Terry et al., 1991; Sze et al., 1996).

ALZHEIMER'S DISEASE

Alzheimer's disease is an age-associated disorder that affects 7–10% of individuals >65 years of age and 35–40% of individuals >85 years of age. Two genetic pat-

Pharmacological Treatment of Alzheimer's Disease: Molecular and Neurobiological Foundations,
Edited by Brioni and Decker
ISBN 0-471-16758-4   © 1997 Wiley-Liss, Inc.

terns have been demonstrated: inheritance of mutations in autosomal-dominant familial cases and inheritance of allele type in late-onset cases. The majority of early-onset cases of AD are familial and inherited as an autosomal-dominant disorder. Mutations have been identified in several genes that cosegregate with affected members of familial AD (FAD) pedigrees. The first FAD mutations were identified in the amyloid precursor protein (APP) (Chartier-Harlin et al., 1991; Goate et al., 1991; Hendricks et al., 1992; Mullan et al., 1992). At least 13 different missense mutations have been identified in a gene designated presenilin 1 (PS1), located on chromosome 14. Mutations in the PS2 (STM2) gene, localized on chromosome 1, have been reported to cause autosomal-dominant AD in Volga German kindreds and in an Italian pedigree (St. George-Hyslop et al., 1992; Alzheimer's Disease Collaborative Group, 1995; Levy-Lahad et al., 1995a, b; Li et al., 1995; Rogaev et al., 1995; Sherrington et al., 1995). In addition, inheritance of a particular allele of the apolipoprotein E (apoE) gene is associated with increased risk for late-onset FAD.

Encoded by alternatively spliced mRNA, PS1 is an integral membrane protein predicted to contain between seven (Sherrington et al., 1995) and nine (Slunt et al., 1995) transmembrane helices. The majority of FAD-linked mutations occur within or immediately adjacent to the predicted transmembrane domains (Alzheimer's Disease Collaborative Group, 1995; Sherrington et al., 1995). The absence of deletions or truncation mutations in PS1 suggests that early-onset FAD in affected pedigrees is caused not by a loss of function but, rather, by polypeptides acquiring a deleterious property. Recent studies of fibroblasts obtained from carriers of PS1 mutations suggest that secretion of the Aβ1-42/43 species may be elevated as compared to cells from unaffected family members (Scheuner et al., 1995). Similarly, individuals with PS1 mutations, relative to noncarriers, show elevated levels of plasma Aβ1-42/43 (Song et al., 1995), the form of Aβ that appears to be particularly important in the deposition of amyloid. The media of cultured fibroblasts and plasma obtained from affected members of chromosome-1-linked Volga kindreds show elevations in Aβ1-42/43 relative to noncarriers (D. Selkoe, personal communication). In concert, these investigations are consistent with the idea that mutations in PS1/PS2 influence APP processing to promote the formation of highly amyloidogenic Aβ species.

A member of the APP/amyloid precursorlike protein (APLP 1 and 2) gene family, APP is the precursor of Aβ peptides, composed of 28 amino acids of the ectodomain and 11–14 amino acids of the adjacent transmembrane domain of APP (Glenner and Wong, 1984a, b; Selkoe et al., 1987). In some cases of FAD, missense mutations result in a substitution of the normal valine residue at position 717 (of APP-770) with either isoleucine, glycine, or phenylalanine (Chartier-Harlin et al., 1991; Goate et al., 1991). In two large, related, early-onset AD families from Sweden, a double mutation at codons 670 and 671 results in a substitution of the normal Lys–Met dipeptide to Asn–Leu (Mullan et al., 1992). In another family, affected individuals with presenile dementia and cerebral hemorrhages have a mutation at codon 692 of APP (substitution of glycine for alanine) (Hendricks et al., 1992). Moreover, in hereditary cerebral hemorrhage with amyloid, Dutch-type (HCHWA-D), an APP mutation leading to a Glu–Gln substitution at position 693 is associated with amyloid deposition in blood vessels (Levy et al., 1990).

The mechanisms whereby APP mutations influence precursor processing and contribute to Aβ production have been clarified by in vitro assays and cellular transfection approaches. Cells that express APP harboring the "Swedish" substitutions secrete higher levels of Aβ1-42-containing peptides as compared to cells expressing wild-type (wt) constructs (Citron et al., 1992; Cai et al., 1993; Suzuki et al., 1994). In HCHWA-D, an APP mutation leading to a Glu–Gln substitution at position 693 (corresponding to amino acid 22 of Aβ) is associated with amyloid deposition around blood vessels; in vitro studies indicate that Aβ peptides containing this mutation are more prone to aggregate into fibrils. Cells that express APP harboring the Ala–Gly substitution at amino acid 692 (Hendricks et al., 1992) reveal that α-secretase processing of this mutant polypeptide is inefficient and that secreted Aβ species exhibit considerable microheterogeneity, including the appearance of more hydrophobic species (Haass et al., 1994). Significantly, cells that express APP harboring 717 mutations do not secrete higher levels of Aβ but do secrete a higher fraction of longer Aβ peptides (i.e., extending to Aβ residue 42) relative to cells that express wt APP (Suzuki et al., 1994). The finding that APP harboring 717 mutations is processed to generate higher levels of longer Aβ peptides is of considerable interest because recent physicochemical studies have indicated that Aβ1–42 and/or Aβ1–43, rather than Aβ1–40, may provide a nidus for nucleation-dependent amyloidogenesis (Jarrett and Lansbury, 1993). The observation that APP mutations in early-onset FAD flank or reside within the Aβ sequence indicates that the altered processing of APP is central to the formation of amyloid.

Inheritance of the apoE4 allele (chromosome 19) is a risk factor for late-onset FAD and sporadic AD (Corder et al., 1993; Gomez-Isla et al., 1996). At the apoE locus, three alleles are known: apoE3 has a cysteine at position 112 and an arginine at position 158; apoE4 has arginine at both positions; and apoE2 has cysteine at both positions. The apoE3 allele is most common in the general population (frequency of 0.78); the allelic frequency of apoE4 is 0.14. However, in clinic-based studies, patients with late-onset disease (>65 years of age) have an apoE4 allelic frequency of 0.50. Thus, the presence of apoE4 is associated with an increased incidence of AD (Saunders et al., 1993; Gomez-Isla et al., 1996). The mechanisms whereby the apoE-allele-type influences the risk for late-onset disease are not known.

ANIMAL MODELS

This review focuses on models that reproduce some features of AD, concentrating on species that develop age-associated AD-like abnormalities spontaneously and on mice that express wt or mutant transgenes.

Aged Animals

Although several aged rodent species develop age-associated behavioral deficits and a variety of neurochemical (or neurotransmitter/receptor) brain abnormalities, for the most part, rodents do not spontaneously exhibit the structural/biochemical lesions of AD. However, a variety of breeds of dogs (>18 years of age) develop parenchymal and intravascular deposits of Aβ (Wisniewski et al., 1970, 1990; Okuda et al., 1994). To our knowledge, NFT have not been identified in the aged canine brain. In contrast, bears ranging from >20–30 years of age and sheep (>5–10 years of age) show NFT-like abnormalities similar to those occurring in humans with AD (Nelson et al., 1994; Nelson and Saper, 1995). For example, the brain of one aged Asiatic brown bear showed NFT composed of straight 10- to 16-nm filaments immunoreactive with antibodies directed against phosphorylated epitopes of neurofilaments (NF) and A68/tau. An aged polar bear had numerous senile plaques but no NFT.

Aged monkeys show behavioral and brain abnormalities similar to those occurring in aged humans and individuals with AD (Wisniewski and Terry, 1973a; Bartus et al., 1978, 1979; Goldman-Rakic and Brown, 1981; Struble et al., 1982, 1985; Kitt et al., 1984; Selkoe et al., 1987; Walker et al., 1987, 1988b, 1990; Abraham et al., 1989; Rapp and Amaral, 1989; Wenk et al., 1989; Cork et al., 1990; Heilbroner and Kemper, 1990; Bachevalier et al., 1991; Beal et al., 1991; Martin et al., 1991). With a life span of 37–40 years, rhesus monkeys *(Macaca mulatta)* develop cognitive and memory deficits at the end of the second decade (Presty et al., 1987; Rapp and Amaral, 1989, 1991; Bachevalier et al., 1991; Rapp et al., 1994; Walker, 1994). These deficits become more evident after the midtwenties and progress with increasing age (Presty et al., 1987; Walker et al., 1988b; Bachevalier et al., 1991). Chronological peers show significant differences in performance on behavioral tasks. These variations in performance among aged animals and among tasks are similar to those observed in aged humans.

Aged nonhuman primates develop many of the brain abnormalities observed in older humans (Wisniewski and Terry, 1973a, b; Goldman-Rakic and Brown, 1981; Struble et al., 1982, 1985; Kitt et al., 1984; Selkoe et al., 1987; Walker et al., 1987; 1988a, 1990; Abraham et al., 1989; Wenk et al., 1989; Heilbroner and Kemper, 1990; Cork et al., 1990; Beal et al., 1991; Martin et al., 1991; Poduri et al., 1994; Rapp et al., 1994; Walker, 1994). At ~20–25 years of age, rhesus monkeys show enlarged neurites (i.e., distal axons, nerve terminals, dendrites) and diffuse Aβ deposits in the cortical parenchyma as well as congophilic angiopathy involving cerebral blood vessels (Wisniewski and Terry, 1973a; Struble et al., 1982, 1985; Selkoe et al., 1987; Walker et al., 1987, 1988a; Cork et al., 1990). Neurites, derived from cholinergic, monoaminergic, serotoninergic, GABAergic, and peptidergic populations of neurons (Kitt et al., 1984; Struble et al., 1984, 1985; Walker et al., 1985, 1987, 1988a) accumulate a variety of constituents, including degenerating membranous elements, straight filaments, and a variety of protein markers (Martin et al., 1991, 1994). In individual plaques, neurites are often surrounded by abnormal neuropils that contain Aβ immunoreactivity; their processes may serve as one source for some of the Aβ deposited in the brains of these aged animals. Reactive astrocytes and microglia may also participate in the formation of Aβ (Miyakawa et al., 1992; Martin et al., 1994).

In some older animals, cell bodies in some large cortical neurons exhibit phosphorylated epitopes of NF proteins and A68 (tau) immunoreactivities. In one 34-

year-old animal, a significant number of argyrophilic NFT were associated with abnormal patterns of immunoreactivity for tau, A68, and phosphorylated NF as well as the presence of unusual straight filaments similar to those occurring in neurons that show paired helical filaments in cases of AD. These observations suggest that the formation of NFT is a relatively late-stage event in aged monkeys.

Some older monkeys show decreased concentrations of cholinergic and monoaminergic markers in certain regions of cortex (Goldman-Rakic and Brown, 1981; Wenk et al., 1989; Beal et al., 1991). Alterations in several neurotransmitter systems are believed to contribute to behavioral/cognitive impairments in some aged animals. The presence of neurotransmitter abnormalities is likely to be related to synaptic pathology in aged monkeys (Martin et al., 1994). The distributions and severities of various lesions differ among animals of the same age; presumably, variations in the performance of individual animals on specific behavioral tasks are related to patterns of these lesions in different animals. Aged monkeys may reproduce the cognitive/memory deficits and cellular pathology that occur in individuals with AD; however, because these animals are rare and often cost prohibitive, it is important to develop a small animal model of AD.

The establishment of colonies of transgenic mice that show features of AD will allow a significant number of animals to be available for in vitro and in vivo studies. This approach has proved successful in modeling: Gerstmann–Sträussler–Scheinker syndrome (prion proteins with missense mutation); FAD (APP with mutation); familial amyotrophic lateral sclerosis (superoxide dismutase 1 with missense mutation); and spinocerebellar atrophy (Ataxin-1 with expanded repeats) (Hsiao et al., 1990; Gurney et al., 1994; Prusiner and Hsiao, 1994; Burright et al., 1995; Games et al., 1995; Ripps et al., 1995; Wong et al., 1995).

Transgenic Mice

Transgenic strategies provide a powerful method to examine the causative links between mutations in specific genes and abnormalities in behavior–brain biology.

Over the past several years, scientists in universities, biotechnology companies, and the pharmaceutical industry have used several APP-expressing transgenic strategies to try to produce a genetic model of APP-linked FAD. Because we have reviewed this area elsewhere (Price and Sisodia, 1994), we focus on several recent studies.

Scientists at Exemplar (Burlington, Massachusetts) and Athena Neurosciences (South San Francisco, California) (Games et al., 1995) used a transgene construct in which the platelet derived growth factor (PDGF) β-promotoer drove a human APP minigene encoding the FAD-linked APP (717V→F) mutation; the construct contained portions of APP introns 6–8, which allow alternative splicing of exons 7 and 8. Southern blots disclosed ~40 copies of the mutant transgene inserted at a single site and transmitted in a stable fashion. Levels of human APP mRNA and protein were significantly greater than endogenous levels. Transcripts encoding the three major splicing variants of APP were demonstrable with an ~5:5:1 ratio of 770:751:695 isoforms (Rockenstein et al., 1995), and levels of the transgene product were ~4–5 times higher than endogenous mouse APP (D. Games, personal communication; Games et al., 1995). A 4-kD Aβ-immunoreactive peptide was identified in the brains of these animals. After 8 months of age, Aβ deposits, ranging from diffuse irregular types to compacted plaques with cores, were seen in hippocampus, corpus callosum, and cerebral cortex. Amyloid deposits, stained by the thioflavin, Congo Red, and Bielschowsky methods, increased in number over time. Many plaques showed glial fibrillary acid protein-positive astrocytes as well as microglial cells. Although neurites were distorted and often were present in proximity to plaques, tau-positive neurites and NFT were not present. Animals are said to show behavioral abnormalities and decreased synaptophysin immunoreactivity in hippocampus (D. Games, personal communication). Quantitative estimates of loss of synapses and neuronal numbers in specific cell groups have not been published.

Features of the Exemplar/Athena effort that underlie the impressive neuropathological phenotypes are not fully understood but may include high levels of multiple isoforms of APP transgene products and the expression of the construct in an outbred strain that may be more prone to the development of Aβ deposits. It remains to be determined whether the Exemplar/Athena mice will recapitulate all of the behavioral, pathological, and biochemical features of AD.

Hsiao et al. (1995) produced multiple lines of transgenic FVB mice that express a variety of wt and mutant human and mouse APP transgenes placed under the transcriptional control of the hamster prion gene promotor (Scott et al., 1992). Mice with >20 copies produced 1–5 times endogenous levels of APP and exhibited a variety of behavioral abnormalities including neophobia, seizures, and impaired spatial alterations. Diminished glucose utilization was evident in cortical-limbic areas, and in these brain regions there was significant gliosis but no Aβ deposition or obvious neuronal loss. A similar neurological disorder was observed in older nontransgenic FVB mice, and the presence of the APP transgene appeared to accelerate this age- and strain-related phenotype, which is associated with premature death.

Despite relatively high levels of expression, transgenic FVB/N mice do not appear to develop the same types of AD-related pathologies as observed in the Exemplar mice. Immunocytochemical studies of FVB/N transgenics suggest high levels of neuronal expression in nearly all regions of the brain similar to the transgene expression reported for the Exemplar mice. The two most noteworthy differences between the FVB/N and Exemplar mice are the strains of mice used as transgene hosts and the APP isoforms encoded by each transgene. The Exemplar mice were created in hybrid strains consisting of a mixture of Swiss Webster, C57BL/6J, and DBA/2J, whereas FVB/N mice are inbred. It is not yet known whether the strain background significantly contributed to the pathology, but it is noteworthy that the phenotypes observed in FVB/N mice expressing APP transgenes under the control of the Syrian hamster prion promoter do not occur when the same transgenes are introduced into C57BL/6J mice and expressed at similar or higher levels. These latter data demonstrate that the responses of different inbred strains to genetic lesioning show significant differences. Whether C57BL/6J mice expressing high levels of these APP transgenes will develop AD-related pathology remains to be determined.

In addition to differences in the host background, the Exemplar study used a transgene construct that generated APP-770, APP-751, and APP-695 isoforms in a 5:5:1 ratio (Rockenstein et al., 1995). In contrast, APP transgenes tested in the FVB/N mice encoded APP-695 cDNA. Hence, it is uncertain whether the expression of APP isoforms containing the Kunitz-type protease domains (APP-770 and APP-751) predispose to Aβ deposition.

In a parallel strategy, Lamb and colleagues (1993) used lipid-mediated transfection to introduce an ~650-kb yeast artificial chromosome (YAC) containing the entire unrearranged 400-kb wt APP gene into embryonic stem cells. Embryonic stem cells that expressed human APP were then introduced into mouse blastocytes to generate chimeric mice (Lamb et al., 1993). Subsequent breeding efforts resulted in mice that harbor human sequences in the germline. In these animals, levels of expression of the human transgene-encoded mRNA and protein in brain and peripheral tissues are ~70% the levels of endogenous APP; the splicing pattern of human APP transcripts parallels the stoichiometry of spliced products derived from the endogenous mouse APP gene. At two years of age, mice that express wt APP-YAC have not developed disease.

The collective experience in generating animal models of human neurological disease (Gurney et al., 1994; Games et al., 1995; Wong et al., 1995) suggests that it is important to achieve high levels of expression of the mutant transgene in nervous tissue if mice are to develop phenotypes that resemble those occurring in human diseases.

In addition, it is now increasingly apparent that the strain of mouse may have a significant influence on the phenotypic responses of these animals to specific transgenes. Although the Exemplar data suggest that hybrid mixtures of different strains of mice may increase the potential to generate pathology similar to that occurring in AD, the complex genetic backgrounds of these animals instill increased complexity into studies to define behavioral abnormalities and, moreover, may increase the variability of phenotypic responses. The homogeneity of inbred strains reduces these latter complications, but it is well established that the responses of different inbred strains of mice to genetic lesioning can vary considerably. Thus, it may be necessary to assess the responses of several different inbred strains before identifying animals that recapitulate AD-related phenotypes.

CONCLUSIONS

Perhaps the most promising avenue of future investigations of animal models of AD will involve mating transgenic mice that express PS1/PS2 harboring FAD-linked mutations with mice that express APP. The utility of the prion protein and PDGF promoter vectors to drive high levels of transgenic expression is well documented, and we anticipate that mice overproducing PS1/PS2 can be generated. The availability of transgenic mice expressing APP and PS1, as well as mice in which these loci have been disrupted by gene-targeting strategies, will undoubtedly provide the best opportunity to clarify the contributions and potential interactions of PS1/PS2 and APP to the pathogenesis of AD.

ACKNOWLEDGMENTS

The authors thank Drs. Michael K. Lee, Philip C. Wong, Linda C. Cork, Gopal Thinakaran, Cheryl A. Kitt, Lary C. Walker, Gary L. Wenk, Molly V. Wagster, Robert G. Struble, M. Flint Beal, Mortimer Mishkin, Jocelyn Bachevalier, Neal G. Copeland, and Nancy A. Jenkins who made major contributions to some of the original work cited in this review.

This work was supported by grants from the U.S. Public Health Service (AG 05146 and NS 20471) as well as the American Health Assistance Foundation, the Develbiss Fund, the Alzheimer's Foundation, and the Claster family. Dr. Price is the recipient of a Leadership and Excellence in Alzheimer's Disease (LEAD) award (AG 07914) and a Javits Neuroscience Investigator Award (NS 10580).

REFERENCES

Abraham CR, Selkoe DJ, Potter H, Price DL, Cork LC (1989): α_1-Antichymotrypsin is present together with the β-protein in monkey brain amyloid deposits. Neuroscience 32:715–720.

Alzheimer's Disease Collaborative Group (1995): The structure of the presenilin 1 *(S182)* gene and identification of six novel mutations in early onset AD families. Nature Genet 11:219–222.

Bachevalier J, Landis LS, Walker LC, Brickson M, Mishkin M, Price DL, Cork LC (1991): Aged monkeys exhibit behavioral deficits indicative of widespread cerebral dysfunction. Neurobiol Aging 12:99–111.

Bartus RT, Dean RL, III, Fleming DL (1979): Aging in the rhesus monkey: Effects on visual discrimination learning and reversal learning. J Gerontol 34:209–219.

Bartus RT, Fleming D, Johnson HR (1978): Aging in the rhesus monkey: Debilitating effects on short-term memory. J Gerontol 33:858–871.

Beal MF, Walker LC, Storey E, Segar L, Price DL, Cork LC (1991): Neurotransmitters in neocortex of aged rhesus monkeys. Neurobiol Aging 12:407–412.

Burright EN, Clark HB, Servadio A, Matilla T, Feddersen RM, Yunis WS, Duvick LA, Zoghbi HY, Orr HT (1995): *SCA1* transgenic mice: A model for neurodegeneration caused by an expanded CAG trinucleotide repeat. Cell 82:937–948.

Cai X-D, Golde TE, Younkin SG (1993): Release of excess amyloid β protein from a mutant amyloid β protein precursor. Science 259:514–516.

Chartier-Harlin M-C, Crawford F, Houlden H, Warren A, Hughes D, Fidani L, Goate A, Rossor M, Roques P, Hardy J, Mullan M (1991): Early-onset Alzheimer's disease caused by mutations at codon 717 of the β-amyloid precursor protein gene. Nature 353: 844–846.

Citron M, Oltersdorf T, Haass C, McConlogue L, Hung AY, Seubert P, Vigo-Pelfrey C, Lieberburg I, Selkoe DJ (1992): Mutation of the β-amyloid precursor protein in familial Alzheimer's disease increases β-protein production. Nature 360:672–674.

Corder EH, Saunders AM, Strittmatter WJ, Schmechel DE, Gaskell PC, Small GW, Roses AD, Haines JL, Pericak-Vance MA (1993): Gene dose of apolipoprotein-E type 4 allele and the risk of Alzheimer's disease in late onset families. Science 261:921–923.

Cork LC, Masters C, Beyreuther K, Price DL (1990): Development of senile plaques. Relationships of neuronal abnormalities and amyloid deposits. Am J Pathol 137:1383–1392.

Evans DA, Funkenstein HH, Albert MS, Scherr PA, Cook NR, Chown MJ, Hebert LE, Hennekens CH, Taylor JO (1989): Prevalence of Alzheimer's disease in a community population of older persons. Higher than previously reported. JAMA 262:2551–2556.

Games D, Adams D, Alessandrini R, Barbour R, Berthelette P, Blackwell C, Carr T, Clemens J, Donaldson T, Gillespie F, Guido T, Hagopian S, Johnson-Wood K, Khan K, Lee M, Leibowitz P, Lieberburg I, Little S, Masliah E, McConlogue L, Montoya-Zavala M, Mucke L, Paganini L, Penniman E, Power M, Schenk D, Seubert P, Snyder B, Soriano F, Tan H, Vitale J, Wadsworth S, Wolozin B, Zhao J (1995): Alzheimer-type neuropathology in transgenic mice overexpressing V717F β-amyloid precursor protein. Nature 373: 523–527.

Glenner GG, Wong CW (1984a): Alzheimer's disease: Initial report of the purification and characterization of a novel cerebrovascular amyloid protein. Biochem Biophys Res Commun 120:885–890.

Glenner GG, Wong CW (1984b): Alzheimer's disease and Down's syndrome: Sharing of a unique cerebrovascular amyloid fibril protein. Biochem Biophys Res Commun 122: 1131–1135.

Goate A, Chartier-Harlin M-C, Mullan M, Brown J, Crawford F, Fidani L, Giuffra L, Haynes A, Irving N, James L, Mant R, Newton P, Rooke K, Roques P, Talbot C, Pericak-Vance M, Roses A, Williamson R, Rossor M, Owen M, Hardy J (1991): Segregation of a missense mutation in the amyloid precursor protein gene with familial Alzheimer's disease. Nature 349:704–706.

Goldman-Rakic PS, Brown RM (1981): Regional changes of monoamines in cerebral cortex and subcortical structures of aging rhesus monkeys. Neuroscience 6:177–187.

Gomez-Isla T, West HL, Rebeck GW, Harr SD, Growdon JH, Locascio JJ, Perls TT, Lipsitz LA, Hyman BT (1996): Clinical and pathological correlates of apolipoprotein E ε4 in Alzheimer disease. Ann Neurol 39:62–70.

Gurney ME, Pu H, Chiu AY, Dal Canto MC, Polchow CY, Alexander DD, Caliendo J, Hentati A, Kwon YW, Deng H-X, Chen W, Zhai P, Sufit RL, Siddique T (1994): Motor neuron degeneration in mice that express a human Cu, Zn superoxide dismutase mutation. Science 264:1772–1775.

Haass C, Hung AY, Selkoe DJ, Teplow DB (1994): Mutations associated with a locus for familial Alzheimer's disease result in alternative processing of amyloid β-protein precursor. J Biol Chem 269:17741–17748.

Heilbroner PL, Kemper TL (1990): The cytoarchitectonic distribution of senile plaques in three aged monkeys. Acta Neuropathol 81:60–65.

Hendricks L, van Duijn CM, Cras P, Cruts M, Van Hul W, van Harskamp F, Warren A, McInnis MG, Antonarakis SE, Martin J-J, Hofman A, Van Broeckhoven C (1992): Presenile dementia and cerebral haemorrhage linked to a mutation at codon 692 of the β-amyloid precursor protein gene. Nature Genet 1:218–221.

Hsiao KK, Borchelt DR, Olson K, Johannsdottir R, Kitt C, Yunis W, Xu S, Eckman C, Younkin S, Price D, Iadecola C, Clark HB, Carlson G (1995): Age-related CNS disorder and early death in transgenic FVB/N mice overexpressing Alzheimer amyloid precursor proteins. Neuron 15:1203–1218.

Hsiao KK, Scott M, Foster D, Groth DF, DeArmond SJ, Prusiner SB (1990): Spontaneous neurodegeneration in transgenic mice with mutant prion protein. Science 250:1587–1590.

Jarrett JT, Lansbury PT, Jr. (1993): Seeding "one-dimensional crystallization" of amyloid: A pathogenic mechanism in Alzheimer's disease and scrapie? Cell 73:1055–1058.

Kitt CA, Walker LC, Molliver ME, Price DL (1989): Serotoninergic neurites in senile plaques in cingulate cortex of aged nonhuman primate. Synapse 3:12–18.

Kitt CA, Struble RG, Cork LC, Mobley WC, Walker LC, Joh TH, Price DL (1985): Catecholaminergic neurites in senile plaques in prefrontal cortex of aged nonhuman primates. Neuroscience 16:691–699.

Kitt CA, Price DL, Struble RG, Cork LC, Wainer BH, Becher MW, Mobley WC (1984): Evidence for cholinergic neurites in senile plaques. Science 226:1443–1445.

Lamb BT, Sisodia SS, Lawler AM, Slunt HH, Kitt CA, Kearns WG, Pearson PL, Price DL, Gearhart JD (1993): Introduction and expression of the 400 kilobase *precursor amyloid protein* gene in transgenic mice. Nature Genet 5:22–30.

Levy E, Carman MD, Fernandez-Madrid IJ, Power MD, Lieberburg I, van Duinen SG, Bots GTAM, Luyendijk W, Frangione B (1990): Mutation of the Alzheimer's disease amyloid gene in hereditary cerebral hemorrage, Dutch type. Science 248:1124–1126.

Levy-Lahad E, Wasco W, Poorkaj P, Romano DM, Oshima J, Pettingell WH, Yu C-E, Jondro PD, Schmidt SD, Wang K, Crowley AC, Fu Y-H, Guenette SY, Galas D, Nemens E, Wijsman EM, Bird TD, Schellenberg GD, Tanzi RE (1995a): Candidate gene for the chromosome 1 familial Alzheimer's disease locus. Science 269:973–977.

Levy-Lahad E, Wijsman EM, Nemens E, Anderson L, Goddard KAB, Weber JL, Bird TD, Schellenberg GD (1995b): A familial Alzheimer's disease locus on chromosome 1. Science 269:970–973.

Li J, Ma J, Potter H (1995): Identification and expression analysis of a potential familial Alzheimer disease gene on chromosome 1 related to *AD3*. Proc Natl Acad Sci U S A 92:12180–12184.

Martin LJ, Pardo CA, Cork LC, Price DL (1994): Synaptic pathology and glial responses to neuronal injury precede the formation of senile plaques and amyloid deposits in the aging cerebral cortex. Am J Pathol 145:1358–1381.

Martin LJ, Sisodia SS, Koo EH, Cork LC, Dellovade TL, Weidemann A, Beyreuther K, Masters C, Price DL (1991): Amyloid precursor protein in aged nonhuman primates. Proc Natl Acad Sci U S A 88:1461–1465.

Miyakawa T, Katsuragi S, Yamashita K, Ohuchi K (1992): Morphological study of amyloid fibrils and preamyloid deposits in the brain with Alzheimer's disease. Acta Neuropathol 83:340–346.

Mullan M, Crawford F, Axelman K, Houlden H, Lillius L, Winblad B, Lannfelt L (1992): A pathogenic mutation for probable Alzheimer's disease in the APP gene at the N-terminus of β-amyloid. Nature Genet 1:345–347.

Nelson PT, Saper CB (1995): Ultrastructure of neurofibrillary tangles in the cerebral cortex of sheep. Neurobiol Aging 16:315–323.

Nelson PT, Greenberg SG, Saper CB (1994): Neurofibrillary tangles in the cerebral cortex of sheep. Neurosci Lett 170:187–190.

Okuda R, Uchida K, Tateyama S, Yamaguchi R, Nakayama H, Goto N (1994): The distribution of amyloid beta precursor protein in canine brain. Acta Neuropathol 87:161–167.

Poduri A, Gearing M, Rebeck GW, Mirra SS, Tigges J, Hyman BT (1994): Apolipoprotein E4 and beta amyloid in senile plaques and cerebral blood vessels of aged rhesus monkeys. Am J Pathol 144:1183–1187.

Presty SK, Bachevalier J, Walker LC, Struble RG, Price DL, Mishkin M, Cork LC (1987): Age differences in recognition memory of the rhesus monkey *(Macaca mulatta)*. Neurobiol Aging 8:435–440.

Price DL, Sisodia SS (1994): Cellular and molecular biology of Alzheimer's disease and animal models. Ann Rev Med 45:435–446.

Prusiner SB, Hsiao KK (1994): Human prion diseases. Ann Neurol 35:385–395.

Rapp PR, Amaral DG (1991): Recognition memory deficits in a subpopulation of aged monkeys resemble the effects of medial temporal lobe damage. Neurobiol Aging 12:481–486.

Rapp PR, Amaral DG (1989): Evidence for task-dependent memory dysfunction in the aged monkey. J Neurosci 9:3568–3576.

Rapp PR, Kansky MT, Roberts JA, Eichenbaum H (1994): New directions for studying cognitive decline in old monkeys. Semin Neurosci 6:369–377.

Ripps ME, Huntley GW, Hof PR, Morrison JH, Gordon JW (1995): Transgenic mice expressing an altered murine superoxide dismutase gene provide an animal model of amyotrophic lateral sclerosis. Proc Natl Acad Sci U S A 92:689–693.

Rockenstein EM, McConlogue L, Tan H, Power M, Masliah E, Mucke L (1995): Levels and alternative splicing of amyloid β protein precursor (APP) transcripts in brains of APP transgenic mice and humans with Alzheimer's disease. J Biol Chem 270:28257–28267.

Rogaev EI, Sherrington R, Rogaeva EA, Levesque G, Ikeda M, Liang Y, Chi H, Lin C, Holman K, Tsuda T, Mar L, Sorbi S, Nacmias B, Piacentini S, Amaducci L, Chumakov I, Cohen D, Lannfelt L, Fraser PE, Rommens JM, St George-Hyslop PH (1995): Familial Alzheimer's disease in kindreds with missense mutations in a gene on chromosome 1 related to the Alzheimer's disease type 3 gene. Nature 376:775–778.

Saunders AM, Strittmatter WJ, Schmechel D, St. George-Hyslop PH, Pericak-Vance MA, Joo SH, Rosi BL, Gusella JF, Crapper-MacLachlan DR, Alberts MJ, Hulette C, Crain B, Goldgaber D, Roses AD (1993): Association of apolipoprotein E allele ε4 with late-onset familial and sporadic Alzheimer's disease. Neurology 43:1467–1472.

Scheuner D, Bird T, Citron M, Lannfelt L, Schellenberg G, Selkoe D, Viitanen M, Younkin SG (1995): Fibroblasts from carriers of familial AD linked to chromosome 14 show increased Aβ production. Soc Neurosci Abstr 21:1500.

Scott MR, Köhler R, Foster D, Prusiner SB (1992): Chimeric prion protein expression in cultured cells and transgenic mice. Protein Sci 1:986–997.

Selkoe DJ, Bell DS, Podlisny MB, Price DL, Cork LC (1987): Conservation of brain amyloid proteins in aged mammals and humans with Alzheimer's disease. Science 235: 873–877.

Sherrington R, Rogaev EI, Liang Y, Rogaeva EA, Levesque G, Ikeda M, Chi H, Lin C, Li G, Holman K, Tsuda T, Mar L, Foncin J-F, Bruni AC, Montesi MP, Sorbi S, Rainero I, Pinessi L, Nee L, Chumakov I, Pollen D, Brookes A, Sanseau P, Polinsky RJ, Wasco W, Da Silva HAR, Haines JL, Pericak-Vance MA, Tanzi RE, Roses AD, Fraser PE, Rommens JM, St. George-Hyslop PH (1995): Cloning of a gene bearing missense mutations in early-onset familial Alzheimer's disease. Nature 375:754–760.

Slunt HH, Thinakaran G, Lee MK, Sisodia SS (1995): Nucleotide sequence of the chromosome 14-encoded *S182* cDNA and revised secondary structure prediction. Amyloid: Int J Exp Clin Invest 2:188–190.

Song X-H, Suzuki N, Bird T, Peskind E, Schellenberg G, Younkin SG (1995): Plasma amyloid β protein (Aβ) ending at Aβ42 (43) is increased in carriers of familial AD (FAD) linked to chromosome 14. Soc Neurosci Abstr 21:1501.

St. George-Hyslop PH, Haines P, Rogaev E, Mortilla M, Vaula G, Pericak-Vance M, Foncin J-F, Montesi M, Bruni A, Sorbi S, Rainero I, Pinessi L, Pollen D, Polinsky R, Nee L, Kennedy J, Macciardi F, Rogaeva E, Liang Y, Alexandrova N, Lukiw W, Schlumpf K, Tanzi R, Tsuda T, Farrer L, Cantu J-M, Duara R, Amaducci L, Bergamini L, Gusella J, Roses A, Crapper McLachlan D (1992): Genetic evidence for a novel familial Alzheimer's disease locus on chromosome 14. Nature Genet 2:330–334.

Struble RG, Price, Jr., Cork LC, Price DL (1985): Senile plaques in cortex of aged normal monkeys. Brain Res 361:267–275.

Struble RG, Hedreen JC, Cork LC, Price DL (1984): Acetylcholinesterase activity in senile plaques of aged macaques. Neurobiol Aging 5:191–198.

Struble RG, Cork LC, Whitehouse PJ, Price DL (1982): Cholinergic innervation in neuritic plaques. Science 216:413–415.

Suzuki N, Cheung TT, Cai X-D, Odaka A, Otvos L, Jr., Eckman C, Golde TE, Younkin SG (1994): An increased percentage of long amyloid β protein secreted by familial amyloid β protein precursor (βAPP$_{717}$) mutants. Science 264:1336–1340.

Sze C-I, Troncoso JC, Kawas CH, Mouton PR, Price DL, Martin LJ (1996): Loss of the presynaptic vesicle protein synaptophysin in hippocampus correlates with early cognitive decline in aged humans, submitted.

Terry RD, Masliah E, Salmon DP, Butters N, DeTeresa R, Hill R, Hansen LA, Katzman R (1991): Physical basis of cognitive alterations in Alzheimer's disease: Synapse loss is the major correlate of cognitive impairment. Ann Neurol 30:572–580.

Walker LC (1994): The senescent primate brain. Semin Neurosci 6:379–385.

Walker LC, Masters C, Beyreuther K, Price DL (1990): Amyloid in the brains of aged squirrel monkeys. Acta Neuropathol 80:381–387.

Walker LC, Kitt CA, Cork LC, Struble RG, Dellovade TL, Price DL (1988a): Multiple transmitter systems contribute neurites to individual senile plaques. J Neuropathol Exp Neurol 47:138–144.

Walker LC, Kitt CA, Struble RG, Wagster MV, Price DL, Cork LC (1988b): The neural basis of memory decline in aged monkeys. Neurobiol Aging 9:657–666.

Walker LC, Kitt CA, Schwam E, Buckwald B, Garcia F, Sepinwall J, Price DL (1987): Senile plaques in aged squirrel monkeys. Neurobiol Aging 8:291–296.

Walker LC, Kitt CA, Struble RG, Schmechel DE, Oertel WH, Cork LC, Price DL (1985): Glutamic acid decarboxylase-like immunoreactive neurites in senile plaques. Neurosci Lett 59:165–169.

Wenk GL, Pierce DJ, Struble RG, Price DL, Cork LC (1989): Age-related changes in multiple neurotransmitter systems in the monkey brain. Neurobiol Aging 10:11–19.

Wisniewski HM, Terry RD (1973a): Reexamination of the pathogenesis of the senile plaque. In Zimmerman HM (ed): "Progress in Neuropathology." New York: Grune & Stratton, pp 1–26.

Wisniewski HM, Terry RD (1973b): Morphology of the aging brain, human and animal. Prog Brain Res 40:167–186.

Wisniewski HM, Wegiel J, Morys J, Bancher C, Soltysiak Z, Kim KS (1990): Aged dogs: An animal model to study beta-protein amyloidogenesis. In Maurer K, Riederer P, Beckmann

H (eds): "Alzheimer's Disease. Epidemiology, Neuropathology, Neurochemistry, and Clinics." Wien: Springer-Verlag, pp 151–168.

Wisniewski H, Johnson AB, Raine CS, Kay WJ, Terry RD (1970): Senile plaques and cerebral amyloidosis in aged dogs. A histochemical and ultrastructural study. Lab Invest 23:287–296.

Wong PC, Pardo CA, Borchelt DR, Lee MK, Copeland NG, Jenkins NA, Sisodia SS, Cleveland DW, Price DL (1995): An adverse property of a familial ALS-linked SOD1 mutation causes motor neuron disease characterized by vacuolar degeneration of mitochondria. Neuron 14:1105–1116.

PART III

ALZHEIMER'S DRUG DISCOVERY AND DEVELOPMENT

Alzheimer's Disease: An International Public Health Problem — Clinical Goals, Strategies, and Outcomes

PETER J. WHITEHOUSE

University Hospitals of Cleveland, Case Western Reserve University, Cleveland, Ohio 44106

INTRODUCTION

Alzheimer's disease and related dementias are public health challenges of global scope. The exciting molecular and systems neurobiological approaches to the development of more effective pharmacological treatments represent the greatest promise for long-term success to international responses to this growing epidemic. This chapter contends, however, that biologically oriented scientists and clinicians need to be more explicit about their therapeutic goals and their strategies for achieving those goals and to be cognizant of the forces that are affecting how scientific progress and clinical care will occur in the countries of the world that are facing dramatic aging of their populations.

Our considerations will begin with a review of the current and projected future impact of dementia on world health followed by a discussion of what appropriate therapeutic goals should be set to meet this enormous challenge. We will then consider the changes occurring in academia, industry, and government that may limit our ability to respond to these goals. A pervasive sense that resources will be increasingly constrained must be met with a desire to look creatively at how we can work smartly with new organizational strategies and tactics. Finally we will look at the international dimensions of these challenges, focusing on the development of more effective interventions for these devastating diseases.

Pharmacological Treatment of Alzheimer's Disease: Molecular and Neurobiological Foundations,
Edited by Brioni and Decker
ISBN 0-471-16758-4 © 1997 Wiley-Liss, Inc.

SOCIAL IMPERATIVE OF DEMENTIA

Understanding the scope of the public health challenge is important for motivating government, industry, and private foundations to rise to the challenge of dementia. So far, the focus on the public health problems of Alzheimer's disease (AD) has concentrated primarily on the Atlantic rim in North America and Europe because of the greater recognition of this type of dementia, the greater number of epidemiological studies, and the size of the pharmaceutical market.

In the United States it is estimated that 3–4 million individuals are affected by AD. The prevalence at age 65 is approximately 1%; however, the chance of getting AD increases dramatically as one ages, approaching 50% by the age of 80, according to some studies. Thus, in the United States alone the number of AD victims is expected to grow to 12–15 million by the middle of the next century as a result of our aging population.

Similar population forces are evident in Europe, particularly in countries such as in Scandinavia where the population has aged rapidly. In the European Union 18% of people were over the age of 60 in 1990, a percentage expected to rise to 30% in 2030. The old-old (over 80) will double from 3% currently in the same time span (*Economist*, 1996).

In 1945, Japan had an average life expectancy comparable to that of Western countries at the turn of the century. Japan has aged rapidly over 50 years to have the most long-lived population in the world. In addition the birth rate in Japan is low, beneath so-called replacement levels, so that the ratios of active workers to retirees in the future will cause significant social, economic, and political strain. This dramatic graying of their population is rapidly causing tremendous strain on health care services for the elderly, inspiring a national government strategic plan to increase community services called the Golden Plan. Moreover, these trends have encouraged a focus on degenerative diseases in Japanese science enterprise. Japanese policymakers have recently recognized that AD, in addition to stroke, is a common cause of dementia in their country.

The populations of India, China, and other countries with enormous populations are aging at a similarly rapid rate. If war or other diseases such as AIDS do not alter this shift in demographics, these countries will face enormous numbers of elderly and therefore many demented patients in the decades to come. In 15 years there will be 400 million individuals over 60 in poor countries, double the number in rich countries. As seen in the improvement of health and nutrition, a rapid aging of the population incurs problems of an imbalance with birth rates because of government-supported limitations in the number of children (*Economist*, 1996).

THERAPY FOR AD

Enamored by the exciting efforts to find a cure for AD, we have not thoroughly analyzed our therapeutic goals and tried to understand how we might achieve them with greater efficiency. Moreover, it is becoming clear that biological interventions will be part of new, rapidly evolving health systems that will include new psychosocial therapeutic options as well.

Certain principles should underlie an analysis of therapeutic goals. The goals should be patient-, family-, and society-driven, not the province of one particular discipline or profession. Efforts should be made to develop goals and assessment techniques that span different health care settings. Goals should be specific to stages of disease but not based exclusively on a biological medical model.

Type of Therapies

Alzheimer's disease therapies have been thought of as either symptomatic or disease course altering. Neurotransmitter system drugs such as cholinesterase inhibitors may provide some temporary relief to patients by improving symptoms. A different approach is needed in preventing the progressive loss of neurons and synapses, which is presumably the foundation of progressive deterioration of cognition. Attempts to develop therapies to change a disease course are divided into those based on an understanding of pathogenesis (e.g., amyloid formation) and those that apply knowledge of neuronal viability without necessarily understanding why neurons die in a particular disorder (e.g., growth factors).

Symptomatic Therapy

Cholinesterase inhibitors have been the most successful symptomatic therapies in AD. Building on the observations of neuronal loss in the basal forebrain (Whitehouse, 1995) and detrimental effects on cognition of anticholinergic drugs, physostigmine was shown to have short-term effects. Tacrine has now been approved in over a dozen countries, and other cholinesterases such as E2020 (Eisai), ENA 713 (Sandoz), and metriphonate (Bayer)—to mention a few—are showing promising results. Receptor-specific agonists such as xanomeline (Lilly) may represent the next generation of cholinomimetic therapies. The critical issues for all these drugs will be the balance between efficacy and safety.

A relatively neglected area of symptomatic treatment has been the noncognitive or behavioral symptom. Patients with dementia frequently have symptoms such as agitation, depression, and psychosis. These symptoms are treatable with currently available neuroleptics and antidepressants, but better approaches are needed.

Slowing Progression

Neurons eventually die in the brains of patients with AD. A second generation of therapy would go beyond symptomatic drugs and prevent this cell degeneration. A variety of mechanisms have been proposed for cell death in the central nervous system (CNS), including excitotoxic damage, calcium accumulation, and dysfunction in growth factors. Nerve growth factors (NGF) illustrate the general principles behind this approach, although the therapeutic trials with intraventricular mouse NGF in Sweden have unfortunately been disappointing. In animals NGF prevents experimental damage to the cholinergic basal forebrain and improves learning and memory in such experimental paradigms. Other oral-administered agents such as deprenyl (Somerset) and acetyl carnitine (Sigma Tau) are being tested in AD subjects to try to slow progression (Whitehouse, 1995).

Prevention

An understanding of pathogenesis might lead to discussions about not only arresting progression but also intervening early in the disease to prevent the onset of the disorder. Prevention strategies can be divided into primary, secondary, and tertiary strategies, depending on whether the disease is already present and active or not. Presumably treatments to slow or prevent progression would have more profound effects on health care costs than just symptomatic treatments.

The useful clinical concept of excess disability (the presence of a coexisting illness, such as pneumonia, that temporarily makes cognitive impairment worse) reinforces the idea that many preventive techniques can be used to maintain the patient's function.

Quality of Life

There is growing recognition that in trials of therapeutic interventions in AD, targeted therapeutic outcomes need to consider quality of life (QOL) (Annas, 1995; Birren et al., 1991; Deimling et al., 1989; DeJong, 1989; Hurley et al., 1992; Katz, 1987; Kerner et al., 1995; Kiyak et al., 1991; Lane et al., 1987; Lawton et al., 1994a; Lawton, 1994b; Mendez et al., 1990; Neuhauser et al., 1995; Ripich et al., 1994; Teri and Logson, 1991; Whitehouse and Rabins, 1992; Wilson and Cleary, 1995; WHO-100, 1995). QOL includes physical and mental health, function, social relationships, and subjective well-being. It is a controversial concept in that it is broad and hopelessly vague. QOL can be measured using both objective (i.e., externally rated) and subjective (self-rated) means. It is obvious that patients with severe dementia are impaired concerning their ability to make subjective judgments about their own QOL, but we have not even begun to explore the range of those abilities in mild to moderate dementia. Moreover, improving caregiver QOL is an important goal for therapeutic interventions as well.

The study of QOL in dementia is important because of its ties to pharmacoeconomics. A variety of techniques can be used to examine costs and benefits of therapeutic interventions. For chronic disease cost–utility seems most appropriate for many circumstances. In this approach individuals or groups are asked to assign weights to the value of certain outcomes. These utility weights can be compared with costs using so-called QUALYS (quality-adjusted life years). Such pharmacoeconomic studies are likely to play an increasingly important role even in phase III studies of antidementia drugs.

Stage-Specific Goals

The goals of therapy in many diseases are stage-specific, and this should be true in AD. Goals for mildly affected individuals or even presymptomatic individuals will be clearly different from those for a severely demented patient who can no longer recognize family members. There needs to be serious consideration given to end-of-life care in dementia because quality of death is as important a consideration as quality of life.

Organizational Efforts to Examine Therapeutic Goals

National Alzheimer's Advisory Panel   In the United States, the National Alzheimer's Advisory Panel exists to provide advice to Congress and to the Secretary of the Department of Health and Human Services. This group is currently reviewing therapeutic goals in AD and is examining goals that may be appropriate for different stages of severity of dementia. Its efforts are an attempt to examine goals across different disciplines and to remain focused on patient- and family-centered as well as culturally sensitive outcomes. Subgroups are examining not only goals to improve cognition but also approaches to noncognitive symptoms. Moreover, assessment of the effects of interventions on activities of daily living and quality of life will be considered.

Regulatory Bodies   The clearest guides to goals for biological therapy are the statements by regulatory bodies, such as the U.S. Food and Drug Administration (FDA) and the European Medicines Evaluation Agency (EMEA), about the criteria that need to be satisfied before a drug is approved. These guidelines, which exist in draft status, focus on the effects of a drug on the cognition and global status of an individual patient. For example, unofficial FDA guidelines suggest that a cognition-enhancing drug should improve performance on an objective psychometric test as well as a measure of clinical meaningfulness, such as a clinician's global impression of change (Leber, 1990).

Guidelines on how to demonstrate slowed progression of disease have not been established by any group. The complex design issues facing us are how to differentiate between a prolonged symptomatic benefit and a disease-course-altering effect. Moreover, attention has been focused almost exclusively on cognitive symptoms, without recognition that noncognitive symptoms such as agitation, psychosis, and depression significantly contribute to the problems of patients and families.

Outcomes Research Approaches   The Agency for Health Care Policy and Research (AHCPR), a government organization in the United States, has programs to develop so-called PORTS (Patient Outcome Research Teams) that systematically examine the available literature to evaluate the efficacy of interventions currently available. AHCPR also integrates this information into guidelines for practicing physicians and other health care providers. Guidelines will be emerging shortly concerning the early recognition of dementia.

At the time of this writing, a Fall 1996 conference on new approaches to outcomes assessment in AD was being planned by the AHCPR, the National Alzheimer's Association, the National Institute of Aging, the National Alzheimer's Advisory Panel, the Department of Health and Human Services, and several other U.S. organizations. The conference will attempt to bring together communities that have not yet communicated with one another, namely the AD intervention community and experts on outcomes assessments, who have worked in different disease areas. For example, a number of PORTS have reported work in conditions such as schizophrenia. The focus of the conference will be on developing new directions for assessing biological and behavioral interventions.

STRATEGIES FOR RESEARCH AND DEVELOPMENT

In most countries, efforts to develop more effective interventions for AD patients and their families involve academia, government, and industry in cooperative relationships. All these sectors are being affected dramatically by major social and economic forces, which are causing profound rethinking about the purpose and goals of organizations and the mechanisms for achieving their missions.

Academia

In most countries, academic health centers are the sites of fundamental biological discoveries and the clinical testing of new interventions, but these centers are under considerable financial stress. Reductions in research and clinical revenues are occurring because of major changes in the health care system, driven in large part by the increased number of elderly patients. These changes are threatening the ability of academic centers to successfully accomplish their integrated missions of research, education, service, just at the time when closer coordination among these mission components is needed (Fox, 1995; King's Fund, 1992; London's Health Service, 1992; *Science,* 1996).

Government

Many government funding agencies are reducing both intramural and extramural support for research, or at least reducing rates of growth (Abelson, 1995; Byerly and Pielke, 1995; Roush, 1995; Press, 1995). For example, in the United States, concerns have been raised about the role of the National Institutes of Health in clinical research (Kelly, 1995).

Research dollars invested in AD represent a much smaller percentage of the economic impact of the disease on the world's population than for many other disorders, such as cancer. Increased public advocacy efforts are needed to keep this point in the public mind.

Lay Organizations

In the United States, the National Alzheimer's Association has been an effective lobby for increasing dollars for research. This organization has faced the difficult challenge of advocating for health care change necessary to better care for those with the disorder today, as well as arguing for funds for future research. A worrisome sign is that the National Alzheimer's Advisory Panel, which has been in existence now for almost a decade, is at risk for being terminated.

Internationally, AD lay organizations have organized into a confederation called Alzheimer's Disease International, headquartered in London, which may prove to be an effective organization for global advocacy. Over the last several years, local and national Alzheimer's associations in the United States and in the United Kingdom and Italy have increased their public policymaking efforts with some success.

Industry

For the past several years, support for medical research from the pharmaceutical and biotechnology industries has exceeded that from the National Institutes of Health. However, the pharmaceutical industry faces growing pressure from health care providers to reduce the cost of medications, and as a result its commitment to research and development is in jeopardy (Gambardella, 1992; Omta et al., 1994; Taggart, 1993). This is particularly true in fields such as neuroscience, which is viewed by many prominent companies as a major potential area for contributing socially and economically. Nevertheless, it is one that represents an enormous challenge and needs long-term investment.

In 1993, the U.S. Office of Technology Assessment (a government office that has since been eliminated, perhaps unwisely, by budget cutting) issued a report entitled *Pharmaceutical Research and Development: Cost, Risks and Rewards.* It emphasized the costs and risks associated with research and development in the pharmaceutical industry. In 1990 dollars, the cost of developing the average drug was estimated at almost \$200 million. The average drug produced a 4% surplus, so research and development can still be a profitable venture. However, we must be concerned that the pharmaceutical industry will diminish if the rewards of investing in research and development cannot be realized.

Conflicts of Interest

More effective interactions among academic health centers, government, and industry will be necessary to develop more effective therapeutic intervention programs. However, measures must be taken to preserve society's trust in the scientific enterprise (Whitehouse and Morris, 1996).

An example is the formulation of guidelines for investigators who receive monies from federal sources. Regulations have required that all recipients of grant monies must establish conflict of interest committees to review the relationships a federal grant recipient has with business. These federal guidelines give considerable flexibility to the institution receiving the funds regarding how to define potential conflicts of interest. However, in general, a close relationship such as owning stock in a business is considered more significant than, for example, receiving a consulting fee.

It remains to be seen whether these guidelines serve their purpose of maintaining public trust but not impeding scientific progress. More empirical studies of relationships between academic and industry are needed to examine what kinds of relationships are productive, profitable, and yet principled. In addition to these empirical studies, some further conceptual thought is necessary concerning conflict of interest. As suggested above, collaborations between academia, government, and industry seem desirable, and perhaps potential conflicts of interest should not be avoided. Perhaps they should even be encouraged. The key is trust. As Fukuyama (1995) has stressed, trust is an essential building block of the economic well-being of a country.

APPROACHES FOR THE FUTURE

New models for collaboration between private organizations, academia, government, and industry are clearly needed. The Reagan Institute in the United States, recently developed by the National Alzheimer's Association, may represent one such interesting organizational vehicle. One component of the Reagan Institute that should become more important is the electronic distribution of information to individuals with similar goals in order to support grant review and collaborations between academia and industry.

No longer can we afford the old model of basic science in which inquiry is driven by the curiosity of individual investigators without adequate consideration of the long-term implications of research for clinical care. We must reconsider the commonly expressed opinion that basic science will benefit humankind in some unpredictable and unspecified time. We need to understand better how fundamental knowledge can be converted into practical interventions.

In many countries, major national efforts are underway to reconsider how research and development will be guided in the future and how the creation of new knowledge can be integrated into health care systems. For example, the National Academy of Science (1995) in the United States has just reviewed federal research and development efforts. Its report, *Allocating Federal Funds for Science and Technology*, was developed by the Committee on Criteria for Federal Support of Research and Development. This report represents the most fundamental exploration of federal research and development policy ever conducted. Thirteen recommendations are presented that focus on making the allocation process more systematic and comprehensive. The total funds spent on true research and development is identified, ensuring that excellent scientific input is provided in the process of allocation and choice of projects, and improving federal management of research and development efforts. One interesting revelation in the report is that much of what is considered research and development by the federal government is not viewed as such by this committee, for example, later development of large-scale projects.

Similarly, a government report was published several years ago in the United Kingdom (Chancellor of the Duchy of Lancaster, 1993). It called for major changes in the structure of science and a renewed focus on the impact of science on quality of life and the economic well-being of citizens of the United Kingdom.

In the United States, there are major issues to face about federal research and development in health care. For example, what is the role of the National Institutes of Health in its intramural programs and its support of clinical research? How can programs be better coordinated across institutions?

CHANGES IN THE HEALTH CARE SYSTEM

Scientists and clinicians in the United States are aware of major changes in our health care system, merely by being citizens and paying attention to our own health insurance. Much of the economic strain on the health care system is driven by two factors, the rapid introduction of technology and the aging of our population. Fundamental changes are also at work in many other countries, and they show similar features. In many countries the educational system has not produced the kind of health care providers necessary to support the health of populations. We have too many specialists and not enough generalists.

It is not yet clear whether managed competition or capitation represents a universal evolution of health care in countries other than the United States. It is clear, however, that there have been shifts in the balance between government and private roles in health care organizations, and not just in the United States.

In the United States, the predominant change in health care is a move from fee for service to capitation. In this environment, health maintenance organizations (HMOs) have become more dominant, and companies have become more dominant as payers in the health care system. Nevertheless, through Medicare and Medicaid the federal government plays an important role in financing health care, and it is contributing to the drive toward a capitated system.

This capitated system is revealing the deficiencies in the health care providers that we currently train. It is also raising serious questions about the value of new technology and interventions. No longer can this technology be introduced and paid for without serious thought to its contribution to the quality of care.

Pharmaceutical companies are reacting to the changes in health care systems in many dramatic ways. Some companies, such as Merck and Lilly, are developing relationships with health care organizations. The critical challenge will be to get new drugs on formularies, particularly when they are more expensive than older medications. Pharmaceutical companies are also beginning to consider whether they should be more than purveyors of pills. A number of companies are developing disease state management or health prevention programs. In some circumstances, companies are actually providing comprehensive services to patients with disease, such as Lilly for patients with diabetes. Thus, pharmaceutical companies may become competitors with other components of the health care system for providing integrated care.

It seems clear that in the future we will have a different health care system, probably one that is capitated and better integrated. Unified financing information and case management systems will bind together more components of the health care system. Clearly, the artificial separations between acute care (i.e., hospitals and physicians' offices) and chronic care (i.e., community and long-term institutional care) need to be eliminated in the United States and other countries in order to provide comprehensive care networks.

GLOBAL ISSUES

As emphasized in the previous sections of this chapter, many forces altering science and health care are common to the major developed nations. This recognition of common problems is occurring at a time when studies in modern molecular genetics and neurobiology are being conducted collaboratively in laboratories around the world. The promise of neuroscience for developing effective therapies has never been greater. Excitement is shared around the world, but clinicians and scientists are facing major challenges in how to take advantage of these scientific opportunities, obtain adequate resources, and develop means for applying their discoveries more rapidly in clinical practice.

To many it is most exciting to search for new scientific discoveries, such as those in molecular biology, that offer great promise for developing medication more effectively. It is also important, however, to look at the systemic and management aspects of scientific research. Scientific advancement and the solution of clinical problems will always require individual creativity and scientific discovery, but improvements in the processes by which we conduct science will also improve our productivity and our ability to improve the quality of people's lives (Pollner, 1992; National Academy of Sciences, 1995; Chancellor of the Duchy of Lancaster, 1993).

International Conference on Harmonization

Road blocks to scientific collaboration exist at many different levels of drug development. In the increasingly conflict-ridden and competitive environment of science and health care, we must seek win–win situations that can be viewed as advantageous to all parties. One such opportunity is the standardization of drug development processes. The International Conference on Harmonization (ICH), primarily a group of government regulators, has been meeting for several years to make the submission of new drug applications more consistent across national boundaries. Although this has been a slow process, the group is making progress in bringing harmonization to the regulatory mechanics in the United States, Japan, and the European Union.

International Working Group on Harmonization of Dementia Drug Guidelines

Because the ICH has not been examining disease-specific areas, the International Working Group on the Harmonization of Dementia Drug Guidelines (IWGHDDG) has been formed. Dementia drug development is in the early stages, and there is considerable variability among nations. The primary purpose of the IWGHDDG is to examine existing and proposed guidelines for drug development in dementia and make it easier to conduct multinational, multisite studies in dementia.

Leading academics, representatives from the pharmaceutical industry, and regulators from around the world are reviewing guidelines from Japan, Canada, United States, and Europe. Working subgroups have been established to examine specific differences in proposed guidelines as well as conceptual issues important for future studies. These subgroups focus on instrumentation (e.g., objective psychometric tests and clinical global tests) and new topics such as activities of daily living and quality of life. Attention is being paid to broad issues, such as cultural differences, that are important in designing multinational drug studies.

The IWGHDDG is also considering fundamental ethical issues that affect the development of medications for AD. The problem of conflict of interest was mentioned above. In multisite, multinational studies, some agreement must be reached about the appropriate relationships between industry and the academic sites. For example, should we prohibit consulting by the academic investigator while a study is underway? Another important issue is the nature of informed consent and cognitive impairment. How do we get appropriate informed consent to make sure that participation in research is voluntary, though the patient is perhaps unable to understand the process and make decisions? Moreover, different medications have been approved in different countries, and there are different cultural attitudes toward medications. The role of placebos is an issue to resolve.

As of this writing, the most recent meeting of the IWGHDDG occurred in Osaka in July 1996 as part of the Fifth International Alzheimer's Disease and Related Disorders Conference. There we continued our focus on European guidelines and paid special attention to the situation in Japan. The Japanese Ministry of Health and Welfare expressed its intention to revise the guidelines for development of drugs for vascular disease and to develop specific guidelines in the area of AD and vascular dementia.

CONCLUSION

Those of us who are neuroscientists see that the understanding of brain dysfunction in dementia truly has increased over the last several decades. We also have an uneasy sensation that the environment in which we are conducting our science has changed dramatically. Thus, for those who are interested in improving the quality of life of AD patients and their families, it is imperative to pay attention to the broader policy and social forces. These are the factors that will affect scientists and clinicians alike in their ability to accomplish their work. We need to look at these changes positively, as opportunities for examining our scientific processes and organizations, particularly the way in which we transfer technology into the clinical arena.

REFERENCES

Abelson PH (1995): Science and technology policy. Science 267:435.

Annas GJ (1995): Reframing the debate on health care reform by replacing our metaphors. N Engl J Med 332(11):744–747.

Birren JE, Lubben JE, Rowe CJ, Deutchman DE (1991). "The Concept and Measurement of Quality of Life in the Frail Elderly." San Diego: Academic Press.

Byerly R Jr, Pielke R Jr (1995): The changing ecology of United States science. Science 269:1531–1532.

Chancellor of the Duchy of Lancaster (1993): Realising our potential: "A strategy for science, engineering and technology." Presented to Parliament by the Chancellor of the Duchy of Lancaster by Command of her Majesty. London: HMSO.

Deimling GT, Bass DM, Townsend AL, Noelker LS (1989): Care-related stress: A comparison of spouse and adult-child caregivers in shared and separate households. J Aging Health 1:76–82.

DeJong R (1989). Measurement of quality of life changes in patients with Alzheimer's disease. Clin Ther 11(4).

Economist (1996): Survey: The economics of ageing. Economist. New York: Economist Newspaper Group.

Fox KC, Holden C (1995): Careers '95: The future of the Ph.D. Science 270:141–146.

Fukuyama F (1995): "Trust: A study of the social virtues and the creation of prosperity." New York: Free Press.

Gambardella A (1992): Competitive advantages from in-house scientific research: The US pharmaceutical industry in the 1980s. Res Policy 21:391–407.

Hurley AC, Volicer BJ, Hanarahan PA, House S, Volicer L (1992): The assessment of discomfort in advanced Alzheimer's patients. Res Nurs Health, 15:369–377.

Katz S (1987): The science of quality of life. J Chron Dis 6:459–463.

Kelly WN, Randolph MA (1995): From the Institute of Medicine: Careers in clinical research: Obstacles and opportunities. JAMA 273:1–12.

Kerner DN, Patterson MB, Thomas L, Kaplan RM (1995): Validity of the Quality of Well-Being Scale for patients with Alzheimer's disease. Annual Meeting Supplement Posters D035-D038 S171:D037.

King's Fund (1992): King's Fund Commission on the Future of London's Acute Health Services, London Health Care 2010: Changing the future of services in the capital. London: King's Fund London Initiative.

Kiyak H, Asuman, Teri L, Borson S (1991): Physical and functional health assessment in normal aging and in Alzheimer's disease: Self-reports vs family reports. Gerontologist 34(3):324–330.

Lane DA (1987): Utility, decision, and quality of life. J Chron Dis 40(6):585–591.

Lawton MP (1994b): Quality of life in Alzheimer's disease. Alzheimer's Dis Assoc Disord 8(3):138–150.

Lawton MP, van Haitsma K, Klapper J (1994): A balanced stimulation and retreat program for a special care dementia unit. Alzheimer's Dis Assoc Disord 8:S133–S138.

Leber P (1990): Guidelines for the Clinical Evaluation of Antidementia Drugs: First Draft. U.S. Food and Drug Administration: Washington, D.C.

London's Health Service (1992): "Report of the Inquiry into London's Health Service, Medical Education and Research." Presented to the Secretaries of State for Health and Education by Sir Bernard Tomlinson. London: HMSO Publications.

Mendez MF, Martin RJ, Smith KA, Whitehouse PJ (1990): Psychiatric symptoms in Alzheimer's disease. J Neuropsych Clin Neurosci 2:228–33.

National Academy of Science (1995): National Academy of Sciences, National Academy of Engineering, Institute of Medicine, National Research Council Reports (1995): "Allocating Federal Funds for Science and Technology." Committee on Criteria for Federal Support of Research and Development. Washington, D.C.: National Academy Press.

Neuhauser D, McEachern JE, Headrick L (1995). "Clinical CQ1: A Book of Readings." Oakbrook, IL: Joint Commission on Accreditation of Healthcare Organizations.

Omta SWF, Bouter LM, van Engelen JML (1994): Managing industrial pharmaceutical R&D. A comparative study of management control and innovative effectiveness in European and Anglo-American companies. R&D Management 24(4):303–315.

Pollner F (1992): The "strategic plan:" Mixing salesmanship and science. J NIH Res 4:33–37.

Press F (1995): Needed: Coherent budgeting for science and technology. Science 270:1448–1450.

Ripich DN, Petrill SA, Whitehouse PJ, Ziol EW (1994): Gender differences in language in AD patients: A longitudinal study. Neurology 45(2):229–301.

Roush W (1995): R&D impact: A numbers game? Science 270:1748–1749.

Taggart J (1993): "The World Pharmaceutical Industry." London and New York: Routledge.

Teri L, Logson RG (1991): Identifying pleasant activities for Alzheimer's disease patients: The Pleasant Events Schedule-AD. Gerontologist 31:124–127.

U.S. Office of Technology Assessment Summary Report (1993): *Pharmaceutical Research and Development: Costs, Risks and Rewards.* Washington D.C.: Government Printing Office.

Whitehouse PJ (1995): Future prospects for Alzheimer's disease therapy: Ethical and policy issues for the international community. Acta Neurol Scand 165:145–149.

Whitehouse PJ, Morris JC (1996): Disclosure of financial interest: A new policy for Alzheimer disease and associated disorders. Alzheimer's Dis Assoc Disord 10(1):1–2.

Whitehouse PJ, Rabins PV (1992): Quality of life and dementia. Alzheimer's Dis Assoc Disord 6(3):135–137.

WHO-100 (1995): The World Health Organization Quality of Life-100, Division of Mental Health World Health Organization CH-1211 Geneva 27, Switzerland.

Wilson IB, Cleary PD (1995): Linking clinical variables with health-related quality of life: A conceptual model of patient outcomes. JAMA 273(1).

CHAPTER 15

Use of CSF-Based Markers in the Diagnosis of Alzheimer's Disease

PETER SEUBERT, DOUGLAS GALASKO, and MICHAEL A. BOSS

Athena Neurosciences, Inc., 800 Gateway Boulevard, South San Francisco, California 94080 (P.S.); Department of Neurosciences, University of California at San Diego and Veteran's Affairs Medical Center, San Diego, California 92161 (D.G.); Athena Diagnostics, Inc., Four Biotech Park, 377 Plantation Street, Worcester, Massachusetts 01605 (M.A.B.)

NEED FOR AN ACCURATE DIAGNOSTIC TEST FOR ALZHEIMER'S DISEASE

Alzheimer's disease (AD) is the fourth leading cause of death in the United States, afflicting an estimated 4 million Americans. Currently, approved therapies are only moderately effective in a fraction of those affected with AD. It is often asked why then should one develop a diagnostic test for a currently incurable, and largely untreatable, ailment. We offer several arguments to support the need for such a test.

In the diagnostic evaluation for dementia and AD, the clinician combines inclusionary and exclusionary features to determine the presence of "probable" AD. The inclusionary elements come from history, cognitive testing, and neuroimaging, while exclusionary features are sought by history, examination, cognitive testing, and laboratory tests for metabolic causes of dementia. Although AD is the most common cause of dementia in the elderly, accounting for about 60–80% of cases, many other conditions can cause or contribute to dementia. The only way to confirm AD is by demonstrating the signature lesions of plaques and tangles in the brain examined at biopsy or autopsy. Although the ultimate accuracy of the clinical diagnosis, calibrated against autopsy, may be high (>85%) in expert hands, studies that have attained this degree of accuracy have usually entailed a more extensive evaluation than that typical of routine clinical practice. The diagnostic evaluation of

Pharmacological Treatment of Alzheimer's Disease: Molecular and Neurobiological Foundations,
Edited by Brioni and Decker
ISBN 0-471-16758-4   © 1997 Wiley-Liss, Inc.

dementia often requires several visits, and its accuracy is enhanced by follow-up to demonstrate that the dementia progresses over time. In the presence of potential causes of dementia other than AD or of atypical clinical features, the diagnosis of AD is more difficult. This uncertainty is captured by clinical categories such as possible AD (representing atypical AD or dementia thought to be primarily due to AD in the presence of one or more additional conditions that can contribute to dementia) and mixed dementia (AD with vascular dementia). Very mild dementia is another elusive area requiring considerable clinical judgment, as evidenced by terms such as mild cognitive impairment, age-associated memory impairment, and patients "at risk" for AD, which describe patients with memory complaints, many of whom will progress to develop overt AD. A tool such as a laboratory test that supported the clinical diagnosis of AD would be of value in enhancing diagnostic accuracy and making the workup more efficient.

As many of the other chapters in this volume detail, new therapeutic options in the treatment of AD are apt to emerge in the next few years. The key to the success of many of these approaches is to accurately identify the patient who will benefit from the drug as early in the course of disease as possible, before extensive neurodegeneration has occurred. It is likely that these therapies will only slow and not reverse the degenerative process. The challenge to the researcher is to devise tests that identify patients as early as or earlier than the present-day physician can. In addition these test must be extremely specific, given the prognostic and psychological implications of a diagnosis of AD, and ideally not be cross-reactive for similarly presenting dementias (e.g., multi-infarct dementia, and Lewy body variant of AD).

Diagnostic indicators of AD, depending on their nature, may have added use beyond the initial identification of afflicted individuals. Many of the therapeutic approaches now under investigation are aimed at arresting the suspected pathological processes and the ultimate loss of synapses and neurons occurring in AD. Biomarkers that directly reflect these destructive processes may also have utility as surrogate measures for drug efficacy. Serial measurements of biomarkers are then likely to become an important component of clinical trials in AD as a means to demonstrate a drug effect. Finally, it is increasingly apparent that, despite its relatively uniform pathological profile, Alzheimer's disease is a heterogeneous disorder with a multitude of genetic and other factors at work. Age of onset and rate of progression in AD vary widely. Conceivably, biological markers may help to explain some of the variability of onset and course. Whether a patient's responsiveness to a particular therapy also can be predicted based on one or several biomarkers also deserves to be explored.

THE PRACTICALITY OF A CSF-BASED AD DIAGNOSTIC TEST

Despite the imaginative efforts of many, AD diagnostics based on peripheral fluids and cells [reviewed in Scott (1993)] have met with, as yet, limited success. Until such efforts yield the requisite specificity/sensitivity for clinical utility, we are left with markers measured in the cerebrospinal fluid (CSF), which have, as will be discussed, yielded the most promising results. There remains in the lay community a psychological concern surrounding the drawing of CSF, despite the proven utility and safety of this procedure, which has been in use for over 100 years. Although technically more demanding than drawing blood, the lumbar puncture is a minimally invasive outpatient procedure that is used routinely as an aid to neurological diagnosis in a host of conditions, ranging from acute disorders such as meningitis to chronic conditions such as multiple sclerosis. Serious complications of lumbar puncture are extremely rare and the procedure is usually well tolerated.

The most significant adverse effect associated with the procedure is postlumbar puncture headache (PLPH), which is estimated to occur in 10% of cases in the general population. PLPH is thought to occur due to lowering of CSF pressure after the lumbar puncture (LP) from persistent leakage of CSF at the site of puncture. The risk of headache may be reduced by using small-caliber needles to perform lumbar puncture, by cautioning patients against physical activity during the day following the procedure, and possibly by maintaining patients recumbent for an hour after the procedure. Interestingly, the incidence of PLPH appears to be much lower in demented subjects. In a large study of 395 demented subjects, only 2% developed PLPH (Blennow et al., 1993). This has been similar to our own experience in that PLPH is less common in elderly or demented subjects. Furthermore, in another large study (Hindley et al., 1995) fully 92% of elderly subjects (mean age 72 years) agreed to a second LP, demonstrating the acceptability of the procedure. Thus, while not trivial, lumbar punctures in elderly demented patients are a relatively straightforward procedure and, as we will discuss, the potential information gained outweighs the minimal discomfort involved.

CSF MARKER STUDIES: STUDY DESIGN CONSIDERATIONS

Many factors can potentially cloud the interpretation and utility of CSF markers as aids to the diagnosis of AD. Several of these are peculiar to CSF. For example, the concentrations of most proteins in CSF are much lower than those typical of serum; therefore assays for CSF markers relevant to dementia often need to be able to detect very low levels of the substance of interest. For some CSF constituents, assays must be quantitative in a range of picograms to low nanograms per milliliter, which poses many technical challenges. Some substances show concentration gradients in CSF, usually associated with higher levels in the CSF obtained at the beginning of the draw compared to those later aliquots of CSF. Accompanying aging and dementia, brain volume decreases and CSF volume correspondingly increases. This relative dilution of CSF constituents may lower the concentration of markers, which may need to be corrected for by normalizing levels of the marker against CSF total protein.

Further considerations are whether the assay is affected by contamination of CSF by blood during lumbar puncture, or by freezing or prolonged storage of CSF prior to the assay. The levels of some CSF metabolites, for example, monoamines, are influenced by diet, physical activity, and time of day. It is prudent to examine the test–retest reliability of the CSF measurement by performing serial lumbar punctures on a group of patients.

A variety of medical conditions unrelated to dementia may affect the composition of CSF and levels of the marker under study. These include lumbar spine degenerative disease, peripheral neuropathy, acute and chronic inflammatory and infectious CNS conditions, destructive lesions such as stroke, and medications with potential CNS actions. Since the coexistence of these conditions in elderly patients may influence the specificity of the diagnostic test, their effects on the marker need to be characterized.

Finally, many details are important in designing a study to demonstrate that a marker has diagnostic utility for AD. Since the clinical diagnosis of AD carries an element of inaccuracy, patients in marker studies should be diagnosed as accurately as possible by rigorously applying clinical research criteria to achieve a "gold standard" for comparison. Ideally, patients should be followed to demonstrate that they have progressive dementia and to obtain autopsy confirmation of AD in at least some individuals. The severity of dementia should be assessed to determine whether the marker is sensitive to all stages of AD. Control subjects need to be chosen carefully to show that the marker distinguishes patients with AD from other patient groups, namely nondemented individuals of comparable age, patients with other dementias, and patients with other neurodegenerative diseases.

While this list of possible confounds seems daunting, addressing these issues is critical in the evaluation of the true potential of a CSF-based diagnostic marker for AD.

NEUROTRANSMITTERS AND NEUROPEPTIDES AS POTENTIAL MARKERS OF AD

Research in this area has been fully covered in a recent review (Van Gool and Bolhuis, 1991) and will only be summarized here.

After decreased levels of several neurotransmitters and neuropeptides were found in the brains of patients with AD, similar patterns were sought in CSF. The earliest and most robust neurochemical marker of AD was a striking deficiency in markers of cholinergic neurotransmission. Decreased levels of key metabolic and biosynthetic enzymes for acetylcholine (ACh), namely acetylcholinesterase (AChE) and choline acetyltransferase (ChAT), were found in the cortex of AD patients and correlated with the severity of dementia assessed close to the time of death (Perry et al., 1978). ACh levels in CSF are very low, since this molecule is cleaved by cholinesterases that are present in abundance in CSF. Although levels of ACh in CSF do not satisfactorily separate subjects with AD from controls, within the AD group there is a correlation between these levels and cognitive test scores (Davis et al., 1982). Most studies of cholinergic markers in CSF have focused on the more stable enzymes involved in the metabolism of this neurotransmitter. Several clinical studies of AChE activity in CSF have been carried out. These have shown no difference, or at best a slight decrease in AChE levels or activity in AD compared to nondemented elderly subjects, with a great deal of overlap (Atack et al., 1988a, Elble et al., 1987; reviewed by Van Gool and Bolhuis, 1991). Furthermore, measures of AChE activity did not separate patients with early AD from controls. Studies of choline acetyltransferase (CAT) and of choline have also been unrevealing. Cerebrospinal fluid ACh markers therefore do not appear to have a role in the diagnosis of AD.

Levels of several aminergic markers are unchanged or slightly decreased in the brain in AD. As an index of CNS dopaminergic activity, CSF studies have focused on homovanillic acid (HVA), a stable metabolite of dopamine. Although some studies found decreased HVA in CSF of AD patients relative to controls, many have found no difference. In one study, CSF levels of HVA were decreased only in AD patients with Parkinsonian signs (Kaye et al., 1988). Other amine markers have been measured in CSF, notably serotonin [5-hydroxytryptophan (5HT)] and its metabolite 5-hydroxyindole acetic acid (5-HIAA). Findings varied between studies but overall showed decreases in 5HT with no change in 5-HIAA in AD compared to controls (Sofic et al., 1989; Tohgi et al., 1992). Reduction of HVA and 5-HIAA in AD are evident mainly in patients with moderate to severe dementia (Blennow et al., 1991). The norepinephrine marker 3-methoxy-4-hydroxyphenylglycol (MHPG) also did not show changes in CSF in AD. Chromogranin A is a protein stored and released with catecholamines, whose levels in CSF are thought to reflect the activity of mainly noradrenergic neurons in the brain. Although levels appeared to be decreased in the CSF of patients with Parkinson's disease, there was no change in AD compared to controls (O'Connor et al., 1993).

Various amino acids have been measured in CSF. Excitatory amino acids related to glutamate have been identified as important neurotransmitters, which may be capable of causing neuronal death under circumstances when their levels are increased. Studies have not found any significant difference between AD and control CSF levels of glutamate or any other amino acid (e.g., Pomara et al., 1992).

Neuropeptides act as neurotransmitters in many regions of the brain and show changes in AD compared to controls. Many neuropeptides are detectable in CSF, including somatostatin, neuropeptide Y, α-melanocyte-stimulating hormone (MSH), and corticotropin-releasing factor (CFR). Of these, somatostatin has been the most widely studied in CSF, prompted by the finding of a marked decrease in somatostatin levels in the brain in AD. CSF studies have shown a slight decrease (about 20%) in somatostatin levels between AD patients and controls, with much overlap (e.g., Atack et al., 1988b). None of the other neuropeptides examined has proven useful in distinguishing AD patients from controls.

PATHOLOGY-RELATED PROTEINS EXAMINED FOR DIAGNOSTIC UTILITY IN AD

A logical step in the search for CSF-based markers of AD is to examine the levels of proteins that are pathologically altered in the AD brain. The protein constituents of plaques and tangles suggest many candidate leads.

Neuronal Thread Protein

Ozturk et al. (1989) made the observation that areas of the brain affected with a high burden of AD pathology showed increased staining with antibodies against pancreatic thread protein, and subsequently it was shown that brain expressed a related protein termed "neuronal thread protein" (NTP). An initial report showed that NTP was elevated in the CSF of AD subjects compared to subjects with multiple sclerosis and to middle-aged nondemented controls (de la Monte et al., 1992). A later study (Blennow, et al., 1995b) found a substantial degree of overlap between AD and control levels of NTP in CSF. Interestingly, there was a strong correlation between levels of NTP and albumin levels in CSF, leading the authors to conclude that much of the NTP immunoreactivity in CSF was likely due to leakage from serum across the blood–brain barrier (BBB).

This raises an important theoretical and practical point. Whether the BBB is altered in AD is contentious, but there is agreement that aging is likely associated with a degree of breakdown of the BBB and with attendant increased BBB leakage. Thus, studies of proteins that occur systemically in serum at higher concentrations than in the CSF must also consider to what extent each protein normally crosses the BBB and whether its elevation in an age-associated condition such as AD reflects nonspecific compromise in the BBB rather than an association with disease. On a practical level, it is important first to ensure that the CSF sample assayed is free of blood contamination. Simultaneous measurement of the protein of interest and of albumin, both in serum and CSF, analogous to the immunoglobulin G (IgG) index used in the diagnosis of multiple sclerosis, would be the most accurate way to assess whether intra-CNS production or passage from serum to CSF is responsible for elevated values.

α-1 Antichymotrypsin

A number of proteins, more familiar for their roles in the body's acute inflammatory response, have been found in the senile plaques of AD, suggesting that proteins involved in this process may be useful diagnostically for AD. The observations that the acute-phase protease inhibitor α-1-antichymotrypsin (α-ACT) is a component of senile plaques (Abraham et al., 1988) prompted several groups to investigate its potential utility in the diagnosis of AD. The results of several recent studies of CSF levels of α-ACT have been mixed, showing either an increase (Matsubara et al., 1990; Shinohara et al., 1991; Licastro et al., 1995) or no change (Pirttila et al., 1994; Delamarche et al., 1991; Nakamura et al., 1994) in AD.

Furthermore these studies disagree as to whether serum and CSF α-ACT levels are related, an important point in light of the above discussion of BBB leakage. There are several further possible explanations for the lack of agreement among studies. The studies used different assays, some of which were barely sensitive enough to quantify CSF α-ACT. Studies did not report on factors such as medication use or coincident inflammatory conditions, either of which could influence serum α-ACT and therefore CSF α-ACT. In addition, some of the positive studies had only small numbers of subject samples. It appears that controversy in this area will persist.

Clq

The complement component Clq, which can be detected in senile plaques (Ishii and Haga, 1984), showed a decrease in the CSF of AD subjects compared to controls (Smyth et al., 1944). This is somewhat surprising as it might be expected that complement proteins would be elevated in the postulated inflamed state of the AD brain. Smyth et al. (1994) attribute this decrease to increased complement consumption, due to deposition or destruction. The levels of Clq were further found to correlate with the severity of cognitive impairment, with lower levels in moderate and severe dementia. At present the utility of this marker is unclear, as it was not very successful in identifying AD patients with mild dementia.

Interleukins

Interleukins (IL) may act as mediators of tissue damage in inflammatory conditions and may be produced by activated cells in the brain. Although altered levels of expression of various interleukins have been found in the brain in AD, leading to speculation that they may be mediators of tissue damage in AD, CSF studies of IL-1 (Pirtilla et al., 1994) and IL-6 (Yamada et al., 1995) did not find significant differences between AD and control subjects.

Ubiquitin

Ubiquitin is a protein of the heat shock family and plays an important role in protein folding and in the targeting of abnormal proteins for degradation. While the ubiquitin pathway itself does not appear to be abnormal in AD, ubiquitinated proteins such as tau (see below) may be markers of cellular damage. Paired helical filament (PHF) preparations isolated from AD brain possess conjugates immunoreactive with both tau and ubiquitin (Mori et al., 1987) antibodies. Wang et al. (1991) examined CSF samples using a competitive enzyme-linked immunosorbent assay (ELISA) based on an antibody to conjugated ubiquitin (the antibody was raised against PHF and recognized ubiquitin conjugated proteins) as well as an assay that detected both conjugated and free ubiquitin. The two assays yielded similar results. These authors found reasonable sensitivity and specificity for the diagnosis of AD in this study (both about 80%) with the admitted caveats that the CSF samples were not collected by any uniform protocol and that the assay was technically "difficult to control." The authors reiterate the point that one must scrupulously exclude blood from the CSF sample when measuring this marker.

More recent reports on CSF ubiquitin neither strongly support nor refute these findings. It has been observed that Creutzfeldt–Jakob disease patients show extremely high levels (>10 times the control mean) of ubiquitin immunoreactivity in CSF (Manaka et al., 1992). Further studies with the conjugation-dependent antibody did not achieve the high sensitivity and specificity initially reported, but it is unclear if this result is due to the composition of the neurological control group or to the use of postmortem (ventricular) CSF (Kudo et al., 1994). By using ratios of

CSF to serum ubiquitin levels, Blennow et al. (1994a) showed that the majority of AD and vascular dementia cases were elevated relative to controls and concluded this measure may have potential as a non-disease-specific marker for cerebral degeneration. In any event, further study will be necessary to determine real clinical potential of this measure.

Apolipoprotein E

The recent discovery that apolipoprotein E (apoE) genotype is linked to late-onset AD, with the E4 allele increasing the risk of developing AD (Strittmatter et al., 1993) has focused much attention on this lipoprotein. ApoE is made by astrocytes in the brain (Pitas et al., 1987), and since these cells undergo hyperplasia in AD, one might expect CSF apoE to increase. ApoE is also deposited in AD brain (Namba et al., 1991). Somewhat surprisingly, two studies have reported a reduction of CSF apoE in AD (Blennow et al., 1994b; Lehtimaki et al., 1995). While the difference between AD and controls was rather modest in the study of Lehtimaki et al. (1995), Blennow et al. (1994b) found virtually no overlap between levels in AD patients and normal controls. However, patients with frontal lobe dementia had a similar decrease in CSF apoE, shedding doubt on the specificity of the finding for AD. The severity of dementia in the AD patients was not reported. Neither study reported the apoE genotypes of subjects, which may have been a factor associated with variation in levels of CSF apoE, since apoE3 and E4 have different affinities for binding to receptors. A third CSF study (Carlsson et al., 1991) did not provide information on AD but showed that acute and chronic inflammatory disorders of the CNS led to an increase in CSF apoE. Clearly, more work is needed to clarify whether CSF apoE is a clinically useful marker in AD.

Apolipoprotein J

Apolipoprotein J, also known as clusterin or SP40, 40 is found in senile plaques (McGeer et al., 1992) and can bind to the amyloid β-peptide (Aβ) (Golabek et al., 1995). Levels of apoJ and its mRNA are increased in the brain in AD (Oda et al., 1994). When CSF apoJ was measured by ELISA, only a very slight increase on average was found in AD compared to controls (Choi-Miura et al., 1992).

Amyloid Precursor Protein

The discovery that the amyloid found in AD brain is derived from a larger precursor protein (Kang et al., 1987) led to several investigations of the precursor's potential as a diagnostic marker in AD (Palmert et al., 1990; Prior et al., 1991; Henriksson et al., 1991; Van Nostrand et al., 1992; Nakamura et al., 1994). One cannot necessarily make a better case for whether amyloid precursor protein (APP) would be expected to increase (it is a reactive protein in astrocytes and fragments of the protein are deposited in excess in AD brain) or decrease (loss of neurons would remove a major cellular source of APP production) in the CSF. In fact, most studies report a decrease in the CSF APP levels of AD subjects. The question is whether this result is clinically useful. The overlap observed by most researchers between AD and control CSF APP values is rather large. However, Van Nostrand et al. (1992) using a unique monoclonal antibody assay observed a more discriminative result. The severity of dementia in this study was not reported, so it is unclear if this assay will be useful in detecting AD in its early stages. The reasons for the discrepancies among studies will need to be determined and further work is necessary to show whether this assay will have utility in the relevant patient groups of importance (e.g., early dementias, non-AD dementias). Finally, APP exists in several isoforms due to both splicing variations and posttranslational modifications [Seubert et al. (1993) and reviewed in Selkoe (1994)]. While some studies have begun to explore these variables with limited success, it is unclear if their measure improves the utility of this analyte to the differential diagnosis of AD. For instance, one study found increased CSF levels of APP containing the Kunitz-type protease inhibitor (KPI) inhibitor in AD in comparison to multi-infarct dementia (MID) and nondemented controls, although the levels overlapped for over half of the AD patients; too few controls were studied to determine whether APP-KPI increased with aging (Urakami et al., 1992).

Amyloid β-Peptide

Aβ, a peptide of approximately 4 kD, is the principle component of the amyloid found in senile plaque cores and cerebrovasculature in AD (Glenner and Wong, 1984; Masters et al., 1985). Although it forms highly insoluble deposits in AD, Aβ exists in a soluble physiological form in the CSF, predominantly as a 40-amino-acid peptide ($A\beta_{40}$), produced in small amounts by cells expressing APP (Seubert et al., 1992; Shoji et al., 1992). The unambiguous demonstration of Aβ in CSF was cause for optimism since a key component of one of the pathological hallmarks of AD was now measurable. Despite results reporting some correlation of Aβ levels with dementia severity (Nitsch et al., 1995), the clinical utility of this measure has been disappointing. In our laboratories, and others, virtual complete overlap is observed in AD versus control subjects' CSF Aβ levels (Nakamura et al., 1994; Motter et al., 1995; Southwick et al., 1996). While these findings were disappointing, several intriguing observations (see below) soon revealed that Aβ peptides with varying lengths at their carboxy-termini are very different in many key properties, prompting closer examination of this area.

Amyloid β_{42}-Peptide

Several pieces of evidence implicate Aβ peptides extending to 42 amino acids in length as important participants in AD pathology. Biophysically, $A\beta_{42}$ is more prone to aggregation and precipitation than $A\beta_{40}$ in vitro (Jarrett et al., 1993). Studies have implicated increases in the ratio of the soluble forms of $A\beta_{42}$:$A\beta_{40}$ as critical in the etiology of several familial AD subtypes that include mutations not only to those in the APP gene itself (Suzuki et al., 1994) but to other recently identified loci as well (Scheuner et al., 1995). Thus, small disturbances in this balance may be sufficient to bring on the disease at a relatively early age. Also, Iwatsubo et al., (1994) showed, by immunocytochemical methods, striking differences in the deposition patterns of $A\beta_{40}$ versus $A\beta_{42}$. Specifically, $A\beta_{42}$ seems to deposit initially in diffuse plaques and makes up the bulk of parenchymal amyloid. These results are consistent with ELISA measures of AD brain samples (Gravina et al., 1995).

We developed an ELISA to measure specifically $A\beta_{42}$ in CSF, which is sensitive enough to detect levels of the order of picograms per milliliter (Motter et al., 1995). $A\beta_{42}$ was found to account for about 10% of the total $A\beta$ found in CSF. When we compared patients with AD, other dementias, and neurodegenerative disorders with cognitively normal age-matched controls, we found that the AD patients had significantly lower concentrations of $A\beta_{42}$ in CSF (Figure 1). Levels of the total $A\beta$, reflecting mainly species that end at position 40, did not differ among the groups. In the AD subjects, levels of $A\beta_{42}$ did not correlate significantly with age, duration of dementia, or the degree of cognitive impairment. The important point to note from these data is that normal levels of $A\beta_{42}$ are indicative of the absence of AD.

Our current hypothesis is that the decrease in CSF $A\beta_{42}$ in AD is related to plaque burden. Plaques may themselves sequester $A\beta_{42}$, diminishing its release into CSF. As plaques progressively enlarge, their volume increases exponentially, making them an efficient sink for binding $A\beta_{42}$. In the AD brain the transport or clearance of $A\beta_{42}$ from areas of its production may be impaired, leading to increased local elevation of $A\beta_{42}$ concentrations that strongly favor deposition in the parenchyma. If our interpretation is correct that CSF $A\beta_{42}$ concentration is inversely related to plaque burden, and if plaque burden is a precursor of dementia, then CSF $A\beta_{42}$ would be expected to have predictive value in asymptomatic individuals. One way of testing this hypothesis is to follow the elderly controls in our studies; we would predict that subjects who have shown decreased (or low normal) levels of $A\beta_{42}$ would have an increased risk of manifesting symptoms of AD upon follow-up.

Tau

In 1993, Vandermeeren and colleagues published a report measuring tau levels in the CSF of AD patients and in a number of other conditions. This seminal work received surprisingly little attention at the time, largely because recognition of its practical value required careful analysis by the reader. While these authors reported that several subjects with other conditions also had elevated tau in their CSFs, the false positives were almost all conditions extremely unlikely to be confused with AD such as encephalitis, amyotrophic lateral sclerosis (ALS), and other acute conditions. We subsequently built an immunoassay to measure tau, using a pair of monoclonal antibodies that recognized all six isoforms of human tau regardless of their phosphorylation state. In two published studies, we have replicated the finding that tau is elevated in the CSF in AD (Vigo-Pelfrey et al., 1995; Motter et al., 1995). Our experience echoed that of Vandermeeren and co-workers (1993) in that some

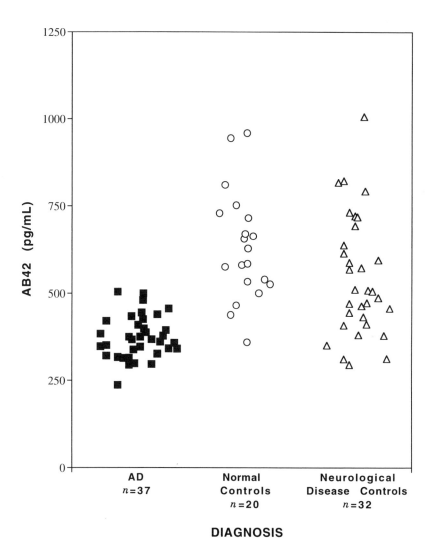

DIAGNOSIS

FIGURE 1. CSF $A\beta_{42}$ is decreased in AD. Levels of $A\beta_{42}$ were determined by ELISA. In this study AD subjects were classified as mild to moderately demented (MMSE mean = 17.5 ± 7.1) and were community dwelling with an average age of 70 ± 9.1. Neurological disease controls had a variety of conditions including frontal lobe dementia, depression, vascular dementia, Parkinson's disease, and several others. This group had an average MMSE of 23 ± 8.2 and an average age of 66 ± 9.1 years. The normal control group was neurologically and cognitively normal and of an average age of 70 ± 6.2. The average $A\beta42$ value of the AD group (383 ± 76 pg/mL) was significantly different ($p < 0.0001$) than either the neurological disease (543 ± 177 pg/mL) or normal control (632 ± 156 pg/mL) groups. Figure reproduced from Motter, et al. (1995) with permission.

AD patients failed to show an increase in CSF tau, while a few controls with other neurological disorders had high tau levels.

During 1995, six additional publications have also confirmed this finding (Jensen et al., 1995; Hock et al., 1995; Arai et al., 1995; Mori et al., 1995; Munroe et al., 1995; Tato et al., 1995), using three different ELISA assays and independent subject populations that in sum represent 1000 individuals, over 300 of whom had been diagnosed with AD. Considering the available scatter plot data published in total, and excluding subjects under the age of 60 plus subjects with infections or acute conditions (who are unlikely to be a relevant confounding group in the diagnosis of AD), over 50% of AD subjects have elevated levels of tau compared to <6% of other neurological disease subjects (undoubtedly contaminated with concurrent AD as noted by the authors in these studies) and <0.5% of normal controls (Table 1). If one compares AD with elderly normal controls alone, increased CSF tau identifies an even higher proportion of affected subjects. Aside from the global agreement among these studies that CSF tau is elevated in AD, several facts are worth discussing. In both the Arai and co-workers (1995) and Motter and co-workers (1995) studies, no significant correlation between disease severity and tau level was detected. In Figure 2, the CSF tau levels of subjects from the Motter et al. (1995) study are shown. As can be seen, an elevation of tau CSF above 312 pg/mL was a fairly certain indicator of AD and roughly two thirds of the AD subjects surpassed this cutoff. The Mini-Mental State Examina-

TABLE 1. Subjects Testing Positive for CSF Tau[a]

Study	AD	OD	CON
Vandermeeren et al. (1993)	13/27	2/25	0/51
Vigo-Pelfrey et al. (1995)	28/71	4/84	0/26
Mori et al. (1995)	12/14	0/14	0/36
Jensen et al. (1995)	14/21	2/31	0/30
Munroe et al. (1995)	9/24	2/39	0/14
Motter et al. (1995)	22/37	1/32	1/20
Arai et al. (1995)	41/70	6/51	0/19
Totals	139/264	17/286	1/196
Percent	53	5.9	0.5

[a]Summary of published CSF Tau studies. Subjects were classified as probable AD (AD), other disease condition (OD), or control (CON) according to authors of each study. "Positive" results were determined by analysis of published scatter plots of values, using cutoffs optimized for specificity for AD. Patients who were young (<60 years old) or with acute/infectious conditions were excluded from the analysis. No published scatter plot data from Hock et al. (1995) or Tato et al. (1995) were available. Over half of the AD subjects demonstrate elevated levels of tau, compared to less than 1% of the normal controls.

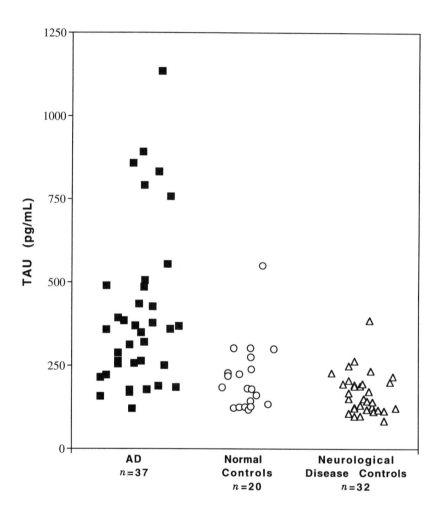

DIAGNOSIS

FIGURE 2. CSF tau is increased in AD. CSF from subjects described in Figure 1 were assayed for tau concentration. Tau levels in AD subjects averaged 407 ± 241 pg/mL, which is significantly higher ($p > 0.001$) than either the neurological diseases control (168 ± 63 pg/mL) or normal control (212 ± 102 pg/mL) groups. Figure reproduced from Motter et al. (1995), with permission.

tion (MMSE) scores and duration of the disease were compared to the tau levels of the AD subjects and found not to correlate significantly (Figures 3 and 4). In fact, we have observed that early-stage AD patients (MMSE 21–29) also show elevated tau (Galasko et al., 1996; Riemenschneider et al., 1996). What this suggests is that tau elevation may be present as early as or even before the expert clinician can make the diagnosis of AD. It will be very exciting to test subjects in even earlier stages, when dementia per se is not present, to see if tau is elevated and predictive of the imminent onset of symptomatology. At present we do not

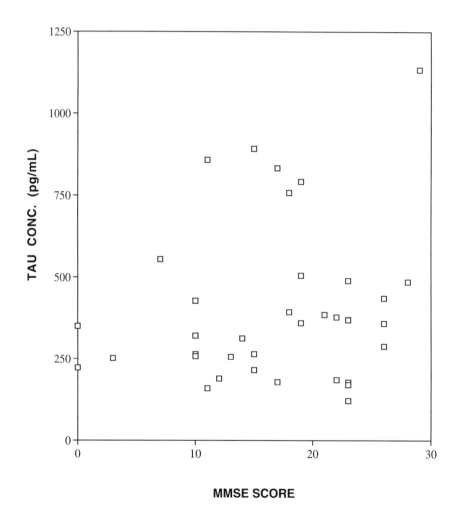

MMSE SCORE

FIGURE 3. Lack of correlation of mini-mental state examination scores with tau levels. MMSE scores were plotted against tau levels for the AD subjects described in Figures 1–3. No significant correlation was detected. One interpretation of this data is that tau elevation persists throughout the course of disease.

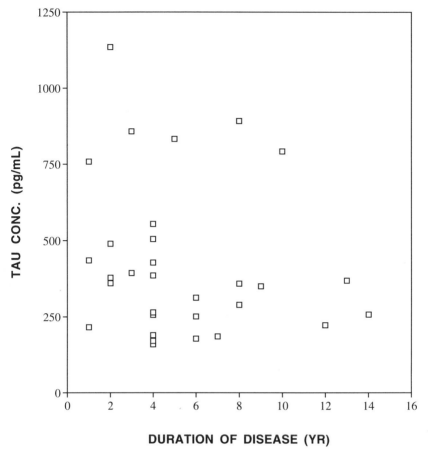

FIGURE 4. Lack of correlation between duration of AD and tau levels. The estimated duration of dementia due to AD was plotted versus tau levels for the AD subjects described in Figure 1–3. No significant relationship was found. These data further support the persistance of the tau elevation in the disease.

know how early the tau increase occurs; however, since false positives in cognitively normal elderly are rare, we infer that the interval is not likely to be very long.

In addition, other conditions that can be confused clinically with AD, including depression, frontal lobe dementias, and Lewy body disease, generally do not show increased CSF in tau. In the published experience with CSF tau, patients with neurological and neurodegenerative conditions that would not be mistaken for AD usually show low CSF tau, with some exceptions. From the literature and our own published observations, increased levels of tau occur in some cases of stroke (especially if the lumbar puncture is performed within weeks of the event), ALS, multi-infarct dementia, Creutzfeld-Jakob disease, peripheral neuropathy, and brain damage due to acute carbon monoxide poisoning. These exceptions accounted for fewer than 5% of neurological controls in the published studies, and it should be emphasized that concomitant AD was not definitively ruled out in these cases. It should also be noted that not all AD subjects show elevated levels of tau. Studies are in progress to determine if antemortem tau levels relate to postmortem pathology. For example, CSF tau levels seem to correlate with NFT counts (Galasko et al., 1995) but less strongly with plaque counts. Interestingly several demented patients with normal tau levels turned out to have the Lewy body variant of AD, in which lower NFT counts are usually seen.

Since PHF tau is extensively phosphorylated, much of the research surrounding tau and PHF formation has concentrated in this area [reviewed in Trojanowski and Lee, (1994)]. In the non-AD human brain multiple potential phosphorylation sites are apparently not phosphorylated, in contrast to the phosphorylation observed on PHF tau. This would suggest that phosphorylated tau measurements in CSF might be of even more utility than a "pan-tau" assay. Certain lines of evidence actually argue against this approach. First, the phosphorylation state of normal human brain tau is actually fairly extensive, when examined in biopsied specimens. The lack of phosphorylation previously detected is largely due to dephosphorylation occurring during the postmortem interval (Matsuo et al. (1994). Also, elevation of tau in non-AD CSF samples is unusual, so determining the phosphorylation state of CSF tau is unlikely to add specificity to the test.

Use of Combined Measures

It is unlikely any single test will, with perfect specificity, correctly identify all AD patients regardless of disease stage. Simultaneous measure of multiple analytes may improve the specificity and/or sensitivity over that of a single test either by providing a second positive indication of the presence of AD or, as will be described below, by identifying individuals who do not have the disease.

In our own research we have utilized the simultaneous measure of tau and $A\beta_{42}$. A plot of combined data from Figures 1 and 2 is shown in Figure 5. The plot can be subdivided into four quadrants using marker value cutoffs optimized for specificity as shown. Use of the combined measures allows accurate classification of more subjects than either one alone. For example, subjects with normal tau levels, which includes several AD subjects, can be further resolved by the use of $A\beta_{42}$ levels. Note that the upper left quadrant of Figure 5 (normal tau, normal $A\beta_{42}$) is virtually free of AD subjects. Thus, while an elevated tau level indicates AD is very likely, a normal tau level alone does not rule out AD unless combined with a normal level of $A\beta_{42}$. Similarly, the ability of low $A\beta_{42}$ levels to dictate a diagnosis of AD is enhanced when combined with an elevated tau measure. Sixty percent of the subjects in this study were classified into a quadrant that yields diagnostic information (the upper-left or lower-right quadrants). At this point we have neither the longitudinal nor the pathological data to explain why some subjects are not classified definitively by these tests, although speculations have been presented above and are under active investigation.

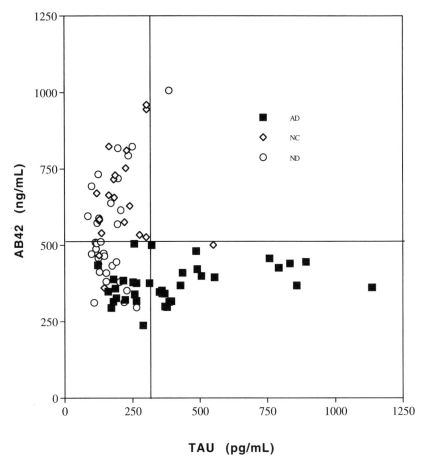

FIGURE 5. Combined measure of tau and $A\beta_{42}$. The data from Figures 1 and 2 are combined. Cutoff lines were drawn for optimal specificity for AD. Note that only a single non-AD subject is in the lower-right quadrant (1/22) and that the upper-left quadrant is exclusively non-AD subjects. Combined use of measures allows accurate classification of more subjects than either measure alone. Figure reproduced from Motter et al. (1995), with permission.

FUTURE CONSIDERATIONS

As stated earlier, the goal of discovering biomarkers for the differential diagnosis of AD is to assist the clinician in determining the cause of cognitive decline in a presenting patient. Current research is providing rational assays that are promising in this task. While certain of these tests, alone or in combination, approach the clinician's level of accuracy of diagnosis, future research will be challenged to prove whether these tests can predict the imminent onset of AD before extensive synaptic loss or neurodegeneration has occurred. As stressed in the beginning of this review, early identification of the AD patients most likely to benefit from treatment is critical as therapeutic options become available. If the present CSF markers for AD truly reflect the process of plaque deposition, tangle formation, and/or synaptic loss, then one would predict these markers to have utility in identifying the early-stage patient as well as in monitoring the efficacy of various therapies targeted against these destructive processes.

REFERENCES

Abraham CR, Selkoe DJ, Potter H (1988): Immunochemical identification of the serine protease inhibitor α1-antichymotrypsin in the brain amyloid deposits of Alzheimer's disease. Cell 52:487–501.

Arai H, Terajima M, Miura M, Higuchi S, Muramatsu T, Machida N, Seiki H, Takase S, Clark CM, Lee V M-Y, Trojanowski JQ, Sasaki A (1995): Tau in cerebrospinal fluid: A potential diagnostic marker in Alzheimer's disease. Ann Neurol 38:649–652.

Atack J, May C, Kaye J, Kay AD, Rapoport SI (1988a): Cerebrospinal fluid cholinesterases in aging and in dementia of the Alzheimer type. Ann Neurol 23:161–167.

Atack JR, Beal MF, May C, Kay JA, Mazurek MF, Kay AD, Rapoport SI (1988b): Cerebrospinal fluid somatostatin and neuropeptide Y Concentrations in aging and in dementia of the Alzheimer type with and without extrapyramidal signs. Arch Neurol 435:269–274.

Blennow K, Wallin A, Agren H, Spenger C, Siegfried J, Vanmechelen E (1995a): Tau protein in cerebrospinal fluid: A biochemical marker for axonal degeneration in Alzheimer's disease? Mol Chem Neuropathol 26:231–245.

Blennow K, Wallin A, Chong JK (1995b): Cerebrospinal fluid "neuronal thread protein" comes from serum by passage over the blood-brain barrier. Neurodegeneration 4:187–193.

Blennow K, Davidsson P, Wallin A, Gottfries CG, Svennerholm L (1994a): Ubiquitin in cerebrospinal fluid in Alzheimer's disease and vascular dementia. Internal Psychoger 6:13–22.

Blennow K, Hesse C, Fredman P (1994b): Cerebrospinal fluid apolipoprotein E is reduced in Alzheimer's disease. Neuroreport 5:2534–2536.

Blennow K, Wallin A, Häger O (1993): Low frequency of post-lumbar puncture headache in demented patients. Acta Neurol Scand 88:221–223.

Blennow K, Wallin A, Gottfries CG, Lekman A, Karlsson I, Skoog I, Svennerholm L (1991): Significance of decreased lumbar CSF levels of HVA and 5-HIAA in Alzheimer's disease. Neurobiol Aging 13:107–113.

Carlsson J, Armstrong VW, Reiber H, Felgenhauer K, Seidel D (1991): Clinical relevance of the quantification of apolipoprotein E in cerebrospinal fluid. Clin Chem Acta 196: 167–156.

Choi-Miura NH, Ihara Y, Fukuchi K, Takeda M, Nakano Y, Tobe T, Tomita M (1992): SP-40, 40 is a constituent of Alzheimer's amyloid. Acta Neuropathol (Berl) 83:260–264.

Davis KL, Hsieh JY-K, Levy MI (1982): Cerebrospinal fluid acetylcholine, choline, and senile dementia of the Alzheimer's type. Psychopharmacol Bull 18:193–195.

de la Monte SM, Volicer L, Hauser SL, Wands JR (1992): Increased levels of neuronal thread protein in cerebrospinal fluid of patients with Alzheimer's disease. Ann Neuronal 32:733–742.

Delamarche C, Berger F, Gallard L, Pouplard-Barthelaix A (1991): Aging and Alzheimer's disease: Protease inhibitors in cerebrospinal fluid. Neurobiol Aging 12:71–74.

Elble R, Giacobini E, Scarsella GF (1987); Cholinesterases in cerebrospinal fluid. Arch Neurol 44:403–407.

Galasko D, Clark C, Chang L, Miller B, Green RC, Motter R, Seubert P (1996): Cerebrospinal fluid levels of tau protein are increased early in the course of Alzheimer's disease. Neurology (in press).

Galasko D, Hansen L, Vigo Pelfrey C, Schenk D, Seubert P (1995): Antemortem CSF tau is related to neuronal pathology at autopsy in Alzheimer's disease (Abst.) Soc Neurosci 581.8.

Glenner GG, Wong CW (1984): Alzheimer's disease: Initial report of the purification and characteristics of a novel cerebrovascular amyloid protein. Biochem Biophys Res Comm 120:885–890.

Golabek A, Marques MA, Lalowski M, Wisniewski T (1995): Amyloid β binding proteins in vitro and in normal human cerebrospinal fluid. Neurosci Lett 191:79–82

Gravina SA, Ho L, Eckman CB, Long KE, Otvos Jr. L, Younkin LH, Suzuki N, Younkin SG (1995): Amyloid β protein (Aβ) in Alzheimer's disease brain: Biochemical and immunocytochemical analysis with antibodies specific for forms ending at Aβ_{40} or Aβ42(43). J Biol Chem 270:7013–7016.

Henriksson T, Barbour RM, Braa S, Ward P, Fritz LC, Johnson-Wood K, Chung HD, Burke W, Reinikainen KJ, Riekkinen P, Schenk DB (1991): Analysis and quantitation of the β-amyloid precursor protein in the cerebrospinal fluid of Alzheimer's disease patients with a monoclonal antibody-based immunoassay. J Neurochem 56:1037–1042.

Hindley NJ, Jobst KA, King E, Barnetson L, Smith A, Haigh AM (1995): High acceptability and low morbidity of diagnostic lumbar puncture in elderly subjects of mixed cognitive status. Acta Neurol Scand 91:405–411.

Hock C, Golombowski S, Naser W, Müller-Spahn (1995): Increased levels of τ protein in cerebrospinal fluid of patients with Alzheimer's disease-correlation with degree of cognitive impairment. Ann Neurol 37:414–415.

Ishii T, Haga S (1984): Immuno-electron microscopic localization of complements in amyloid fibrils of senile plaques. Acta Neuropath (Berl) 63:296–300.

Iwatsubo T, Odaka A, Suzuki N, Mizusawa H, Nukina N, Ihara Y (1994): Visualization of Aβ42(43) and Aβ40 in senile plaques with end-specific Aβ monoclonals: Evidence that an initially deposited species is Aβ42(43). Neuron 13:45–53.

Jarrett JT, Berger EP, Lansbury Jr. PT (1993). The carboxy terminus of the β amyloid protein is critical for the seeding of amyloid formation: implications for the pathogenesis of Alzheimer's disease. Biochemistry 32:4693–4697.

Jensen M, Basun H, Lannfelt L (1995): Increased cerebrospinal fluid tau in patients with Alzheimer's disease. Neurosci Lett 186:189–191.

Kang J, Lemaire HG, Unterbeck A, Salbaum JM, Masters CL, Grzeschik K-H, Multihaup G, Beyreuther K, Müller-Hill B (1987): The precursor of Alzheimer's disease amyloid A4 protein resembles a cell surface receptor. Nature 325:733–736.

Kaye JA, May C, Daly E, Atack JR, Sweeney DJ, Luxenberg JS, Kay AD, Kaufman S, Milstein S, Friedland RP, Rapoport SI (1968): Cerebrospinal fluid monoamine markers are decreased in dementia of the Alzheimer type. Neurology 88:554–557.

Kudo T, Iqbal K, Ravid R, Swaab D, Brundke-Iqbal (1994): Alzheimer disease: Correlation of cerebro-spinal fluid and brain ubiquitin levels. Brain Res 639:1–7.

Lehtimäki T, Pirtilliä T, Mehta PD, Wisniewski HM, Frey H, Nikkari T (1995): Apoliprotein E (ApoE) polymorphism and its influence on ApoE concentrations in the cerebrospinal fluid in Finnish patients with Alzhemier's disease. Hum Genet 95:39–42.

Licastro F, Parnetti L, Morina MC, Davis LJ, Cucinotta D, Gaiti A, Senin U (1995): Acute phase reactant α1-antichymotrypsin is increased in cerebrospinal and serum of patients with probable Alzheimer disease. Alzheimer Dis Assoc Disorder 9:112–118.

Manaka H, Kato T, Kurita K, Katagiri T, Shikama Y. Kujirai K, Kawanami T, Suzuki Y, Nihei K, Sasaki H (1992): Marked increase in cerebrospinal fluid ubiquitin in Creutzfeld-Jacob disease. Neurosci Lett 139:47–49.

Masters CL, Simms G, Weinman A, Multhaup G, McDonald BL, Beyreuther K (1985): Amyloid plaque protein in Alzheimer's disease and Down's syndrome. Proc Natl Acad Sci U S A 82:4245–4269.

Matsubara E, Hirai S, Amari M, Shoji M, Yamaguchi H, Okamoto K, Ishiguro K, Harigaya Y, Wakabayashi (1990): α1-Antichymotrypsin as a possible marker for Alzheimer-type dementia. Ann Nuerol 28:561–567.

Matsuo ES, Shin R-W, Billingsley ML, Van de Voorde A, O'Connor M, Trojanowski JQ, Lee V M-Y (1994): Biopsy-derived adult human brain tau is phosphorylated at many of the same sites as Alzheimer's disease paired helical filament tau. Neuron 13:989–1002.

McGeer PL, Kawamata T, Walker DG (1992): Distribution of clusterin in Alzheimer brain tissue. Brain Res 579:337–341.

Mori H, Hosoda K,Matsubara E, Nakamoto T, Furiya Y, Endoh R, Usami M, Shoji M, Maruyama S, Hirai S (1995): Tau in cerebrospinal fluids: Establishment of the sandwich ELISA with antibody specific to the repeat sequence in tau. Neurosci Lett 186:181–183.

Mori H, Kondo J, Ihara Y (1987): Ubiquitin is a component of paired helical filaments in Alzheimer's disease. Science 235:1641–1644.

Motter R, Vigo-Pelfrey C, Kholodenko D, Barbour R, Johnson-Wood K, Galasko D, Chang L, Miller B, Clark C, Green R, Olson D, Southwick P, Wolfert R, Munroe B, Lieberburg I, Seubert P, Schenk D (1995): Reduction of β-amyloid peptide 42 in the cerebrospinal fluid of patients with Alzheimer's disease. Ann Neurol 38:643–648.

Munroe WA, Southwick PC, Chang I, Scharre DW, Echols Jr. CL, Fu Pc, Whaley JM, Wolfert RL (1995): Tau protein in cerebrospinal fluid as an aid in the diagnosis of Alzheimer's disease. Ann Clin Lab Sci 25:207–217.

Nakamura T, Shoji M, Harigaya Y, Wantanabe M, Hosoda K, Cheung TT, Shaffer LM, Golde TE, Younkin LH, Younkin SG, Hirai S (1994): Amyloid β protein levels in cerebrospinal fluid are elevated in early-onset Alzheimer's disease. Ann Neurol 36:903–911.

Namba Y, Tomonaga M, Kawasaki H, Otomo E, Ikeda K (1991): Apolipoprotein E immunoreactivity in cerebral amyloid deposits and neurofibrillary tangles in Alzheimer's disease and Kuru plaque amyloid in Creutzfeld-Jakob disease. Brain Res 531:163–166.

Nitsch RM, Rebeck GW, Deng M, Richardson UI, Tennis M, Schenk DB, Vigo-Pelfrey C, Lieberburg I, Wurtman RJ, Hyman BT, Growden JH (1995): Cerebrospinal fluid levels of amyloid β-protein in Alzheimer's disease: Inverse correlation with severity of dementia and effect of apolipoprotein E genotype. Ann Neurol 37:512–518.

O'Connor DT, Cervenka HJ, Stone RA, Parmer RJ, Franco-Bourland RE, Madrazo I, Langlais P (1993): Chromogranin A immunoreactivity in human cerebrospinal fluid: Properties, relationship to noradrenergic neuronal activity, and variation in neurologic disease. Neurosciences 56:999–1007.

Oda T, Pasinetti GM, Osterburg HH, Anderson C, Johnson SA, Finch CE (1994); Purification and characterization of brain clusterin. Biochem Biophys Res Comm 204: 1131–1136.

Ozturk M, de la Monte SM, Gross J, Wands JR (1989): Elevated levels of an exocrine pancreatic secretory protein in Alzheimer's disease brain. Proc Natl Acad Sci U S A 86:419–423.

Palmert MR, Usiak M, Mayeux R, Raskind M, Tourtellotte WW, Younkin SG (1990): Soluble derivatives of the β amyloid protein precursor in cerebrospinal fluid: Alterations in normal aging and in Alzheimers' disease. Neurology 40:1028–1034.

Perry EK, Tomlinson BE, Blessed G, Bergmann K, Gibson PH, Perry RH (1978): Correlation of cholinergic abnormalities with senile plaques and mental test scores in senile dementia. Br Med J 2:1457–1459.

Pirttila T, Mehta PD, Frey H, Wisniewski HM (1994): α1-Antichymotrypsin and IL-1β are not increased in CSF or serum in Alzheimer's disease. Neurobiol Aging 15:313–317.

Pitas RE, Boyles JK, Lee SH, Foss D, Mahley RW (1987): Astrocytes synthesize apolipoprotein E and metabolize apoplipoprotein E-containing lipoproteins. Biochem Biophys Acta 917:148–161.

Pomara N, Singh R, Deptula D, Chou JC-Y, Schwartz M, LeWitt P (1992): Glutamate and other CSF amino acids in Alzheimer's disease. Am J Psych 149:251–254.

Prior R, Mönning U, Schreiter-Gasser U, Weidemann A, Blennow K, Gottfries CG, Masters CL, Beyreuther K (1991): Quantitative changes in the amyloid βA4 precursor protein in Alzheimer cerebrospinal fluid. Neurosci Lett 124:69–73.

Riemenschneider M, Buch K, Schmolke M, Kurz A, Guder WG (1996): Cerebrospinal protein tau is elevated in early Alzheimer's disease. Neurosci Lett 212:209–211.

Scheuner D, Bird T, Citron M, Lannfelt L, Schellenberg G, Selkoe DJ, Viitanen M, Younkin SG (1995): Fibroblasts from carriers of familial AD linked to chromosome 14 show increased Aβ production. Soc Neurosci Abs 589.10.

Scott RB (1993): Extraneuronal manifestations of Alzheimer's disease. J Am Geriatr Soc 41:268–276.

Selkoe DJ (1994): Cell biology of the amyloid β-protein precursor and the mechanism of Alzheimer's disease. Ann Rev Cell Biol 10:373–403.

Seubert P, Oltersdorf T, Lee MG, Barbour R, Blomquist C, Davis DL, Bryant K, Fritz LC, Galaski D, Thal LJ, Lieberburg I, Schenk DB (1993): Secretion of β-amyloid precursor protein cleaved at the amino terminus of the β-amyloid peptide. Nature 361:260–263.

Seubert P, Vigo-Pelfrey C, Esch F, Lee M, Dovey H, Davis D, Sinha S, Schlossmacher M, Whaley J, Swindlehurst C, McCormack R, Wolfert R, Selkoe D, Lieberburg I, Schenk D (1992): Isolation and quantification of soluble Alzheimer's β-peptide from biological fluids. Nature 359:325–327.

Shinohara Y, Yamamoto M, Ohsuga H, Ohsuga S, Akiyama K, Yoshii F, Tsuda M, Kamiguchi H, Yamamura M (1991): Alpha-1-antichymotrypsin and antitrypsin in CSF of patients with Alzheimer-type dementia. In Iqbal K, McLachlan DRC, Winblad B, Wisniewski HM (eds): "Alzheimer's Disease: Basic Mechanisms, Diagnosis and Therapeutic Strategies" New York: Wiley, pp 541–545.

Shoji M, Golde TE, Ghiso J, Cheung TT, Estus S, Shaffer LM, Cai X-D, McKay DM, Tintner R, Frangione B, Younkin SG (1992): Production of the Alzheimer amyloid β protein by normal proteolytic processing. Science 258:126–129.

Smyth MD, Cribbs DH, Tenner AJ, Shankle WR, Dick M, Kesslak JP, Cotman CW (1994): Decreased levels of Clq in cerebrospinal fluid of living Alzheimer patients correlate with disease state. Neurobiol Aging 15:609–614.

Sofic E, Fritze J, Schnaberth G, Bruck J, Riederer P (1989): Biogenic amines and their metabolites in neurodegenerative diseases. J Neuro Trans 1:131–132.

Southwick P, Yamagata SK, Echols CL, Higson GJ, Neynaber SA, Parson RE, Munroe WA (1996): Assessment of amyloid β protein in cerebrospinal fluid as an aid in the diagnosis of Alzheimer's disease. J Neurochem 66:259–265.

Strittmatter WJ, Saunders AM, Schmechel D, Pericak-Vance M, Enghild J, Salvesen GS, Roses AD (1993): Apolipoprotein E: High avidity binding to β-amyloid and increased frequency of type 4 allele in late-onset familial Alzheimer disease. Proc Natl Acad Sci U S A 90:1977–1981.

Suzuki N, Cheung TT, Cai X-D, Odaka A, Otvos L, Eckman C, Golde TE, Younkin SG (1994): An increased percentage of long amyloid β protein secreted by familial amyloid β protein precursor (βAPP_{717}) mutants. Science 264:1336–1340.

Tato RE, Frank A, Hernanz A (1995): Tau concentrations in cerebrospinal fluid of patients with dementia of the Alzheimer type. J Neruol Neurosurg Psych 59:280–283.

Tohgi H, Abe T, Takahashi S, Kumura M, Takahashi J, Kikuchi T (1992): Concentrations of serotonin and its related substances in the cerebrospinal fluid in patients with Alzheimer's type dementia. Neurosci Lett 141:9–12.

Trojanowski JQ, Lee VM-Y (1994): Phosphorylation of neuronal cytoskeletal proteins in Alzheimer's disease and Lewy body dementias. Am N Y Acad Sci 747:92–109.

Urakami K, Takahashi K, Saitoh H, Okada A, Nakamura S, Tanaka S, Kitaguchi N, Tokushima Y, Yamamoto S (1992): Amyloid β protein precursors with kunitz-type protease inhibitor domains and acetylcholinesterase in cerebrospinal fluid from patients with dementia of the Alzheimer type. Acta Neurol Scand 85:343–346.

Van Gool WA, Bolhuis PA (1991): Cerebrospinal fluid markers of Alzheimer's disease. J Am Geriatr Soc 39:1025–1039.

Van Nostrand WE, Wagner SL, Shankle WR, Farrow JS, Dick M. Rozemuller JM, Kuiper MA, Wolters EC, Zimmerman J, Cotman CW, Cunningham DD (1992): Decreased levels of soluble amyloid β-protein precursor in cerebrospinal fluid of live Alzheimer disease patients. Proc Natl Acad Sci U S A 89:2551–2555.

Vandermeeren M, Mercken M, Vanmechelen E, Six J, Van de Voorde A, Martin J-J, Cras P (1993): Detection of τ proteins in normal and Alzheimer's disease cerebrospinal fluid with a senstivie sandwich enzyme-linked immunosorbent assay. J Neurochem 61: 1828–1834.

Vigo-Pelfrey C, Seubert P, Barbour R, Blomquist C, Lee M, Lee D, Coria F, Chang L, Miller B, Lieberburg I, Schenk D (1995): Elevation of microtubule-associated protein tau in the cerebrospinal fluid of patients with Alzheimer's disease. Neurology 45:788–793.

Wang GP, Iqbal K, Bucht G, Winblad B, Wisniewski HM, Grundke-Iqbal I (1991): Alzheimer's disease: Paired helical filament immunoreactivity in cerebrospinal fluid. Acta Neuropathol 82:6–12.

Yamada K, Kono K, Umegaki H, Yamada K, Iguchi A, Fukatsu T, Nakashima N, Nishiwaki H, Shimada Y, Sugita Y, et al. (1995): Decreased interleukin-6 level in the cerebrospinal fluid of patients with Alzheimer type dementia. Neurosci Lett 186:219–221.

CHAPTER 16

Considerations for Clinical Trials in Alzheimer's Disease

NEAL R. CUTLER and JOHN J. SRAMEK

California Clinical Trials, Beverly Hills, California 90211

INTRODUCTION

Controlled clinical trials provide a scientifically sound mechanism for the investigation of promising new compounds for the treatment of Alzheimer's disease (AD). Adherence to rigorous methods in study design and execution are essential to ensure that promising compounds are given the opportunity to display potential efficacy. This chapter will discuss many of the elements that contribute to successful clinical research in Alzheimer's disease. First we review the process of patient assessment and subject selection, considering the difficulty of diagnosing AD, the heterogeneity of the AD population, the prevalence of multiple morbidity in the elderly, and the wide range of disease severity. We then discuss important elements to consider in study design and execution, including sample size, patient compliance, and informed consent. Several types of trial end points are presented and evaluated.

PATIENT ASSESSMENT: SELECTING AD PATIENTS FOR CLINICAL TRIALS

Subject selection is one of the most important variables in planning a successful clinical trial. It demands scrupulous attention, both in early phases assessing safety and tolerance and in later phases evaluating efficacy. Careful subject selection will not only help ensure sound data, but will also minimize safety risks posed to study participants (Darragh et al., 1985). The potential risks to subjects can be minimized

Pharmacological Treatment of Alzheimer's Disease: Molecular and Neurobiological Foundations,
Edited by Brioni and Decker
ISBN 0-471-16758-4   © 1997 Wiley-Liss, Inc.

even in phase I trials, during which humans are first exposed to a given study compound. One review of 157 phase I trials involving 1325 normal volunteers noted no serious side effects related to drug administration (Johansson et al., 1984). Another analysis of data from 331 researchers involving 133,000 subjects in many protocols over a 3-year period reported that injuries occurred in only 3.7% of subjects, and of those injuries, 1% (49 subjects) were fatal or permanently disabling (Cardon et al., 1976). Achieving these impressive statistics is the result of continued efforts to ensure patient safety.

A major tool in optimizing subject selection is the careful definition of inclusion/exclusion criteria. These criteria define the types of patients to be enrolled, delineating characteristics necessary for a subject's inclusion in or exclusion from the trial. Such guidelines tend to become more stringent as understanding of the disease being studied increases. They require consideration of the following factors.

Diagnostic Criteria

The most important characteristic of patients in an AD drug trial is presence of Alzheimer's disease, yet AD is difficult to diagnose with absolute certainty while a patient is alive. Investigators must make every effort to include only those patients who meet accepted diagnostic criteria for AD and exclude those who have secondary causes of dementia. Particular attention should be paid to identifying subjects with diseases that are often misdiagnosed as AD, including Parkinson's disease, multi-infarct dementia, and brain tumor. To accurately evaluate the effects of a compound on the progression of AD, such patients need to be excluded from enrollment in the trial.

Even the most conscientious efforts at clinical diagnosis are inevitably imprecise. It has been estimated that in patients enrolled in AD clinical trials, diagnostic accuracy is only 75–80% (Reines, 1989). Although a number of sets of criteria can be used to establish the presence of dementia, only a few have met with widespread acceptance. Diagnostic validity is enhanced by using the *Diagnostic and Statistical Manual* (DSM; now in its fourth edition) of the American Psychiatric Association, the tenth edition of the International Classification of Diseases (ICD-10), and/or the NINCDS-ADRDA criteria for AD (APA, 1994; World Health Organization, 1992; McKhann et al., 1984; Amaducci et al. 1990).

In our own trials, the diagnosis of probable AD has been most frequently determined by clinical evaluation and by NINCDS-ADRDA and DSM criteria. The NINCDS-ADRDA document defines dementia as progressive and global memory loss accompanied by deterioration of other intellectual functions including deficits in at least two of the following areas: language use, perception, motor skills, learning ability, problem solving, abstract thought, and judgment. Alzheimer's disease is then defined as the condition of having dementia with onset between ages 40 and 90, and absence of systemic or other brain diseases that could account for dementia, and a lack of disturbance in consciousness. Generally, progressive memory deterioration and declines in other cognitive functions must have been observed or documented for a year or more.

A number of cognitive function tests and scales for the assessment of AD are also frequently administered with particular scores required for inclusion in the study population. Such tests can be administered and scored by independent investigators to minimize bias. Several of the more common rating/staging instruments and typical cutoff scores for patient inclusion include:

- Folstein Mini-Mental State Examination (MMSE) score between 12 and 26 (Folstein et al., 1975)
- Global Deterioration Scale (GDS) score of 3–5 (Reisberg et al., 1982)
- Hamilton Depression Scale score less than 18 (Hamilton, 1960)
- Wechsler Adult Intelligence Scale (WAIS), Vocabulary Subtest, scaled score of 9 or higher (Stone et al., 1988)
- Modified Hachinski ischemia scale score of 4 or less (Rosen et al., 1980).

Patients should be excluded from participation if any part of their physical or neurological examinations, as well as laboratory analyses, show any abnormalities that might indicate alternate causes for whatever dementia is suffered by the patient. Computerized tomography scans or magnetic resonance imaging scans within one year of enrollment must be compatible with probable AD and can be used to detect exclusionary characteristics such as intracranial mass lesions, potential or extant tumors, or signs of vascular dementia. Chest X-rays can identify other disqualifying criteria, including aneurysms and malignancies. Furthermore, because some central nervous system (CNS) active compounds (including some cholinergics) can reduce seizure threshold, patients with underlying seizure disorders must be excluded, and consequently, an electroencephalogram with hyperventilation should be performed. A patient history is another source of information, acquired from medical records and from the subject, family members, or caregivers. For AD patients, a responsible caregiver must be available, not only to answer inquiries during subject screening but also to administer study medication during outpatient portions of the study.

Homogeneity of Study Population

Investigators should attempt to enroll a homogenous group of patients to minimize variance introduced by outside factors. This greatly improves the validity of statistical analyses. As early as phase I trials, information can be collected that reflects not only the safety profile of the compound but also the potential effect of the drug on the cognitive capacity of patients. If the entry criteria are not tightly defined, however, the study population may be so heterogenous that results are much less valuable. For example, if patients with other dementing disorders besides AD were to be included, a potentially effective AD compound might appear to be ineffective since it would not necessarily have an effect in the patients with other disorders. At the other extreme, if criteria are too restrictive, investigators may have difficulty enrolling an adequate number of subjects into the trial.

One factor that can influence the heterogeneity of the study population is patient age. Early investigational drug studies in most diseases generally exclude elderly subjects for several reasons. First, young healthy subjects are easier to recruit. More importantly, however, older subjects respond differently to compounds than do younger populations because of pharmacokinetic, homeostatic, and other alterations that occur with physiological aging. These changes tend to cause a greater number of adverse effects associated with drug use, making early trials in elderly populations less safe than in young populations. Despite these complications, AD trials must include aged populations early on in clinical trials. While young volunteers can serve as subjects early in the investigational process, it is important to test the drug in elderly populations—both healthy and with AD—as early as possible to accurately show the drug's effects on the target population.

Unfortunately, the elderly population that makes up the large majority of AD patients tends to be more heterogenous than younger populations. It has been suggested that even patients who meet commonly accepted diagnostic criteria for AD and have no other exclusionary disorders comprise a heterogeneous population according to neuropsychological, clinical, neuropathologic, and neurochemical parameters (Siegfried, 1991). As a result, when utilizing random samples in clinical trials that evaluate possible AD compounds, the resulting data may not reveal subpopulations of diseased patients for whom the agent may be most appropriate. Subtle drug effects in particular subgroups may be lost when patient characteristics are diverse.

Another concern associated with age that can affect heterogeneity is that AD patients tend to differ according to their age at onset of AD. Patients with early disease onset tend to have fewer neuropathologic and neurochemical changes (e.g., neurotransmitter and neuropeptide deficiencies, decreased concentrations of plaques and tangles) than do patients with late-onset AD. While it remains unknown whether this phenomenon is related to the disease process itself or to individual differences, it may influence a subject's response to CNS-active compounds (Cutler, 1989; Cutler et al., 1991).

Multiple Diseases/Medications

Many elderly patients with AD have secondary diseases ranging from hypertension, atherosclerosis, osteoarthritis, and osteoporosis to diabetes, stroke, and cancer. Most of these illnesses require one or more medications. As we have noted, adverse drug reactions generally tend to be up to three times higher in the elderly than in younger subjects, and the risks of these responses increase with polypharmacy (Nolan and O'Malley, 1988a,b). Elderly subjects tend to exhibit a greater sensitivity to CNS-active drugs and are more likely to show adverse effects from these compounds. Such increased sensitivity is attributed to changes in patient parameters such as cardiac index, renal function, basal metabolic rate, vital capacity, tissue perfusion, and end-organ receptor changes associated with aging.

One disease to be considered in AD drug trials is depression. Depression can influence both physiological as well as psychological response to the treatment compound and is of particular concern in tests of CNS-active drugs. The Cornell Scale for Depression in Dementia, which utilizes information from caregivers and a patient interview, has been found to be a reliable and sensitive rating scale for evaluating the severity of depression in patients being considered for entry into AD drug trials (Alexopoulos et al., 1988). The Hamilton Depression Rating Scale is also frequently used, though it is not as specific to AD as the Cornell scale since it measures characteristics such as insomnia and retardation that are not applicable to AD due to sleep–wake reversal in demented patients (Cutler, 1989). The utility of the Hamilton scale has also been questioned because it requires the subject to have sufficient cognitive capacity and judgment to respond to questions associated with affect and ideation and thus may not be a valid tool in assessing patients with moderate to severe dementia (Alexopoulos et al., 1988).

The preponderance of concomitant diseases and medications complicates recruitment of patients for AD trials. As a general rule, protocols should not allow use of concomitant medications that could potentiate the effects of the compound being tested or mask the evaluation of adverse events. This restriction would therefore exclude patients with a large number of specific diseases since it might endanger patient safety were patients to temporarily discontinue regular medications. Furthermore, the potential for adverse drug reactions increases exponentially as more drugs are administered, regardless of age. Therefore, drugs are best studied as monotherapy, and particularly in the United States, protocols usually attempt to achieve this goal. Of course, it is not always possible to do so since as many as 87% of elderly subjects are taking other medications (Alexopoulos et al., 1988), with some studies placing the mean number of prescribed medications at two to three per individual (Nolan and O'Malley, 1988b). Researchers must also keep in mind that if investigational drugs are ultimately approved and widely prescribed, they will often be taken concomitantly with previously excluded medications by patients with multiple disorders. Nevertheless, it remains important to exclude patients with certain clinically significant diseases in the testing process for AD compounds, at least through the early part of phase II, either because of increased risk to the patient or because these concomitant diseases are likely to confound test results. Concomitant medical disorders commonly listed as exclusion criteria include the presence of significant cardiovascular, thyroid, hepatic, renal, pulmonary, gastrointestinal illness, other central nervous system disorders (particularly stroke), or any other disorder (or its drug treatment) that could interfere with the absorption, distribution, metabolism, or excretion of the study compound.

After initial safety and efficacy trials, phase III trials may use less stringent criteria in patient selection. This ensures that the drug will be tested in a population that is more representative of the one that will eventually take the marketed compound, should the compound make it that far. This helps to characterize side effect profiles in patients on multiple medications as well as determine long-term effects.

Disease Severity

AD is a chronic, progressive disease, and subjects lie on a continuum of disease severity. It is possible that particular compounds may have greater potential for efficacy at one part of the severity spectrum than another. Thus, data derived from patients with mild dementia may not be predictive of drug activity in patients with severe disease, and vice versa. In a study of the centrally active calcium channel blocker nimodipine, for example, those patients with mild AD (as indicated by a high MMSE score) exhibited less clear-cut response to nimodipine than did those with severe AD (Cutler, 1993). Thus, it is important to determine disease severity in enrolled patients, and to take this information into account when response and outcome data are evaluated, especially for CNS-active drugs. Degree of dementia, in fact, may be an exclusionary criteria: if patients are severely demented, they may be incapable of comprehending and/or adhering to instructions about taking the study compound as defined in the protocol or in following directions during evaluative tests administered to assess drug efficacy.

To complicate matters, disease severity can change during the course of a clinical trial. Although investigators might carefully diagnose each subject as he or she is enrolled in the trial, disease progression does occur, and its rate will vary from individual to individual. AD drugs are generally considered successful if they arrest progression of the disease, enabling drug-treated patients to remain at a particular severity of dementia while the cognitive abilities of placebo-treated patients continue to deteriorate over the course of a drug trial. For example, in one of the large studies of tacrine, the statistically significant advantage of tacrine seen after 6 weeks of treatment was based not on improvement in tacrine patients per se, but on the significantly smaller decline on the Alzheimer's Disease Assessment Scale (ADAS; Rosen et al., 1984) seen in tacrine patients as compared to placebo patients (0.7 points compared to 3.8 points) (Davis et al., 1992). In cases like this, it is worthwhile to determine whether a drug's efficacy is observed only at particular disease stages or at all stages in the course of the illness. While there is no consensus on the best instrument for assessing severity of disease, a number of scales are available to evaluate degrees of cognitive deficit and are specific for dementia syndromes. These include the MMSE, the ADAS, and GDS, the Mattis Dementia Scale (Mattis, 1976), the Nurses' Observation Scale for Geriatric Patients (NOSGER; Spiegel et al., 1991), the Sandoz Clinical Assessment-Geriatric (Venn, 1983), the Clinical Dementia Rating scale (CDR; Berg, 1988), and the Blessed Memory Information Concentration Test (Blessed et al., 1968). Another useful test not specific to dementia is the Computerized Neuropsychological Test Battery (CNTB; Veroff et al., 1991).

STUDY DESIGN AND EXECUTION

Trial Design

The simplest design for a clinical trial is a parallel group design in which patients are randomly assigned to receive either study medication (one or more dose groups can be used) or placebo. The major disadvantage of this design is that the potential lack of homogeneity between groups necessitates the use of large numbers of patients. These studies are also performed double blind, meaning that neither the patient nor the persons responsible for treatment (including both investigators and drug company personnel) know whether a patient is receiving placebo or experimental treatment.

Outcome objectives must be clearly defined in the protocol prior to conducting a trial. As mentioned earlier, in AD the absence of disease progression may be viewed as a positive outcome. Regardless of the level of "improvement" designated as positive, however, instruments for measuring efficacy must be selected relatively early on in trial deisgn.

Another important consideration is the number of treatment arms that will be incuded. Often more than one active treatment arm is used, with several dose levels of the compound being studied represented. This permits characterization of the side effect profile at different doses relative to the benefits incurred at each dose. Beneficial effects of many drugs in development for AD appear to begin at dosages close to those at which potentially significant side effects occur. An accurate determination of the maximum tolerated dose is essential *prior to efficacy studies* to avoid a no-effect dose.

Sampling Considerations

Sampling issues are very important to a successful clinical trial. There should be no significant demographic or baseline study rating differences between treatment groups, a condition that generally occurs when patients are randomly assigned to study treatment. In instances where baseline data could be easily skewed by relatively few outliers, it may be wise either to control the range of inclusion criteria or to stratify entry into the study at randomization to study medication to ensure statistically equivalent cells.

Sample size is a second critical issue. Producing meaningful and scientifically valid conclusions about the effect of the study drug relative to placebo requires a sampling strategy that is based on accepted statistical practice and adheres to principles of power analysis. Power analysis determines how many patients will be necessary to identify a statistically significant effect in the compound, taking into account the types of statistical tests to be used, the level of heterogeneity in the patients to be studied (greater heterogeneity generally requires a larger number of patients), and the expected magnitude of the treatment's effect. It is important to clarify the goals of a study early on and make sure that the questions asked, statistical techniques utilized, and sample design are all in conjunction. As the questions a study addresses become more complex, more patients will be needed in order to assure that an adequate statistical assessment of efficacy can be undertaken.

Attrition is another factor that can influence statistical validity of results, especially in studies of longer duration. Sample sizes diminish as patients leave a study, either of their own volition—because they fail to see improvement in their symptoms or experience adverse events—or as deemed necessary by the investigator for health, safety, compliance, or other reasons. If the sample becomes too small, entire studies can be compromised, particularly when analyzing last observation carried forward (LOCF) results. U.S. federal guidelines for evaluating drug efficacy require that all patients who enter the randomization phase of a trial be incuded in the final analysis, and that, should they drop out early, their last observation be utilized. When attrition is substantial (>30%) or where a sample is very small, an analysis using LOCF may produce results that do not accurately reflect the efficacy of a drug, limiting the credibility of final results (Merz, 1994). Even where sample sizes are large, results can be seriously compromised by relatively few early discontinuations, which often occur when patients experience poor tolerance of a first dose. If the study involves several dose levels of the compound, and there is sufficient reason to believe that dropouts will be higher in one of the arms (e.g., because of adverse events), then the study should be adequately powered to compensate for this eventuality.

Attrition is doubly problematic when large numbers of individuals drop out from a single treatment group, whether active drug or placebo. Even aside from its statistical importance, it is essential to collect clear data on why individuals leave a study to understand efficacy, safety, and tolerance parameters of an investigational compound.

Patient Compliance

To ensure validity of results in a clinical trial, drugs must be taken according to protocol specifications. Departures from these guidelines by subjects can invalidate study findings, undermining accurate evaluation of the compound being tested (Spilker, 1987). A patient assigned to an active drug group who exhibits poor compliance might achieve outcomes similar to patients in the placebo group, diminishing the likelihood that differences between populations will be detectable (Meinert and Tonascia, 1986). Some subjects will inevitably fail to adhere to the therapy prescribed for them regardless of safeguards set up to prevent this. While some noncompliance is related to intentional noncooperation, it may also be associated with poor patient understanding of the dosage schedule, adverse effects, or difficulty in swallowing large pills. In fact, it is unrealistic to presume that perfect compliance is possible, except perhaps when compounds are administered on an inpatient basis by a member of the research team. Compliance will also vary with dose regimen; perfect compliance is more difficult to achieve with drugs that require dosing three or four times a day than with drugs that require dosing only once or twice a day. Studies have shown that elderly populations tend to comply poorly with drug regimens in general, with one investigation indicating that 59% of participating outpatients over the age of 60 take medications improperly (Shaw, 1982). In AD subjects, declines in cognitive abilities can interfere further with adherence to study protocols. It is therefore critical to enlist the aid of caregivers in ensuring compliance with drug administration schedules and availability of transportation to clinic visits.

Noncompliance can also be minimized by making special efforts during recruitment. Subjects and caregivers should be told why cooperation is important, and should be told the precise dosage schedule repeatedly until the patient and caregiver both comprehend it thoroughly. During subsequent patient visits to the clinic, the patient should bring his or her medication along, so remaining pills can be counted to help determine whether the dosage schedule has been followed. Inquiries should also be made of the subject and caregiver regarding whether the patient has adhered to the assigned drug regimen; this can often be done unobtrusively as part of routine questioning about adverse effects (Pocock, 1983). Some investigators have further improved patient adherence by having drugs delivered daily to patients' homes, by telephoning the patient each time a dosage is supposed to be taken, or by supplying the patient with a preset alarm that rings when medicine should be taken (Spilker, 1987).

Informed Consent

Impaired cognitive function can interfere not only with compliance but also with a subject's capacity to provide informed consent. The U.S. federal government mandates that all subjects participating in clinical trials give both oral and written consent prior to enrollment. Potential risks and benefits of enrollment in the research project, as well as screening tests and the process of randomization, must be explained to patients in layman's language as part of the informed consent process. Care should be taken in enrolling AD subjects in clinical investigations, as the elderly in general are a vulnerable population, and the presence of AD or another dementing illness calls for additional precautions. Experienced staff members should be capable of evaluating whether the older patient has the capacity for assimilating study-related information. Does the subject comprehend the difference between an investigational drug trial and typical medical treatment? Does he or she need the consent form read aloud and seem capable of asking questions to ensure full understanding of the document? AD subjects should offer their own informed consent when possible, although third parties—such as family members, close friends, or caregivers—may need to be brought into the process to play an advocacy role on the patient's behalf. When a third party has assumed power of attorney or legal guardianship of the AD patient, he or she must provide additional consent for the patient.

All protocols and informed consent forms must be reviewed and approved by an Institutional Review Board (IRB) (in the United States) or a comparable Ethics Committee (in the United Kingdom) before initiation of the study. These groups must include members from several disciplines with at least one nonscientist and at least one member not affiliated with the institution that will be conducting the trial. As the major ethical overseer of the clinical trial, the IRB will require the investigator to submit progress reports on the trial and information on any serious or unexpected events that arise during the clinical trial.

Protocols take special care to specify the population to be tested. In phase I trials, normal volunteers are used most often, though there is growing acceptance of the use of patients with the target disease to test safety in the appropriate population. This is especially useful in illnesses where patients may process drugs differently than normal volunteers, including Alzheimer's disease. Indeed, it would be unethical to expose normal volunteers to the drugs used to treat certain disorders (e.g., cancer) (Cutler et al., 1994; Cutler and Sramek, 1995a,b).

These and other considerations are frequently built into the protocol. Even so, it is important for the investigator to stay alert for any events that might compromise the ethical conduct of a trial, since the investigator has a responsibility to inform patients of any relevant information that comes up during a trial that might affect informed consent. The investigator must also take care to train staff members who will be conducting various aspects of the protocol to make sure they maintain acceptable ethical standards. They must also be sure to preserve the blind element of the study and conduct ratings/assessments without bias.

Responses to Consider in Establishing Trial End Points

Many a compound in development as a treatment for Alzheimer's disease has been promising in animal models only to prove disappointing when tested in humans. To date, no animal model is close enough to the disease for predictions to be reliable. Drug development therefore must rely on clinical studies to reveal the true value of a new compound. One difficulty stems from the limitations of primary end point measures, which currently remain based on clinical assessment. A biologically based secondary end point would be less subjective and more useful. Thus, investigators are seeking surrogate markers that could provide additional useful information in the drug development process. To be truly useful, a surrogate marker should have five essential characteristics: first, its response should be linked logically to the primary end point (clinical improvement) on solid theoretical ground (e.g., mediated by a relevant receptor). Second, there should be validation that the change in the surrogate marker is correlated with or is predictive of meaningful changes in the primary end point. Third, the surrogate marker should be quantifiable with adequate precision and a high level of reproducibility. Fourth, the marker should be relatively inexpensive; and fifth, there must be easy access to its use.

Central End-Organ Response. Measures of brain structure, such as computed tomography (CT) and magnetic resonance imaging (MRI) are useful in the diagnosis of AD but have little application in measuring drug response, since the primary structural defects of AD, amyloid plaques and neurofibrillary tangles, are not visible using these techniques. Therefore investigators have turned to functional measures of disease.

Metabolic measures have shown some utility in AD research. Positron emission tomography (PET) and single-photon-emission computerized tomography (SPECT) may be used to obtain quantitative measures of regional cerebral blood flow (rCBF), regional cerebral metabolic rate of glucose ($rCMR_{glc}$), and regional metabolic rate of oxygen ($rCMRO_2$) from the brains of awake humans [for reviews, see Rapoport (1991) and Weinstein et al. (1993)]. In addition, both PET and SPECT are increasingly being used to image specific neurochemical receptors (Busatto and Pilowsky, 1995). As research tools, these techniques have already provided valuable information in the study of end-organ response to drugs in AD, and they are likely to continue to do so in the future. However, their high cost and limited access render these measures of little use in routine clinical drug development.

Frost (1992) argues that more important advances will come from improvements in "chemical resolution." In particular, several receptor ligands containing radioactive tracers for PET or SPECT scans have become available in recent years [see Herscovitch et al (1990) for a review], and these are likely to have great utility in small-scale pharmacological studies. Several studies in this area have revealed the value of taking multiple end-organ measures to elucidate disease mechanisms and determine the effects of potential treatments. For example, Olson et al. (1992) used psychometric tests, EEG, ^{11}C-butanol PET to image rCBF, and ^{11}C-nicotine PET to image cholinergic nicotinic receptors in a single AD patient being treated with nerve growth factor (NGF). NGF caused marked increases in ^{11}C-nicotine uptake (as compared to a baseline value), which the authors ascribed to increased density of cholinergic nerve terminals and/or to increased numbers of nicotinic binding sites per terminal. There was also a significant increase in CBF, which persisted for 3 months after the conclusion of the treatment, at a time when the effects on ^{11}C-nicotine uptake had disappeared, indicating that the two observations are separate phenomena.

In any case, detailed knowledge of AD disease mechanisms and potential treatments may be advanced significantly by the advent of increased chemical resolution in imaging techniques. It is already possible to image neurotransmitter receptors and uptake sites, and imaging of second-messenger systems may soon be possible. In the foreseeable future it may be possible to image DNA and RNA fragments in vivo. All these techniques may have important applications in AD research, although again, their routine use in clinical drug development will remain limited because of high cost and limited accessibility.

A third functional measure that may have limited utility in AD research is the electroencephalogram (EEG). In moderate and severe AD, the EEG shows significant slowing (Soininen and Riekkinin, 1992). Because EEGs remain largely normal throughout the early stages of disease, they have only limited diagnostic applications. However, EEG slowing, which may reflect the degree of cholinergic deficit (Soininen and Riekkinin, 1992), is predictive of a poorer prognosis. The potential lack of specificity of this measure further limits its utility in selecting patients for drug trials.

Electrical response of the brain may also be measured using evoked potentials (EPs). Goodin et al. (1978) reported that one of the components of the auditory evoked potential (the P300) was significantly delayed in patients with dementia, giving impetus to the use of EPs in AD research. However, delays in P300 latency have also been observed in nondementing disorders such as depression and schizophrenia (Pfefferbaum et al., 1984) and in nondemented elderly subjects (Ford and Pfefferbaum, 1985). Despite these results, EP measures do not appear to provide a reliable approach and their potential as diagnostic tools is low.

Investigators have also sought neurochemical measures of response to compounds developed for AD. Analysis of cerebrospinal fluid (CSF) can provide a valuable end-organ measure in research studies. Many CSF markers have been investigated in AD patients, including neurotransmitters, neuropeptides, amino acids, biopterin, and others. CSF measures that may have potential utility in the differential diagnosis of dementia include reductions in levels of somatostatin and corticotropin-releasing factor (CRF) (Soininen et al., 1981, 1984; Serby et al., 1984; Cutler, 1988; Martinez et al., 1993; Yasuda et al., 1993; Tato et al., 1995). One problem with CSF measures is that lumbar punctures are uncomfortable, inconvenient, and carry with them some (albeit remote), risk of damage to the nervous system, either from infection or from the needle itself. Investigators must verify that diagnosis will be significantly improved by use of the procedure before doctors will be comfortable making it a routine diagnostic or study tool.

Of the biological surrogate end points for AD, functional measures of brain metabolism and receptor distribution seem at present to have the most potential for determining the efficacy and mechanism of action of potential treatments, but their use is primarily limited to research settings. There is currently no ideal measure of central biological function that is valid, quantifiable, quick, or easy to use in routine clinical drug development.

Peripheral End-Organ Response. A second area of research has centered on *peripheral* end-organ responses. Since the brain is the target organ for all potential AD compounds, techniques that measure the response of the brain give the most direct indications of a compound's efficacy and mechanism of action. However, in the absence of an effective measure, responses within peripheral organs and tissues can provide important information. Peripheral measures also have the advantages of being relatively inexpensive and noninvasive and of being easier, in general, to measure. Of course, peripheral measures are only useful to the extent that they are tightly coupled with central measures of interest, and many have been tested only to prove disappointing.

One of the primary strategies for pharmacological intervention in AD involves offsetting the deficits of the central cholinergic system by inhibiting acetylcholinesterase (AChE) activity. It would be useful to be able to assess the central activity of these compounds. The most obvious way involves the withdrawal of CSF, but this is highly impractical in studies involving large numbers of subjects. For this reason, a reliable peripheral marker of central AChE activity is desirable.

Human blood has long been known to contain high levels of cholinesterase activity (Galehr and Plattner, 1928), though the function of this activity remains unclear. Withdrawal of blood is routine, and assays for cholinesterase activity in plasma and erythrocytes are relatively simple and straightforward. Therefore, if a consistent relationship could be established between cholinesterase inhibition in the brain and cholinesterase inhibition in one or more blood components, blood cholinesterase assays would constitute a reliable and practical marker for central cholinesterase activity. Evidence for this relationship has been mixed, with some studies showing reliable correlations (Nordgren et al., 1978; Hallack and Giacobini, 1986, 1987, 1989; Sherman and Messamore, 1989; Thomsen et al., 1989, 1991) and others showing correlations to be unreliable (Comroe et al., 1946; Grob et al., 1947; Gershon and Shaw, 1961; Sherman et al., 1987; Becker and Giacobini, 1988).

We therefore cannot recommend uncritical reliance on blood cholinesterase measurements as a marker of AChE inhibition in the brain. However, with attention to a number of methodological issues and cautious interpretation, blood cholinesterase measurements may yet be a reasonable index of central AChE inhibition. Attempts should be made to differentiate AChE from butyrylcholinesterase (BuChE), as AChE inhibition is more meaningful biologically. Separating erythrocytes from plasma provides a good first approximation at such a differentiation, since AChE is the predominant enzyme in erythrocytes and BuChE is the predominant enzyme in plasma (St. Clair et al., 1986; Barr et al., 1988; Sirviö et al., 1989). But there are small amounts of AChE in plasma and BuChE in erythrocytes, so if accurate quantitative results are needed, techniques that specifically measure one or the other enzyme should be employed. These techniques include the use of specific inhibitors or highly discriminating monoclonal antibodies (Siegel et al., 1966; Mikalsen et al., 1986). Furthermore, when assaying for cholinesterase, care should be taken to avoid washing or dilution of the sample if at all possible, because of evidence that a loosely bound pool of reversible inhibitor may be removed in the process (Thomsen et al., 1988; Moriearty and Becker, 1992).

Certain other factors must be kept in mind when interpreting blood cholinesterase data. The relationship between central and peripheral AChE inhibition varies from drug to drug, so it is unlikely that there will ever be an equation to predict central AChE inhibition from erythrocyte AChE inhibition. Even within a single cholinesterase inhibitor, the relationship between central and peripheral inhibition depends on a number of factors, such as mode of administration, acute versus chronic dosing, time after dose, and interindividual differences.

Despite all these caveats, we believe that it is possible that further research may allow erythrocyte AChE inhibition to be used as a marker of brain inhibition. If detailed pharmacokinetic studies of cholinesterase inhibitors included explicit attempts to establish a relationship between the two measures, it might be possible to derive a formula to predict central AChE inhibition from erythrocyte AChE inhibition, provided that the drug was administered in a specified dosing regimen and pharmacokinetic measures were done at specified time points after the dose.

We recently investigated a novel peripheral measure: serum amylase as a marker for the maximum tolerated dose of a muscarinic agonist. We conducted a phase I safety/tolerance study of xanomeline tartrate, an agonist that shows a high affinity for the M1 muscarinic receptor (Sramek et al., 1995). Although the compound has high affinity for the predominantly centrally located M1 receptor, lower affinity binding at other muscarinic sites, including M3 receptors of the pancreas and salivary glands, also occurs. Therefore we examined serum amylase, fractionated into pancreatic and salivary enzymes, as a potential marker of the maximum tolerated dose of xanomeline tartrate as determined by clinical safety evaluations. We found a trend for increased salivary amylase in the highest dosage tested, though the difference was not statistically significant due to the small sample size. One subject with moderate hypersalivation and other intolerable adverse effects at the highest dosage showed a fourfold increase in salivary amylase levels from baseline. If these increases in salivary amylase are due to M3 mediated effects, this suggests that at higher doses, specificity for the M1 receptor may begin to disappear. Though further research is necessary to determine the value of this assay, we concluded that elevated salivary amylase may signal the lower end of the intolerable spectrum for xanomeline.

Neuropsychological Response. Because biological markers have proven so difficult to develop, neuropsychological assessment tools continue to be the mainstay of drug response assessment. They measure improvements in neuropsychological functioning produced by experimental drugs and play a critical role in screening and selection of subjects for participation in clinical drug trials. In addition to their routine purpose of aiding in the selection of demented subjects, such assessments sometimes assist in the more specific objective of selecting subjects with a particular range of severity of dementia.

Unfortunately, the evaluation tools conventionally used to assess changes in neuropsychological function in AD drug studies are not designed well for these goals. The two most universally used tests are the Mini-Mental State Examination (MMSE; Folstein et al., 1975), used for screening and staging, and the Alzheimer's Disease Assessment Scale (ADAS; Rosen et al., 1984), used to measure efficacy. They have significant limitations, particularly in the assessment of patients in the early stages of disease, and as a result, there may be significant errors in subject selection and an insensitivity to drug effects.

While the MMSE has been shown to be an excellent screening instrument in epidemiologic studies of dementia, it has demonstrated deficiencies in the selection and staging of individual subjects. It is a short assessment, concentrating on cognitive dysfunction, and evaluating recent memory, attention, concentration, naming, repetition, comprehension, ideational praxis, constructional praxis, and the capacity to create a sentence. While originally designed to document cognitive change and screen large numbers of subjects, the MMSE is also frequently used to stratify and stage patients according to disease severity for studies of CNS compounds. A perfect score on the MMSE is 30; a score of 26 or less is often used as an inclusion criterion in dementia studies, while a score of 27 or above is used to exclude subjects. A study comparing the MMSE to the Global Deterioration Scale (GDS; Reisberg et al., 1982) in normal elderly subjects and AD patients found a strong relationship between the two tests; however, the range of scores on the MMSE that corresponded to moderate cognitive decline/mild AD on the GDS (stage 4) was 16–23, leading to the conclusion that subjects with MMSE scores greater than 23 cannot be classified as having true AD. Another study reported a false-positive rate of 39% and a false-negative rate of 5% when MMSE cutoff values were 23/24 (Anthony et al., 1982).

The ADAS is the most widely used test battery for measuring drug responsiveness in AD. Designed to measure deficits associated specifically with AD, this instrument evaluates both cognitive and noncognitive dysfunctions in diseased patients, including language, memory, and spatial capacity. The 45-min-long, 21-item test includes word recall and word recognition tasks, other cognitive tasks, and assessment of noncognitive behaviors. The ADAS is not sensitive to mild impairment, however, reducing its potential applications in drug studies that include subjects with mild dementia. Furthermore, it is complex to administer and score, and training of examiners to administer the ADAS is difficult, resulting in standardization problems in multicenter trials. It does, however, have two distinct advantages over other assessment instruments used previously in geriatric psychopharmacologic research: sensitivity to a broader range of severity of dementia and specificity regarding the major dysfunctions characteristic of people with AD.

There are several instruments designed to assess specific functions that may be lost in AD. For instance, in the Benton Visual Retention Test (Benton, 1974), visual memory and constructional praxis ability are measured; the subject is shown cards on which geometric figures of varying complexity appear, after which he or she attempts to reproduce the figures on a sheet of paper. The Buschke Selective Reminding Procedure (Buschke, 1973) is a short-term memory test; it involves reading a list of words to a subject, whereupon he or she repeats those words that are recalled. Some conventional tests are designed as rating scales and screening instruments to specifically measure dementia, and are often used for staging the severity of AD. The Mattis Dementia Rating Scale (Mattis, 1976) measures the primary cognitive deficits of AD and consists of five subscales: attention, initiation and perseveration, construction, conceptualization, and memory. The Blessed Dementia Rating Scale (Blessed et al., 1968) is composed of two parts: a series of questions that assess cognitive function, and a questionnaire that determines the patient's daily-living capabilities; combined scores from these sections provide an overall dementia score. Studies have demonstrated a correlation between the Blessed scale and the neuropathological markers (neurofibrillary tangles, neuritic plaques) of AD.

Because of limitations of existing measures in neuropsychopharmacologic research, we have developed the Computerized Neuropsychological Test Battery (CNTB; Veroff et al., 1991), a new instrument for measuring cognitive function in clinical drug trials of CNS compounds. It evaluates a number of neuropsychological functions: motor speed, information processing rate, attention, verbal and spatial learning, memory and delayed recall, and language and spatial abilities. Broadly comprehensive in the assessment of cognitive functions, its modules are based on established tests—for example, paired associate learning from the Wechsler Memory Scale (Wechsler, 1945), and the Boston Naming Test (Buschke and Fuld, 1974). All are already validated for their sensitivity to changes in neuropsychological functioning associated with focal lesions, aging, AD, and the effect of drugs on the CNS.

The 11 modules of the CNTB are administered in a standardized order and with standardized stimulus durations. Although the computer controls the sequence of administration of the modules and the sequence, pace, and duration of presentation of test stimuli, the CNTB is not an automated test battery. Instead, the computer maximizes ease of administration and serves as an "expert system," assisting the technician administering the test by presenting stimuli, pacing the reading of word lists, and timing responses. For test subjects, their tasks are no more complex and the response demands no more difficult or technical than in traditional tests. In some modules (the word-list learning and paired associate learning modules), the technician reads the words to the subject as they appear on the computer screen, and the subject responds verbally; in other modules (reaction time, visual matching, visual memory), the subject views the visual stimuli as they appear on the computer screen and responds by pointing or striking a single key. No subjective observer judgment is required. All responses are recorded and scored in the computer in a standardized manner; for each subject on each module, the computer calculates means, standard deviations, and percentages of types of responses.

The CNTB has demonstrated a broader range of sensitivity, including the ability to detect even mild impairment. It is more comprehensive in its assessment of a variety of neuropsychological functions, including evaluation of reaction time and information-processing speed; this permits not only improved analysis of specific drug effects, but it also allows a broader range of applications in drug research of other neurologic disorders, such as multi-infarct dementia and Parkinson's disease. The CNTB has multiple forms, proven validity, and excellent test–retest and alternate form reliability. In addition, the CNTB has practical advantages over conventional tests. As a computer-assisted battery, training of technicians is simple, as are test administration and data scoring, collection, and analysis.

The CNTB is now being used to evaluate drug efficacy in clinical trials (e.g., Sudilovsky et al., 1993; Fleishaker et al., 1993; Cutler et al., 1993; Cutler et al., 1996; Shrotriya et al., submitted). These trials have confirmed the validity of the battery itself in detecting cognitive impairment and have also shown the CNTB to be more consistently sensitive across a range of disease severity than other assessments. The CNTB has provided reliable measures for pharmacologic agents that may have efficacy in AD (Cutler et al., 1996). The CNTB continues to show excellent test–retest and alternate form reliability and adaptability to multicenter trials.

To improve AD drug study research, efforts must be made to reduce errors in subject selection. When designing and choosing neuropsychological screening instruments, the intent should be to minimize the number of dementia subjects missed during the patient selection process, while eliminating enrollment of normals in the trial. Supplementary neuropsychological tests should be used in addition to the MMSE to enhance accuracy of subject selection.

Attention must also be directed toward the neuropsychological measures of efficacy as the primary end-organ response in clinical trials. With these tools, researchers should be able to assess changes in mildly impaired subjects. They also need comprehensive assessments of function to understand the mechanisms of drug action and far wider application to other neurological diseases besides AD. The tests should be easy to administer and score, and standardization should be possible for multicenter clinical trials.

SUMMARY

In planning clinical trials for Alzheimer's disease, patient selection must be carefully considered to ensure that treatments will be effective in the desired population, and studies should be designed with the unique characteristics of the Alzheimer's patient population firmly in mind. The quest for a cure for Alzheimer's disease will no doubt continue for some time. Nevertheless, comprehensive research that incorporates meticulous attention to detail in the conduct of clinical trials should ultimately lead to breakthroughs that will permit development of truly effective treatments.

REFERENCES

Alexopoulos GS, Abrams RC, Young RC, Shamoian CA (1988): Cornell scale for depression in dementia. Biol Psychiatry 23:271–284.

Amaducci L, Angst J, Bech P (1990): Consensus conference on the methodology of clinical trials of "nootropics," Munich, June 1989: Report of the Consensus committee. Pharmacopsychiatry 23:171–175.

American Psychiatric Association (1994): "Diagnostic and Statistical Manual of Mental Disorders," 4th ed., Washington D.C.: American Psychiatric Press.

Anthony JC, LeResche L, Niaz U, von Korff MR, Folstein MF (1982): Limits of the Mini-Mental State as a screening test for dementia and delirium among hospital patients. Psycholog Med 12:397–408.

Barr RD, Koekebakker M, Lawson AA (1988): Acetylcholinesterase in the human erythron. II. Biochemical assay. Am J Hematol 28:260–265.

Becker RE, Giacobini E (1988): Mechanisms of cholinesterase inhibition in senile dementia of the Alzheimer type: Clinical, pharmacological, and therapeutic aspects. Drug Dev Res 12:163–195.

Benton AL (1974): "The Revised Visual Retention Test," 4th ed. New York: Psychological Corporation.

Berg L (1988): Clinical dementia rating (CDR). Psychopharmacol Bull 24:627.

Blessed G, Tomlinson BE, Roth M (1968): The association between quantitative measures of dementia and senile change in the cerebral grey matter of elderly subjects. Br J Psychiatry 114:797–811.

Busatto GF, Pilowsky LS (1995): Neuroreceptor mapping with in-vivo imaging techniques; Principles and applications. Br J Hosp Med 53:309–313.

Buschke H (1973): Selective reminding for analyses of memory and learning. J Verbal Learn Verbal Behav 12:543–549.

Buschke H, Fuld PA (1974): Evaluating storage, retention, and retrieval in disordered memory and learning. Neurology 24:1019.

Cardon PV, Dommel FW, Trumble RR (1976): Injuries to research subjects—a survey of investigators. N Engl J Med 295:650–654.

Comroe JH, Todd J, Koelle GB (1946): The pharmacology of di-isopropyl fluorophosphate (DFP) in man. J Pharmacol Exp Ther 87:281–290.

Cutler NR, Veroff AE, Bodick NC, Offen WW, Sramek JJ (1996): Cognitive improvement in Alzheimer's Disease: use of the CNTB in a trial of xanomeline. Biol Psychiatry 39:660.

Cutler NR (1993): Results of American studies on treatment of primary degenerative dementia with nimodipine. Talk presented at a symposium entitled "Calcium, Brain Function, and Dementia: Treatment Implications" at the Bayer Satellite to the 6th Congress of the International Psychogeriatric Association, Berlin, Germany, September 5, 1993.

Cutler NR (1989): Fundamental considerations in evaluating CNS-active compounds for Alzheimer's disease. Brain Dysfunction 2:211–216.

Cutler NR (1988): Utility of biological markers in the evaluation and diagnosis of Alzheimer disease. Brain Dysfunction 1:12–31.

Cutler NR, Sramek JJ (1995a): Scientific and ethical concerns in clinical trials in Alzheimer's patients: The bridging study. Eur J Clin Pharmacol 48:421–428.

Cutler NR, Sramek JJ (1995b): The target population in phase I clinical trials of cholinergic compounds in Alzheimer's disease: The role of the "bridging study." Alzheimer Dis Assoc Disord 9:139–145.

Cutler NR, Shrotriya RC, Sramek JJ, Veroff AE, Seifert RD, Reich LA, Hironaka DY (1993): The use of the Computerized Neuropsychological Test Battery (CNTB) in an efficacy and safety trial of BMY 21,502 in Alzheimer's disease. Ann N Y Acad Sci 695:332–336.

Cutler NR, Sramek JJ, Veroff AE (1994): "Alzheimer's Disease: Optimizing Drug Development Strategies." Chichester, England: Wiley.

Cutler NR, Sramek JJ, Narang PK (1991): Geriatrics: Clinical trials in an aging population. J Clin Res Pharmacoepidemiol 5:241–253.

Darragh A, Kenny M, Lambe R, Brick I (1985): Sudden death of a volunteer. Lancet 1:93–94.

Davis KL, Thal LJ, Gamzu ER, Davis CS, Woolson RF, Gracon SI, Drachman DA, Schneider LS, Whitehouse PJ, Hoover TM, Morris JC, Kawas CH, Knopman DS, Earl NL, Kumar V, Doody RS, Tacrine Collaborative Study Group (1992): A double-blind, placebo-controlled multicenter study of tacrine for Alzheimer's disease. N Engl J Med 327:1253–1259.

Fleishaker JC, Sisson TA, Sramek JJ, Conrad J, Veroff AE, Cutler NR (1993): Psychomotor and memory effects of two adinazolam formulations assessed by a computerized neuropsychological test battery. J Clin Pharmacol 33:463–469.

Folstein M, Folstein S, McHugh R (1975): Mini-Mental State: A practical method for grading the cognitive state of patients for the clinician. J Psychiatr Res 12:189–198.

Ford JM, Pfefferbaum A (1985): Age-related changes in event-related potentials. Adv Psychophysiol 1:301–339.

Frost JJ (1992): Receptor imaging by positron emission tomography and single-photon emission computed tomography. Invest Radiol 27(Suppl 2):S54–S58.

Galehr O, Plattner F (1928): Uber das Schicksal des Acetylcholins im Blute. Pflugers Arch 218:488–505.

Gershon S, Shaw FH (1961): Psychiatric sequelae of chronic exposure to organophosphorous insecticides. Lancet 24:1371–1374.

Goodin DS, Squires KC, Starr A (1978): Long latency event-related components of the auditory evoked potential in dementia. Brain 101:635–648.

Grob D, Lilienthal JL, Harvey AM, Jones BF (1947): The administration of di-isopropyl fluorophosphate (DFP) to man. I. Effect on plasma and erythrocyte cholinesterase; general systemic effects; use in study of hepatic function and erythropoiesis; and some properties of plasma cholinesterase. Bull John Hopkins Hosp 81:217–244.

Hallack M, Giacobini E (1989): Physostigmine, tacrine and metrifonate: the effect of multiple doses on acetylcholine metabolism in rat brain. Neuropharmacology 28(3):199–206.

Hallack M, Giacobini E (1987): A comparison of the effects of two inhibitors on brain cholinesterase. Neuropharmacology 26(6):521–530.

Hallack M, Giacobini E (1986): Relation of brain regional physostigmine concentration to cholinesterase activity and acetylcholine and choline levels in rat. Neurochem Res 11(7):1037–1048.

Hamilton M (1960): A rating scale for depression. J Neurol Neurosurg Psychiatry 23:56–62.

Herscovitch P, Carson RE, Zunkeler B, Jacobs G, Plascjak P (1990): A method for rapid repeat measurements of regional cerebral blood flow (rCBF) with positron emission tomography (PET) and O-15 water. Soc Neurosci Abstr 16:23.

Johansson G, Ablad B, Hansson E (1984): Prediction of adverse drug reactions in clinical practice from animal experiments and phase I–III studies. In Bostrom H, Ljungstedt N (eds): "Detection and Prevention of Adverse Drug Reactions (Skandia International Symposium." Stockholm: Almqvist and Wiskell International.

Martinez M, Frank A, Hernanz A (1993): Relationship of interleukin-1 beta and beta 2-microglobulin with neuropeptides in cerebrospinal fluid of patients with dementia of the Alzheimer type. J Neuroimmunol 48:235–240.

Mattis S (1976): Mental status examination for organic mental syndrome in the elderly patient. In Bellack R, Karasu B (eds): "Geriatric Psychiatry." New York: Grune & Stratton.

McKhann G, Drachman D, Folstein M, Katzman R, Price D, Stadlan EM (1984): Clinical diagnosis of Alzheimer's disease: Report of the NINCDS-ADRDA work group under the auspices of Department of Health and Human Services Task Force on Alzheimer's disease. Neurology 34:939–944.

Meinert CL, Tonascia S (1986): "Clinical Trials: Design, Conduct and Analysis." New York: Oxford University Press.

Merz WA (1994): Placebo response in panic disorder: a review. Eur Psychiatry 9:123–127.

Mikalsen A, Andersen RA, Alexander J (1986): Use of ethopropazine and BW 284C51 as selective inhibitors for cholinesterases from various species. Comp Biochem Physiol C83:447–449.

Moriearty PL, Becker RE (1992): Inhibition of human brain and RBC acetylcholinesterase (AChE) by heptylphysostigmine (HPTL). Meth Find Exp Clin Pharmacol 14:615–621.

Nordgren I, Bergstrom M, Holmstedt B, Sandoz M (1978): Transformation and action of metrifonate. Arch Toxicol 41:31–41.

Nolan L, O'Malley K (1988a): Prescribing for the elderly. Part I. Sensitivity of the elderly to adverse drug reactions. J Am Geriatr Soc 36:142–149.

Nolan L, O'Malley K (1998b): Prescribing for the elderly. Part II. Prescribing patterns: Differences due to age. J Am Geriatr Soc 36:245–254.

Olson L, Nordberg A, von Holst H, Backman L, Ebendal T, Alafuzoff I, Amberla K, Hartvig P, Herlitz A, Lilja A (1992): Nerve growth factor affects ^{11}C-nicotine binding, blood flow, EEG, and verbal episodic memory in an Alzheimer patient (case report). J Neural Transm [P-D Sect] 4:79–95.

Pfefferbaum A, Wenegrat BG, Ford JM, Roth WT, Koppel BS (1984): Clinical application of the P3 component of event-related potentials, II: Dementia, depression and schizophrenia. Electroencephalogr Clin Neurophysiol 59:104–124.

Pocock SJ (1983): "Clinical Trials: A Practical Approach." Chichester, England: Wiley.

Rapoport SI (1991): Positron emission tomography in Alzheimer's disease in relation to disease pathogenesis: a critical review. Cerebrovasc Brain Metab Rev 3: 297–335.

Reines SA (1989): Early clinical trials in Alzheimer's disease: Selection and evaluation of drug candidates. In Iqbal K, Wisniewski HM, Winblad B (eds): "Alzheimer's Disease and Related Disorders." New York: Alan R. Liss.

Reisberg B, Ferris SH, DeLeon MJ, Crook T (1982): The Global Deterioration Scale for assessment of primary degenerative dementia. Am J Psychiatry 139: 1136–1139.

Rosen WG, Mohs RC, Davis KL (1984): A new rating scale for Alzheimer's disease. Am J Psychiatry 141:1356–1364.

Rosen WG, Terry RD, Fuld PA, Katzman R, Peck A (1980): Pathological verification of ischemic score in differentiation of dementias. Ann Neurol 7:485–488.

Serby M, Richardson SB, Twente S, Siekierski J, Corwin J, Rotrosen J (1984): CSF somatostatin in Alzheimer's disease. Neurobiol Aging 5:187–189.

Shaw PG (1982): Common pitfalls in geriatric drug prescribing. Drugs 23:324–328.

Sherman KA, Messamore E (1989): Cholinesterase inhibitor therapy for Alzheimer dementia: What do animal models tell us? Prog Clin Biol Res 17:1209–1222.

Sherman KA, Kumar V, Ashford JW, Murphy JM, Elble RJ, Giacobini E (1987): Effect of oral physostigmine in senile dementia patients: Utility of blood cholinesterase inhibition and neuroendocrine responses to define pharmacokinetics and pharmacodynamics. In Strong R, (ed): "Central Nervous System Disorders Of Aging: Strategies for Intervention," Vol. 33. New York: Raven Press, pp 71–90.

Shrotriya RC, Cutler NR, Sramek JJ, Veroff AE, Hironaka DY (in press): An efficacy and safety trial of BMY 21,502 in Alzheimer's disease. Ann Pharmacother.

Siegel GJ, Lehrer GM, Silides D (1966): The kinetics of cholinesterases measured fluorometrically. J Histochem Cytochem 14:473–478.

Siegfried KR (1991): Methodology of clinical trials with anti-dementia compounds. In Hindmarch I, Hippius H, Wilcock GK (eds): "Dementia: Molecules, Methods and Measures." Chichester: Wiley.

Sirviö J, Kutvonen R, Koininen H, Hartikainen P, Riekkinen PJ (1989): Cholinesterases in the cerebrospinal fluid, plasma, and erythrocytes of patients with Alzheimer's disease. J Neural Transm 75:119–127.

Soininen H, Riekkinin PJ Sr (1992): EEG in diagnostics and follow-up of Alzheimer's disease. Acta Neurol Scand Suppl 139:36–39.

Soininen HI, Jolkkonen JT, Reinikainen KJ, Halonen TO, Riekkinen PJ (1984): Reduced cholinesterase activity and somatostatin-like immunoreactivity in the cerebrospinal fluid of patients with dementia of the Alzheimer's type. J Neurol Sci 63:167–172.

Soininen H, MacDonald E, Rekonen M, Riekkinen PJ (1981): Homovanillic acid and 5-hydroxyindoleacetic acid levels in cerebrospinal fluid of patients with senile dementia of Alzheimer type. Acta Neurol Scand 64:101–107.

Spiegel R, Brunner C, Ermini-Funfschilling D, Monsch A, Notter M, Puxty J, Tremmel L (1991): A new behavioral assessment scale for geriatric out- and in-patients: the NOSGER (Nurses' Observation Scale for Geriatric Patients). JAGS 39:339–347.

Spilker B (1987): "Guide to Planning and Managing Multiple Clinical Studies." New York: Raven Press.

Sramek JJ, Hurley DJ, Wardle TS, Satterwhite JH, Hourani J, Dies F, Cutler NR (1995): The safety and tolerance of xanomeline tartrate in patients with Alzheimer's disease. J Clin Pharmacol 35:800–806.

St. Clair DM, Brock DJH, Barron L (1986): A monoclonal antibody technique for plasma and red cell acetylcholinesterase activity in Alzheimer's disease. J Neurol Sci 73:169–176.

Stone BJ, Gray JW, Dean RS, Wheeler TE (1988): An examination of the Wechsler Adult Intelligence Scale (WAIS) subtests from a neuropsychological perspective. Int J Neurosci 40:31–39.

Sudilovsky A, Cutler NR, Sramek JJ, Wardle T, Veroff AE, Mickelson W, Markowitz S, Repetti S. (1993): A pilot clinical trial of the angiotension converting enzyme inhibitor ceranapril in Alzheimer's disease. Alzheimer Dis Assoc Disord 7:105–111.

Tato RE, Frank A, Hernanz A (1995): Tau protein concentrations in cerebrospinal fluid of patients with dementia of the Alzheimer type. J Neurol Neurosurg Psychiatry 59:280–283.

Thomsen T, Kaden B, Fischer JP, Bickel U, Barz H, Gusztony G, Cervos-Navarro J, Kewitz H (1991): Inhibition of acetylcholinesterase activity in human brain tissue and erythrocytes by galanthamine, physostigmine and tacrine. Eur J Clin Chem Clin Biochem 29:487–492.

Thomsen T, Kewitz H, Pleul O (1989): A suitable method to monitor inhibition of cholinesterase activities in tissues as induced by reversible enzyme inhibitors. Enzyme 42:219–224.

Thomsen T, Kewitz H, Pleul O (1988): Estimation of cholinesterase activity (EC 3.1.1.7; 3.1.1.8) in undiluted plasma and erythrocytes as a tool for measuring *in vivo* effects of reversible inhibitors. J Clin Chem Clin Biochem 26:469–475.

Venn RD (1983): The Sandoz Clinical Assessment-Geriatric (SCAG) scale. Gerontology 29:185–189.

Veroff AE, Cutler NR, Sramek JJ, Prior PL, Mickelson W, Hartman JK (1991): A new assessment tool for neuropsychopharmacologic research: The computerized neuropsychological test battery. J Geriatr Psychiatr Neurol 4:211–217.

Wechsler D (1945): A standardized memory scale for clinical use. J Psychol 19:87–95.

Weinstein HC, Scheltens P, Hijdra A, van Royen, EA (1993): Neuro-imaging in the diagnosis of Alzheimer's disease. II. Positron and single photon emission tomography. Clin Neurol Neurosurg 95:81–91.

World Health Organization (1992): "International Statistical Classification of Diseases and Related Health Problems: ICD-10," Geneva: World Health Organization.

Yasuda M, Minamitani N, Maeda K (1993): Peptide histidine methionine in cerebrospinal fluid of patients with senile dementia of the Alzheimer type. Jpn J Psychiatry Neurol 47:85–90.

CHAPTER 17

Cholinesterase Inhibition in the Treatment of Alzheimer's Disease: Further Evaluation of the Clinical Effects of Tacrine

STEPHEN I. GRACON and WILLIAM G. BERGHOFF

Parke-Davis Pharmaceutical Research, Division of Warner-Lambert Company, Ann Arbor, Michigan 48105

INTRODUCTION

The impetus for the clinical evaluation of tacrine as a treatment for Alzheimer's disease (AD) was provided by emergence of the cholinergic hypothesis (Davies and Maloney, 1976; Davies, 1981; Bartus et al., 1982) and reports of modest effects with another cholinesterase inhibitor, physostigmine, in patients with AD (Davis and Mohs, 1982; Mohs et al., 1985; Stern et al., 1988). Optimism about the possibility that tacrine represented a breakthrough treatment for AD was generated by a 1986 *New England Journal of Medicine* article by Summers and colleagues and the accompanying, enthusiastic editorial (Davis and Mohs, 1986; Summers et al., 1986).

The treatment effects seen in subsequent large-scale clinical trials of tacrine were more modest than the dramatic effects reported by Summers. However, tacrine (Cognex) was approved for marketing in the United States based upon efficacy demonstrated in two randomized, double-blind, placebo-controlled studies, one of 12-weeks' duration at doses up to 80 mg/day, and one of 30-weeks' duration at doses up to 160 mg/day (Farlow et al., 1992; Knapp et al., 1994).

This chapter summarizes efficacy and safety data and analyses that have been completed during the 2 years following approval of tacrine in the United States. It begins with a review of treatment expectations in AD, followed by a reexamination of the results of the 30-week study.

Pharmacological Treatment of Alzheimer's Disease: Molecular and Neurobiological Foundations,
Edited by Brioni and Decker
ISBN 0-471-16758-4   © 1997 Wiley-Liss, Inc.

More tangible evidence of tacrine's beneficial effects is provided by long-term (2-year) follow-up of patients from the 30-week study, which showed a reduced risk for nursing home placement among patients who achieved higher tacrine doses. The results of the 30-week study and 2-year follow-up are then reevaluated in light of the emerging evidence of the role of apolipoprotein E (apoE) in AD. Finally, the benefits and risks of tacrine treatment are put into perspective based on this additional information.

TREATMENT EXPECTATIONS IN ALZHEIMER'S DISEASE

Alzheimer's disease is a heterogeneous disease, clinically, genetically, pathologically, and biochemically (Alhainen and Riekkinen, 1993). Diagnosis is based on the exclusion of other possible causes of dementia and is more difficult in the early stages of the disease. The overall accuracy of diagnosis is 80–90% among experienced clinicians. The variability in clinical presentation, rate of disease progression, and performance on psychometric tests makes it difficult to demonstrate significant treatment effects. Not all patients would be expected to respond to a single treatment, and the degree of benefit may vary depending on genetic factors as well as severity of illness and underlying neuroanatomic, biochemical, and neurotransmitter pathologies. A fundamental issue associated with the evaluation of potential treatments for AD is establishing realistic expectations for treatment effects.

Patients with AD show a progressive loss of cognitive function beginning with seemingly benign memory lapses and culminating in severe dementia involving all domains of cognitive function. Decline is punctuated intermittently by behavioral problems of varying severity. Figure 1 shows the progressive deterioration in Mini-Mental State Examination (MMSE; Folstein et al., 1975) score over time. Superimposed are five hypothetical responses to an effective treatment for AD (Feldman and Gracon, 1996).

Treatment A represents an agent that delays the onset of cognitive and functional decline in patients with a known risk for the development of AD. The ability to define the "at-risk" population and the rate of conversion from risk to diagnosis currently limit the usefulness of this research strategy. However, recent reports on a possible association of apoE genotype with onset of AD have raised hopes for a mechanism by which to affect the onset of disease (Poirier et al., 1993; Saunders et al., 1993). Most researchers recognize the major benefit of such a treatment: a delay in the onset of disease, thus maintaining functional independence long enough to allow individuals at risk to live out their natural life span without the debilitating effects of cognitive and functional decline. It is this approach, emphasizing maintenance of functional independence and community care, that has the greatest implications for patients, caregivers, and society.

Treatment B represents a curative agent, which restores a patient to his or her premorbid level of performance. The magnitude of the treatment effect would be a function of the severity of impairment at the start of treatment: the more impaired the patient, the larger the treatment effect. Given the underlying neuropathology

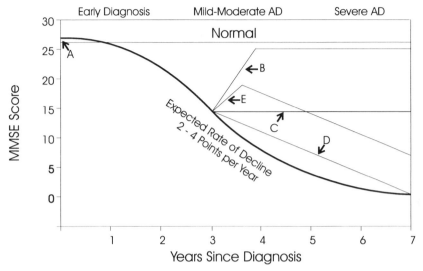

FIGURE 1. Hypothetical treatment responses to an effective treatment for AD.

present in even mildly impaired patients, it is unrealistic to expect this type of response with any agent currently being investigated.

Treatment C represents an agent that abruptly halts decline. Assuming 100% effectiveness at all stages of the illness, the magnitude of the treatment effect would be a function of the duration of study. For example, based on a worsening of three points per year on the MMSE in untreated patients, a recognizable treatment effect (i.e., a 1.5-point difference between treatment groups) would not be apparent until a patient had been treated for 6 months, and the effect would be judged clinically important only if it was also recognizable on a clinician-rated global assessment.

Treatment D represents an agent that does not halt disease progression. However, the gradual separation between treated patients and those who remain untreated suggests a symptomatic effect on the rate of decline.

Finally, treatment E shows the effect that might be expected with a cholinesterase inhibitor or cholinergic agonist: a modest improvement both from baseline and relative to placebo. Improvement would result from potentiation of the remaining cholinergic neurons and thus would vary with both disease severity and the degree of underlying neuropathology. Given enough time and assuming there is no effect on the underlying neuropathologic process, all patients would eventually decline.

Clearly, an ideal drug would completely reverse the disease process and restore patients to their premorbid level of functioning. However, given the current body of knowledge, a drug that delays disease onset may be a more realistic goal. Despite intense efforts among researchers to discover such agents, we appear to be a long way—10 years or more—from providing these types of restorative or preventive therapies. Today, physicians must be satisfied to optimize the use of symptomatic treatments, which can themselves provide major benefits.

RESULTS OF CLINICAL TRIALS: ADDITIONAL ANALYSES OF THE 30-WEEK STUDY

Effects on Cognitive Function, Clinical Assessments, and Behavior

Decline in cognitive function is the cardinal symptom of AD, and a beneficial treatment effect on cognitive function is today a *sine qua non* of efficacy for an antidementia drug. The cognitive subscale of the Alzheimer's Disease Assessment Scale (ADAS-Cognitive) was developed to provide a comprehensive assessment of cognitive function in patients with AD. It was designed to be sensitive both cross sectionally and longitudinally over a broad range of disease severity (Rosen et al., 1984).

Concurrent with the clinical development of tacrine, regulatory agencies worldwide were formulating guidelines for the assessment of antidementia drugs. Concern was raised about the possibility of showing an effect on a highly sensitive test of cognitive function that may have little impact on or relevance, in terms of daily function, to the patient, caregiver, or physician.

Regulatory agencies have reached a consensus that demonstration of efficacy must include significant effects on both cognitive function and a clinician-rated global assessment or an assessment of activities of daily living or behavior. Tacrine has shown significant effects in all four areas (Farlow et al., 1992; Knapp et al., 1994; Kauffer et al., 1996): cognitive function as assessed by the ADAS-Cognitive and MMSE; global assessment on the Clinical Global Impression of Change (CGIC; Clinical Global Assessment, 1976), Clinician Interview-Based Impression of Change (CIBIC; Knopman et al., 1994), and Global Deterioration Scale (GDS; Reisberg et al., 1982); activities of daily living as assessed by the Progressive Deterioration Scale (PDS; DeJong et al., 1989) and Physical Self-Maintenance Scale (PSMS; Lawton and Brody, 1969); and behavior as assessed by the Neuropsychiatric Inventory (NPI; Cummings et al. 1994). The following section provides a more detailed look at correlations between global assessments and tacrine's effects on cognitive function, clinical assessments, and behavior.

ADAS-Cognitive Factor Analysis

The factor structure of the ADAS-Cognitive has been evaluated by Kim et al. (1994) in a study of linopirdine by Olin and Schneider (1995) based on the 30-week study, and by Talwalker et al. (1996) using data from both the 12- and 30-week studies. Each of these groups found that the individual items comprising the ADAS-Cognitive project onto the domains of memory, language, and praxis, with the heaviest weighting toward memory.

Olin and Schneider (1995) reported significant effects for tacrine-treated patients versus placebo in all three domains, further supporting the robust nature of tacrine's treatment effects. Placebo-treated patients showed worsening on each of the domain scores, while patients taking tacrine improved. All three domains were sensitive to longitudinal changes in placebo-treated patients and to the treatment effects of tacrine as assessed by analysis of covariance for each ADAS-Cognitive factor. Olin and Schneider conclude: "The cholinesterase inhibitor tacrine has broad effects on cognition." Future analyses of these data should examine differential effects of tacrine treatment on each factor.

Correlations with Clinical Assessments

The robust nature of tacrine's treatment effect was confirmed by significant correlations between clinician global ratings and changes in cognitive function scores, caregiver ratings, and activities of daily living among both placebo and tacrine-treated groups in the 30-week study (Table 1) (Knopman et al., 1994). In particular, the week 30 ratings on the CIBIC and Final Comprehensive Consensus Assessment (FCCA; Knopman et al., 1994) correlated with week 30 change scores on the ADAS-Cognitive, MMSE, PSMS, Instrumental Activities of Daily Living (IADL; Lawton and Brody, 1969), PDS, CGIC, and GDS.

This method of analysis has limitations because change scores include within-subject variability, which is capable of reducing their reliability (Knopman et al., 1994). However, these change scores correspond clearly to the concept of change in CIBIC and FCCA. There were modest but statistically significant correlations in the appropriate direction ($p < 0.01$, adjusted for multiplicity), providing further evidence of the clinical relevance of the response detected on the CIBIC and FCCA.

The CIBIC rating is based entirely on information obtained in a one-on-one interview between the clinician and patient without caregiver input or reference to psychometric test scores. The FCCA rating also is based on an interview, but the clinician may consult the caregiver, family, or clinic staff and review the patient's performance on activities of daily living scales.

The modest degree of correlation serves to confirm that the measures are independent even though there are some overlapping features. Significantly higher levels of correlation given the modest effect size would bring into question the independence of the measures, their ability to capture different elements of patient performance, and the integrity of the study. The CIBIC and FCCA therefore provide an assimilation by the clinician of all clinically relevant information, based only on an interview for the CIBIC and including caregiver input for the FCCA.

The PDS was developed specifically for assessing activities of daily living and quality of life for patients with AD and their caregivers and provides the most comprehensive assessment of activities of daily living (Table 2) (DeJong et al., 1989). The PDS was significantly correlated with the CIBIC and FCCA and was most highly correlated with the caregiver's global rating.

Effects of Tacrine on Behavioral Changes in AD

The noncognitive features of AD and behavioral problems (delusions, personality and emotional changes, dysphoria, anxiety, and agitation) increase caregiver burden as well as the need for nursing home placement (Cohen et al. 1993). These symptoms are disturbing to the caregiver and difficult to predict and treat. Kaufer et al. (1996) recently reported on their experience in the amelioration of

TABLE 1 Study 970-61: Correlations Between CIBIC, FCCA, PDS, Caregiver-CGIC, and Other Scales on Change from Baseline to Week 30 for the Evaluable Population

(Pearson Correlation Coefficients)

	ADAS-Cognitive	ADAS-Noncognitive	MMSE	PSMS	IADL	PDS	CIBIC	C-CGIC	FCCA	GDS
CIBIC										
Placebo										
r^2	0.391	0.092	−0.407	0.219	0.186	−0.271	—	−0.317	0.907	0.375
p	<0.001[a]	0.328	<0.001[a]	0.020	0.050	0.004[a]	—	<0.001[a]	<0.001[a]	<0.001[a]
Tacrine										
r^2	0.342	0.145	−0.381	0.365	0.356	−0.411	—	−0.446	0.893	0.467
p	<0.001[a]	0.081	<0.001[a]	<0.001[a]	<0.001[a]	<0.001[a]	—	<0.001[a]	<0.001	<0.001[a]
FCCA										
Placebo										
r^2	0.424	0.086	−0.421	0.293	0.150	−0.332	0.907	−0.365	—	0.345
p	<0.001[a]	0.362	<0.001[a]	0.002[a]	0.115	<0.001[a]	<0.001[a]	<0.001[a]	—	<0.001[a]

Tacrine										
r^2	0.384	0.225	−0.403	0.370	0.363	−0.502	0.893	−0.550	—	0.589
p	<0.001[a]	0.006[a]	<0.001[a]	<0.001[a]	<0.001[a]	<0.001[a]	<0.001[a]	<0.001[a]	—	<0.001[a]
PDS										
Placebo										
r^2	−0.165	−0.146	0.228	−0.469	−0.515	—	−0.271	0.564	−0.332	−0.004
p	0.089	0.122	0.017	<0.001[a]	<0.001[a]	—	0.004[a]	<0.001[a]	<0.001[a]	0.710
Tacrine										
r^2	−0.271	−0.271	0.228	−0.249	−0.557	—	−0.411	0.610	−0.502	−0.365
p	0.001[a]	<0.001[a]	0.006[a]	0.003[a]	<0.001[a]	—	<0.001[a]	<0.001[a]	<0.001[a]	<0.001[a]
C-CGIC										
Placebo										
r^2	−0.180	−0.109	0.189	−0.357	−0.263	0.564	−0.317	—	−0.365	−0.136
p	0.064	0.249	0.048	<0.001[a]	0.006[a]	<0.001[a]	<0.001[a]	—	<0.001[a]	0.159
Tacrine										
r^2	−0.229	−0.258	0.300	−0.280	−0.384	0.610	−0.446	—	−0.550	−0.355
p	0.006[a]	0.002[a]	<0.001[a]	<0.001[a]	<0.001[a]	<0.001[a]	<0.001[a]	—	<0.001[a]	<0.001[a]

[a] $p < 0.01$.

TABLE 2   Content Areas for Progressive Deterioration Scale Questionnaire Items

Dressing	Handling money, checkbook, etc.
Eating habits	Household chores
Normal daily precautions	Tools, household implements
Remembering placements/placing appropriately	Work/hobbies
Comfort in unusual setting	Social interactions/meaningful conversation
Independent travel/finding way home	Current events
Telling time	Driving
Telephoning	

behavioral symptoms in patients with AD receiving tacrine in an open-label setting. The NPI was the primary outcome measure (Cummings et al., 1994). The NPI is a validated, caregiver-based questionnaire that assesses the frequency and severity of 10 behaviors: delusions, hallucinations, agitation/aggression, depression/dysphoria, anxiety, elation/euphoria, apathy, disinhibition, irritability, and aberrant motor behavior.

Patient scores on the NPI improved significantly from baseline and, more importantly, showed a dose–response relationship. Target symptoms of anxiety, apathy, hallucinations, aberrant motor behavior, and disinhibition were most responsive to tacrine treatment. In patients who also showed improved cognitive function based on MMSE scores, the most improved behavioral symptom was apathy. The greatest response was among patients with MMSE scores of 14–21 at baseline.

LONG-TERM EFFECTS OF TACRINE ON DISEASE MILESTONES AND EFFICACY ASSESSMENTS

The most important question arising from the controlled studies was whether the acute, symptomatic effects of tacrine treatment observed over 30 weeks translated into effects on long-term outcomes of the natural history of AD such as burden of care, nursing home placement, and mortality. Figure 2 shows a schematic representation of the natural history of AD (Feldman and Gracon, 1996). MMSE score is used as a surrogate of disease severity, and disease milestones are indicated.

Almost 75% of patients in the United States will eventually enter a nursing home with an average stay of more than 3 years (Welch et al., 1992). Although nursing home placement may be a somewhat imprecise end point, it is a major decision point in patient management. Duration of illness, cognitive function, activities of daily living, and severity of behavioral symptoms are important risk factors for nursing home placement and are good indicators for the severity of illness and level of care burden for the caregiver.

Patients who completed the 30-week double-blind study and those who terminated early were eligible to receive long-term, open-label tacrine treatment at the discretion of the study physician in consultation with the family.

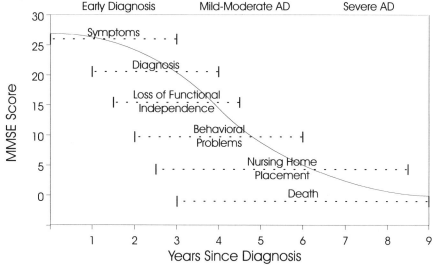

FIGURE 2. The natural history of AD.

Approximately 2 years after the last patient completed the double-blind phase, the protocol was amended to allow collection of follow-up information on nursing home placement and mortality. Attempts were made, through the study centers, to contact the families of all 663 patients who originally entered the study. Data were collected to determine whether patients continued to take tacrine and at what daily dose; and whether they were living at home, in a nursing home, or had died (Knopman et al., 1996).

Patients and Methods

Follow-up data on nursing home placement were available for 595 (90%) of the 663 patients randomized to treatment in the 30-week study. Forty-three patients were lost to follow-up; date of nursing home entry was unknown for 8 patients; residential status was unknown for 5; and 12 patients were in an assisted-care facility prior to randomization in the 30-week study. Mortality data were available for all 663 patients who entered the study, 81 of whom had died.

Data were analyzed by logistic regression. Nursing home placement and mortality were analyzed first at the end of double-blind treatment (week 30). Follow-up data were then analyzed based on patients' treatment status: all patients by last tacrine dose taken regardless of time off drug prior to follow-up ("all patients"); patients who were on tacrine at follow-up or who had been off drug for 60 days or less prior to an event, by last dose taken ("on tacrine"). The "on tacrine" results are presented here because all patients continued to have adequate caregiver support, and the only obvious potential source of bias was patients' ability to tolerate gastrointestinal side effects. The results of both analyses were, however, consistent.

TABLE 3   Study 970-61: Logistic Regression Analysis of Nursing Home Placement or Mortality at Week 30

Comparison	Odds Ratio	95% CI	Difference Favors	p Value
80 mg/day vs. placebo[a]	1.1	[0.3, 3.8]	80 mg/day	0.833
120 mg/day vs. placebo	1.6	[0.6, 4.1]	120 mg/day	0.338
160 mg/day vs. placebo	2.8	[1.0, 7.8]	160 mg/day	0.046[b]

[a]The sample size for the 80-mg/day treatment group was considerably smaller, approximately one-third that of the placebo group.
[b]$p < 0.05$.

Nursing Home Placement and Mortality at Week 30

At the end of the 30-week double-blind period, there was evidence of a trend toward a reduced probability of nursing home placement or death with increasing tacrine dose, which was statistically significant at 160 mg/day tacrine (Table 3).

Results: Nursing Home Placement and Mortality for Patients on Tacrine at Follow-up

The "on tacrine" analysis of nursing home placement included data for 320 patients, and the analysis of mortality included data for 308. Screening characteristics and follow-up data for these patients are in Tables 4 and 5, respectively.

Analyses of the follow-up data indicated that the probability of nursing home placement was significantly reduced for patients taking tacrine at doses > 80 mg/day when compared to patients who were taking tacrine 80 mg/day or less. A trend toward reduced mortality was seen for patients taking >120 mg/day versus ≤ 80 mg/day (Table 6; Figures 3 and 4). Fewer than 10% of tacrine-treated patients died. Therefore, estimates and significance levels for analyses of mortality should be interpreted with caution as they may be highly influenced by one or two events.

Kaplan-Meier estimates of the 25th percentile for nursing home placement (Table 5) were 303 days for patients with a dose of 20 to ≤80 mg/day, 747 days for patients with a dose of >80 to ≤120 mg/day, and 742 days for patients with a dose of >120 to ≤160 mg/day. This represents a significant delay in time to institutionalization of slightly more than 400 days, as indicated by dashed lines in Figure 3.

The long-term follow-up of patients who participated in the 30-week high-dose study is the most important new efficacy information available for tacrine since approval. Because it is observational data, it warrants critical review. In the absence of randomization, there is always concern of potentially biased results or conclusions.

The major interpretative difficulty is that the treatment assignment was not random or blinded. As such, a bias could have produced these results by segregating patients on the basis of tolerance. Patients who were destined to decline more

TABLE 4 Study 970-61: Screening Characteristics for Patients Included in Follow-up Analyses of NHP and Mortality, Patients on Tacrine by Dose (mg/day)

Characteristic	NHP N = 320			Mortality N = 308		
	>20 to ≤80 N = 102	>80 to ≤120 N = 96	>120 to ≤160 N = 122	>40 to ≤80 N = 97	>80 to ≤120 N = 88	>120 to ≤160 N = 123
Sex, N (%)						
Male	45 (44)	53 (55)	72 (59)	38 (39)	47 (53)	74 (60)
Female	57 (56)	43 (45)	50 (41)	59 (61)	41 (47)	49 (40)
p Value		0.014			<0.001	
Age, yr						
Mean	73.1	72.5	71.8	73.4	72.4	72.1
SD	8.0	7.8	7.8	8.4	8.1	7.5
Range	50–95	52–86	53–87	50–95	52–85	54–87
p Value		0.353			0.221	
MMSE						
Mean	17.9	18.5	19.3[a]	17.9[a]	19.2[b]	19.4[c]
SD	5.4	4.6	5.1	5.7	5.3	5.1
Range	10–29	10–27	3–28	5–29	4–29	3–28
p Value		0.361			0.262	

(Continued)

TABLE 4 (*Continued*)

Characteristic	NHP N = 320			Mortality N = 308		
	>20 to ≤80 N = 102	>80 to ≤120 N = 96	>120 to ≤160 N = 122	>40 to ≤80 N = 97	>80 to ≤120 N = 88	>120 to ≤160 N = 123
GDS						
Mean	4.56	4.44	4.52	4.60	4.36	4.50
SD	0.86	0.97	0.90	0.87	0.91	0.91
Range	3–6	2–6	2–6	3–6	2–6	2–6
p Value		0.269			0.055	
PSMS						
Mean	8.5	8.1	7.6	8.5	7.8	7.5
SD	3.1	3.0	2.4	3.2	2.7	2.1
Range	6–23	6–20	6–17	6–23	6–19	6–15
p Value		0.021			0.006	
IADL						
Mean	15.3	13.7[b]	13.8	15.3	13.4[b]	13.9
SD	6.0	5.6	5.5	6.0	5.8	5.5
Range	4–28	3–28	2–27	4–28	3–28	2–27
p Value		0.019			0.008	

The N for some parameters was less than the total N, because some patients were missing screening or follow-up values: NHP: [a]N = 119; [b]N = 95. Mortality: [a]N = 96; [b]N = 87; [c]N = 119.

TABLE 5 Study 970-61: Follow-up Data for Patients Included in Analyses of NHP and Mortality, Patients on Tacrine by Dose (mg/day)

Characteristic	NHP N = 320			Mortality N = 308		
	>20 to ≤80 N = 102	>80 to ≤120 N = 96	>120 to ≤160 N = 122	>40 to ≤80 N = 97	>80 to ≤120 N = 88	>120 to ≤160 N = 123
Time off tacrine						
Mean	8	5	4	7	4	4
SD	16	13	10	14	14	12
Median	0	0	0	0	0	0
Range	0–55	0–58	0–51	0–60	0–58	0–58
p Value		0.003			0.001	
Cumulative days of tacrine exposure						
Mean	466	603	637	468	634	651
SD	256	202	157	283	187	157
Median	484	659	664	576	687	669
Range	14–897	94–896	149–925	1–897	107–896	43–925
p Value		<0.001			<0.001	
At follow-up						
Institutionalized or dead	46 (45)	21 (22)	26 (21)	13 (13)	9 (10)	7 (6)
Days to event						
Range	15–863	138–841	172–772	113–755	133–726	258–671
25th percentile[a]	303	747	742	—	—	—
On other investigational medications						
Yes	0 (0)	0 (0)	0 (0)	0 (0)	0 (0)	0 (0)
Not stated	4 (4)	3 (3)	0 (0)	13 (13)	3 (3)	1 (1)
p Value		0.137			0.002	

[a]Kaplan-Meier estimates.

TABLE 6 Study 970-61: Logistic Regression Analysis of NHP and Mortality at Follow-up, by Tacrine Dose (mg/day) for Patients Who Were on Tacrine

Comparison	Odds Ratio	95% CI	Difference Favors	p Value
NHP				
>80 to ≤ 120 vs. 20 to ≤ 80	2.7	[1.4, 5.2]	>80 to ≤ 120	0.003
>120 to ≤ 160 vs. 20 to ≤ 80	2.8	[1.5, 5.2]	>120 to ≤ 160	0.001
Mortality				
>80 to ≤ 120 vs. 20 to ≤ 80	1.3	[0.5, 3.3]	>80 to ≤ 120	0.602
>120 to ≤ 160 vs. 20 to ≤ 80	2.6	[0.9, 7.1]	>120 to ≤ 160	0.063

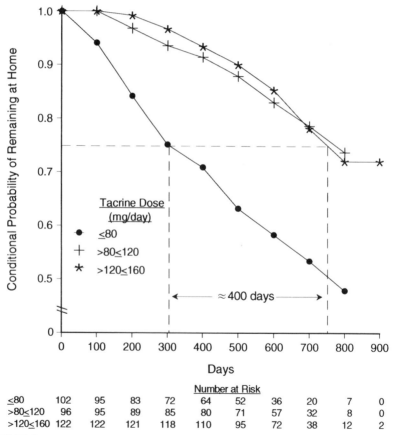

FIGURE 3. 30-Week study: Probability of remaining at home, patients on tacrine by dose (From Cox Proportional Hazards Regression).

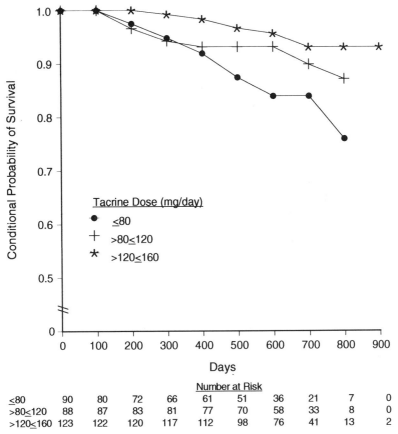

FIGURE 4. 30-Week study: Probability of survival, patients on tacrine by dose (From Cox Proportional Hazards Regression).

slowly could also have been the ones who could titrate to and tolerate higher tacrine doses. Therefore, these patients would have had a better outcome regardless of treatment compared with those who were more frail and could neither tolerate tacrine treatment nor be maintained at home. A related source of bias may be that patients with good social support systems, which are necessary for the four times daily dosing and frequent lab testing, may have self-selected to produce the result. Neither of the above alternative explanations can be totally refuted with the present data but are unlikely given that this analysis of patients who continued to take tacrine demonstrated a significant delay in time to nursing home placement on the same order of magnitude as other analyses.

Horwitz et al. (1990) outlined principles designed to increase the scientific value of observational studies. These include comparison of results and estimated effect sizes from observational studies with those from randomized controlled trials, careful patient selection and characterization, consideration of the reference time point used in analyses, adjustments for baseline comparability of patient populations, and balance in predictors of disease progression. The analyses of follow-up data satisfied all these criteria. Patients who participated in the randomized, double-blind, placebo-controlled studies of tacrine were carefully selected according to NINCDS criteria for a diagnosis of probable AD (McKhann et al., 1984) and were mildly to moderately impaired at baseline based on MMSE scores of 10–26, inclusive. Patients treated with tacrine showed improved cognitive function, global ratings, and activities of daily living compared with those on placebo. Because these end points are relevant to the natural history of AD, robust effects on these measures should be expected to produce effects on longer-term end points such as nursing home placement. Significant effects were seen in the 30-week placebo-controlled study, which were consistent with analyses of long-term follow-up. Consideration of reference time points and predictors of disease progression as well as adjustments for baseline comparability did not alter the results.

Knopman et al. (1996) conclude that there is an association between high-dose tacrine treatment and a reduced risk of nursing home placement and mortality. The most likely explanation is a salutary effect of tacrine on the symptoms of AD rather than a selection bias. The authors conclude that to establish causality would require a long-term, multiyear, prospective, randomized trial, the ethics of which demand alternative approaches.

EFFECT OF THE APOLIPOPROTEIN E (APOE) ALLELE ON TREATMENT RESPONSE TO TACRINE

ApoE is a polymorphic plasma protein involved in lipid transport. Three alleles designated $\epsilon2$, $\epsilon3$, and $\epsilon4$ result in three homozygous and three heterozygous genotypes (Poirier et al., 1993). The presence of the $\epsilon4$ allele has been identified as a risk factor for late-onset familial and sporadic AD (Saunders et al., 1993). However, its role in the pathogenesis of AD is not clear. Poirier and co-workers (1993) suggested that defects in reinnervation and synaptic plasticity in relation to apoE genotype may result in an exacerbation of the normal age-related decline in cell number and lipid content, particularly in areas of the cerebral cortex. These findings may also have implications for determining the effectiveness of cholinomimetic treatments in AD (Poirier, 1994).

ApoE genotype was determined for 572 of the 663 patients (86%) who participated in the 30-week study (data on file). The main effects of the $\epsilon4$ allele on the week 30 observed cases population and placebo-treated patients alone were examined. In addition, analyses of the primary efficacy outcome measures (ADAS-Cognitive, CIBIC, FCCA) and long-term data on nursing home placement and mortality were repeated, adjusting for apoE genotype and for patients with and without an $\epsilon4$ allele.

Analyses of the main effects of $\epsilon4$ suggested that patients without an $\epsilon4$ allele declined at a faster rate than patients with the allele. Tacrine was effective in both populations; however, the magnitude of the drug–placebo difference was consistently but not statistically significantly larger in patients without an $\epsilon4$ allele. Results of analyses of nursing home placement showing a reduced rate of placement for patients achieving higher tacrine doses were more significant in favor of a dose–response to tacrine when apoE genotype was considered than when it was not. No statistically significant effect of tacrine was seen on mortality when analyses were adjusted for apoE genotype.

These results suggest that rates of cognitive decline differ based on apoE genotype. These differences are not trivial given the magnitude of the treatment effects seen to date, and apoE genotype should be considered in analyses of efficacy data for any antidementia agent.

SUMMARY OF SAFETY INFORMATION

The following sections provide a brief review of tacrine's safety profile in patients with AD based on clinical studies, a treatment IND (TIND), and 2-year postmarketing experience.

Adverse Event Profile

During clinical development, including a TIND in the United States, over 12,000 patients were treated with tacrine. Ninety-nine percent of patients in clinical trials were over 50 years of age, and 56% were over 70. In the TIND, 75% of patients were over 70 years of age. In the first 2 years following marketing approval in the United States, an estimated 200,000 patients were treated.

The adverse event profile established during clinical trials (Table 7) remained consistent as more patients were exposed to tacrine. The most frequent adverse events continued to be elevated liver transaminase levels, followed by dose-related peripheral cholinergic effects primarily affecting the gastrointestinal tract (nausea, vomiting, diarrhea, dyspepsia, anorexia).

REASSESSMENT OF THE BENEFITS AND RISKS OF TACRINE TREATMENT

Tacrine appears to be a symptomatic treatment, and it is important for patients to remain on tacrine to maintain benefit. It is expected that over the long-term patients will decline, and at some point the family will likely decide whether to continue treatment. This is an intensely personal decision, which often occurs when the caregiver no longer can cope with the burden of care and is considering placing the patient in a nursing home.

Long-term data show that patients who continue tacrine treatment have some preservation of basic and instrumental activities of daily living relative to patients who stop treatment. Even these small benefits can make a huge difference in a caregiver's ability to continue to care for the patient at home.

TABLE 7 Adverse Events Reported by ≥ 2% of Patients Who Received Tacrine According to the Recommended Regimen Compared with All Patients Who Received Tacrine During Clinical Studies

	Recommended Regimen		All Patients[a]
	Placebo	Tacrine	Total Tacrine
Adverse Event	N = 342	N = 634	N = 2706
Tacrine-associated events[b]			
Elevated transaminases	1.5%	29.0%	23.5%
Nausea and/or vomiting	8.5	28.1	28.6
Diarrhea	5.3	15.6	14.4
Dyspepsia	6.4	9.0	9.0
Myalgia	5.3	8.5	7.5
Anorexia	3.2	8.5	9.3
Rash[c]	5.3	7.3	7.3
Ataxia	3.5	5.7	7.6
Flatulence	1.5	3.5	3.7
Weight decrease	1.2	3.3	4.1
Tremor	0.6	2.2	2.8

[a]All patients who received tacrine during clinical trials.
[b]Probability of occurrence significantly higher during tacrine treatment than placebo treatment ($p < 0.05$, log-rank chi-square test).
[c]Includes COSTART terms rash, rash-erythematous, rash-maculopapular, urticaria, petechial rash, rash-vesiculobullous, and pruritus.

The risks of tacrine treatment are small relative to its potential benefits. But achieving optimal treatment response requires an accurate diagnosis, careful dose-titration, and transaminase monitoring.

Alzheimer's disease is a devastating illness for which tacrine is an effective symptomatic treatment. It is important that physicians provide their patients the best available treatments in the best environment possible. Simply raising awareness of the illness, removing the stigma of diagnosis, and offering social, moral, and pharmacologic support is a great deal more than has previously been possible.

REFERENCES

Alhainen K, Riekkinen Sr PJ (1993): Discrimination of Alzheimer patients responding to cholinesterase inhibitor therapy. Acta Neurol Scand 149(Suppl):16–21.

Bartus RT, Dean RL, Beer B, Lippa AS (1982): The cholinergic hypothesis of geriatric memory dysfunction. Science 217:408–417.

Clinical Global Assessment Scale (CGI) (1976): In Guy W (ed): "ECDEU Assessment Manual for Psychopharmacology." Rockville, MD: U.S. Dept of Health, Education, and Welfare, National Institute of Mental Health, pp 218–222.

Cohen CA, Gold DP, Shulman KI, Wortley JT, McDonald G, Wargon M (1993): Factors determining the decision to institutionalize dementing individuals: A prospective study. Gerontologist 33:714–720.

Cummings JL, Mega M, Gray K, Rosenberg-Thompson S, Carusi DA, Gornbein J (1994): The neuropsychiatric inventory: Comprehensive assessment of psychopathology in dementia. Neurology 44:2308–2314.

Davies P (1981): Theoretical treatment possibilities for dementia of the Alzheimer type: The cholinergic hypothesis. In Crook T, Gershon S (eds): "Strategies for the Development of an Effective Treatment for Senile Dementia." Madison, CT: Mark Powley Associates, pp 19–35.

Davies P, Moloney AJF (1976): Selective loss of central cholinergic neurons in Alzheimer's disease. Lancet 2:1043.

Davis KL, Mohs RC (1986): Cholinergic drugs in Alzheimer's disease. N Engl J Med 315:1286–1287.

Davis KL, Mohs RC (1982): Enhancement of memory processes in Alzheimer's disease with multiple-dose intravenous physostigmine. Am J Psychiatry 139:1421–1424.

DeJong R, Osterlund OW, Roy GW (1989): Measurement of quality-of-life changes in patients with Alzheimer's disease. Clin Ther 11:545–554.

Farlow M, Gracon SI, Hershey LA, Lewis KW, Sadowsky CH, Dolan-Ureno J (1992): A controlled trial of tacrine in Alzheimer's disease. JAMA 268:2523–2529.

Feldman H, Gracon S (1996): Alzheimer's disease: Symptomatic drugs under development. In Gauthier S (ed): "Clinical Diagnosis and Management of Alzheimer's Disease." London:Martin Dunitz Ltd, pp 239–259.

Folstein MF, Folstein SE, McHugh PR (1975): Mini-mental state: A practical method for grading the cognitive state of patients for the clinician. J Psychiat Res 12:189–198.

Horwitz RI, Viscoli CM, Clemens JD, Sadock RT (1990): Developing improved observational methods for evaluating therapeutic effectiveness. Am J Med 89:630–638.

Kaufer DI, Cummings JL, Christine D (1996): Effect of tacrine on behavioral symptoms in Alzheimer's disease: An open-label study. J Geriatr Psychiatry Neurol 9:1–6.

Kim YS, Nibbelink DW, Overall JE (1994): Factor structure and reliability of the Alzheimer's Disease Assessment Scale in a multicenter trial with linopirdine. J Geriatr Psychiatry Neurol 7:76–86.

Knapp MJ, Knopman DS, Solomon PR, Pendlebury WW, Davis CS, Gracon SI (1994): A 30-week randomized controlled trial of high-dose tacrine in patients with Alzheimer's disease. JAMA 271:985–991.

Knopman D, Schneider L, Davis K, Talwalker S, Smith F, Hoover T, Gracon S (1996): Long-term tacrine (Cognex) treatment: Effects on nursing home placement and mortality. Neurology 47:166–177.

Knopman DS, Knapp MJ, Gracon SI, Davis CS (1994): The clinical interview-based impression (CIBI): A clinician's global change rating scale in Alzheimer's disease. Neurology 44:2315–2321.

Lawton MP, Brody EM (1969): Assessment of older people: Self-maintaining and instrumental activities of daily living. Gerontologist 9:176–186.

McKhann G, Drachman D, Folstein M, Katzman R, Price D, Stadlan EM (1984): Clinical diagnosis of Alzheimer's disease: Report of the NINCDS-ADRDA work group. Neurology 34:939–944.

Mohs RC, Davis BM, Johns CA, Mathé AA, Greenwald BS, Horvath TB, Davis KL (1985): Oral physostigmine treatment of patients with Alzheimer's disease. Am J Psychiatry 142:28–33.

Olin JT, Schneider LS (1995): Assessing response to tacrine using the factor analytic structure of the Alzheimer's Disease Assessment Scale (ADAS)—cognitive subscale. Int J Geriatr Psychiatry 10:753–756.

Poirier J (1994): Apolipoprotein E in animal models of CNS injury and in Alzheimer's disease. Trends Neurosci 17:525–530.

Poirier J, Davignon J, Bouthillier D, Kogan S, Bertrand P, Gauthier S (1993): Apolipoprotein E polymorphism and Alzheimer's disease. Lancet 342:697–699.

Reisberg B, Ferris SH, De Leon MJ, Crook T (1982): The Global Deterioration Scale for assessment of primary degenerative dementia. Am J Psychiatry 139:1136–1139.

Rosen WG, Mohs RC, Davis KL (1984): A new rating scale for Alzheimer's disease. Am J Psychiatry 141:1356–1364.

Saunders AM, Strittmatter WJ, Schmechel D, St. George-Hyslop PMH, Pericak-Vance MA, Joo SH, Rosi BL, Gusella JF, Crapper-MacLachlan DR, Alberts J, Hulette C, Crain B, Goldgaber D, Roses AD (1993): Association of apolipoprotein E allele ϵ4 with late-onset familial and sporadic Alzheimer's disease. Neurology 43:1467–1472.

Stern Y, Sano M, Mayeux R (1988): Long-term administration of oral physostigmine in Alzheimer's disease. Neurology 38:1837–1841.

Summers WK, Majovski LV, Marsh GM, Tachiki K, Kling A (1986): Oral tetrahydroaminoacridine in long-term treatment of senile dementia, Alzheimer type. N Engl J Med 315:1241–1245.

Talwalker S, Overall JE, Srirama MK, Gracon SI (1996): Cardinal features of cognitive dysfunction in Alzheimer's disease: A factor-analytic study of the Alzheimer's Disease Assessment Scale. J Geriatr Psychiatry Neurol 9:39–46.

Welch HG, Walsh JS, Larson EB (1992): The cost of institutional care in Alzheimer's disease: Nursing home and hospital use in a prospective cohort. J Am Geriatr Soc 40:221–224.

CHAPTER 18

Development of Muscarinic Agonists for the Symptomatic Treatment of Alzheimer's Disease

JUAN C. JAEN and ROY D. SCHWARZ

Parke-Davis Pharmaceutical Research, Division of Warner-Lambert Company, Ann Arbor, Michigan 48105

INTRODUCTION

Alzheimer's disease (AD) is an age-related neurodegenerative disorder characterized by a progressive loss of cognitive function. Within the brain, neurofibrillary tangles and amyloid-containing plaques are hallmarks of this disorder and their presence provides definitive confirmation of AD at the time of autopsy. Degeneration of discrete neuronal populations is also characteristic of AD (Whitehouse et al., 1982). The loss of histochemical markers for forebrain cholinergic neurons has been a reproducible finding, and this loss has been correlated with diminished cognitive function and the severity of the neuropathological markers (Perry et al., 1978; Bartus et al., 1982; Whitehouse and Au, 1986). The so-called *cholinergic hypothesis* of AD is based on these and similar observations. Drawing on the successful use of dopaminergic agents in Parkinson's disease to compensate for the loss of *substantia nigra* dopaminergic input to the striatum, a logical corollary of the *cholinergic hypothesis* is that various therapies aimed at enhancing cholinergic neurotransmission should provide at least symptomatic improvement in AD patients (Jaen et al., 1992).

Many direct and indirect pharmacologic approaches possess the ability to increase brain cholinergic tone. Greatest attention has focused over the past decade on acetylcholinesterase inhibitors (AChEIs), muscarinic agonists, and acetylcholine (ACh) releasing agents. Other indirect cholinomimetic approaches include high-

Pharmacological Treatment of Alzheimer's Disease: Molecular and Neurobiological Foundations,
Edited by Brioni and Decker
ISBN 0-471-16758-4   © 1997 Wiley-Liss, Inc.

dose ACh precursor therapy (e.g., choline, lecithin), prolyl endopeptidase (PEP) inhibitors, thyrotropin-releasing hormone (TRH) analogues, and galanin receptor antagonists. Agents that simply amplify the endogenous level of cholinergic activity may become less effective as the disease progresses and cholinergic neuronal loss is more pronounced. On the other hand, postsynaptic muscarinic receptors appear to remain intact in postmortem AD brain (Mash et al., 1985; Pearce and Potter, 1991). Thus activation of these receptors with muscarinic agonists should diminish the cognitive impairment associated with cholinergic neuron loss. However, recent reports raise the possibility that the concentration of m1 and m4 receptors (which together make up much of what is defined as the pharmacological M_1 receptor, see below) may be decreased in AD brain (Flynn et al., 1995). In spite of these reservations, the rationale for evaluating muscarinic agonists in AD patients is a very strong one, and it has received significant clinical attention over the past decade.

FIRST-GENERATION MUSCARINIC AGONISTS

Several muscarinic agonists were expediently evaluated in AD patients following the observation of cholinergic neuron loss in AD brain (Figure 1). These *first-generation* muscarinic agonists were not specifically designed for use in AD. They were generally products of natural origin (arecoline, pilocarpine) or older pharmacological agents that had been designed for other uses (bethanechol, oxotremorine). The results of these early clinical trials were consistently disappointing. Administration of these compounds was associated with a high incidence of parasympa-

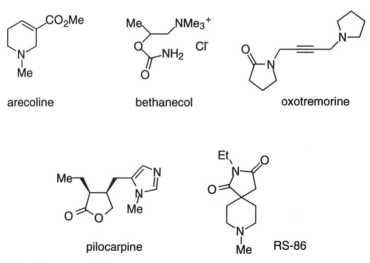

FIGURE 1. Structures of first-generation muscarinic agonists: arecoline, bethanechol, oxotremorine, pilocarpine, and RS-86.

thetic side effects (hypersalivation, nausea, diarrhea, lachrimation, increased urination, etc.). Additionally, these first-generation compounds generally possessed poor oral bioavailabilities, short duration of action, and other pharmacokinetic limitations.

Arecoline is a naturally occurring cholinomimetic, displaying activation of muscarinic (Marmé, 1890) and nicotinic receptors (von Euler et al., 1945) Its memory-enhancing activity has been demonstrated in animals and humans (Haroutunian et al., 1985; Sitaram et al., 1978; Christie et al., 1981). Unfortunately, the methyl ester functionality of arecoline is rapidly hydrolyzed in vivo to the biologically inactive arecaidine by esterases (Patterson and Kosh, 1993; Sethy and Francis, 1990), which severely limits the utility of this agent, particularly by the oral route of administration. Intravenous infusions of arecoline were shown to produce positive cognitive effects in small groups of AD patients. However, even by the intravenous route, the short half-life of arecoline makes it clinically unacceptable (Christie et al., 1981; Tariot et al., 1988; Raffaele et al., 1991; Soncrant et al., 1993).

Bethanechol is a close analogue of the muscarinic/nicotinic agonist carbachol. The quaternary ammonium nature of this compound makes it very unlikely to cross the blood–brain barrier. While preliminary observations of AD patients treated with intraventricular infusions of the muscarinic agonist bethanechol suggested some clinical improvement, the results from subsequent studies were more equivocal. Most patients tolerated the surgery quite well; however, the limited clinical efficacy observed in the early trials and the invasive nature of the surgical procedure did not justify continued evaluation of bethanechol (Harbaugh et al., 1989, 1984; Gauthier et al., 1986; Penn et al., 1988). Out of seven AD patients treated orally with oxotremorine, a synthetic muscarinic agonist, five showed unexpected depressive reactions, and no conclusions on the cognitive performance of this agonist could be reached (Davis et al., 1987). Oral doses of pilocarpine, with and without lecithin, produced no positive effects in four AD patients (Caine, 1980). Unlike the very small numbers of patients that were involved in the aforementioned studies, almost 500 AD patients were treated with RS-86, a synthetic spiro-piperidyl compound with cholinomimetic activity in animals. While some individuals showed positive responses, the majority either showed no effect or were unable to continue dosing due to troublesome cholinergic side effects (Wettstein and Spiegel, 1984; Bruno et al., 1986; Hollander et al., 1987; Mouradian et al., 1988).

As indicated above, demonstrating clinical efficacy with first-generation muscarinic agonists was largely unsuccessful. While in some cases the clinical trials were flawed (e.g., too few patients or poor outcome measures utilized), all of these compounds produced dose-limiting peripheral cholinergic side effects at doses equal to or below those required to produce some cognitive improvement. In addition, they also suffered from limited oral activity, poor biodistribution, limited CNS penetration, or short duration action. In order to overcome these limitations, it was soon suggested in the late 1980s that muscarinic agonists with good CNS permeability and a high degree of selectivity for brain receptors would be ideal candidates for AD therapy. Muscarinic receptors were initially divided into subtypes according to classical pharmacologic methods (see below). Brain muscarinic receptors are assumed to be predominantly of the M_1 subtype, particularly those in cortical and hippocampal areas, two brain regions associated with learning and memory, while peripheral tissues (smooth muscle and glandular tissue in particular) are associated primarily with muscarinic receptors of the M_2 and M_3 subtypes. Unwanted peripheral side effects generally stem from activation of these latter receptors. Thus, a selective M_1 muscarinic agonist should be clinically efficacious in AD at doses lower than those producing dose-limiting peripheral cholinergic side effects (Davis et al., 1995).

CHARACTERIZATION OF MUSCARINIC RECEPTOR SUBTYPES

Multiple subtypes of muscarinic receptors were originally characterized pharmacologically through the use of selective antagonists. In receptor binding and second messenger studies, M_1 receptors show high affinity and sensitivity to the atypical muscarinic antagonist pirenzepine and 4-DAMP (4-diphenylacetoxy-N-methylpiperidine methiodide), while M_2 receptors show low affinity and sensitivity to pirenzepine and higher affinity and sensitivity to such compounds as AF-DX 116 and methoctramine. Additionally, receptors of the M_3 subtype are more sensitive to p-F-HHSiD (para-fluorohexahydrosiladifenidol) and 4-DAMP and possess lower affinity for pirenzepine and AF-DX116. An M_4 receptor has been postulated, but there are no selective agonists/antagonists for this receptor subtype (Nathanson, 1987; Hulme et al., 1990; Caulfield, 1993).

The existence of five muscarinic receptor subtypes (m1–m5) as five distinct gene products was identified through the use of molecular cloning techniques (Caulfield, 1993). The porcine cortical m1 receptor was the first muscarinic receptor to be cloned, followed shortly thereafter by the successful cloning of the porcine m2 receptor from the heart (Kubo et al., 1986a,b). Three additional receptors from both rat and human (m3–m5), were subsequently cloned, sequenced, and expressed (Bonner et al., 1987, 1988; Peralta et al., 1987a,b). It now appears that the four pharmacologically defined receptors (M_1–M_4) correspond fairly closely to the receptors defined on the basis of molecular genetics (m1–m4). The m5 receptor remains largely uncharacterized since there are no subtype-selective agonists/antagonists, and convincing data for direct measurement of receptor protein in brain is lacking.

The use of stably transfected clonal cell lines has helped to identify signal transduction pathways associated with the five subtypes, whereby receptor occupation by agonists results in the activation of specific second messengers. In most neuronal cells, m1, m3, and m5 receptors appear to be positively coupled to phospholipase C (PLC) resulting in both the formation of diacylglycerol, which subsequently activates protein kinase C (PKC), and also the release of inositol trisphosphate (IP_3), which in turn liberates free, intracellular calcium. Other effects mediated by these three receptors include activation of calcium-dependent potassium and chloride currents, inhibition of m-currents, the release of arachidonic acid, and the stimulation of cAMP levels (Jones, 1993). In contrast, the primary transduction pathway of m2 and m4 receptors involves negative coupling to adenylyl cyclase. Additional events mediated by m2 and m4 receptors include the stimulation of an inward rectifying current, inhibition of calcium currents, and the activation of cation conductances (Peralta et al., 1988; Jones, 1993).

LOCALIZATION OF MUSCARINIC RECEPTOR SUBTYPES IN THE CNS

Radioligand binding studies, autoradiography, and the immunological measurement of receptor proteins by the use of subtype-selective antibodies have all contributed to the mapping of muscarinic receptors in the central nervous system (CNS). Additionally, the use of Northern blot analysis and in situ hybridization techniques have allowed the localization of brain mRNAs encoding these receptors to also be accurately determined. Within the brain, m1 receptors are widely distributed, with highest concentrations detected in the cerebral cortex, hippocampus, and striatum; the cortex and hippocampus are two brain areas intimately involved in memory and learning processes. While best described peripherally in the heart, m2 receptors are predominant in brainstem regions (e.g., pons, medulla), suggestive of a role in vegetative functions and are also found in cerebellum, hypothalamus, and thalamus. The density of m3 receptors appears to be relatively low across all brain areas examined, making it difficult to determine function, while m4 receptors are in highest abundance in the striatum, with lower levels in the cortex, hippocampus, and thalamus. The high level in the striatum strongly suggests a role for m4 receptors in motor control. There seems to be some debate on whether m5 receptor protein has been accurately measured in the CNS, but m5 mRNA has been detected in the substantia nigra, an area rich in dopamine neuronal cell bodies, suggesting that m5 receptors may be involved in the control of dopamine release and/or synthesis (Brann et al., 1988; Levey et al., 1991; Li et al., 1991; Wall et al., 1991; J Wei et al., 1994).

CHARACTERIZATION OF RECEPTOR SUBTYPE SELECTIVITY FOR MUSCARINIC AGONISTS

A major issue in the development of new muscarinic agents is the question of accurately defining receptor subtype selectivity for a given compound. Different groups have used a variety of techniques and assays to determine selectivity. Receptor binding assays using high-affinity antagonist ligands (e.g., ^{3}H-QNB, ^{3}H-NMS) in transfected cells clearly define the subtype selectivity of novel muscarinic antagonists (Dorje et al., 1991). In most cases, these results are identical to those obtained in tissue bath preparations. However, there are some major exceptions. For example, pirenzepine, which is the definitive antagonist used to pharmacologically define M_1 receptors, shows only a three- to fourfold separation between m1 and m4 receptors using membranes from transfected Chinese hamster ovary (CHO) cells (Buckley et al., 1989). Thus, the M_1 classification may actually correspond to the sum of m1 and m4 receptor activity. For muscarinic agonists, whole-cell receptor binding studies in transfected cells expressing the cloned human receptor subtypes, using ^{3}H-NMS as the ligand, allowed compounds to be classified into one of two groups: group I agonists (AF-102B, arecoline, BM-5, and RS-86), which show no difference in affinity between receptor subtypes, and group II agonists (carbachol, L-670, 207, McN-A-343, oxotremorine, and pilocarpine), which show some selectivity between specific pairs of subtypes (selectivity defined as more than threefold difference in binding affinity). However, no agonist tested was truly subtype selective using binding as the only criterion (Schwarz et al., 1993). Additionally, examination of a novel series of oxime agonists showed that binding greatly underestimated subtype selectivity compared to results obtained in functional second-messenger assays (Jaen et al., 1995).

Measuring the production of second messengers or other cellular events associated with receptor activation may be the most definitive means currently available to define the true subtype selectivity of muscarinic agonists. Second-messenger assays have been successfully used to measure agonist-stimulated phosphatidylinositol (PI) hydrolysis associated with m1, m3, and m5 receptors, and inhibition of forskolin-stimulated cyclic adenosine monophosphate (cAMP) accumulation with m2 and m4 receptors. Estimates of the subtype selectivity of arecoline, carbachol, oxotremorine, and pilocarpine have been presented, but as noted below are confused by the variable number of spare receptors present for each subtype and to the sensitivity of the separate assays used to measure these two second messengers (Schwarz et al., 1993). Lazareno et al. (1993) have successfully used measurement of ^{35}S-GTP-γ-S binding and ^{32}P-GTP hydrolysis [guanidinyl triphosphate (GTP)ase activity] to characterize muscarinic agonists. This technique has the advantage of using a single assay across all five receptor subtypes, regardless of which G-protein the receptor is coupled to. Another method to functionally assess compounds is the use of receptor selection and amplifcation technology (R-SAT). This technology is based on the observation that expression of PI-linked receptors (m1, m3, and m5) induce agonist-dependent foci formation in NIH 3T3 cell cultures. Coexpression with the enzyme marker β-galactosidase allows the increase in cell proliferation to be monitored spectrophotometrically with an appropriate substrate. For those receptors negatively coupled to adenylyl cyclase, additional coexpression with the chimeric G-protein Gq-I5 allows coupling to the PI pathway and subsequent foci formation with agonist application (Brauner Osborne et al., 1995; Burstein et al., 1995).

The major caveat to using functional measures as a means of defining receptor subtype selectivity is that the total number of receptors and types of G-proteins present for each cell line expressing an individual subtype is absolutely critical (Richards and van Giersbergen, 1995). In cells with a large receptor reserve (i.e., a high number of spare receptors), both full and partial agonists will produce marked effects, while in cells with a low receptor reserve only full agonists will elicit a response (Richards, 1991). Since both potency and efficacy are affected by receptor number, compounds could appear to be functionally subtype selective when they are not, if there are unequal numbers of spare receptors in the various recombinant cell lines. Equal numbers of receptors can be genetically engineered into each cell line, or agents such as propylbenzylcholine mustard (PrBCM) can be used to irreversibly alkylate receptors, in order to achieve a desired level of receptors (Schwarz et al., 1993; Wang and El-Fakahany, 1993).

SECOND-GENERATION MUSCARINIC AGONISTS

We utilize the term *second-generation* muscarinic agonists to refer to those agents that were developed specifically for the treatment of AD. These agents have seen various levels of success in overcoming the pharmacokinetic and nonselectivity problems of the first-generation compounds, which are those that predate the cholinergic hypothesis of AD (Bartus et al., 1982). Several second-generation muscarinic agonists are in advanced stages of clinical or late-preclinical evaluation, such as milameline, xanomeline, YM796, AF-102B, WAL-2014, and PD 151832, the structures of which are illustrated in Figure 2 (Eglen and Watson, 1996).

MILAMELINE (CI-979/RU35926)

Milameline is a muscarinic agonist with a novel profile that overcomes the major limitations of first-generation agonists (Schwarz et al., Davis et al., 1995). The compound is a tetrahydropyridine oxime structurally related to the naturally occurring muscarinic agonist arecoline. The *O*-methyl aldoxime moiety provides a bio-

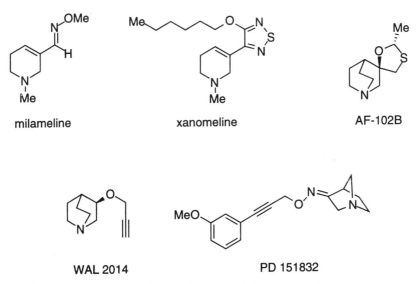

FIGURE 2. Structures of second-generation muscarinic agonists: milameline, xanomeline, AF-102B, WAL 2014, and PD 151832.

logically stable bioisostere for the acetate group of ACh or arecoline's methyl ester (Toja et al., 1991). In vitro, milameline binds to muscarinic receptors in rat brain tissue with EC_{50} values of 3.1 and 2.1 μM when using the antagonist ligands [³H]QNB and [³H]pirenzepine, and $EC_{50} = 20.4$ nM with the agonist ligand [³H]CMD (cis-methyldioxolane) (Schwarz et al., 1991; Toja et al., 1991). In transformed CHO cells expressing human muscarinic receptors (CHO-Hm1–CHO-Hm5), milameline displayed equal affinity for the five receptor subtypes (Sedman et al., 1995). Little or no binding was observed to a number of other CNS neurotransmitter receptors, and there was no inhibition of acetylcholinesterase. Milameline is a partial muscarinic agonist in human neuroblastoma SK-N-SH cells, stimulating PI hydrolysis to about 35% of the efficacy of the full agonist carbachol. Low micromolar potency and efficacy similar to that in the SK-N-SH cells was observed for the stimulation of PI hydrolysis in CHO-Hm1 and CHO-Hm3 cells was well as the inhibition of forskolin-stimulated cAMP accumulation in CHO-Hm2 and CHO-Hm4 cells (Davis et al., 1995). Like other muscarinic agonists, milameline decreased the release of [³H]ACh from rat brain slices, the result of its interaction with putative presynaptic m2 autoreceptors. All functional responses were blocked by muscarinic antagonists, such as scopolamine or atroprine.

An additional in vitro observation, which may have implications for the effects of milameline on AD progression, is that milameline enhances the release of soluble amyloid precursor protein (APP) from CHO-Hm1 and CHO-Hm3 cells (Emmerling et al., 1995). Activation of cell-surface receptors that are positively coupled to PLC, including m1 and m3 muscarinic receptors, results in an increased release of soluble APPs (Nitsch et al., 1992; Hung et al., 1993). The inverse relationship between production of soluble APP and formation of the β-amyloid peptide suggests that milameline may have a similar effect on APP processing *in vivo*, and thus its effects on AD may go beyond symptomatic improvement to actually having some beneficial influence on disease progression.

In both rodents and nonhuman primates, milameline showed excellent CNS penetration and potent oral activity, with a duration of action exceeding 2 hr. Central muscarinic activity in rats was demonstrated in a variety of tests. Spontaneous swimming activity was decreased at doses between 1 and 3.2 mg/kg taken orally (po), while scopolamine-induced swimming activity was blocked in a dose-dependent manner, with an $ED_{50} = 0.32$ mg/kg subcutaneous (sc). Core body temperature was lowered upon acute dosing (0.32 mg/kg, po) with slightly smaller decreases observed upon daily administration for 14 days. Using the hydrogen clearance technique, local cortical blood flow was increased in the frontal cortex of awake, unrestrained rats at doses of 1.0 mg/kg sc and higher; the duration of action of milameline in this model depended on the dose administered and persisted beyond 120 min at a dose of 10 mg/kg po. Cholinomimetics produce a characteristic decrease in the total power of electroencephalographic (EEG) activity with arousal marked as a shift to low voltage, desynchronized fast-wave activity. In rats, milameline produced such a pattern at doses of 0.1–1.0 mg/kg (po and sc), while in rhesus monkeys this effect was produced at doses of 0.01 mg/kg [intramuscularly (im)] and greater (Schwarz et al., 1991; Davis et al., 1995).

The in vivo effects of milameline on cognitive performance are best demonstrated in rodents. In a lesion-induced impairment model, basal forebrain cholinergic neurons in rats were destroyed with bilateral injections of the excitotoxin ibotenic acid. Using a modified Morris water maze task as a measure of spatial working memory, lesioned rats treated with either 0.1 or 0.32 mg/kg sc of milameline acquired this task more quickly than did control lesioned rats receiving saline. This increase in spatial performance is presumed to be associated with a restoration of cholinergic function upon administration of the agonist (Davis et al., 1995). Additionally, milameline (0.22–0.5 mg/kg po), given 10 min before 0.1 mg/kg sc scopolamine, was able to partially attenuate the amnesic effects of the muscarinic antagonist in rats performing a radial arm maze task (M'Harzi et al., 1995).

Milameline, in a manner consistent with its in vitro activity, produces peripheral side effects in animals that are consistent with activation of peripheral muscarinic receptors such as lacrimation, salivation, urination, diarrhea, bradycardia, and increased pulmonary resistance. In rodents, side effects become more severe as the dose increased. In a model of gastrointestinal function, both stomach emptying and intestinal propulsion were increased in rats, with a minimally effective dose of 0.8 mg/kg po. Significant side effects in monkeys were noted at 0.17 mg/kg, im, but appeared to be reduced in severity with repeated administration. These peripheral side effects for both species diminished in severity and frequency with repeated administration, while central efficacy was maintained. Thus, unlike earlier agents (e.g., oxotremorine, RS-86), which showed side effects at doses below those activating CNS receptors, milameline produced peripheral effects at doses above those at which the desired central effects were observed (Schwarz et al., 1991).

In phase I trials conducted in normal healthy subjects, milameline was well tolerated at single and multiple doses up to 1.0 mg. Peripheral cholinergic signs (sweating, hypersalivation, and increased urinary frequency) were observed at 0.5 and 1.0 mg. Dose-limiting gastrointestinal signs (stomach pain, emesis) were found at the 2 mg/q6h (every 6 hours) dose and all adverse effects resolved when milameline was discontinued. In aged normal volunteers and patients with probable AD, gradual dose escalation extended the tolerated daily dose to 3 mg (Sedman et al., 1995; Stramek et al., 1995b). Milameline has recently completed its first phase II multicenter clinical trial, and the results of this study will be presented later in 1997.

XANOMELINE

Xanomeline (also known as LY246708) is a second-generation muscarinic agonist with a structure based on arecoline, in which the labile ester functionality has been replaced with a bioisoteric 1, 2, 5-thiadiazol-3-yl ring (Sauerberg et al., 1992a,b; Mitch et al., 1993, 1995; Bymaster et al., 1994; Shannon et al., 1994a). The ability of xanomeline to displace radiolabeled agonist and antagonist ligands from M_1 receptors (brain hippocampal and cortical membranes) with high and equal affinity ([^{3}H]oxotremorine, $IC_{50} = 3-10$ nM; [^{3}H]pirenzepine, $IC_{50} = 5-10$ nM) is consistent with the profile of a low-efficacy partial M_1 agonist (Shannon et al., 1994b). The weaker potency for displacement of [^{3}H]QNB from M_2 receptors (brain stem) (IC_{50} = 70 nM) suggests a slight preference for binding to M_1 versus M_2 muscarinic receptors.

As indicated in a previous section, in vitro binding studies are not particularly well suited for the assessment of the true subtype selectivity of muscarinic agonists (Schwarz et al., 1993). Thus, the functional M_1 selectivity of xanomeline has been further evaluated with the help of isolated issue preparations. Agonist effects were noted in the rabbit vas deferens (M_1 receptors) with an EC_{50} = 0.006 nM. A far greater concentration (EC_{50} = 2μM) was required to activate M_2 receptors (guinea pig atria) (Shannon et al., 1994b). Xanomeline induced the dose-dependent contraction of guinea pig ileum (EC_{50} = 9 nM), an effect that is primarily mediated by M_3 muscarinic receptors. Thus, these in vitro tissue studies suggest a muscarinic receptor subtype selectivity profile of $M_1 > M_3 > M_2$.

The use of cell lines expressing cloned muscarinic receptor subtypes is particularly useful to better define the selectivity of muscarinic agonists, including the intrinsic activity at the various receptor subtypes. Even so, the ease of activation of cloned receptors is greatly dependent on the cell lines expressing them. For example, xanomeline is uniquely efficacious at activating m1 receptors expressed in CHO cells (EC_{50} = 0.004 μM; full agonist) but weaker and less efficacious when the m1 receptors are expressed in BHK cells (EC_{50} = 21 μM; 72% of carbachol's maximal effect) (Shannon et al., 1994b). The extreme potency of the compound on CHO-m1 cells is probably best explained by the high receptor reserve of these cells (Bymaster et al., 1994). Comparing the effects of xanomeline across human muscarinic m1–m5 receptors expressed in various cell lines, xanomeline displays the following subtype selectivity profile; m1 > m5 ≥ m4 ≥ m2 > m3 (Shannon et al., 1994b). Some discrepancy is seen between the subtype selectivity determined in tissue preparations and cell lines.

Activation of m1 and m3 muscarinic receptors results in an increased release of soluble APPs (Nitsch et al., 1992). Xanomeline produces a concentration-dependent increase in APPs secretion from CHO-Hm1 cells, with an EC_{50} of about 10 nM and a maximal effect comparable to the nonselective muscarinic agonist carbachol (Eckols et al., 1995). The intriguing implication of this observation is that m1 muscarinic agonists might interfere with β-amyloid peptide formation in AD brain.

Very few reports exist on the effects of xanomeline on animal behavior or cognitive performance. This is in contrast to the multiple reports that exist on acetylcholinesterase inhibitors and various other muscarinic agonists. A series of elegant neurochemical measurements in rat brain provide supporting evidence for the activation of central M_1 receptors following oral administration of the compound (Bymaster et al., 1994). Oral doses between 10 and 60 mg/kg produce pronounced increases in striatal dopamine release (as measured by levels of its metabolite DOPAC), consistent with activation of m1 receptors on dopaminergic nerve terminals, although the contribution of m4 receptors to this effect cannot be ruled out (Levey, 1993). Xanomeline also produces an increase in striatal acetylcholine levels, suggestive of M_2 receptor activation (Bymaster et al., 1994). The magnitude of this M_2 effect is smaller than that produced by the nonselective muscarinic agonist oxotremorine.

In clinical trials, healthy young adults were more tolerant of single and multiple doses of xanomeline than healthy elderly volunteers (Lucas et al., 1995a,b). In the latter group, the maximum tolerated dose (MTD) was 50 mg three times a day, at which dose patients experienced diarrhea, nausea, vomiting, diaphoresis, and hypotension (Sramek et al., 1995a). A double-blind, placebo-controlled bridging study was conducted to evaluate the safety and tolerance of xanomeline in Alzheimer's disease patients (Sramek et al., 1995a; Cutler et al., 1995). A total of 48 patients [58–85 years old, Mini Mental State Examination (MMSE) scores between 10 and 26] were administered fixed doses of xanomeline ranging from 25 to 115 mg, po) three times a day for 7 days. The MTD was found to be 100 mg three times per day (associated with typical parasympathetic adverse events such as mild-to-moderate nausea, vomiting, incontinence of stool, diarrhea, diaphoresis, lacrimation, hypersalivation, and tremors). This MTD in Alzheimer's patients was twice the MTD reported in healthy elderly volunteers, consistent with the greater tolerance of Alzheimer's patients to the side effects of other muscarinic agonists (Sedman et al., 1995). Xanomeline is extensively metabolized following oral administration, displaying a large first-pass effect. This may account for the large intra- and interindividual variability observed in several of the human studies.

A recent multicenter double-blind, placebo-controlled study with 300 AD patients evaluated three dose levels of xanomeline (25, 50, and 75 mg, three times per day). The 75-mg dose was found to produce moderate improvement relative to placebo on several scales (Bodick et al., 1994, 1995). The parasympathetic nature of the observed adverse events suggests that the degree of M_1 selectivity seen in preclinical models does not translate into a significant therapeutic margin in the clinic. Xanomeline is reported to continue in clinical development, but a new transdermal formulation has replaced the initial oral formulation, as a possible solution to the pharmacokinetic limitations of the compound.

Replacement of the thiadiazole ring (ester bioisotere) of xanomeline with other, similar heterocycles, such as isothiazole, oxadiazole, or pyrazine, result in the loss of muscarinic activity (Sauerberg, 1992a). Interestingly, tetrahydropyridyl-oxazole compounds structurally related to xanomeline have been described as potent muscarinic antagonists (Mitch et al., 1994), illustrating how the intrinsic activity of muscarinic agonists can be greatly affected by relatively minor structural changes (Moos et al., 1992).

YM796

YM796 is a bicyclic spiro-piperidinyl compound, structurally related to the classical muscarinic agonist RS-86. Problems associated with a poor pharmacokinetic profile and a very small therapeutic window have limited the clinical use of RS-86 (Hollander et al., 1987). The rationale for the design of YM796 seems to have been the desire to maintain the rigid nature of the compound, in order to promote receptor subtype selectivity, while at the same time exploring structural variations that might lead to an improved pharmacokinetic profile. Other investigators have used a similar approach to design various other analogues of RS-86 (Ishihara et al., 1992; Tsukamoto et al., 1995, 1993).YM796 contains one asymmetric center, and as such can exist in two enantiomeric forms. Most of the muscarinic pharmacology resides in the $(-)$-enantiomer, and in fact $(-)$-YM796 is the substance that is being developed clinically.

Both enantiomers of YM796 bind to muscarinic receptors from rat cerebral cortex ([^{3}H]pirenzepine binding; M_1 receptors) with K_i values of 1.6 and 5.1 μM for the $(-)$ and $(+)$-enantiomers, respectively. PI hydrolysis in rat hippocampal preparations is stimulated by $(-)$-YM796, but with relatively low intrinsic activity (Hidaka et al., 1991).

The relative affinity of both enantiomers of YM796 for cloned rat m1 and m2 muscarinic receptors (expressed in a murine fibroblast B82 cell line) was evaluated using [^{3}H]$(-)$-methylquinuclidinyl benzilate as the radioligand. Both enantiomers displayed relatively similar affinities for binding to a given receptor subtype, and both of them showed a slight preference for binding to m1 over m2 receptors [K_i values for $(-)$-YM796: m1: 16.4 μM; m2: 52 μM]. In second-messenger assays performed on the same transfected cells, $(-)$-YM796 displayed partial agonism at m1 receptors (about 33% of carbachol's maximal effect; $EC_{50} = 26.5$ μM), but this compound displayed no effects on m2 receptors up to the highest tested concentration of 1 mM. The $(+)$-enantiomer was essentially inactive against both receptor subtypes (Wei et al., 1992). These results highlight once again the danger of relying on binding affinities for assessing the receptor subtype selectivity of muscarinic agonists (Schwarz et al., 1993). Because of its partial agonist character at m1 receptors, $(-)$-YM796 may be less likely than other, full agonists to produce down-regulation and desensitization of these receptors when administered to cholinergically impaired subjects (HB Wei et al., 1994).

In the pithed rat model, $(-)$-YM796 produced a dose-dependent increase in heart rate [$ED_{50} = 385$ μg/kg, intravenously (iv)] which was blocked by the M_1-selective muscarinic antagonist pirenzepine, but not by the M_2-selective antagonist methoctramine (Kasai et al., 1992).

The behavioral effects of $(-)$-YM796 have been evaluated in various animal models. Passive avoidance models of learning have been frequently used to evaluate the effects of cholinomimetics and other types of cognition enhancing drugs. The learning impairment produced in mice by the muscarinic antagonist scopolamine (1 mg/kg sc) was reversed by $(-)$-YM796 at doses between 0.03 and 1.0 mg/kg po, with the maximal benefit observed at 0.3 mg/kg. A similar improvement in passive avoidance behavior was noted in senescence-accelerated mice, a genetic model of cholinergic hypofunction (Suzuki et al., 1995a,b). In an electrolytically induced model of cholinergic deficiency (the rat nucleus basalis magnocellularis lesion model), $(-)$-YM796 improved performance in passive avoidance and Morris water maze tests, at doses between 0.016 and 0.25 mg/kg po (Wanibuchi et al., 1990, 1991).

$(-)$-YM796 significantly attenuates the cognitive impairment induced by focal cerebral ischemia in rats. Oral administration of $(-)$-YM796 for several days after a middle cerebral artery occlusion, at doses between 0.1 and 1 mg/kg, improved learning in a passive avoidance task. This effect was mediated by muscarinic receptor activation, as it could be blocked by the M_1 muscarinic antagonist pirenzepine (Yamaguchi et al., 1995).

The potential of $(-)$-YM796 for producing various typically cholinergic side effects was evaluated in mice (Wanibuchi et al., 1994). Mouse core-body temperature dropped ($2°C$ at a dose of 44 mg/kg; pronounced increase in salivary secretion was noted at 22 mg/kg). No tremors were produced up to the highest dose tested of 128 mg/kg po. These doses are significantly higher than those required to produce cognitive improvement and suggest the existence of a wide therapeutic window.

$(-)$-YM796 has been advanced into clinical study for the treatment of Alzheimer's disease. The compound was reported to be in phase 2 human trials in 1992 in Japan and Germany (*Scrip*, 1995b).

AF-102B

Under the premise that a conformationally rigid compound would be desirable for providing selectivity between muscarinic receptor subtypes, AF-102B was designed and synthesized with results from receptor binding and functional assays providing evidence for M_1 selectivity (Fisher et al., 1986). AF-102B binds to muscarinic receptors with a K_i of 5.0 μM in rat brain tissue using [^{3}H]-QNB and shows an agonist-like shift in the presence of a nonhydrolyzable GTP analogue (Fisher et al., 1989). Additional binding studies with [^{3}H]pirenzepine, and [^{3}H]CMD in rat cortical and cerebellar tissues, suggested selectivity for M_1 receptors (Fisher et al., 1991a,b; Iga et al., 1991). However, displacement of [^{3}H]NMS binding using CHO cells transfected with the human muscarinic receptor subtypes show no subtype selectivity (Schwarz et al., 1993).

In functional second-messenger assays using rat m1- and m3-transfected CHO cells, AF-102B stimulated PI hydrolysis in CHO-Rm1 cells as a weak partial agonist (25% of carbachol stimulation) but did not produce such an effect in the CHO-Rm2 cells. In contrast, AF-102B acted as a full agonist on CHO-Rm1 cells in its ability to elevate intracellular calcium levels. Forskolin-stimulated cAMP accumulation was only partially reduced in PC12 cells, which possess predominantly m4 receptors (Fisher et al., 1991a and 1994). It is unknown to what extent the possible variations in receptor reserve across these cell lines may have contributed to the selectivity profile obtained for AF-102B (Schwarz et al., 1993).

Additional in vitro observations that support the M_1 character of AF-102B are effects on neurotransmitter release from rat hippocampal and striatal synaptosomes, which is preferentially controlled by M_1 heteroreceptors rather than M_2 autoreceptors (Ono et al., 1988); the ability to induce pirenzepine-sensitive depolarizations of isolated rabbit superior cervical ganglia (Mochida et al., 1988); and finally the blockade of calcium-dependent potassium currents underlying slow after-hyperpolarization (Fisher et al., 1991a).

Other in vitro effects have also been observed with AF-102B. It showed a neurotrophic-like effect (indicated by neurite outgrowth) in PC12 cells transfected with m1 receptors (PC12M1), an effect that was synergistic with that of nerve growth factor (NGF). AF-102B also stimulated secretion of soluble APPs in these same PC12M1 cells. This effect appeared to be as potent as that of carbachol, as judged by the decline in membrane-associated APPs, and the enhanced secretion of APPs was potentiated by NGF, further illustrating the interaction between m1 receptor activation and NGF, beyond the phenotype effects on neurite outgrowth (Gurwitz et al., 1993; Fisher et al., 1994). These in vitro observations, if observed in vivo, might positively impact disease progression in AD.

In vivo, AF-102B has shown positive behavioral effects in a large number of animal models: (a) AF-102B improved performance in rodents treated with the cholinotoxin AF-64A, as measured in a step-through passive avoidance task, an 8-arm radial maze task, a T-maze task, and in the Morris water maze (MWM). Repetitive administration of AF-102B to the test animals did not diminish the efficacy of AF-102B in the MWM test, indicating that tolerance to the drug had not occurred. (b) AF-102B reversed the amnesia produced in rats and mice by scopolamine in passive avoidance task. (c) AF-102B significantly improved the performance of aged rats in MWM and 8-arm radial maze tasks. (d) AF-102B reversed memory impairments in a two-way shuttle avoidance task and passive avoidance task following electrolytic lesioning of rat basal forebrain neurons. (e) AF-102B enhanced the performance of C57BL/10 mice (hippocampally deficient) in the MWM test. And (f) AF-102B improved retention in a delayed match-to-sample procedure performed in squirrel monkeys (Fisher et al., 1991).

AF-102B produces typical cholinergic side effects (e.g., salivation, lacrimation, and diarrhea). However, these occur at doses that are $10-100$ times higher than those producing positive effects on cognitive performance. Unwanted central effects (e.g., tremors, hypothermia, and purposeless chewing) also show this same degree of separation from the desired cognitive effects. This separation has been attributed to the preferential M_1 nature of this compound (Fisher et al., 1991a).

Phase I and II clinical trails have been performed in both Japan and the United States. No data has appeared in the literature concerning these trials; however, there is some information from a single-blind, placebo-controlled, parallel-group study from Israel. Doses of 20, 40, and 60 mg, 3 times per day, with 2-week placebo lead-in and lead-out phases, were administered to 43 mild to moderately severe AD patients. A significant effect of AF-102B on ADAS cognitive and word recognition scales was found at 40 and 60 mg, with caregivers also noting improvement. The compound was well tolerated with only one dropout due to adverse effects, which were cholinergic in nature (e.g., salivation and diaphoresis). Further clinical trials in AD patients are anticipated (Fisher et al., 1994).

WAL 2014

This compound is the R-($-$) enantiomer of a simple quinuclidininyl ether derivative (see Figure 2). Although its pharmacological profile has not been extensively discussed in the literature, the existing report provides a general outline (Ensinger et al., 1993). WAL 2014 displays no muscarinic receptor subtype binding selectivity (various rat tissue preparations). The functional m1 selectivity of WAL 2014 was evaluated in CHO-Hm1 and CHO-Hm3 cells. The compound is a partial agonist at m1 receptors, about 10 times weaker in potency than carbachol, and a weak partial agonist at m3 receptors. In isolated tissue preparation (rabbit vas deferens, M_1; guinea pig atrium, M_2; guinea pig ileum, M_3), WAL 2014 displays full agonism at M_1 receptors, with approximately 30-fold weaker potency than carbachol. At M_2 and M_3 receptors, WAL 2014 is a weak partial agonist, requiring a concentration about four times higher than that required to produce a half-maximal M_1 response (Ensinger et al., 1993).

The pithed rat and the Thiry fistula dog ileal motility suppression models were used to evaluate the selective M_1 effects of WAL 2014 in vivo (Ensinger et al., 1993). Results from both models are consistent with a preferential activation of M_1 over M_2 and M_3 receptors, at least in the peripheral organs. Evidence of CNS penetration comes in the form of an increase in EEG theta power level following intravenous doses of $1-10$ mg/kg, an effect typical of central cholinomimetic agents. Both the EEG and the pithed rat effects are observed in the same intravenous dose range, which may be suggestive of good CNS penetration. However, other authors have suggested that the EEG effects of cholinergic agents may be primarily mediated by M_2 receptors (Davis et al., 1993). There are no published reports on the oral bioavailability of WAL 2014 in animals, or its efficacy in any animal models of cognition.

The human safety and tolerability of WAL 2014 has been evaluated in young healthy male volunteers. Two single-blind, single-dose safety studies were conducted which together explored the dose range $0.5-160$ mg po. The studies indicated that WAL 2014 is rapidly absorbed, with an absolute oral bioavailability $\geq 70\%$ (Adamus et al., 1995). Increased salivation was noted at single doses of 40 mg and higher. Other typical parasympathetic side effects, which were observed at doses of 100 mg and higher, included urination, lacrimation, gastrointestinal effects, sweating, nausea, and so forth. Cardiovascular side effects included slight tachycardia and systolic hypertension at doses of 80 and 120 mg and higher, respectively. Evaluation of the clinical efficacy of WAL 2014 in demented patients is currently under way in Germany (*Scrip*, 1995a).

FUTURE OF MUSCARINIC AGONIST THERAPY IN ALZHEIMER'S DISEASE

The promise of a meaningful cholinergic treatment for AD that existed in the mid-1980s never fully materialized. The initial excitement soon gave way to the realization that, in order to obtain the full potential of cholinergic therapy, agents would need to produce significant activity in the CNS without dose-limiting parasympathetic side effects, and they would need to possess a pharmacokinetic profile that allowed for convenient oral dosing of the patients. In general, the cholinomimetic agents that existed in the mid-1980s, the first-generation compounds, had not been optimized for these parameters and consistently failed to demonstrate efficacy in AD when taken to the clinic. Thus far, only one first-generation cholinomimetic, the AChE inhibitor tacrine, has been granted regulatory approval in the United States for the treatment of AD (*Scrip,* 1992).

Various strategies have been pursued to design second-generation cholinomimetics, primarily muscarinic agonists and AChE inhibitors. While the latter fall outside the scope of this chapter, the reader is referred to several recent reviews (Jaen and Davis, 1993). In the area of muscarinic agonists, most of the novel design ideas originated from naturally occurring compounds (e.g., arecoline, pilocarpine, etc.) and proceeded in the direction of bioisosteric replacement of biologically unstable moieties (such as the ester group in arecoline, which was replaced with an oxime and a thiadiazole in milameline and xanomeline, respectively) and the introduction of structural elements that would enhance their M_1 (or m1) subtype selectively. In most cases, this selectivity was achieved not by affecting binding affinities to the various receptor subtypes, but rather by adjusting the intrinsic activity of the compounds for the various receptor subtypes and/or optimization of the partitioning of the drug into the desired biological compartment (the brain) (Bromidge et al., 1992; Moltzen and Bjornholm, 1995). Several second-generation muscarinic agonists are presently in very advanced stages of clinical evaluation in AD patients. Some of the most prominent ones (milameline, xanomeline, YM796, AF-102B, etc. have been reviewed here, but several others (thiopilocarpine, SKB-202026, SR 46559, etc.) are also thought to be in the clinic (Eglen et al., 1996). Needless to say, several of these compounds will never make it out of the clinical obstacle course. However, early indications are that several of them are better tolerated and possess better pharmacokinetic characteristics than their first-generation progenitors (Sedman et al., 1995; Sramek et al., 1995a; Adamus et al., 1995). On the other hand, at the present time relatively little information has been disclosed regarding the clinical efficacy of these compounds and expectations still remains high.

Predicting the future is always a difficult task, but one may speculate on the future directions of muscarinic agonist research, both preclinically and clinically. At the preclinical level, various groups and pharmaceutical companies continue the quest for yet better pharmacokinetic profiles and greater m1 selectivity. One such effort has resulted in the identification of PD151832, a somewhat unusual bicyclic oxime structure that was designed in our laboratories and that appears to be a very selective m1/m4 agonist (i.e., truly selective M_1 agonist) in vitro, possesses oral efficacy in animal models of cognition, and displays a very large separation between central efficacy and dose-limiting side effects (Jaen et al., 1995).

A set of recent preclinical observations that may have dramatic clinical consequences deal with the possible link between muscarinic receptor pharmacology and Alzheimer's disease progression. The first of these observations deals with the increased production of soluble APP and reduction in β-amyloid peptide (β/A4) levels observed in vitro as a result of m1 or m3 receptor activation (Nitsch et al., 1992; Buxbaum et al., 1992; Hung et al., 1993). Although these effects have not been confirmed in vivo yet, they are nevertheless suggestive of a greater role for muscarinic agonist therapy in AD than just simple cognitive enhancement. More work needs to be done in animal models (e.g., APP transgenic mice) to firm up this possibility. However, the real challenge in evaluating the cholinomimetic–disease progression link will be posed to clinicians, who no doubt will have to modify their current protocols to measure not only short-term cognitive improvement but also effects on disease progression.

In conclusion, muscarinic pharmacology has come a long ways in the past 15 years. Since the days of intracerebral infusions (bethanechol) and plasma half-lives of less than 15 min (arecoline), several orally active, CNS permeable, centrally selective muscarinic agonists have been designed specifically for the treatment of AD. It should not be much longer before the results are in for several of these compounds, at which point we will all be able to judge the soundness of the muscarinic corollary to the *cholinergic hypothesis of AD*.

REFERENCES

Adamus WS, Leonard JP, Tröger W (1995): Phase I clinical trials with WAL 2014, a new muscarinic agonist for the treatment of Alzheimer's disease. Life Sci 56:883–890.

Bartus RT, Dean RL, Beer B, Lippa AS (1982): The cholinergic hypothesis of geriatric memory dysfunction. Science 217:408–417.

Bodick NC, Offen W (1995): Xanomeline: The first study of the safety and efficacy of an M_1 agonist in mild and moderate Alzheimers disease. Eur. Neuropsychopharmacol. 5:Abs. S-16-4.

Bodick NC, DeLong AF, Bonate PL, Gillespie T, Henry DP, Satterwhite JH, Lucas RA, Heaton J, Carter GV, Farde L, Cutler NR, Sramek JJ, Seifert RD, Conrad JJ, Wardle TS (1994): Xanomeline, a specific M_1 agonist: Early clinical studies. In Giacobini E, Becker R (eds): "Alzheimer Disease: Therapeutic Strategies." Boston: Birkhauser, pp. 234–238.

Bonner TI, Young AC, Brann MR, Buckley NJ (1988): Cloning and expression of the human and rat m5 muscarinic receptor genes. Neuron 1:403–410.

Bonner TI, Buckley J, Young A, Brann MR (1987): Identification of a family of muscarinic receptor genes. Science 237:527–532.

Brann MR, Buckley NI, Bonner TI (1988): The striatum and cerebral cortex express different muscarinic receptor mRNAs. FEBS Lett 230:90–94.

Brauner Osborne H, Ebert B, Brann MR, Falch E, Krogsgaard Larsen P (1995): Annulated heterocyclic bioisosteres of norarecoline. Synthesis and molecular pharmacology at five recombinant human muscarinic acetylcholine receptors. J Med Chem 38:2188–2195.

Bromidge SM, Brown F, Cassidy F, Clark MSG, Dabbs S, Hawkins J, Loudon JM, Orlek BS and Riley GJ (1992): A novel and selective class of azabicyclic muscarinic agonists incorporating an N-methoxy imidoyl halide or nitrile functionality. Bioorg Med Chem Lett 2:791–796.

Bruno G, Mohr E, Gillespie M, Fedio P, Chase TN (1986): Muscarinic agonist therapy of Alzheimer's disease. A clinical trial of RS-86. Arch Neurol 43:659–661.

Buckley NJ, Bonner TI, Buckley CM, Brann MR (1989): Antagonist binding properties of five cloned muscarinic receptors expressed in CHO-K1 cells. Mol Pharmacol 35: 469–476.

Burstein ES, Spalding TA, Hill Eubanks D, Brann MR (1995): Structure-function of muscarinic receptor coupling to G proteins. Random saturation mutagenesis identifies a critical determinant of receptor affinity for G proteins. J Biol Chem 270:3141–3146.

Buxbaum JD, Oishi M, Chen, HI, Pinkas-Kramarski R, Jaffe EA, Gandy SE, Greengard P (1992): Cholinergic agonists and interleukin-1 regulate processing and secretion of the Alzheimer β/A4 protein precursor. Proc Natl Acad Sci 89:10075–10078.

Bymaster FP, Wong DT, Mitch CH, Ward JS, Calligaro DO, Schoepp DD, Shannon HE, Sheardown MJ, Olesen PH, Suzdak PD, Swedberg MD, Sauerberg P (1994): Neurochemical effects of the M_1 muscarinic agonist xanomeline (LY246708/NNC11-0232). J Pharmacol Exp Ther 269:282–289.

Caine ED (1980): Cholinomimetic treatment fails to improve memory disorders. N Engl J Med 303:585–586.

Caulfield MP (1993): Muscarinic receptors—characterization, coupling, and function. Pharmacol Therap 58:319–379.

Christie JE, Shering A, Ferguson J, Glen AI (1981): Physostigmine and arecoline: Effects of intravenous infusions in Alzheimer presenile dementia. Br J Psychiatry 138:46–50.

Cutler NR, Sramek JJ, Seifer RD, Conrad JI, Wardle TS (1995): The safety and tolerance of xanomeline tartrate, an M_1-specific cholinergic agonist, in patients with Alzheimers disease .I. In Hanin, Yoshida, Fisher (eds): "Alzheimers and Parkinsons Diseases." New York: Plenum, pp 479–482.

Davis KL, Hollander E, Davidson M, Davis BM, Mohs RC, Horvath TB (1987): Induction of depression with oxotremorine in patients with Alzheimer's disease. Am J Psychiatry 144:468–471.

Davis RE, Doyle PD, Carroll RT, Emmerling MR, Jaen JC (1995): Cholinergic therapies for Alzheimer's disease. Palliative or disease altering? Arzneimittelforschung 45:425–431.

Davis R, Raby C, Callahan MJ, Lipinski W, Schwarz R, Dudley DT, Lauffer D, Reece P, Jaen J, Tecle H (1993): Subtype selective muscarinic agonists: Potential therapeutic agents for Alzheimer's disease. Prog Brain Res 98:439–445.

Dorje F, Wess J, Lambrecht G, Tacke R, Mutschler E, Brann MR (1991): Antagonist binding profiles of five cloned human muscarinic receptor subtypes. J Pharmacol Exp Ther 256:727–733.

Eckols K, Bymaster FP, Mitch CH, Shannon HE, Ward JS, DeLapp NW (1995): The muscarinic agonist xanomeline increases soluble amyloid precursor protein release from Chinese Hamster Ovary-m1 cells. Life Sci 57:1183–1190.

Eglen RM, Watson N (1996): Selective muscarinic receptor agonists and antagonists. Pharmcaol Toxicol 78:59–68.

Emmerling MR, Moore CJ, Coyle PD, Carroll RT, Davis RE (1995): Cell surface receptor mediated control of amyloid precursor protein secretion: Involvement of pleiotropic signal transduction cascades. In Hanin, Yoshida, Fisher (eds). "Alzheimer's and Parkinson's Diseases." New York: Plenum, pp 131–139.

Ensinger HA, Doods HN, Immel-Sehr AR, Kuhn FJ, Lambrecht G, Mendla KD, Müller RE, Mutschleer E, Sagrada A, Walther G, Hammer R (1993): WAL2014—A muscarinic agonist with preferential neuron-stimulating properties. Life Sci 52:473–480.

Fisher A, Heldman E, Gurwitz D, Haring R, Karton Y, Meshulam H, Pittel Z, Marciano D, Marcovitch I, Brandeis R (1994): Selective signaling via novel muscarinic agonists: Implication for Alzheimer's disease treatments and clinical update. In Giacobini E, Becker R (eds): "Alzheimer Disease: Therapeutic Strategies." Boston: Birkhauser, pp 219–223.

Fisher A, Brandeis R, Karton I, Pittel Z, Gurwitz D, Haring R, Sapir M, Levy A, Heldman E (1991a): ($\pm$)-cis-2-methyl-spiro(1,3-oxathiolane-5,3′)quinuclidine, an M_1 selective cholinergic agonist, attenuates cognitive dysfunctions in an animal model of Alzheimer's disease. J Pharmacol Exp Ther 257:392–403.

Fisher A, Haring R, Gurwitz D, Fraser CM, Pittel Z, Heldman E, Karton I, Brandeis R, Barak D (1991b): New muscarinic agonists with special emphasis on AF102B. In Becker R, Giacobini E (eds): "Cholinergic Basis for Alzheimer Therapy." Boston: Birkhauser, pp 354–362.

Fisher A, Brandeis R, Pittel Z, Karton M, Sapir S, Dachir A, Levey A, Heldman E (1989): ($\pm$)-cis-2-methyl-spiro(1,3-oxathiolane-5,3′)quinuclidine (AF102B): A new M_1 agonist attenuates dysfunctions in AF-64A-treated rats. Neurosci Lett 102:325–331.

Fisher A, Brandeis R, Pittel Z, Karton I, Sapir M, Dacher S, Levy A, Mizobe F, Heldman E (1986): A new M_1 agonist with potential application in Alzheimer's disease. Neurosci Abstr 13:657.

Flynn DD, Ferrari-DiLeo G, Mash DC, Levey AI (1995): Differential regulation of molecular subtypes of muscarinic receptors in Alzheimer's disease. J Neurochem 64: 1888–1891.

Gauthier S, Leblanc R, Robitaille Y, Quirion R, Carlsson G, Beaulieu M, Bouchard R, Dastoor D, Ervin F, Gauthier L (1986): Transmitter-replacement therapy in Alzheimer's disease using intracerebroventricular infusions of receptor agonists [published erratum appears in Can J Neurol Sci 1987 May; 14(2):189]. Can J Neurol Sci 13:394–402.

Gurwitz D, Haring R, Pinkas-Kramarski R, Stein R, Fisher A (1993): Neurotropic-like effects of AF102B, and M_1-selective muscarinic agonist, in PC12 cells transfected with M_1 muscarinic receptors. Neurosci Abstr 19:1767.

Harbaugh RE, Reeder TM, Senter HJ, Knopman DS, Baskin DS, Pirozzolo F, Chui HC, Shetter AG, Bakay RA, Leblanc R, Watson RT, DeKosky ST, Schmitt FA, Reed SL, Johnston JT (1989): Intracerebroventricular bethanechol chloride infusion in Alzheimer's disease. Results of a collaborative double-blind study. J Neurosurg 71:481–486.

Harbaugh RE, Roberts DW, Coombs DW, Saunders RL, Reeder TM (1984): Preliminary report: Intracranial cholinergic drug infusion in patients with Alzheimer's disease. Neurosurgery 15:514–518.

Haroutunian V, Barnes E, Davis KL (1985): Cholinergic modulation of memory in rats. Psychopharmacology 87:266–271.

Hidaka K, Nakamura Y, Akiho H, Harada M, Wanibuchi F, Tsukamoto S, Usuda S (1991): In vitro pharmacology of YM796: A novel, potent and selective M_1 agonist. J Neurochem 57(Suppl):S92.

Hollander E, Davidson M, Mohs RC, Horvath TB, Davis BM, Zemishlany Z, Davis KL (1987): RS86 in the treatment of Alzheimer's disease: Cognitive and biological effects. Biol Psychiatry 22:1067–1078.

Hulme EC, Birdsall NJM, Buckley NJ (1990): Muscarinic receptor subtypes. Ann Rev Pharmacol Toxicol 30:633–673.

Hung AY, Haass C, Nitsch RM, Qiu WQ, Citron M, Wurtman RJ, Growdon JH, Selkoe DJ (1993): Activation of protein kinase C inhibits cellular production of the amyloid β-protein. J Biol Chem 268:22959–22962.

Iga Y, Ogane N, Saito Y, Samuraizono S, Kawanishi G (1991): AF102B: Preclinical experience. In Becker R, Giacobini E. (eds): "Cholinergic Basis for Alzheimer Therapy." Boston: Birkhauser, pp 363–369.

Ishihara Y, Yukimasa H, Miyamoto M, Goto G (1992): Central cholinergic agents. III. Synthesis of 2-alkoxy-2,8-diazaspiro[4.5]decane-1,3-diones as muscarinic agonists. Chem Pharm Bull 40:1177–1185.

Jaen JC, Davis RE (1993): Cholinergic therapies for Alzheimer's disease: Acetylcholinesterase inhibitors of current clinical interest. Curr Opin Invest Drugs 2:363–377.

Jaen J, Barrett S, Brann M, Callahan M, Davis R, Doyle P, Eubanks D, Lauffer D, Lauffer L, Lipinski W, Moreland D, Nelson C, Raby C, Schwarz R, Spencer C, Tecle H (1995): In vitro and in vivo evaluation of the subtype selective muscarinic agonist PD151832. Life Sci 56:845–852.

Jaen JC, Johnson G, Moos WH (1992): Cholinomimetics and Alzheimer's disease. Bioorg Med Chem Lett 2:777–780.

Jones SVP (1993): Muscarinic receptor subtypes: Modulation of ion channels. Life Sci 52:457–464.

Kasai C, Hanayama M, Sato S, Taguchi K, Hidaka K, Asano M (1992): Determination of muscarinic agonist potencies of YM796, a novel, potent, and selective M_1 agonist, in a pithed rat preparation. Jpn J Pharmacol 58(Suppl):388P.

Kubo T, Fukuda K, Mikami A, Maeda A, Takahashi H, Mishina M, Haga K, Ichiyama A, Kangawa K, Kojima M, Matsuo H, Hirose T, Numa S (1986a): Cloning, sequencing and expression of complementary DNA encoding the muscarinic acetylcholine receptor. Nature 323:414–416.

Kubo T, Maeda A, Sugimoto K, Akiba I, Mikami A, Takahashi H, Haga T, Haga K, Ichiyama A, Kangawa K, Matsuo H, Mishina M, Hirose T, Numa S (1986b): Primary structure of porcine cardiac muscarinic acetylcholine receptor deduced from the cDNA sequence. FEBS Lett 209:367–372.

Lazareno S, Farries T, Birdsall NJ (1993): Pharmacological characterization of guanine nucleotide exchange reactions in membranes from CHO cells stably transfected with human muscarinic receptors m1–m4. Life Sci 52:449–456.

Levey AI (1993): Immunological localization of m1–m5 muscarinic acetylcholine receptors in peripheral tissues and brain. Life Sci 52:441–448.

Levey AI, Kitt CA, Simonds WF, Price DL, Brann MR (1991): Identification and localization of muscarinic acetylcholine receptor proteins in brain with subtype-specific antibodies. J Neurosci 11:3218–3226.

Li M, RP Yasuda, Wall SJ, Wellstein A, Wolfe BB (1991): Distribution of m2 muscarinic receptors in rat brain using antisera selective for m2 receptors. Mol Pharmacol 40:28–35.

Lucas RA, Heaton J, Carter GV, Satterwhite H (1995a): Single and multiple dose safety, pharmacodynamics and pharmacokinetics of xanomeline, a novel muscarinic M_1 agonist in healthy male subjects. In I Hanin, Yoshida, Fisher (eds): "Alzheimers and Parkinsons Diseases." New York: Plenum, pp 469–473.

Lucas RA, Heaton J, Carter CG, Satterwhite H (1995b): Safety, tolerance, and pharmacokinetics of xanomeline tartrate: A novel muscarinic M_1 agonist in healthy elderly subjects. In I Hanin, Yoshida, Fisher (eds): "Alzheimers and Parkinsons Diseases." New York: Plenum, pp 475–478.

Marmé W (1890): Arecanusse. Therap Monatsh 4:291.

Mash DC, Flynn DD, Potter LT (1985): Loss of M_2 myscarine receptors in the cerebral cortex in Alzheimer's disease and experimental denervation. Science 228:1115–1117.

M'Harzi M, Palou AM, Oberkander C, Barzaghi F (1995): Antagonism of scopolamine-induced memory impairments in rats by the muscarinic agonist RU 35926 (CI-979). Pharmacol Biochem Behav 51:119–124.

Mitch CH, Bymaster FP, Calligaro DO, Quimby SJ, Schoepp DD, Wong DT, Shannon HE (1994): Muscarinic antagonist activity of 3-(5-alkoxy-oxazol-2-yl)-1,2,5,6-tetrahydropyridines. Bioorg Med Chem Lett 4:1721–1724.

Mitch CH, Bymaster FP, Calligaro DO, Quimby SJ, Sawyer BD, Shannon HE, Ward JS, Olesen PH, Sauerberg P, Sheardown MJ, Suzdak PD (1995): Xanomeline: A potent and selective M_1 muscarinic agonist in vitro. In I. Hanin, Yoshida, Fisher (eds): "Alzheimers and Parkinsons Diseases" New York: Plenum, pp 457–461.

Mitch CH, Bymaster FP, Calligaro DO, Quimby SJ, Sawyer BD, Shannon HE, Ward JS, Olesen PH, Sauerberg P, Sheardown MJ, Suzdak PD (1993): Hexyloxy-TZTP: A potent and selective M_1 agonist in vtiro. Life Sci 52:550.

Mochida S, Mizobe F, Fisher A, Kawanishi G, Kobayashi H (1988): Dual synaptic effects of activating M_1 muscarinic receptors in superior cervical ganglia of rabbits. Brain Res 455:9–17.

Moltzen EK, Bjornholm B (1995): Medicinal chemistry of muscarinic agonists: Developments since 1990. Drugs Future 20:37–54.

Moos WH, Bergmeier SC, Coughenour LL, Davis RE, Hershenson FM, Kester JA, McKee JS, Marriott JG, Schwarz RD, Tecle H, Thomas AJ (1992): Cholinergic agents: Effect of methyl substitution in a series of arecoline derviatives on binding to muscarinic acetylcholine receptors. J Pharm Sci 81:1015–1019.

Mouradian MM, Mohr E, Williams JA, Chase TN (1988): No response to high-dose muscarinic agonist therapy in Alzheimer's disease. Neurology 38:606–608.

Nathanson NM (1987): Molecular properties of the muscarinic acetylcholine receptor. Ann Rev Neurosci 10:195–236.

Nitsch RM, Slack BE, Wurtman RI, Growdon JH (1992): Release of Alzheimer amyloid precursor derivatives stimulated by activation of muscarinic acetylcholine receptors. Science 258:304–307.

Ono S, Saito Y, Ohgane N, Kawanishi G, Mizobe F (1988): Heterogeneity of muscarinic autoreceptors and heteroreceptors in the rat brain: Effects of a novel M_1 agonist. AF102B. Eur J Pharmacol 155:77–84.

Patterson TA, Kosh JW (1993): Elucidation of the rapid in vivo metabolism of arecoline. Gen Pharmacol 24:641–647.

Pearce B, Potter LT (1991): Coupling of m1 muscarinic receptors to G-proteins in Alzheimer's disease. Alzheimer's Dis Assoc Disord 5:163–172.

Penn RD, Martin EM, Wilson RS, Fox JH, Savoy SM (1988): Intraventricular bethanechol infusion for Alzheimer's disease: Results of double-blind and escalating-dose trials. Neurology 38:219–222.

Peralta EG, Ashkenazi A, Winslow JW, Ramachandran J, Capon DJ (1988): Differential regulation of PI hydrolysis and adenylyl cyclase by muscarinic receptor subtypes. Nature 334:434–437.

Peralta EG, Ashkenazi A, Winslow JW, Smith DH, Ramachandran J, Capon DJ (1987a): Distinct primary structures, ligand-binding properties and tissue-specific expression of four human muscarinic acetylcholine receptors. EMBO J 6:3923–3929.

Peralta EG, Winslow JW, Peterson GL, Smith DH, Ashkenazi A, Ramachandran J, Schimerlick MI, Capon DJ (1987b): Primary structure and biochemical properties of an M_2 muscarinic receptor. Science 236:600–605.

Perry EK, Tomlinson BE, Blessed G, Bergmann K, Gibson P, Perry RH (1978): Correlation of cholinergic abnormalities with senile plaques and mental test scores in dementia. Br Med J 2:1457–1459.

Raffaele KC, Berardi A, Morris PP, Asthana S, Haxby JV, Schapiro MB, Rapoport SI, Soncrant TT (1991): Effects of acute infusion of the muscarinic cholinergic agonist arecoline on verbal memory and visuo-spatial function in dementia of the Alzheimer type. Prog Neuropsychopharmacol Biol Psychiatry 15:643–648.

Richards MH (1991): Pharmacology and second messenger interactions of cloned muscarinic receptors. Biochem Pharmacol 42:1645–1653.

Sauerberg P, Olesen PH, Suzdak PD, Sheardown MJ, Mitch CH, Quimby SJ, Ward JS, Bymaster FP, Sawyer BD, Shannon HE (1992a): Synthesis and structure-activity relationships of heterocyclic analogues of the functional M_1 selective muscarinic agonist hexyloxy-TZTP. Bioorg Med Chem Lett 2:809–814.

Richards MH, van Giersbergen PLM (1995): Human muscarinic receptors expressed in A9L and CHO cells: Activation by full and partial agonists. Br J Pharmacol 114:1241–1249.

Sauerberg P, Olesen PH, Nielsen S, Treppendahl S, Sheardown M, Honoré T, Mitch CH, Ward JS, Pike AJ, Bymaster FP, Sawyer BD, Shannon HE (1992b): Novel functional M_1 selective muscarinic agonists. Synthesis and structure-activity relationships of 3-(1,2,5-thiadiazolyl)-1,2,5,6-tetrahydro-1-methylpyridines. J Med Chem 35:2274–2283.

Schwarz RD, Davis RE, Jaen JC, Spencer CJ, Tecle H, Thomas AJ (1993): Characterization of muscarinic agonists in recombinant cell lines. Life Sci 52:465–472.

Schwarz RD, Coughenour LL, Davis RE, Dudley DT, Moos WH, Pavia MR, Tecle H (1991): Novel muscarinic agonists for the treatment of Alzheimer's disease. In Becker R, Giacobini E (eds): "Cholinergic Basis for Alzheimer Therapy." Boston: Birkhauser, pp 347–353.

Scrip (1995a): 2028:8.

Scrip (1995b): 2082:9.

Scrip (1992): 1770:29.

Sedman AJ, Bockbrader H, Schwarz RD (1995): Preclinical and phase I clinical characterization of CI-979/RU35926, a novel muscarinic agonist for the treatment of Alzheimer's disease. Life Sci 56:877–882.

Sethy VH, Francis JW (1990): Pharmacokinetics of muscarinic cholinergic drugs as determined by ex vivo (^{3}H]-oxotremorine-M binding. J Pharmacol Methods 23:285–296.

Shannon HE, Bymaster FP, Calligaro DO, Greenwood B, Mitch CH, Sawyer BD, Ward JS, Wong DT, Olesen PH, Sheardown MJ, Swedberg MDB, Suzdak PD, Sauerberg P (1994a): Xanomeline: A novel muscarinic receptor agonist with functional selectivity for M1 receptors. J Pharmacol Exp Ther 269:271–281.

Shannon HE, Bymaster FP, Calligaro DO, Greenwood B, Mitche CH, Ward JS, Sauerberg P, Olesen P, Sheardown M, Swedberg MDB, Suzdak PD (1994b): Xanomeline: An efficacious and specific M_1 receptor agonist—preclinical update. In Giacobini E, Becker R (eds): "Alzheimer Disease: Therapeutic Strategies, " Birkhauser, Boston, pp 229–233.

Sitaram N, Wiengartner H, Gillin JC (1978): Human serial learning: enhancement with arecoline and choline and impairment with scopolamine. Science 201:274–276.

Soncrant TT, Raffaele KC, Asthana S, Berardi A, Morris PP, Haxby JV (1993): Memory improvement without toxicity during chronic, low dose intravenous arecoline in Alzheimer's disease. Psychopharmacology 112:421–427.

Sramek JJ, Hurley DJ, Wardle TS, Satterwhite JH, Hourani J, Dies F, Cutler NR (1995a): The safety and tolerance of xanomeline tartrate in patients with Alzheimer's disease. J Clin Pharmacol 35:800–806.

Sramek JJ, Sedman AJ, Reece PA, Hourani J, Bockbrader H, Cutler NR (1995b): Safety and tolerability of CI-979 in patients with Alzheimer's disease. Life Sci 57:503–510.

Suzuki M, Yamaguchi T, Ozawa Y, Iawi A, Yamamoto M (1995a): Effect of YM796, a novel muscarinic agonist, on the impairment of passive avoidance response in senescence-accelerated mice. Pharmacol Biochem Behav 51:623–626.

Suzuki M, Yamaguchi T, Ozawa Y, Ohyama M, Yamamoto M (1995b): Effects of (−)-S-2,8-dimethyl-3-methylene-1-oxa-8-azaspiro[4.5]decane L-tartrate monohydrate (YM796), a novel muscarinic agonist, on disturbance of passive avoidance learning behavior in drug-treated senescence-accelerated mice. J Pharmacol Exp Ther 275:728–736.

Tariot PN, Cohen RM, Welkowitz JA, Sunderland T, Newhouse PA, Murphy DL, Weingartner H (1988): Multiple-dose arecoline infusions in Alzheimer's disease. Arch Gen Psychiatry 45:901–905.

Toja E, Bonetti C, Butti A, Hunt P, Fortin M, Barzaghi F, Formento ML, Maggioni A, Nencioni A, Galliani G (1991): 1-Alkyl-1, 2, 5, 6-tetrahydropyridine-3-carboxaldehyde-O-alkyl-oximes: a new class of potent orally active agonists related to arecoline. Eur J Med Chem Chim Ther 26:853–868.

Tsukamoto S, Nagaoka H, Igarashi S, Wanibuchi F, Hidaka K, Tamura T (1995): Synthesis and structure-activity studies of a series of 1-oxa-2,8-diazaspiro[4.5]decan-3-ones and related compounds as M_1 muscarinic agonists. Chem Pharm Bull 43:1523–1529.

Tsukamoto S, Ichihara M, Wanibuchi F, Usuda S, Hidaka K, Harada M, Tamura T (1993): Synthesis and structure-activity studies of a series of spirooxazolidine-2,4-diones: 4-oxa analogues of the muscarinic agonist 2-ethyl-8-methyl-2,8-diazaspiro[4.5]decane-1, 3-dione. J Med Chem 36:2292–2299.

von Euler US, Domeji B (1945): Nicotine-like actions of arecoline. Acta Pharmacol 1:263–269.

Wall SJ, Yasuda RP, Hory F, Flagg S, Martin BM, Ginnis EI, Wolfe BB (1991): Production of antisera selective for m1 muscarinic receptors using fusion proteins: Distribution of m1 receptors in rat brain. Mol Pharmacol 39:643–649.

Wang SZ, El-Fakahany EE (1993): Application of transfected cell lines in studies of functional receptor subtype selectivity of muscarinic agonists. J Pharmacol Exp Ther 266: 237–243.

Wanibuchi F, Nishida T, Yamashita H, Hidaka K, Koshiya K, Tsukamoto S, Usuda S (1994): Characterization of a novel muscarinic receptor agonist, YM796: Comparison with cholinesterase inhibitors in in vivo pharmacological studies. Eur J Pharmacol 265: 151–158.

Wanibuchi F, Konishi T, Hidaka K, Akiho H, Nakamura Y, Takahashi K, Tsukamoto S, Usuda S (1991): Muscarinic activity of a novel M_1 agonist, YM796 and its optical isomer. Soc Neurosci Abtr 488.5.

Wanibuchi F, Konishi T, Harada M, Terai M, Hidaka K, Tamura T, Tsukamoto S, Usada S (1990): Pharmacological studies on novel muscarinic agonists, 1-oxa-8-azapiro[4.5]decane derivatives YM796 and YM954. Eur J Pharmacol 187:479–486.

Wei J, Walton EA, Milici A, Buccafusco JJ (1994): m1–m5 Muscarinic receptor distribution in rat CNS by RT-PCR and HPLC. J Neurochem 63:815–821.

Wei HB, Yamamura HI, Roeske WR (1994): Down-regulation and desensitization of the muscarinic M1 and M2 receptors in transfected fibroblast B82 cells. Eur J Pharmacol 268:381–391.

Wei HB, Roeske WR, Lai J, Wanibuchi F, Hidaka K, Usuda S, Yamamura HI (1992): Pharmacological characterization of a novel muscarinic partial agonist, YM796, in transfected cells expressing the m1 and m2 muscarinic receptor gene. Life Sci 50:355–363.

Wettstein A, Spiegel R (1984): Clinical trials with the cholinergic drug RS 86 in Alzheimer's disease (AD) and senile dementia of the Alzheimer type (SDAT). Psychopharmacology 84:572–573.

Whitehouse PJ, Au KS (1986): Cholinergic receptors in aging and Alzheimer's disease. Prog Neuropsychopharmacol Biol Psychiatry 10:665–676.

Whitehouse P, Price D, Strubble R, Clark A, Coyle J, DeLong M (1982): Alzheimer's disease and senile dementia: Loss of neurons in the basal forebrain. Science 215:1237–1239.

Yamaguchi T, Suzuki M, Yamamoto M (1995): YM796, a novel muscarinic agonist, improves the impairment of learning behavior in a rat model of chronic focal cerebral ischemia. Brain Res 669:107–114.

CHAPTER 19

Neuronal Nicotinic Receptors: Potential Treatment of Alzheimer's Disease with Novel Cholinergic Channel Modulators

MICHAEL W. DECKER and JORGE D. BRIONI

Neuroscience Discovery, Abbott Laboratories, Abbott Park, Illinois 60064-3500

INTRODUCTION

Twenty years ago, decreases in the activity of the synthetic and degradative enzymes for acetylcholine (ACh)—choline acetyltransferase and acetylcholinesterase—were found in the cortex and hippocampus of brains from patients dying with Alzheimer's disease (AD) (Bowen et al., 1976; Davies and Maloney, 1976; Perry et al., 1977). Subsequently, the cause of this reduced cholinergic input to cortex and hippocampus was identified as cholinergic cell loss and cell shrinkage in the nucleus basalis of Meynart (NBM) and the medial septal area/diagonal band of Broca (Coyle et al., 1983; Whitehouse et al., 1982). Cholinergic hypofunction is still the most consistent neurotransmitter abnormality associated with AD.

The apparent relationship between cholinergic hypofunction and cognitive decline coupled with early pharmacological data in humans and in experimental animals indicating a role for ACh in cognitive function suggested that cognitive dysfunction in AD might be a cholinergic-related disorder (Bartus et al., 1982; Coyle et al., 1983). Experiments in rodents appeared to support an important role for these forebrain cholinergic systems in cognitive function, as several studies demonstrated deficits in learning and memory in animals subjected to lesions of either the NBM or the septal area (Decker et al., 1992a; Dekker et al., 1991; Gray and McNaughton, 1982; Olton, 1990). These studies established the importance of cholinergic dys-

Pharmacological Treatment of Alzheimer's Disease: Molecular and Neurobiological Foundations,
Edited by Brioni and Decker
ISBN 0-471-16758-4   © 1997 Wiley-Liss, Inc.

function in the cognitive deficits observed in AD and also provided animal models for testing compounds that might be useful in treating the cognitive symptomatology of the disorder. Although subsequent work has greatly modified our view of the role of ACh in cognitive function (Fibiger, 1991; Gallagher and Colombo, 1995; Voytko et al., 1994) (see also Chapters 4 and 5), the cholinergic hypothesis is still an important driving force in developing palliative treatments for AD.

The cholinergic hypothesis of AD provides the theoretical underpinnings of many of the attempts to treat this disorder. Early rational approaches to developing potential treatments attempted to augment cholinergic function. This general approach arose out of the successful treatment of dopaminergic hypofunction in Parkinson's disease (PD) with L-DOPA, the precursor for dopamine (DA). The administration of choline, a precursor for ACh, was not a notable success in treating AD (Bartus et al., 1982); and alternative attempts to enhance cholinergic function have included treatment with drugs that inhibit AChE [e.g., Tacrine; see Chapter 17), agents that increase the release of ACh [e.g., linopirdine (Brioni et al., 1993)], and compounds that stimulate muscarinic cholinergic receptors (see Chapter 18). This latter approach does not depend on potentiation of ongoing activity and thus does not rely on the existence of intact presynaptic elements to produce increased cholinergic tone, which might be important in advanced AD where cholinergic neurons are devastated. A direct agonist approach, however, does not mimic the spatial and temporal qualities of phasic release of ACh observed under normal conditions (Sarter et al., 1990).

Interestingly, although both nicotinic and muscarinic receptors have been recognized for decades, muscarinic agents were predominant in the first efforts to treat AD. In part, this was because muscarinic receptors are much more abundant in the brain than are nicotinic cholinergic receptors (nAChRs) (Araujo et al., 1990); in fact, it has only recently been widely accepted that nAChRs are important in brain function. In addition, it was well established that muscarinic blockade impaired function on cognitive tests in humans (Christensen et al., 1992; Drachman, 1977) as well as in experimental animals (Bartus and Johnson, 1976; Caulfield et al., 1983; Decker et al., 1990; Eckerman et al., 1980; Flood and Cherkin, 1986; Rush, 1988), supporting the idea that muscarinic neurotransmission was important for cognitive function. Finally, because of toxic and adverse effects of $(-)$-nicotine itself, the therapeutic potential of nicotinic agents has not been extensively explored.

A reevaluation of the therapeutic potential of treatments targeting nAChRs is required for several reasons. First, involvement of nicotinic cholinergic neurotransmission in cognitive function now appears to be supported by pharmacological studies in experimental animals and in humans, as nAChR agonists and antagonists can improve and impair cognitive performance, respectively. Second, nAChR stimulation is capable of releasing a variety of neurotransmitters often found to be reduced in AD, including ACh itself. Third, nicotinic mechanisms participate in the neurogenic control of local cerebral blood flow, which is impaired in AD. Fourth, possible neuroprotective properties of nicotinic agents are supported by work with several *in vitro* and *in vivo* models and by the clinical observation that long-term use of nicotine (i.e., smoking) is negatively correlated with risk for AD (Duijn and Hofman, 1991; Lee, 1994). Finally, it is now understood that several nAChR subtypes are differentially expressed in the brain, ganglia, and neuromuscular junction, receptor diversity that makes it possible to develop agents that will be more selective, and potentially safer, than $(-)$-nicotine itself.

NOVEL CHOLINERGIC CHANNEL MODULATORS

Molecular biological and biochemical studies of the nAChRs in the last decade have established that nAChRs are pentameric structures composed of various α, β, γ, and δ subunits that form different channels with unique electrophysiological properties. The nAChR located in the neuromuscular junction composed of $\alpha1\beta1\delta\gamma$ subunits has been extensively characterized and has served as a model system for the study of a number of ligand-gated ion channels (Galzi et al., 1991). Although it is not yet clear which subunit combinations form the nAChRs in the peripheral and central nervous system, the pharmacology of the putative nAChR subtypes and the selectivity of the known nAChR ligands is beginning to emerge as these subunits can be transiently or permanently expressed in neuronal and nonneuronal cells.

The nAChR is a protein complex that contains binding sites for ACh (the neurotransmitter) as well as binding sites for other types of drugs, and activation or inhibition of these sites can regulate sodium, potassium, and calcium flux through the cholinergic channels. Classical nAChR ligands [e.g., $(-)$-nicotine and $(-)$-cytisine] bind to the ACh binding site on the α subunit of the receptor, whereas recent evidence suggests that neuronal nAChR function can be enhanced or inhibited via sites distinct from those for $(-)$-nicotine (Williams et al., 1994). Interestingly, the antagonistic actions of $(-)$-cytisine in oocytes expressing the $\alpha3\beta2$ subunit combination and the antagonist effect of $(-)$-nicotine on $\alpha9$ nAChR subunits (Elgoyhen et al., 1994; Luetje and Patrick, 1991) also demonstrate that these ligands are not pure activators of all nAChR subtypes.

In view of the unique pharmacological profile of the classical and novel nAChR ligands and due to the evolving complexity of the neuronal nAChRs, a new nomenclature that accurately reflects the pharmacological diversity has been proposed (Arneric et al., 1995a, 1996). The actions of a larger number of agents, termed cholinergic channel modulators (ChCM), may occur via the selective interaction at the ACh site or by allosteric effects (Lena and Changeux, 1993). In this regard, the effects of the ChCMs could be either facilitatory (cholinergic channel activators, ChCAs) or inhibitory (cholinergic channel inhibitors, ChCIs) (Arneric et al., 1996).

ChCAs may activate the cholinergic channel by binding to the ACh site, as in the case of $(-)$-nicotine, or by activating allosteric sites, as is the case for 2-methylpiperidine and physostigmine. ChCIs may inhibit the effect of ACh at the level of the cholinergic channel by at least three likely mechanisms: (1) competitive antagonism at the ACh site as with dihydro-β-erythroidine (DHβE); (2) ion channel blockade, as in the case of mecamylamine; and (3) noncompetitive allosteric inhibition, as shown with agmatine, chlorpromazine, progesterone, MK-801, substance P, arachidonic acid, barbiturates, and procaine (Brioni et al., 1996b).

Experimental research on nAChR ligands during the last decades has been limited to the assessment of $(-)$-nicotine and other naturally occurring alkaloids, but in recent years major efforts in the medicinal chemistry area have been aimed at developing novel modulators of the cholinergic channel. Among the recently synthesized ChCMs are ABT-418 [(*S*)-3-methyl-5-(1-methyl-2-pyrrolidinyl)isoxazole], A-85380 [3-(2-(*S*)-azetidinylmethoxy)pyridine], SIB-1663 [2,3,3a,4,5,9b-hexahydro-7-methoxy-1H-pyrrolo [3,2-H]isoquinoline], SIB-1765F [3-ethynyl-5-(1-methyl-pyrrolidin-2-yl)-pyridine fumarate], and GTS-21 (2,4-dimethoxybenzilidene anabaseine). Epibatidine [exo-2-(6-chloro-3-pyridil)-7-azabicyclo[2.2.1]heptane] is another novel ligand that was isolated from the Ecuadorian frog *Epipedobates tricolor.* The structural formulas of these ligands are shown in Figure 1.

BIOCHEMICAL PHARMACOLOGY OF nAChRs

Binding Studies

The development of selective high-affinity radioligand binding probes for many of the subunit combinations of the nAChR has lagged behind the rapid advances in the molecular biology of nAChRs. Accordingly, most studies have focused on the interaction of ligands with either the high-affinity $[^3H](-)$-nicotine or $[^3H](-)$-cytisine binding site thought to be associated with the $\alpha4\beta2$ subtype or the high-affinity $[^{125}I]\alpha$-BgT binding site believed to correspond to a site on the $\alpha7$ subtype. The distribution of the $\alpha4\beta2$ subunit combination coincides with the distribution of high-

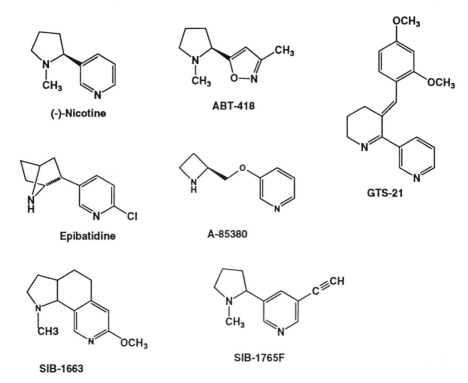

FIGURE 1. Structure of several ChCMs.

affinity nicotine binding sites in rat brain, supporting immunoprecipitation experiments that show that greater than 90% of the high-affinity nicotine binding sites in rat brain can be precipitated by antibodies raised against the $\alpha4$ and $\beta2$ subunits (Flores et al., 1992). A reasonably good correlation also exists between the distribution of $\alpha7$ mRNA, $\alpha7$ protein and that of high-affinity α-BgT binding sites in rodent brain (Clarke et al., 1985; Flores et al., 1992; Seguela et al., 1993). A third distinct population of nAChRs that displays marked selectivity for neuronal bungarotoxin (n-BgT) has more recently been described and may represent receptors containing a combination of $\alpha3$ subunits (Schulz et al., 1991).

Table 1 compares the radioligand binding affinity of a number of ChCMs at the putative $\alpha4\beta2$ and $\alpha7$ receptors in rodent brain, at the human $\alpha4\beta2$ and $\alpha7$ subtypes stably expressed in cell lines, and at the neuromuscular junction $\alpha1\beta1\delta\gamma$ subtype found in *Torpedo* electroplax tissue. Among the ChCMs the rank order of potency at both the rodent and human $\alpha4\beta2$ receptor is A-85380 ($K_i = 0.04$ nM) = ($\pm$)-epibatidine > ($-$)-nicotine > ACh = ABT-418 > GTS-21 > DHβE > MLA (Brioni et al., 1996). DHβE has been shown to be a competitive inhibitor of $[^3H](-)$-cytisine binding to rodent brain (Decker et al., 1995a).

All of the ChCAs display markedly lower affinity for the $[^{125}I]\alpha$-BgT binding site in rodent brain and for the human $\alpha7$ subtype. The rank order of potency at the human $\alpha7$ subtype is MLA ($K_i = 4$nM) > ($\pm$)-epibatidine > A-85380 > GTS-21 > ($-$)-nicotine > ABT-418 > ACh > DHβE. ($\pm$)-Epibatidine is the most potent ChCM at the neuromuscular junction $\alpha1\beta1\delta\gamma$ subtype with a K_i value of 2.7 nM (Sullivan et al., 1994b). A-85380, MLA, and GTS-21 are greater than 100-fold less potent to interact with this subtype (K_i = 350, 1480, and 1500 nM, respectively). DHβE displays a K_i value of 10,000 nM (Decker et al., 1995b), while ABT-418, ACh, and ($-$)-nicotine also display weak affinity for this binding site.

Molecular Biology and Electrophysiology of nAChRs

The identification of 11 nAChR subunit genes in rat, chick, and human brain as well as in sensory tissue provides for a multitude of potential combinations, suggesting that many functional subtypes of neuronal nAChR are possible (Arneric et al., 1995a; Deneris et al., 1991; Elgoyhen et al., 1994; McGehee and Role, 1995; Papke, 1993; Sargent, 1993). Of the neuronal genes, eight ($\alpha2-\alpha9$) code for α subunits and three ($\beta2-\beta4$) encode β subunits (Arneric et al., 1995a; Elgoyhen et al., 1994). Rat, human, and chick nAChR genes of the same name are highly homologous (>70% amino acid identity), suggestive of a common ancestral gene (McGehee and Role, 1995; Sargent, 1993).

Oocyte transfection studies have provided considerable information on the properties of different subunit combinations. Oocytes transfected with pairwise combinations of α and β subunits demonstrate functional responses in confirmation of biochemical data that indicate native nAChRs consist of α/β heteromers (Deneris et al., 1991; McGehee and Role, 1995; Papke, 1993; Sargent, 1993). $\alpha7$, $\alpha8$, and $\alpha9$ gene products differ from other members of the nAChR superfamily in that they can form functional channels in oocytes when expressed as homo-oligomers (Briggs et al., 1995; Elgoyhen et al., 1994; Gerzanich et al., 1994; Seguela et al., 1993).

TABLE 1. Radioligand Binding Properties of Cholinergic Channel Modulators[a]

| | Radioligand Binding Affinity (K_i, nM) | | | | |
| | α4β2 | | α7 | | α1β1δγ |
Compound	Rat Brain	Human K177 Cells	Rat Brain	Human K28 Cells	Torpedo Electroplax
ACh	4	3	>10,000	9,910	>10,000
(−)-Nicotine	1	1	5,000	1,610	>10,000
ABT-418	4.5	6	>10,000	4,000	>10,000
A-85380	0.04	0.04	180	120	350
(±)-Epibatidine	0.04	0.07	120	20	2
SIB-1765F	4	ND	ND	ND	ND
GTS-21	19	23	211	652	1,500
DHβE	24	60	9,000	>10,000	10,000
MLA	2,519	3205	4	10	1,480

[a]ND: not determined. See text for references.

Not all subunit combinations form functional nAChRs. The rat β3 gene in combination with genes for α2, α3, or α4 is unable to form a functional nAChR but may play a regulatory role when coexpressed with α and β subunits (Deneris et al., 1991; McGehee and Role, 1995; Sargent, 1993). Similarly, rat α5 and α6 genes do not participate in the formation of functional nAChR channels when coexpressed with various β subunits but may subserve a regulatory role (McGehee and Role, 1995; Ramirez-Lattore et al., 1993). The existence of regulatory subunits like α5 and β3 provides additional complexity to potential neuronal nAChR subunit combinations and may explain some of the discrepancies in channel properties seen in oocyte expression studies as compared to nAChRs expressed in vivo.

While studies in oocytes have yielded some clues as to the physiological roles of the different nAChR subunits *in vivo*, some caution is required in interpreting these findings because of the atypical nature of the oocyte membrane environment. Accordingly, a number of investigators have sought to establish mammalian cell lines stably expressing defined nAChR subunit combinations. To date, cell lines stably expressing the avian α4β2, rat α3β4, human α4β2, and human α7 (Gopalakrishnan et al., 1995, 1996; Whiting et al., 1992) subtypes have been described. These cell lines have served as valuable systems for investigating the function and regulation of nAChR subtypes and for examining ligand interactions.

(±)-Epibatidine is a very potent agonist at the rodent and human α4β2 subunit combinations either in *Xenopus* oocytes (EC_{50} = 0.016 μM) (Moulton et al., 1996) or stably expressed in a human cell line, K177, (EC_{50} = 0.017 μM) (Gopalakrishnan et al., 1996). It is noteworthy that this agent is a full agonist at the human α4β2 subtype (Gopalakrishnan et al., 1996) but appears to function as a mixed agonist–antagonist at the rodent subtype (Moulton et al., 1996). The rank order of other ChCMs to activate the rodent subtype is ACh (EC_{50} = 2 μM) > (−)-nicotine = ABT-418 > GTS-21 = (±)-anabaseine > (−)-cytisine (EC_{50} > 100μM). ABT-418 (60%), GTS-21 (<5%), (±)-anabaseine (<10%), and (−)-cytisine (<15%) all display less than maximal efficacy relative to ACh to activate the rodent α4β2 subunit combination injected in oocytes. Indeed, it has been demontrated that (−)-cytisine is a potent competitive inhibitor of the rodent α4β2 responses to ACh (IC_{50} = 20 nM) (Papke and Heinemann, 1993). Thus, at rodent α4β2 receptors (−)-nicotine is a full agonist equipotent to ACh whereas(−)-cytisine is a partial agonist. The difference between (−)-cytisine and (−)-nicotine may be related to structural differences and to how the β2 subunit configures a site of agonist interaction in the different conformational states of the receptor.

ABT-418 and (±)-epibatidine are full agonists at the human subtype relative to(−)-nicotine in contrast to their partial efficacy reported at the rat α4β2 subtype (Gopalakrishnan et al., 1996). The rank order of potency at the human subtype is (±)-epibatidine (EC_{50} = 0.016 μM) > (−)-cytisine = A-85380 > (−)-nicotine > ABT-418 > ACh > (+)-nicotine > GTS-21 (EC_{50} > 300 μM) (Briggs et al., 1996; Gopalakrishnan et al., 1996; Sullivan et al., 1996). DHβE is the most potent ChCI at the α4β2 subtype displaying IC_{50} values of 0.05 and 1.87 μM toward the rat and human nAChRs, respectively (Gopalakrishnan et al., 1996; Papke and Heinemann, 1993).

The $\alpha 7$ subunit is capable of forming a functional ion channel when expressed as homo-oligomers in *Xenopus* oocytes (Bertrand et al., 1992; Courturier et al., 1990; Seguela et al., 1993) and transfected cell lines (Gopalakrishnan et al., 1995). As noted earlier, the $\alpha 7$ subunit probably comprises most, if not all, of the high-affinity $[^{125}I]\alpha$-BgT-sensitive nAChRs. Pharmacological and electrophysiological characterization of the $\alpha 7$ subunit expressed in *Xenopus* oocytes and a mammalian cell line (K28) indicate that this receptor desensitizes more rapidly than other nAChRs, is highly sensitive to α-BgT (Courturier et al., 1990; Gopalakrishnan et al., 1995; Seguela et al., 1993), and displays a permeability to Ca^{2+} ions that is significantly greater than those observed for other ligand-gated ion channels including N-methyl-D-aspartate (NMDA) subtype of glutamate receptors (Seguela et al., 1993; Vernino et al., 1992).

The rank order of potency of ChCMs to activate the rodent or human $\alpha 7$ receptor injected into oocytes is $(+)$-anatoxin-a $(EC_{50} = 0.58 \ \mu M) > (\pm)$-epibatidine $> (-)$-cytisine $>$ GTS-21 $> (-)$-nicotine $>$ ABT-418 $>$ ACh. GTS-21 is a relatively potent partial (25%) agonist relative to $(-)$-nicotine at the rodent subtype but displays very weak agonism ($<20\%$) at the human equivalent. Indeed, this ChCM inhibits the channel currents elicited by ACh with an IC_{50} value of 3 μM (Briggs et al., 1995). ABT-418 behaves as either a partial ChCA or mixed ChCA/ChCI relative to ACh for both rat and human $\alpha 7$ receptors (Briggs et al., 1995; Moulton et al., 1996). Methyllycaconitine (MLA) displays marked selectivity toward the $\alpha 7$ subtype, inhibiting the functional responses to ACh with an IC_{50} value of 4 nM (Wonnacott et al., 1993).

nAChR-mediated Release of Neurotransmitters in the Brain

Activation of presynaptic nAChRs leads to the facilitation of the release of several neurotransmitters including dopamine (DA), ACh, norepinephrine (NE), serotonin (5-HT), γ-aminobutyric acid (GABA), and glutamate (Andersen et al., 1971; Beani et al., 1985, 1991; Wonnacott et al., 1990a,b, 1987, 1995). While the subtypes involved in nAChR-mediated release of these neurotransmitters are not firmly established, it appears the effects at distinct subtypes may mediate the release of different neurotransmitters. Thus, several known nAChR ligands selectively release central nervous system (CNS) neurotransmitters, and development of more selective neurotransmitter-releasing agents using this strategy may be possible.

$(-)$-Nicotine stimulates the release of $[^{3}H]$-DA from rat striatal preparations in a stereoselective fashion. $(\pm)$-Epibatidine and A-85380 are the most potent ChCAs to stimulate DA release with EC_{50} values of 0.0008 and 0.0023 μM, respectively (Sullivan et al., 1994, 1996). The rank order of potency of ChCAs to stimulate DA release from rat striatum is $(\pm)$-epibatidine $>$ A-85380 $>$ ACh $= (-)$-nicotine $>$ ABT-418 $>$ SIB-1663 $>$ GTS-21 (Brioni et al., 1996b). Grady and co-workers (1992) have observed a similar rank order of potency of ChCMs to stimulate $[^{3}H]$-DA release from mouse striatal synaptosomes.

Among ChCIs, the rank order of potency to block nAChR-induced release from rat striatal slices is DHβE $(IC_{50} = 0.05 \ \mu M) =$ erysodine $>$ mecamylamine $=$

MLA > chlorisondamine (IC_{50} = 1.3 μM) ~ lobeline (Clarke, 1994; Decker et al., 1995b; Lippiello et al., 1995; Wonnacott et al., 1993, 1990b). DHβE and erysodine are competitive inhibitors of this response while mecamylamine and chlorisondamine behave as noncompetitive channel blockers.

The nAChR subtype(s) mediating the release of DA have not been clearly established. In mice, (−)-nicotine-induced DA release may be mediated via an α3-containing subunit combination, possibly α3β2, on the basis of the ability of n-BgT to block the response (Grady et al., 1992). In rats, a role for an α3-containing subunit combination is suggested by the reports that SIB-1663, a ChCM with reported selectivity toward α3β4 subunits, can stimulate DA release, albeit weakly (Lloyd et al., 1994). The high-affinity binding of (−)-nicotine and other agonists to the putative α4β2 subtype is not a very good predictor of their potency or efficacy to stimulate DA release from striatal preparations (Decker et al., 1995a).

A role for nAChRs in the modulation of ACh release from cortex and hippocampus has been described (Wilkie et al., 1993; Wonnacott et al., 1990b, 1995). While the subtype(s) mediating this effect has not been definitively characterized, recent studies suggest the involvement of the α4β2 subunit combination in the release of ACh from rat hippocampal synaptosomes (Wilkie et al., 1993). A limited number of ChCMs have been evaluated for their ability to stimulate [^{3}H]ACh release from rat hippocampal synaptosomes. (+)-Anatoxin-a is the most potent ChCA with an EC_{50} of 0.14 μM (Thomas et al., 1993), while (−)-nicotine, (−)-cytisine, and ABT-418 display similar potencies (EC_{50} values = 1.7, 3.7, and 3 μM, respectively) (Arneric et al., 1994; Wonnacott et al., 1995). All of the compounds are full agonists to elicit this response. Comparison of the ability of ChCMs to modulate DA and ACh release reveals that while ABT-418 is 10-fold less potent than (−)-nicotine to evoke [^{3}H]-DA release from rat striatal slices, it is equipotent to enhance the release of [^{3}H]ACh from rat hippocampus.

Comparative studies with (−)-nicotine done in vivo also have demonstrated nAChR-mediated release of a variety of neurotransmitters (Benwell and Balfour, 1992; Mitchell, 1993; Ribeiro et al., 1993). However, examination of the potency and efficacy of diverse ChCMs to release CNS neurotransmitters *in vivo* has not been reported yet. These studies would be of critical importance as they would eventually help determine which released neurotransmitters are related to specific behavioral actions of ChCMs.

BEHAVIORAL PHARMACOLOGY OF THE CHOLINERGIC CHANNEL MODULATORS

(−)-Nicotine

The importance of nicotinic cholinergic neurotransmission for normal cognitive function is illustrated by the finding that nAChR blockade can disrupt performance on cognitive tasks. For example, mecamylamine impairs acquisition of avoidance learning, maze learning, and acquisition of spatial information in rodents and disrupts delayed matching-to-sample performance in monkeys and classical conditioning in rabbits (Decker and Majchrzak, 1992; Dilts and Berry, 1967; Elrod et al., 1988; Levin et al., 1987; Oliverio, 1966; Woodruff-Pak et al., 1994b). In these studies involving experimental animals, mecamylamine is more effective in impairing the acquisition of new information than in disrupting retrieval of previously learned information (Decker and Majchrzak, 1992), a pattern of deficits that resembles that found when mecamylamine is given to humans (Newhouse et al., 1994). Moreover, abnormalities of local cerebral blood flow found in AD bear some resemblance to those observed after administration of mecamylamine (Prohovnik, 1990). Until recently, however, mecamylamine was the only nAChR antagonist demonstrated to impair cognitive performance. Attempts to duplicate these effects with the long-lasting blocker, chlorisondamine, have not been successful (Clarke and Fibiger, 1990; Decker and Majchrzak, 1993). Consequently, there has been some reluctance to accept the mecamylamine results as strong evidence for the involvement of nAChRs in cognitive function. For example, the possibility that mecamylamine, which is a channel blocker that acts at NMDA receptor channels at high doses, may impair cognitive performance via effects on glutamatergic neurotransmission must be considered (Clarke and Fibiger, 1990). There is now evidence, however, that at least some of the same cognitive impairments observed with mecamylamine are seen with other nAChR antagonists, such as n-BgT and DHβE, evidence that strengthens the case for the importance of nAChRs in cognitive processes (Curzon et al., 1996; Granon et al., 1995).

The ability of nAChR activation to improve cognitive performance has been demonstrated in a number of reports that (−)-nicotine improves performance in human and in experimental animals. Studies with humans have frequently used smokers as subjects. Although this practice often makes it difficult to determine if the observed improvements are due to true cognitive enhancement or to reduction of withdrawal symptoms, recent studies with minimally deprived smokers suggest that withdrawal symptom relief does not provide a complete account of (−)-nicotine's cognitive-enhancing effects in humans (Rusted et al., 1994; Warburton and Arnall, 1994). Of course, withdrawal effects can be avoided in studies with experimental animals; and although (−)-nicotine-induced improvements in cognitive tasks are not universally observed, a large number of studies have demonstrated that (−)-nicotine can improve performance on a variety of cognitive tasks [for review, see Levin (1992)]. For example, pretraining administration of (−)-nicotine improves retention of inhibitory (passive) shock avoidance training in mice without affecting reactivity to the footshock (Brioni and Arneric, 1993). Similarly, (−)-nicotine administered to rats immediately after inhibitory avoidance training can also enhance retention of the training experience, suggesting that (−)-nicotine's effects on this task may be mediated by effects on memory consolidation processes that take place after the training experience (Decker and Majchrzak, 1993; Haroutunian et al., 1985). (−)-Nicotine's effects are not restricted to aversively motivated tasks, as (−)-nicotine improves the performance of normal rats in the radial arm maze, an appetitively motivated spatial memory task, and enhances delayed matching-to-sample performance in normal monkeys (Buccafusco and Jackson, 1991; Elrod et al., 1988; Levin et al., 1990a).

Or perhaps greater clinical relevance, $(-)$-nicotine can improve performance in models of cognitive impairment. $(-)$-Nicotine ameliorates attentional deficits observed in rats given NBM lesions (Muir et al., 1995) and improves spatial memory task performance of rats with combined lesions of the NBM and the medial septum (Hodges et al., 1991). Spatial learning deficits produced by septal lesions can also be ameliorated by $(-)$-nicotine administration (Decker et al., 1992b); and $(-)$-nicotine can improve the performance of aged animals on learning and memory tasks (Buccafusco and Jackson, 1991; Meguro et al, 1994; Socci et al., 1995; Widzowski et al., 1994). The observation that $(-)$-nicotine can attenuate cognitive deficits found in both aged animals and animals with lesions of the cholinergic basal forebrain provides support for the exploration of the therapeutic potential of nicotinic agents and is consistent with the results of some early trials in humans suggesting that nAChR activation may be useful in the palliative treatment of AD (Jones et al., 1992; Newhouse et al., 1988; Sahakian et al., 1989).

The mechanism underlying nAChR-mediated cognitive enhancement is not clear, but it is possible that release of other neurotransmitters plays a role. As noted earlier, $(-)$-nicotine stimulates the release of DA, NE, 5-HT, and ACh. Many of these same neurotransmitter systems are disrupted in AD and are believed to be important in cognitive processes (Brioni, 1993).

DA release probably plays an important role in a number of $(-)$-nicotine's behavioral effects. For example, DA release is probably the basis for $(-)$-nicotine's stimulant effects on locomotion and may be important in its abuse liability (Clarke, 1990, 1994). DA release may also underlie some of $(-)$-nicotine's cognitive effects. Pretraining administration of $(-)$-nicotine improves retention of inhibitory avoidance, as already noted (Brioni and Arneric, 1993). Interestingly, cytisine, which can also induce DA release, improves performance under these conditions, but lobeline, which does not release DA readily, does not improve performance (Brioni and Arneric, 1993). Moreover, $(-)$-nicotine's effects in this task can be prevented by the DA antagonist, *cis*-flupenthixol (Brioni and Arneric, 1993). Similarly, $(-)$-nicotine's ability to reverse scopolamine-induced inhibitory avoidance deficits can be prevented by DA blockade (Nitta et al., 1994). In addition, mecamylamine-induced impairments of radial maze performance are potentiated by DA antagonists, prevented by D2 agonist treatment, and can be observed after injection into dopaminergic regions [i.e., the substantia nigra and ventral tegmental area (VTA)] (Levin et al., 1994, 1989, 1990b).

Effects on DA cannot account for all of $(-)$-nicotine's cognitive effects, however. Lobeline, an nAChR ligand with minimal potency to release DA (Grady et al., 1992), mimics some of $(-)$-nicotine's cognitive effects (Decker et al., 1993); and as will be discussed below, ABT-418, an nAChR agonist that is less potent than $(-)$-nicotine in releasing DA in vitro, is as potent or more potent than $(-)$-nicotine in improving performance in a variety of cognitive tasks. Similarly, DA release induced by D-amphetamine cannot mimic the improved attentional performance in NBM-lesioned rats produced by $(-)$-nicotine (Muir et al., 1995).

The importance of NE and 5-HT release in $(-)$-nicotine's cognitive effects has not been extensively investigated. The disruptive effects of mecamylamine on radial maze performance can be potentiated by β-adrenergic blockade (Decker, 1992), but neither β-adrenergic blockade nor NE depletion appear to be able to prevent (−)-nicotine-induced enhancement of spatial learning and memory task performance (Gray et al., 1994; Grigoryan et al., 1994). Thus, there is as yet little evidence for the involvement of NE release in (−)-nicotine's cognitive effects. In contrast, there is at least some preliminary evidence that some of the cognitive effects of (−)-nicotine could be mediated by 5-HT release. For example, disruption of serotoninergic neurotransmission can potentiate mecamylamine-induced disruption of water maze performance, and 5-HT depletion can prevent (−)-nicotine-induced enhancement of the performance of septal-lesioned rats (Riekkinen et al., 1994; 1992, 1995).

The ability of (−)-nicotine to stimulate ACh release raises the interesting possibility that nAChR activation could improve cognitive function by increasing ACh release. In this regard, it is notable that (−)-nicotine improves the performance of NBM-lesioned rats on an attentional task, an effect mimicked by cholinesterase inhibition but not by catecholamine release (Muir et al., 1995). If ACh release plays an important role in (−)-nicotine's cognitive effects, it is possible that at least some of the cognitive effects of nAChR activation may be mediated by muscarinic receptors. In support of this idea, (−)-nicotine-induced improvements in delayed matching-to-sample performance in monkeys can be prevented by a dose of muscarinic antagonist that does not by itself affect performance (Terry et al., 1993).

It is entirely possible that different aspects of (−)-nicotine's effects are mediated through the release of different neurotransmitters (Gray et al., 1994); and depending on the complexity of the task, effects on multiple transmitters may be involved. Moreover, many of the behavioral effects of (−)-nicotine may not involve modulatory effect on other neurotransmitter systems. Investigation of the role of transmitter release in the cognitive effects of (−)-nicotine, however, has provided some initial ideas regarding mechanisms involved in these effects. Furthermore, these findings may be useful in elucidating the participation of different nAChR subtypes in cognitive processing, since nAChR-mediated release of different neurotransmitters appears to involve different nAChR subtypes, as discussed earlier.

In addition to the potential for nAChR activation in the palliative treatment of AD, there is some indication that activation of nAChRs may have neuroprotective properties. Preexposure to (−)-nicotine enhances the survival of cell cultures exposed to excitatory amino acids (Akaike et al., 1994; Donnelly-Roberts et al., 1996; Marin et al., 1994). Furthermore, (−)-nicotine can attenuate neuronal loss following knife cuts of the nigral-striatal pathway (Janson et al., 1988). These studies, if confirmed in other models of neurodegeneration, might suggest that nicotinic agents would be useful in slowing neurodegenerative diseases such as AD. An agent with both cognition-enhancing and neuroprotective properties would clearly be superior to one that can only slow the progress of the disease, given that AD cannot currently be diagnosed until after significant cognitive decline has already occurred. Thus, although a compound with only neuroprotective properties might be able to slow further progress of the disease, it would still be important to improve the level of functioning.

Although preclinical work with (−)-nicotine suggests that the compound has some potentially beneficial properties, (−)-nicotine itself has pronounced side-effect liabilities. Many of the beneficial effects of (−)-nicotine are found at doses only slightly below those producing adverse effects; and abuse, cardiovascular, and gastrointestinal liabilities of (−)-nicotine are well documented in humans (Arneric et al., 1995a; Williams et al., 1994). For these reasons, it is important to examine the therapeutic potential of other nAChR ligands. Fortunately, several novel agents have become available for preclinical testing in recent years; some of which are discussed in the following sections.

(±)-Epibatidine

Epibatidine was originally isolated from a frog skin and after the elucidation of its chemical structure, several synthetic pathways have been proposed. (±)-Epibatidine interacts potently with the high-affinity [^{3}H]-nicotine binding site ($K_i = 0.04$ nM), but is 50-fold less potent at α-BgT sites on muscle-type nAChRs and more than 3 orders of magnitude less potent at the α-BgT site present in the brain, the putative $\alpha 7$ subtype ($K_i = 230$ nM). Thus, (±)-epibatidine displays 10- to 100-fold selectivity for the $\alpha 1$ subunit in comparison to the $\alpha 7$ subunit of the nAChR.

The most well-studied property of (±)-epibatidine from the therapeutic point of view is its analgesic-like effect (Badio and Daly, 1994; Qian et al., 1993). (±)-Epibatidine exhibits analgesic-like actions in rodent models (tail-flick, hot-plate, etc.) at doses as low as 25–50 nmol/kg, and this effect appears to be mediated through central nAChRs and not by opioid receptors. (±)-Epibatidine is nearly 100-times more potent than morphine and (−)-nicotine as an analgesic in rodents (Damaj et al., 1994; Sullivan et al., 1994a,b). Doses of (±)-epibatidine that are analgesic also produce hypothermia and reduce locomotor activity in mice, but the time course of (±)-epibatidine's analgesic-like effects and its motor effects can be dissociated (Bannon et al., 1995a).

In rats trained to discriminate (−)-nicotine from saline, (±)-epibatidine induces a full generalization to (−)-nicotine (Figure 2) and is 190-fold more potent than (−)-nicotine (Sullivan et al., 1994a). The enhanced potency of (±)-epibatidine to stimulate DA release agrees well with these in vivo drug discrimination studies. These results suggest that (±)-epibatidine may have addiction liabilities, as both dopamine release and the ability to induce a salient interoceptive cue are characteristic of a wide variety of addictive substances. In this regard, it is important to note that the doses of (±)-epibatidine inducing the cue are significantly lower than those exhibiting analgesic-like properties; so this compound does not represent any improvement in comparison to (−)-nicotine.

In other behavioral tests, (±)-epibatidine impairs retention of the inhibitory avoidance in mice when administered prior to training, an effect that is confounded by a drug-induced reduction in shock sensitivity (Sullivan et al., 1994a); and, unlike (−)-nicotine, (±)-epibatidine does not exhibit anxiolytic-like effects on the elevated plus-maze test (Sullivan et al., 1994b). Further experimentation in this area could clarify the therapeutic potential of (±)-epibatidine-like compounds for the treatment of AD.

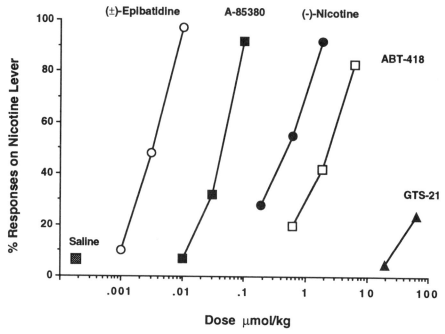

FIGURE 2. Effect of ChCMs in rats trained to discriminate 1.9 μmol/kg (−)-nicotine from saline after systemic injections.

(±)-Epibatidine is the most potent activator of ganglionic and neuromuscular nAChRs described to date, which results in profound hypertension and, eventually, respiratory paralysis as a presumed cause of death. These profound toxicities, its potent nicotine-like cue, and its reduced safety index limit its usefulness as a therapeutic agent at the present time. Medicinal chemistry efforts in this area must achieve selectivity at the level of the nAChR subtypes in order to clarify the therapeutic potential of the (±)-epibatidine analogs for the treatment of AD.

A-85380 is another novel ChCM with high affinity for the α4β2 subunit ($K_i = 0.04$ nM). Its behavioral profile is somewhat similar to (±)-epibatidine as it exhibited analgesic-like actions in the hot-plate (albeit weakly), but it induced the nicotine cue at doses significantly lower than (−)-nicotine (Figure 2). The cardiovascular liabilities of this compound preclude its consideration for clinical evaluation (data not shown).

ABT-418

ABT-418 is an isoxazole isostere of (−)-nicotine (Arneric et al., 1994). This ChCA is a selective activator for the α4β2 subtype relative to the α3 and α7 subtypes as described in the previous sections. In vivo, pretraining administration of ABT-418 enhances retention of inhibitory avoidance training in mice, an effect that is stereoselective and mecamylamine sensitive (Decker et al., 1994a). Improved retention of inhibitory avoidance training is observed in rats with posttraining administration, suggesting that ABT-418 affects memory consolidation processes subsequent to the training experience (Arneric et al., 1995b). In rats with lesions of the medial septum, ABT-418 ameliorates water maze learning deficits (Decker et al., 1994b), an effect that has also been observed with (−)-nicotine (Decker et al., 1992b). Cognition-enhancing effects of ABT-418 are not limited to rodents, as the compound improves the performance of mature adult monkeys in a delayed match-to-sample memory task (Buccafusco et al., 1995). Improved performance with ABT-418 is also observed in aged monkeys whose baseline performance on this task is impaired relative to that of mature adult monkeys (Prendergast et al., submitted). However, the dose of ABT-418 required to improve the performance of aged monkeys is somewhat higher than that required in younger monkeys.

In general, the cognitive effects of ABT-418 are observed at doses comparable to or somewhat lower than the doses at which (−)-nicotine is effective. Profound potency differences between ABT-418 and (−)-nicotine are found in their effects on cerebral blood flow, however. Recent evidence has suggested that some of the cerebral blood flow abnormalities observed in AD patients may be related to degeneration of the basal forebrain (Arneric, 1991; Linville and Arneric, 1991), which appears to be important in the neurogenic control of cerebral circulation. At least some aspects of this control appear to be mediated by nAChRs. For example, (−)-nicotine potentiates increases in cortical blood flow produced by electrical stimulation of the basal forebrain (Arneric, 1991). This same effect is also produced by ABT-418, but at a dose 200 times lower (Decker et al., 1994a). Given that this effect involves potentiation of neurogenic control rather than merely an increase in baseline blood flow suggests that the effect of ABT-418 may be physiologically relevant and that this compound might improve blood flow deficits in AD.

In addition to its cognitive enhancing properties in animal models, ABT-418 exhibits anxiolytic-like actions in the elevated plus-maze model of anxiety in mice and rats (Brioni et al., 1994; Decker et al., 1994a), an effect that persists after a subchronic administration schedule via subcutaneous minipumps (Brioni et al., 1994). ABT-418 was not as efficacious as diazepam in these experimental studies, but a compound with both memory-enhancing and anxiolytic properties might be beneficial for the treatment of AD patients who exhibit periods of anxiety and agitation.

In nicotine-trained rats, ABT-418 is three-fold less potent than (−)-nicotine to induce the nicotine cue (Brioni et al., 1995), and it is also less potent than (−)-nicotine to stimulate dopamine-containing neurons in the ventral tegmental area (Brioni et al., 1995), suggesting than ABT-418 may exhibit less abuse liability in comparison to (−)-nicotine. ABT-418 is also less potent than (−)-nicotine in producing a variety of adverse side effects and accordingly may have an improved safety profile relative to (−)-nicoine (Decker et al., 1994).

ABT-418 has also shown cytoprotective activity. (−)-Nicotine and ABT-418 protect against glutamate-induced toxicity in rat primary cortical cells (Donnelly-Roberts et al., 1996) and in the differentiated human neuroblastoma cell line, IMR 32 (Arneric et al., 1995b). The protective effects of ABT-418 and (−)-nicotine appear to be mediated via an interaction with nAChRs since mecamylamine (10 μM) attenuates these protective effects. Additionally, the cytoprotective effects of these agents are attenuated by nanomolar concentrations of α-BgT and MLA, both selective antagonists of the $\alpha 7$ subtype in this concentration range. The ability of $\alpha 7$ antagonists to prevent the cytoprotective effects of ABT-418 and $(-)$-nicotine would suggest that the agonist/partial agonist activities of these compounds at the $\alpha 7$ subtype may play an important role in the cytoprotective effects.

SIB-1663 and SIB-1765F

SIB-1663 is a ChCM that has low affinity ($IC_{50} = 2000$ nM) for $[^3H](-)$-nicotine binding in rat brain, yet it is selective in its ability to activate the $\alpha 3 \beta 4$ human subtypes expressed in oocytes (Lloyd et al., 1994). In vitro, SIB-1663 induces the release of DA from striatal slices and can also elicit ipsilateral rotations in rats with unilateral 6-OHDA lesions of the nigrostriatal pathway, suggesting that it also causes DA release in vivo. This effect can be blocked by mecamylamine. SIB-1663 also reverses haloperidol-induced catalepsy, an animal model of extrapyramidal motor dysfunction. These properties, as well as the ability to improve retention in a passive avoidance paradigm, suggest that S-1663 may be useful for treating both the motor and cognitive aspects of Parkinson's disease.

SIB-1765F is a novel ChCM with high-affinity ($IC_{50} = 4$ nM) to displace $[^3H](-)$-nicotine binding from rat cortical membranes (Lloyd et al., 1995). It facilitates striatal DA release in vitro and in vivo, and increases NE release from rat hippocampal, thalamic, and prefrontal slices. In behavioral studies, SIB-1765F increased locomotor activity in rats habituated to a test cage and, at high doses (20 mg/kg), induced ipsilateral rotations in rats with unilateral 6-OHDA lesions of the nigrostriatal pathway.

The pharmacological profiles of these two compounds suggest that they may be useful for the management of Parkinson's disease. Data on the abuse potential of these compounds have not been reported yet, and it would be critical to determine if they represent a safer alternative to a nicotine treatment using a patch or gum formulation that has already been considered for Parkinson patients. Similarly, it has been suggested that these compounds improve some measures of cognitive performance in animals, but detailed data are not yet available.

GTS-21

GTS-21 (also known as DMXB) is an analog of anabaseine, an nAChR ligand found in the marine worm, nemertine. Although GTS-21 displays nanomolar affinity for cytisine-labeled sites in rat brain ($IC_{50} = 150$ nM), the compound has only minimal efficacy at $\alpha 4 \beta 2$ subunit combinations expressed in oocytes (de Fiebre et al., 1995; Meyer et al., 1994). In contrast, GTS-21 is a potent but partial agonist (relative to ACh) at $\alpha 7$ receptors expressed in oocytes (de Fiebre et al., 1995). As might be expected of a partial agonist, GTS-21 has antagonist properties at both $\alpha 4 \beta 2$ and at $\alpha 7$ receptors, but this effect may not be the result of competitive inhibition (de Fiebre et al., 1995).

Behavioral testing in experimental animals reveals that GTS-21, like (−)-nicotine, can improve the inhibitory avoidance performance of rats with NBM lesions and enhances the performance of aged rats on a variety of learning and memory tasks (Arendash et al., 1995; Meyer et al., 1994). GTS-21 also improves the performance of aged rabbits on eyeblink conditioning, a classical conditioning task that is impaired in AD patients (Woodruff-Pak et al., 1994a). Consistent with these positive effects in learning and memory tasks, GTS-21 enhances long-term potentiation, a candidate mechanism for memory storage, in hippocampal slices (Hunter et al., 1994). This latter effect is mecamylamine sensitive, suggesting that it is mediated by nAChRs. Where comparisons are possible, GTS-21 appears to be as effective as (−)-nicotine in improving cognitive performance in experimental animals but is somewhat less potent (Arendash et al., 1995; Meyer et al., 1994). GTS-21, however, is considerably less potent than (−)-nicotine in producing a variety of adverse effects in preclinical models and thus may present an improved safety profile (Brioni et al., 1996b; Decker et al., 1995). Similarly, the compound may have reduced addiction liability based on its inability to produce the (−)-nicotine cue in nicotine-trained rats (see Figure 2).

Based on our previous discussion of the potential cytoprotective effects of α7 activation, it is not surprising that cytoprotective properties have been reported for GTS-21. In differentiated PC12 cells, GTS-21 greatly attenuates the reduction in cell number and neurite extention produced by removal of NGF and serum (Martin et al., 1994). This effect can be prevented by mecamylamine, suggesting it is mediated by nAChRs. Whether the neuroprotective actions of GTS-21 are related to inhibition of apoptotic or necrotic mechanisms is unknown at the present time. It has also been reported that twice daily administration of GTS-21 to rats with partial unilateral transection of the fimbria-fornix reduces cell death in the septal area (Martin et al., 1994). This latter interpretation is based on a GTS-21-induced reduction of the difference in cell number between the lesioned and unlesioned side. The possibility that this reduction in side differences resulted from reductions in cell number on the nonlesioned side was not addressed in this preliminary study, so additional in vivo work will be necessary to determine if GTS-21 is truly neuroprotective.

NEW PERSPECTIVES AND CHALLENGES FOR THE NOVEL CHOLINERGIC CHANNEL MODULATORS

Experiments in both laboratory animals and in human subjects support a role for nAChR-mediated neurotransmission in cognitive function, and the observation that Alzheimer's patients have decreased numbers of postsynaptic nAChRs but preserved numbers of postsynaptic muscarinic receptors suggests that nicotinic neurotransmission may be particularly disrupted in AD (Schröder et al., 1991; Whitehouse et al., 1988, 1986). Thus, it is possible that restoration of nicotinic neurotransmission will be useful in treating some of the cognitive deficits of AD. Preliminary evidence suggests that (−)-nicotine itself may have beneficial effects in AD, but the side-effect profile is not favorable. Adverse effects have been observed in acute and chronic treatment studies. For example, a recent experiment in which AD patients were treated with $(-)$-nicotine-containing transdermal patches demonstrated some cognitive benefits but consistent cardiac irregularities resulting from treatment (Wilson et al., 1995). Similarly, studies in animals indicate little separation between doses effective in improving cognitive performance and doses producing adverse effects.

Although a variety of potentially therapeutic actions have been identified for $(-)$-nicotine (Bannon et al., 1995b; Jarvik, 1991), side effects and addiction liabilities have retarded development of this approach. The discovery of distinct nAChR subtypes that may have different roles in the mediation of $(-)$-nicotine's diverse effects suggests that it may be possible to develop selective agents with improved safety profiles and reduced addiction liability. Several of the novel agents described in this review appear to have improved safety profiles, relative to $(-)$-nicotine; and at least two of these agents, ABT-418 and GTS-21, have entered early phases of clinical development. Identification of the native subtypes of nAChRs occurring in brain and the establishment of the physiological and behavioral effects mediated by these subtypes will be an important challenge in the nicotinic area over the next few years. There is already some good evidence that the various effects of nAChR activation are mediated by effects at distinct receptor subtypes. For example, $\alpha 7$ nAChRs do not seem to participate in the expression of the nicotine cue as this behavioral effect is not blocked by the specific $\alpha 7$ antagonist MLA (Brioni et al., 1996a). Once the information on the physiological role of the different putative nAChR subtypes becomes available, it may be possible to take advantage of this receptor diversity for the rational design of novel and selective compounds.

Investigation of the modulatory sites present on the nAChR complex will be another important area for future research. Examination of these sites may lead to the development of compounds that modify ongoing nicotinic neurotransmission, much like the benzodiazepines modulate GABAergic neurotransmission. Compounds with modulatory effects might have improved safety profiles and decreased abuse liability. Moreover, compounds that modulate ongoing activity without directly activating cholinergic channels would be more likely to maintain the spatial and temporal fidelity of normal neurotransmission. If the phasic characteristics of nicotinic neurotransmission are critical for cognitive function, such an agent might be much more effective in AD than a direct agonist.

Several decades have passed since mecamylamine (Inversine) was clinically used as a ganglionic blocking agent for the management of hypertension, but no nAChR ligands have had a significant clinical impact in the CNS area. Although nAChR pharmacology has advanced dramatically over the last few years, much remains to be done. The subunit composition of the native brain nAChRs has to be characterized and the functions of the putative subtypes need to be identified to allow the rational design of subtype-selective compounds. Characterization of the modulatory sites on the receptor complex may provide additional therapeutic opportunities. In order to determine if nAChR ligands might be beneficial for the treatment of CNS disorders, selective ligands that would provide a better safety profile than $(-)$-nicotine itself are needed. The novel ChCMs described in this chapter are the first such tools that will allow the testing of this hypothesis. The preliminary results with clinical tests of $(-)$-nicotine and the entry of two new agents into clinical testing are encouraging events for the field, but important scientific challenges still lie ahead.

REFERENCES

Akaike A, Tamura Y, Yokaota T, Shimohama S, Kimura J (1994): Nicotine-induced protection of cultured cortical neurons against N-methyl-D-aspartate receptor-mediated glutamate cytotoxicity. Brain Res 644:181–187.

Andersen P, Bliss TVP, Skrede KK (1971): Lamellar organization of hippocampal excitatory pathways. Exp Brain Res 13:222–238.

Araujo DM, Lapchak PA, Meaney MJ, Collier B, Quirion R (1990): Effects of aging on nicotinic and muscarinic autoreceptor function in the rat brain: Relationship to presynaptic cholinergic markers and binding sites. J Neurosci 10:3069–3078.

Arendash G, Sengstock G, Sanberg P, Kem W (1995): Improved learning and memory in aged rats with chronic administration of the nicotinic receptor agonist GTS-21. Brain Res 674:252–259.

Arneric SP (1991): New nicotinic agonists and cerebral blood flow. In Becker R, Giacobini E (eds): "Cholinergic Basis for Alzheimer Therapy, Advances in Alzheimer Disease Therapy," Boston: Birkhäuser, pp 386–394.

Arneric SP, Holladay MW, Sullivan JP (1996): Cholinergic channel modulators as a novel therapeutic strategy for Alzheimer's disease. Exp Opin Invest Drugs 5:79–100.

Arneric SP, Sullivan JP, Williams M (1995a): Neuronal nicotinic acetylcholine receptors: Novel targets for CNS therapeutics. In Bloom F, Kupfer D (eds): "Psychopharmacology: Fourth Generation of Progress," New York: Raven Press, pp 95–110.

Arneric SP, Sullivan JP, Decker MW, Brioni JD, Bannon AW, Briggs CA, Donnelly-Roberts D, Radek RJ, Marsh KC, Kyncl J, Williams M, Buccafusco JJ (1995b): Potential treatment of Alzheimer disease using cholinergic channel activators (ChCAs) with cognitive enhancement, anxiolytic-like, and cytoprotective properties. Alzheimer Dis Assoc Disord 9(Suppl 2):50–61.

Arneric SP, Sullivan JP, Briggs CA, Donnelly-Roberts D, Anderson DJ, Raszkiewicz JL, Hughes M, Cadman ED, Adams P, Garvey DS, Wasicak J, Williams M (1994): ABT 418: A novel cholinergic ligand with cognition enhancing and anxiolytic activities: I. In vitro characterization. J Pharmacol Exp Ther 270:310–318.

Badio B, Daly J (1994): Epibatidine, a potent analgetic and nicotinic agonist. Mol Pharmacol 45:563–569.

Bannon AW, Gunther KL, Decker MW (1995a): Is epibatidine really analgesic? Dissociation of the locomotor activity, temperature, and analgesic effects of $(\pm)$-epibatidine. Pharmacol Biochem Behav 51:693–698.

Bannon AW, Decker MW, Williams M, Arneric SP (1995b): Psychotherapeutic potential of selective neuronal nicotinic acetylcholine receptor ligands. In Domino EF (ed): "Brain Imaging of Nicotine and Tobacco Smoking," Ann Arbor: NPP Books, pp 311–334.

Bartus RT, Johnson HR (1976): Short-term memory in the rhesus monkey: Disruption from the anti-cholinergic scopolamine. Pharmacol Biochem Behav 5:39–46.

Bartus RT, Dean RL, Beer B, Lippa AS (1982): The cholinergic hypothesis of geriatric memory dysfunction. Science 217:408–417.

Beani L, Tanganelli S, Antonelli T, Ferraro L, Morari M, Spalluto P, Nordberg A, Bianchi C (1991): Effect of acute and subchronic nicotine treatment on cortical efflux of [³H]-D-aspartate and endogenous GABA in freely moving guinea-pigs. Br J Pharmacol 104: 15–20.

Beani L, Bianchi C, Nilsson L, Nordberg A, Romanelli L, Sivilotti L (1985): The effect of nicotine and cytisine on [³H]-acetylcholine release from cortical slices of guinea-pig brain. Naunyn-Schmiedeberg's Arch Pharmacol 331:293–296.

Benwell MEM, Balfour DJK (1992): The effects of acute and repeated nicotine treatment on nucleus accumbens dopamine and locomotor activity. Br J Pharmacol 105:849–856.

Bertrand D, Bertrand S, Ballivet M (1992): Pharmacological properties of the homomeric α7 receptor. Neurosci Lett 146:87–90.

Bowen DM, Smith CB, White P, Davison AN (1976): Neurotransmitter-related enzymes and indices of hypoxia in senile dementia and other abiotrophies. Brain 99:459–496.

Briggs C, Anderson D, Brioni J, Buccafusco J, Campbell J, Decker M, Donnelly-Roberts D, Gopalakrishnan M, Holladay M, Sullivan J, Arneric S (1996): Functional characterization of the novel nicotinic receptor ligand GTS-21 *in vivo* and *in vitro*. Pharmacol Biochem Behav in press.

Briggs CA, McKenna DG, Piattoni-Kaplan M (1995): Human α7 nicotinic acetylcholine receptor responses to novel ligands. Neuropharmacology 34:583–590.

Brioni JD (1993): Role of GABA during the multiple consolidation of memory. Drug Dev Res 28:3–27.

Brioni JD, Arneric SP (1993): Nicotinic receptor agonists facilitate retention of avoidance training: Participation of dopaminergic mechanisms. Behav Neural Biol 59:57–62.

Brioni JD, Kim DJB, O'Neill AB (1996a): Nicotine CUE: lack of effect of the α7 nicotinic receptor antagonist methyllycaconitine Eur J Pharmacol 301:1–5.

Brioni JB, Decker MW, Sullivan JP, Arneric SP (1996b): The pharmacology of (−)-nicotine and novel cholinergic channel activators. Adv Pharmacol 37:153–213.

Brioni JD, Kim DBJ, Brodie MS, Decker MW, Arneric SP (1995): ABT-418: Discriminative stimulus properties and effect on ventral tegmental cell activity. Psychopharmacology 107:368–375.

Brioni JD, O'Neill AB, Kim DJB, Decker MW, Arneric SP (1994): Anxiolytic-like effects of the novel cholinergic channel activator ABT 418. J Pharmacol Exp Ther 271:353–361.

Brioni JD, Curzon P, Buckley MJ, Arneric SP, Decker MW (1993): Linopirdine (DuP996) facilitates the retention of avoidance training and improves performance of septal-lesioned rats in the water maze. Pharmacol Biochem Behav 44:37–43.

Buccafusco J, Jackson W (1991): Beneficial effects of nicotine administered prior to a delayed matching-to-sample task in young and aged monkeys. Neurobiol Aging 12: 233–238.

Buccafusco J, Jackson W, Terry A, Marsh K, Decker M, Arneric S (1995): Improvement in performance of a delayed matching-to-sample task by monkeys following ABT-418: A novel cholinergic channel activator for memory enhancement. Psychopharmacology 120:256–266.

Caulfield MP, Higgins GA, Straughan DW (1983): Central administration of the muscarinic receptor subtype—selective antagonist pirenzepine selectively impairs passive avoidance learning in the mouse. J Pharm Pharmacol 35:131–132.

Christensen H, Maltby N, Jorm AF, Creasey H, Broe GA (1992): Cholinergic "blockade" as a model of the cognitive deficits in Alzheimer's disease. Brain 115:1681–1699.

Clarke PBS (1994): Nicotine dependence mechanisms and therapeutic strategies. Biochem Soc Symp 59:83–95.

Clarke PBS (1990): Dopaminergic mechanisms in the locomotor stimulant effects of nicotine. Biochem Pharmacol 40:1427–1432.

Clarke PBS, Fibiger HC (1990): Reinforced alternation performance is impaired by muscarinic but not by nicotinic receptor blockade in rats. Behav Brain Res 36:203–207.

Clarke PBS, Schwartz RD, Paul SM, Pert CB, Pert A (1985): Nicotinic binding in rat brain: Autoradiographic comparison of $[^3H]$-acetylcholine, $[^3H]$-nicotine and $[^{125}I]$-α-bungarotoxin. J Neurosci 5:1307–1315.

Courturier S, Bertrand D, Matter JM, Herandez M-C, Bertrand S, Miller N, Valera S, Barkas T, Ballivet M (1990): A neuronal nicotinic acetylcholine receptor subunit (α7) is developmentally regulated and forms a homo-oligomeric ion channel blocked by α-BTX. Neuron 5:847–856.

Coyle J, Price D, DeLong M (1983): Alzheimer's disease: A disorder of cortical cholinergic innervation. Science 219:1184–1190.

Curzon P, Brioni JD, Decker MW (1996): Effect of intraventricular injections of dihydro-β-erythroidine (DHβE) on spatial memory in the rat. Brain Res 714:185–191.

Damaj M, Creasy K, Rosecrans J, Martin B (1994): Pharmacological effects of epibatidine optical enantiomers. Brain Res 664:34–40.

Davies P, Maloney AJ (1976): Selective loss of central cholinergic neurons in Alzheimer's disease. Lancet 25:1403.

de Fiebre CM, Meyer EM, Henry JC, Muraskin SI, Kem WR, Papke RL (1995): Characterization of a series of anabaseine-derived compounds reveals that the 3-(4)-dimethylaminocinnamylidine derivative (DMAC) is a selective agonist at neuronal nicotinic α7/$[^{125}I]$$\alpha$-bungarotoxin receptor subtypes. Mol Pharmacol 47:164–171.

Decker MW (1992): Cholinergic/noradrenergic interactions and memory. In Levin ED, Decker MW, Butcher LL (eds): "Neurotransmitter Interactions and Cognitive Function. Boston: Birkhauser, pp 78–90.

Decker MW, Majchrzak MJ (1993): Effects of central nicotinic cholinergic receptor blockade produced by chlorisondamine on learning and memory performance in rats. Behav Neural Biol 60:163–171.

Decker MW, Majchrzak MJ (1992): Effects of systemic and intracerebroventricular administration of mecamylamine, a nicotinic cholinergic antagonist, on spatial memory in rats. Psychopharmacology 107:530–534.

Decker M, Brioni J, Bannon A, Arneric S (1995a): Diversity of neuronal nicotinic acetylcholine receptors: Lessons from behavior and implications for CNS therapeutics. Life Sci 56:545–570.

Decker MW, Anderson DJ, Brioni JD, Donnelly-Roberts DL, Kang C-H, Piattoni-Paplan M, Swanson S, Sullivan JP (1995b): Erysodine: A competitive antagonist at neuronal nicotinic acetylcholine receptors. Eur J Pharmacol 280:79–89.

Decker MW, Brioni JD, Sullivan JP, Buckley MJ, Radek RJ, Sullivan JP, Buckley MJ, Radek RJ, Raskiewickz JL, Kang CH, Kim DJB, Giardina WJ, Williams M, Arneric SP (1994a): (S)-3-methyl-5-(1-methyl-2-pyrrolidinyl) isoxazole (ABT 418): A novel cholinergic ligand with cognition enhancing and anxiolytic activities: II. In vivo characterization. J Pharmacol Exp Ther 270:319–328.

Decker MW, Curzon P, Brioni JD, Arneric SP (1994b): Effects of ABT 418, a novel cholinergic channel ligand, on learning and memory in septal-lesioned rats. Eur J Pharmacol 261:217–222.

Decker MW, Majchrzak MJ, Arneric SP (1993): Effect of lobeline, a nicotinic receptor agonist, on learning and memory. Pharmacol Biochem Behav 45:571–576.

Decker M, Radek R, Majchrzak M, Anderson D (1992a): Differential effects of medial septal lesions on spatial-memory tasks. Psychobiology 20:9–17.

Decker MW, Majchrzak MJ, Anderson DJ (1992b): Effects of nicotine on spatial memory deficits in rats with spatial lesions. Brain Res 572:281–285.

Decker MW, Tran T, McGaugh JL (1990): A comparison of the effects of scopolamine and diazepam on acquisition and retention of inhibitory avoidance in mice. Psychopharmacology 100:515–521.

Dekker AJ, Connor DJ, Thal LJ (1991): The role of cholinergic projections from the nucleus basalis in memory. Neurosci Biobehav Rev 15:299–317.

Deneris ES, Connolly J, Rogers SW, Duvoisin R (1991): Pharmacological and functional diversity of neuronal nicotinic acetylcholine receptors. Trends Pharmacol Sci 12:34–40.

Dilts SL, Berry CA (1967): Effect of cholinergic drugs on passive avoidance in the mouse. J Pharmacol Exp Ther 158:279–285.

Donnelly-Roberts D, Hu I, Arneric SP, Sullivan JP (1996): In vitro cytoprotective properties of the novel cholinergic channel activator (ChCA), ABT-418. Brain Res 719:36–44.

Drachman DA (1977): Memory and cognitive function in man: Does the cholinergic system have a specific role? Neurology 27:783–790.

Duijn CV, Hofman A (1991): Relation between nicotine intake and Alzheimer's disease. Br Med J 302:1491–1494.

Eckerman DA, Gordon WA, Edwards J, McPhail R, Gage M (1980): Effects of scopolamine, pentobarbital, and amphetamine on radial arm maze performance in the rat. Pharmacol Biochem Behav 12:595–602.

Elgoyhen A, Johnson D, Boulter J, Vetter D, Heinemann S (1994): α9: An acetylcholine receptor with novel pharmacological properties expressed in rat cochlear hair cells. Cell 79:705–715.

Elrod K, Buccafusco JJ, Jackson WJ (1988): Nicotine enhances delayed matching-to-sample performance by primates. Life Sci 43:277–287.

Fibiger H (1991): Cholinergic mechanisms in learning, memory and dementia: A review of recent evidence. Trends Neurosci 14:220–223.

Flood JF, Cherkin A (1986): Scopolamine effects on memory retention in mice: A model of dementia? Behav Neural Biol 45:169–184.

Flores CM, Rogers SW, Pabreza LA, Wolfe BB, Kellar KJ (1992): A subtype of nicotinic cholinergic receptor in rat brain is composed of α4 and β2 subunits and is up-regulated by chronic nicotine treatment. Mol Pharmacol 41:31–37.

Gallagher M, Colombo PJ (1995): Ageing: The cholinergic hypothesis of cognitive decline. Curr Opin Neurobiol 5:161–168.

Galzi J, Revah F, Bessis A, Changeux J (1991): Functional architecture of the nicotinic acetylcholine receptor: From electric organ to brain. Ann Rev Neurosci 31:37–72.

Gerzanich V, Anand R, Lindstrom J (1994): Homomers of α8 and α7 subunits of nicotinic receptors exhibit similar channel but contrasting binding site properties. Mol Pharmacol 45:212–220.

Gopalakrishnan M, Monteggia LM, Anderson DJ, Arneric SP, Sullivan JP (1996): Stable expression, pharmacologic properties and regulation of the human nicotinic acetylcholine α4β2 receptor. J Pharmacol Exp Ther 276:289–297.

Gopalakrishnan M, Buisson M, Touma E, Giordano T, Campbell J, Hu I, Donnelly-Roberts D, Arneric S, Bertrand D, Sullivan J (1995): Stable expression and pharmacological properties of the human α7 nicotinic acetylcholine receptor. Eur J Pharmacol 290:237–246.

Grady S, Marks MJ, Wonnacott S, Collins AC (1992): Characterization of nicotinic receptor-mediated [^{3}H]-dopamine release from synaptosomes prepared from mouse striatum. J Neurochem 59:848–856.

Granon S, Poucet B, Thinus-Blanc C, Changeux JP, Vidal C (1995): Nicotinic and muscarinic receptors in the rat prefrontal cortex: Differential roles in working memory, response selection and effortful processing. Psychopharmacology 119:139–144.

Gray JA, McNaughton N (1982): Comparison between the behavioural effects of septal and hippocampal lesions: A review. Neurosci Biobehav Rev 7:119–188.

Gray JA, Mitchell SN, Joseph MH, Grigoryan GA, Dawe S, Hodges H (1994): Neurochemical mechanisms mediating the behavioral and cognitive effects of nicotine. Drug Dev Res 31:3–17.

Grigoryan GA, Mitchell SN, Hodges H, Sinden JD, Gray JA (1994): Are the cognitive-enhancing effects of nicotine in the rat with lesions to the forebrain cholinergic projections system mediated by an interaction with the noradrenergic system? Pharmacol Biochem Behav 49:511–521.

Haroutunian V, Barnes E, Davies KL (1985): Cholinergic modulation of memory in rats. Psychopharmacology 87:266–271.

Hodges H, Allen Y, Sinden J, Lantos PL, Gray JA (1991): Effects of cholinergic-rich neural grafts on radial maze performance of rats after excitotoxic lesions of the forebrain cholinergic projection system—II. Cholinergic drugs as probes to investigate lesion-induced deficits and transplant-induced functional recovery. Neuroscience 3:609–623.

Hunter B, deFiebre C, Papke R, Kem W, Meyer E (1994): A novel nicotinic agonist facilitates induction of long-term potentiation in the rat hippocampus. Neurosci Lett 168: 130–134.

Janson A, Fuxe K, Agnati L, Katayama I, Harfstrand A, Anderson K, Goldstein M (1988): Chronic nocitine treatment counteracts the disappearance of tyrosine-hydroxylase-immunoreactive nerve cell bodies, dendrites and terminals in the mesostriatal dopamine system of the male rat after partial hemitransection. Brain Res 455:332–345.

Jarvik ME (1991): Beneficial effects of nicotine. Br J Addic 86:571–575.

Jones GMM, Sahakian BJ, Levy R, Warburton DM, Gray JA (1992): Effects of acute subcutaneous nicotine on attention, information processing and short-term memory in Alzheimer's disease. Psychopharmacology 108:485–494.

Lee PN (1994): Smoking and Alzheimer's disease: A review of the epidemiological evidence. Neuroepidemiology 13:131–144.

Lena C, Changeux JP (1993): Allosteric modulations of the nicotinic acetylcholine receptor. Trends Neurosci 16:181–186.

Levin ED (1992): Nicotinic systems and cognitive function. Psychopharmacology 108: 471–431.

Levin ED, Briggs SJ, Christopher NC, Auman JT (1994): Working memory performance and cholinergic effects in the ventral tegmental area and substantia nigra. Brain Res 657:165–170.

Levin ED, Lee C, Rose JE, Reyes A, Ellison G, Jarvik M, Gritz E (1990a): Chronic nicotine and withdrawal effects on radial-arm maze performance in rats. Behav Neural Biol 53:269–276.

Levin ED, McGurk SR, Rose JE, Butcher LL (1990b): Cholinergic-dopaminergic interactions in cognitive performance. Behav Neural Biol 54:271–299.

Levin ED, McGurk SR, Rose JE, Butcher LL (1989): Reversal of a mecamylamine-induced cognitive deficit with the D2 agonist, LY 171555. Pharmacol Biochem Behav 33: 919–922.

Levin ED, Castonguay M, Ellison GD (1987): Effects of the nicotinic receptor blocker, mecamylamine, on radial-arm maze performance in rats. Behav Neural Biol 48:206–212.

Linville DG, Arneric SP (1991): Cortical cerebral blood flow governed by the basal forebrain: Age-related impairments. Neurobiol Aging 12:503–510.

Lippiello PM, Bencherif M, Prince RJ (1995): The Role of desensitization in CNS nicotinic receptor function. In Clarke PBS, Quik M, Adlkofer F, Thurau K (eds): "Effects of Nicotine on Biological Systems," Vol. 11, Basel: Birkhauser, pp 79–85.

Lloyd G, Rao T, Sacaan A, Reid R, Correa L, Whelan K, Risbrough V, Menzaghi F (1995): SIB-1765F a novel nicotinic agonist: Profile in models of extrapyramidal motor dysfunction. Soc Neurosci Abstr 21:11.10.

Lloyd G, McDonald I, Vernier J, Elliott K, Ellis S, Sacaan A, Rao T, Chavez-Noriega L, Johnson E, Velicelebi F, Mengaghi F, Harpold M (1994): Subtype-selective cholinergic ion channel agonists as potential antiparkinson agents. "The Cholinergic Synapse: Structure, Function and Regulation, Baltimore: p 45.

Luetje C, Patrick J (1991): Both α- and β-subunits contribute to the agonist sensitivity of neuronal nicotinic acetylcholine receptors. J Neurosci 11:837–845.

Marin P, Maus M, Desagher S, Glowinski J, Premont J (1994): Nicotine protects cultured striatal neurons against N-methyl-D-aspartate receptor-mediated neurotoxicity. Neuroreport 5:1977–1980.

Martin E, Panickar K, King M, Deyrup M, Hunter B, Wang G, Meyer E (1994): Cytoprotective actions of 2,4-dimethoxybenzylidene anabaseine in differentiated PC12 cells and septal cholinergic neurons. Drug Dev Res 31:135–141.

McGehee DS, Role LW (1995): Physiological diversity of nicotinic acetylcholine receptors expressed by vertebrate neurons. Ann Rev Physiol 57:521–546.

Meguro K, Yamaguchi S, Arai H, Nakagawa T, Doi C, Yamada M, Ikarashi Y, Maruyama Y, Sasaki H (1994): Nicotine improves cognitive disturbances in senscence-accelerated mice. Pharmacol Biochem Behav 49:769–772.

Meyer E, de Fiebre C, Hunter B, Simpkins C, Frauworth N, de Fiebre N (1994): Effects of anabaseine-related analogs on rat brain nicotinic receptor binding and on avoidance behaviors. Drug Dev Res 31:127–134.

Mitchell SN (1993): Role of the locus coeruleus in the noradrenergic response to a systemic administration of nicotine. Neuropharmacology 32:937–949.

Moulton BA, Thinschmidt JS, Quintana R, Meyer EM, Papke RL (1996): The pharmacology of epibatidine and ABT-418 on putative subtypes of rat neuronal nicotinic receptors, submitted.

Muir JL, Everitt BJ, Robbins TW (1995): Reversal of visual attentional dysfunction following lesions of the cholinergic basal forebrain by physostigmine and nicotine but not by the 5-HT3 receptor antagonist, ondansetron. Psychopharmacology 118:82–92.

Newhouse PA, Potter A, Corwin J, Lenox R (1994): Modeling the nicotinic receptor loss in dementia using the nicotinic antagonist mecamylamine: Effects on human cognitive functioning. Drug Dev Res 31:71–79.

Newhouse PA, Sunderland T, Tariot PN, Blumhardt CL, Weingartner H, Mellow A, Murphy DL (1988): Intravenous nicotine in Alzheimer's disease: A pilot study. Psychopharmacology 95:171–175.

Nitta A, Katono Y, Itoh A, Hasegawa T, Nabeshima T (1994): Nicotine reverses scopolamine-induced impairment of performance in passie avoidance task in rats through its action on the dopaminergic neuronal system. Pharmacol Biochem Behav 49:807–812.

Oliverio A (1966): Effects of mecamylamine on avoidance conditioning and maze learning of mice. J Pharmacol Exp Ther 154:350–356.

Olton DS (1990): Dementia: Animal models of the cognitive impairments following damage to the basal forebrain cholinergic system. Brain Res Bull 25:499–502.

Papke R (1993): The kinetic properties of neuronal nicotinic receptors: Genetic basis of functional diversity. Prog Neurobiol 41:509–531.

Papke RL, Heinemann SF (1993): Partial agonists properties of cytisine on neuronal nicotinic receptors containing the beta2 subunit. Mol Pharmacol 45:142–149.

Perry EK, Gibson PH, Blessed G, Perry RH, Tomlinson BE (1977): Neurotransmitter enzyme abnormalities in senile dementia. J Neurol Sci 34:247–265.

Prohovnik I (1990): Muscarinic and nicotinic contributions to the AD cortical perfusion abnormality. Neurobiol Aging 11:262.

Qian C, Li T, Shen TY, Libertine-Garahan L, Eckman J, Biftu T, Ip S (1993): Epibatidine is a nicotinic analgesic. Eur J Pharmacol 250:R13–R14.

Ramirez-Lattore JA, Qu X, Role L (1993): Participation of alpha5 in neuronal nicotinic AChR channels. J Neurosci 13:442–454.

Ribeiro EB, Bettiker RL, Bogdanov M, Wurtman RJ (1993): Effects of systemic nicotine on serotonin release in rat brain. Brain Res 621:311–318.

Riekkinen P, Jr, Riekkinen M (1995): Effects of tetrahydroaminoacridine and nicotine in mucleus basalis and serotonin-lesioned rats. Eur J Pharmacol 279:65–73.

Riekkinen M, Tolonen R, Riekkinen P, Jr. (1994): Interaction between 5-HT$_{1A}$ and nicotinic cholinergic receptors in the regulation of water maze navigation behavior. Brain Res 649:174–180.

Riekkinen P, Jr, M Riekkinen, Sirviö J, Riekkinen P (1992): Effects of concurrent nicotinic antagonist and PCPA treatments on spatial and passive avoidance learning. Brain Res 575:247–250.

Rush DK (1988): Scopolamine amnesia of passive avoidance: A deficit of information acquisition. Behav Neural Biol 50:255–274.

Rusted J, Graupner L, O'Connell N, Nicholls C (1994): Does nicotine improve cognitive function? Psychopharmacology 115:547–549.

Sahakian B, Jones G, Levy R, Gray J, Warburton D (1989): The effects of nicotine on attention, information processing, and short-term memory in patients with dementia of the Alzheimer's type. Br J Psychiatry 154:797–800.

Sargent PB (1993): The diversity of neurona nicotinic acetylcholine receptors. Ann Rev Neurosci 16:403–443.

Sarter M, Bruno JP, Dudchenko P (1990): Activating the damaged basal forebrain cholinergic system: Tonic stimulation versus signal amplification Psychopharmacology 101:1–17.

Schröder H, Giacobini E, Struble RG, Zilles K, Maelicke A (1991): Nicotinic cholinoceptive neurons of the frontal cortex are reduced in Alzheimer's disease. Neurobiol Aging 12: 259–262.

Schulz D, Loring R, Aizenman E, Zigmond R (1991): Autoradiographic localization of putative nicotinic receptors in the rat brain using [^{125}I]neuronal bungarotoxin. J Neurosci 11: 287–297.

Seguela P, Wadiche J, Dineley-Miller K, Dani J, Patrick J (1993): Molecular cloning, functional properties, and distribution of rat brain α7: A nicotinic cation channel highly permeable to calcium. J Neurosci 13:596–604.

Socci DJ, Sanberg PR, Arendash GW (1995): Nicotine enhances Morris water maze performance of young and aged rats. Neurobiol Aging 16:857–860.

Sullivan JP, Donnelly-Roberts D, Anderson DJ, Gopalakrishnan M, Briggs CA, Campbell JE, Piattoni-Campbell M, McKenna DG, Molinari E, Holladay MW, Lin N-H, Arneric SP (1996): A-85380 [3-(2(S)-azetidinylmethoxy) pyridine: In vitro pharmacological properties of a novel 50 pM affinity cholinergic channel ligand. Neuropharmacology in press.

Sullivan J, Briggs C, Donnelly-Roberts D, Brioni J, Radek R, McKenna D, Campbell J, Arneric S, Decker M, Bannon A (1994a): (±)-Epibatidine can differentially evoke responses mediated by putative subtypes of nicotinic acetylcholine receptors (nAChRs). Med Chem Res 4:502–516.

Sullivan J, Decker MW, Brioni JD, Donnelly-Roberts D, Anderson DJ, Bannon AW, Kang C, Adams P, Piattoni-Kaplan M, Buckley MJ, Gopalakrishnan M, Williams M, Arneric SP (1994b): (±)-Epibatidine elicits a diversity of in vitro and in vivo effects mediated by nicotinic acetylcholine receptors. J Pharmacol Exp Ther 271:624–631.

Terry AV, Jr, Buccafusco JJ, Jackson WJ (1993): Scopolamine reversal of nicotine enhanced delayed matching-to-sample performance in monkeys. Pharmacol Biochem Behav 45: 925–929.

Thomas P, Stephens M, Wilkie G, Amar M, Lunt G, Whiting P, Gallaher T, Pereira E, Alkondon M, Albuquerque EX, Wonnacott S (1993): (±)-Anatoxin-A is a potent agonist at neuronal nicotinic acetylcholine receptors. J Neurochem 60:2308–2311.

Vernino S, Amador M, Luetje CW, Patrick J, Dani JA (1992): Calcium modulation and high calcium permeability of neuronal nicotinic acetylcholine receptors. Neuron 8:127–134.

Voytko ML, Olton DS, Richardson RT, Gorman LK, Tobin JR, Price DL (1994): Basal forebrain lesions in monkeys disrupt attention but not learning and memory. J Neurosci 14: 167–186.

Warburton DM, Arnall C (1994): Improvements in performance without nicotine withdrawal. Psychopharmacology 115:539–540.

Whitehouse P, Martino A, Wagster M, Price D, Mayeux R, Atack J, Kellar K (1988): Reductions in [^{3}H]nicotinic acetylcholine binding in Alzheimer's disease and Parkinson's disease. Neurology 38:720–723.

Whitehouse PJ, Martino A, Antuono P, Lowenstein P, Coyle J, Price D, Kellar K (1986): Nicotinic acetylcholine binding sites in Alzheimer's disease. Brain Res 371:146–151.

Whitehouse PJ, Price DL, Struble RG, Clark AW, Coyle JT, DeLong MR (1982): Alzheimer's disease and senile dementia: Loss of neurons in the basal forebrain. Science 215:1237–1239.

Whiting P, Schoepfer R, Lindstrom J, Priestly T (1992): Structural and pharmacological characterization of the major brain nicotinic acetylcholine receptor subtype stably expressed in mouse fibroblasts. Mol Pharmacol 40:463–472.

Widzowski DV, Cregan E, Bialobok P (1994): Effects of nicotinic agonists and antagonists on spatial working memory in normal adult and aged rats. Drug Dev Res 31:24–31.

Wilkie GI, Hutson PH, Stephens MW, Whiting P, Wonnacott S (1993): Hippocampal nicotinic autoreceptors modulate acetylcholine release. biochem Soc Trans 21:429–431.

Williams M, Sullivan J, Arneric S (1994): Neuronal nicotinic acetylcholine receptors. Drug News Perspect 7:205–223.

Wilson AL, Langley LK, Monley J, Bauer T, Rottunda S, McFalls E, Kovera C, McCarten JR (1995): Nicotine patches in Alzheimer's disease: Pilot study on learning, memory and safety. Pharmacol Biochem Behav 51:509–514.

Wonnacott S, Wilkie G, Soliakov L, Whiteaker P (1995): Presynaptic nicotinic autoreceptors and heteroreceptors in the CNS. In Clarke PBS, Quik M, Adlkofer F, Thurau K (eds): "Effects of Nicotine on Biological Systems," Vol. 11, Basel: Birkhauser pp 87–94.

Wonnacott S, Albuquerque EX, Bertrand D (1993): Methyllycaconitine: A new probe that discriminates between nicotinic acetylcholine receptor subclasses. Methods Neurosc 12:263–275.

Wonnacott S, Drasdo A, Sanderson E, Rowell P (1990a): Presynaptic nicotinic receptors and the modulation of transmitter release. In Bock G, Marsh J (eds): "The Biology of Nicotine Dependence," Chichester: Wiley, pp 87–101.

Wonnacott S, Irons J, Rapier C, Thorne B, Lunt GG (1990b): Presynaptic modulation of transmitter release by nicotinic receptors. In Norberg A, Fuxe K, Holmstedt B, Sundwall A (eds): "Progress in Brain Research," Amsterdam: Elsevier, pp 157–163.

Wonnacott S, Fryer L, Lunt G, Freund R, Jungschaffer D, Collins A (1987): Nicotinic modulation of GABAergic neurotransmission in the hippocampus. Soc Neurosci Abstr 17:1352.

Woodruff-Pak D, Li Y, Kem W (1994a): A nicotinic agonist (GTS-21), eyeblink classical conditioning, and nicotinic receptor binding in rat brain. Brain Res 645:309–317.

Woodruff-Pak DS, Li Y-T, Kasmi A, Kem WR (1994b): Nicotinic cholinergic system involvement in eyeblink classical conditioning in rabbits. Behav Neurosci 108:486–492.

CHAPTER 20

Neurotrophic Factors: Potential for Therapeutic Intervention in Alzheimer's

MARY ANN PELLEYMOUNTER and LAWRENCE R. WILLIAMS

Department of Neurobiology, Amgen Inc., 1840 DeHavilland Dr.,
Thousand Oaks, California 91320

INTRODUCTION

Neurotrophic factors can be generally defined as molecules that promote the survival and sustain the differentiated phenotype of neurons (Varon et al., 1984). Nerve growth factor (NGF) was the first neurotrophic factor to be discovered (Levi-Montalcini et al., 1995; Levi-Montalcini, 1982). In the peripheral nervous system, NGF is known to be a target tissue-derived, retrogradely transported, survival-promoting protein critical for the normal development, survival, and homeostasis of sympathetic and sensory neurons (Korsching, 1993). The profound survival-promoting effect of NGF on peripheral neurons led to the speculation that it would similarly affect neurons of the central nervous system (CNS). NGF is now known to act on central as well as peripheral neurons.

NGF is the first member of a defined family of trophic factors known as the neurotrophins; the current members include brain-derived neurotrophic factor (BDNF), neurotrophin-3 (NT-3), NT-4/5, and NT-6 (Thoenen, 1991) [for recent reviews see Lapchak et al. (1993a) and Bothwell (1995)]. NGF is distributed primarily in hippocampus and cortex, with density of mRNA for NGF highest in these areas (Hefti et al., 1989). BDNF is much more widespread, with mRNA expression in hippocampus, cortex, mediolateral thalamus, supramammillary region, medial tuberal nucleus, locus coeruleus, ventrolateral medulla, and the inferior olive complex (Ceccatelli et al., 1991). mRNA for NT3 and NT4/5 is most prominent in the hip-

Pharmacological Treatment of Alzheimer's Disease: Molecular and Neurobiological Foundations,
Edited by Brioni and Decker
ISBN 0-471-16758-4   © 1997 Wiley-Liss, Inc.

pocampus, and in the case of NT3 in the parafloccular lobe of the cerebellum (Cec-catelli et al., 1991; Fischer et al., 1994).

These neurotrophins are known to act via the family of trk tyrosine kinase receptors, that is, trkA, trkB, trkC, and the low-affinity p75 receptor (Chao and Hempstead, 1995; Kaplan et al., 1992; Lamballe et al., 1991; Parada et al., 1992). In the CNS, the expression of trkA, the receptor for NGF, is almost exclusively limited to the cholinergic neurons in the basal forebrain (Korsching et al., 1985; Whittemore and Seiger, 1987; Ferguson et al., 1991; Barker and Murphy, 1992; Venero and Hefti, 1993). Double labeling and co-distribution experiments have shown that the cholinergic neurons of the basal forebrain coincidently express p75 and trkA (Batchelor et al., 1989; Kiss et al., 1988; Woolf et al., 1989; Holtzman et al., 1992; Steininger et al., 1993; Venero et al., 1994; Li et al., 1995; Kordower et al., 1988; Altar et al., 1994b). The low-affinity p75 receptor is more widespread than the trkA receptor, with distribution in areas without dense cholinergic innervation, such as the superior cervical ganglion, the cerebellum, medial vestibular nuclei, and the lateral cochlei (Urschel and Hulsebosch, 1992).

The distribution of cells expressing the receptors specific for the other neurotrophins (i.e., trkB and trkC) is even more widespread, with expression in the olfactory system, neocortex, hippocampus, basal ganglia and basal forebrain, amygdala, thalamus, hypothalamus, substantia nigra and ventral tegmental area (VTA), dorsal raphe, central grey, brainstem orofacial and auditory nuclei, nucleus of the solitary tract, sensory trigeminal nuclei, cerebellum, and spinal cord (Altar et al., 1994c; Merlio et al., 1992). This widespread distribution of trkB and trkC suggests that there is a comparatively large spectrum of central neuronal populations responsive to BDNF, NT-3, and so forth (Escandón et al., 1993; Zhou et al., 1993; Lamballe et al., 1994; Altar et al., 1994b; Middlemas et al., 1991; Klein et al., 1990; Kokaia et al., 1995). In fact, infusions of these neurotrophins, particularly BDNF, has been reported to stimulate or enhance neurochemical markers for catecholaminergic, serotonergic, peptidergic neurons (Martin-Iverson et al., 1994; Altar et al., 1994a; Carnahan and Nawa, 1995; Croll et al., 1994; Nawa et al., 1995; Pelleymounter et al., 1994; Siuciak et al., 1996).

Other novel proteins have been identified that are known to be produced in the brain during development and/or in the adult, and to have neurotrophic activities for specific neuronal populations. These include basic fibroblast growth factor (bFGF) (Blottner and Baumgarten, 1992; Ferguson and Johnson, Jr., 1991; Frim et al., 1993; Lindholm et al., 1994; Louis et al., 1993; Ohsawa et al., 1993) and glial-cell-line-derived neurotrophin factor (GDNF) (Lin et al., 1993). The distribution of bFGF in the adult brain is rather homogeneous (Hefti et al., 1989), whereas GDNF is selectively expressed in the striatum (Blum and Weickert, 1995), septum, thalamus, medulla, and spinal cord (Arenas et al., 1995).

GDNF is one of the most recently discovered centrally active neurotrophic proteins. It was originally identified and purified using assays based on its very potent efficacy in promoting the survival and stimulating the transmitter phenotype of mesencephalic dopaminergic neurons *in vitro* (Lin et al., 1993). GDNF is a glycosylated disulfide-bonded homodimer that has its closest structural homology to the transforming growth factor (TGF)–beta superfamily of neurotrophic proteins (Lin et al., 1933; Krieglstein et al., 1995; Poulsen et al., 1994). In vivo, treatment with exogenous GDNF stimulates the dopaminergic phenotype of substantia nigra neurons and restores functional deficits induced by axotomy or dopaminergic neurotoxins in animal models of Parkinson's disease (Hudson et al., 1995; Beck et al., 1995; Tomac et al., 1995; Hoffer et al., 1994; Gash et al., 1995). Although originally thought to be relatively specific for dopaminergic neurons, at least in vitro, subsequent experiments have found that GDNF has neurotrophic efficacy on brain stem and spinal cord cholinergic motor neurons, both in vivo and in vitro (Oppenheim et al., 1995; Zurn et al., 1994; Yan et al., 1995; Henderson et al., 1994). Evidence is beginning to emerge indicating that GDNF may have a larger spectrum of neurotrophic targets besides mesencephalic dopaminergic and somatic motor neurons (Miller et al., 1994; Yan and Matheson, 1995). In particular, GDNF has recently been reported to have in vivo neurotrophic activity for basal forebrain cholinergic neurons (Williams et al., 1996).

MECHANISM OF ACTION

Although the neurotrophic properties of these proteins have been characterized extensively in vitro and in vivo, very little is known about their specific mechanism(s) of action, that is, how these proteins keep neurons alive and/or protect them against toxic or traumatic injury. The most information is known about the neurotrophin family of proteins (Barker and Murphy, 1992; Maness et al., 1994; Yancopoulos et al., 1990; Barde, 1990; Kaplan et al., 1992). Several laboratories are investigating what second-messenger systems and/or genes (e.g., MAP kinases and immediate early genes) are activated by ligand–receptor interaction (Widmer et al., 1993a; Volonte et al., 1993; Marsh et al., 1993; Knüsel et al., 1992b; Batistatou et al., 1992; Loeb et al., 1992; Stephens et al., 1994). However, the final pathway regulating survival of affected neurons remains to be elucidated.

An intriguing connection is evolving between neurotrophic factors, oxidative stress, apoptosis, and programmed neuronal death. When neurotrophic factors are removed from cultures of trophic factor-dependent neurons (Deckwerth and Johnson, Jr. 1993a,b; Johnson, Jr. et al., 1995; Svendsen et al., 1994; Sofroniew et al., 1993) or neurons are placed under conditions of oxidative stress (Roberts-Lewis et al., 1993; Samples and Dubinsky, 1993; Ratan et al., 1994; Ratan and Baraban, 1994; Whittemore et al., 1994), they undergo a process cell death with the characteristics of apoptotic neuronal death. Apoptosis may in fact be mediated by oxidative stress and free-radical damage (Buttke and Sandstrom, 1994).

One mechanism by which the neurotrophic factors may mediate neuronal survival, at least in part, is by the specific stimulation of endogenous antioxidant enzyme systems (Williams, 1995). Such a stimulation was first described by the laboratory of Perez-Polo, Jackson et al. (1990) found that NGF provided protection of rat pheochromocytoma PC12 cells to oxidative stress induced by hydrogen peroxide. NGF treatment of the cells was found to stimulate the activity of catalase. More recently, Pan et al. (1993) and Sampath et al. (1994) have extended these results to examine glutathione metabolism. They reported that NGF treatment of PC12 cells stimulated glutamylcysteine synthetase activity, the rate-limiting enzyme for glutathione (GSH) synthesis, increased GSH levels by 100%, and stimulated glutathione peroxidase (GSH-Px) and glucose 6-phosphate dehydrogenase activities. In primary cultures of hippocampal or cortical neurons, neurotrophins and FGF protect neurons from death-induced oxidative stress (Zhanga et al., 1993; Cheng and Mattson, 1994; Cheng et al., 1994; Mattson et al., 1995). Nisticò et al. (1991, 1992) examined several antioxidant enzyme activities in young and aged rats in vivo. They found that NGF treatment of aged rats restored the age-related decrease in catalase activity and increased superoxide dismutase (SOD) and GSH-PX activity.

BDNF was reported to protect neuroblastoma cells in culture against toxicity induced by 6-hydroxydopamine and 1-methyl-4phenylpyridinium (MPP+), two dopaminergic toxins believed to act through free-radical mechanisms. Spina et al. (1993) found that the levels of the oxidized form of glutathione were decreased in the BDNF-treated cultures due to an apparent specific stimulation of glutathione reductase enzyme activity; catalase activity was not affected by BDNF treatment.

NEUROTROPHIC FACTORS AND NEURODEGENERATIVE DISEASE

Amyotrophic lateral sclerosis (ALS), Parkinson's disease (PD), and Alzheimer's disease (AD) are major human neurodegenerative disorders, the etiologies for which remain unknown. Although a unique subset of neurons is particularly affected in each of the three diseases, they have several intriguing similarities in the morphological pathologies and biochemical abnormalities associated with each disease. This has led Eisen and Calne (1992), among others (Varon et al., 1984; Williams, 1995; Olanow, 1993; Appel, 1981; Coyle and Puttfarcken, 1993), to speculate that these three diseases share a common etiology. The causative agents or mechanisms hypothesized to underlie the common cause of these diseases include excitatory amino acid toxicity (Eisen and Calne, 1992; Coyle and Puttfarcken, 1993); oxidative stress (Williams, 1995; Ames et al., 1993; Olanow, 1993; Pacifici and Davies, 1991), neurotrophin deficiency (Appel, 1981; Varon et al., 1984; Hefti and Weiner, 1986; Maness et al., 1994), and apoptosis (Su et al., 1994; Cotman et al., 1994; Dragunow et al., 1995). Because the identified neurotrophic factors discussed above are known to affect the neuronal populations that degenerate in ALS, PD, and AD, the neurotrophic factors have been proposed as efficacious therapies for the neurodegenerative diseases (Appel, 1981; Varon et al., 1984). BDNF (Oppenheim et al., 1992b; Sendtner et al., 1992; Oppenheim et al., 1992a) and GDNF (Henderson et al., 1994; Oppenheim et al., 1995; Zurn et al., 1994; Yan et al., 1995) are neurotrophic for spinal motor neurons and have been tested or are being considered for testing in clinical trials for ALS. Similarly, GDNF (Lin et al., 1993; Hudson et al., 1995; Beck et al., 1995; Tomac et al., 1995; Gash et al., 1995) and BDNF (Altar et al., 1994a) are being considered for efficacy trials with Parkinson's disease because of the reported neurotrophic activity they express for mesencephalic dopaminergic neurons.

NEUROTROPHIC FACTORS AND SENILE DEMENTIA OF THE ALZHEIMER'S TYPE

A variety of neuronal populations have been shown to undergo degenerative changes in AD, including neurons from the dorsal raphe, locus coeruleus (Zweig et al., 1988; Zubenko et al., 1988; Hardy et al., 1985), and substantia nigra (Zubenko et al., 1988). Some peptidergic neurons also show degenerative changes in AD, including somatostatin (Beal et al., 1986), corticotropin releasing factor (CRF) and neuropeptide Y (NPY) (Bouras et al., 1986). Finally, several receptor populations appear to decline in some AD patients, including D1 receptors in the putamen and hippocampus (Cortes et al., 1988), hippocampal glutamate metabotropic and AMPA receptors (Dewar et al., 1991), cortical M2 muscarinic receptors (Mash et al., 1985) and cortical nicotinic receptors (Whitehouse et al., 1988; Nordberg and Winblad, 1986). It is interesting to note that there is no evidence to date of a reduction in NGF mRNA (Jette et al., 1994) and only equivicol evidence for a reduction in NFG receptors (Higgins and Mufson, 1989; Goedert et al., 1989) in Alzheimer's patients. There has been one report, however, of a significant reduction in mRNA for BDNF in the hippocampal formation of AD patients (Phillips et al., 1991). Currently, there is no information about the status of NT3, NT4/5, or GDNF in AD patients.

The most consistently observed degeneration and neurochemical dysfunction associated with senile dementia of the Alzheimer's type (SDAT) is in the basal forebrain cholinergic neurons, their projections and terminals (Bartus et al., 1982; Perry et al., 1992; Whitehouse et al., 1982; Katzman, 1986; Coleman and Flood, 1987; Wilcock et al., 1982; Mountjoy, 1986; Reinikainen et al., 1988; Rylett et al., 1983). There are many reports of degenerative changes in cholinergic neurons of the nucleus basalis magnocellularis (nBM), along with reduced choline acetyltransferase and acetylcholinesterase activity, choline uptake, and acetylcholine release [for review, see Hardy et al. (1985)]. One group has found that the most severe and widespread cholinergic degeneration is found in younger AD brains (70–80 years old) and is accompanied by degeneration of several other systems, such as NE, GABA, and somatostatin, whereas patients with later onset AD (90–100 years old) have a more restricted and specific cholinergic neurodegeneration (Rossor et al., 1984).

The consistent and severe degeneration of subcortical cholinergic neurons and their projections to paleo- and neocortex in AD has been associated with the cognitive defects that characterize the disease (Bartus et al., 1982). Likewise, the observations of variable degeneration in noradrenergic and dopaminergic systems have been associated with the affective and psychotic symptoms that are also fairly common in AD (Zubenko and Moossy, 1988). There is considerable interest, therefore, in the potential use of one or more neurotrophic factors for treatment of SDAT, since these proteins have the potential to limit or prevent the degeneration of a variety of target neuronal populations, along with the ability to stimulate neurochemical activity of surviving dysfunctional neurons.

ANIMAL MODELS OF NEUROTROPHIC FACTOR EFFICACY IN SDAT

Most in vivo research modeling neuronal dysfunction associated with SDAT has focused on the basal forebrain cholinergic systems because of the hallmark degeneration of these systems in AD (Hefti, 1994; Olson, 1994). There are two primary projection systems: (i) the projection neurons of the medial septum and diagonal band of Broca (MS/DB) to the hippocampus and (ii) the projection neurons of the nucleus basalis magnocellularis (NBM) to the cerebral cortex and amygdala, see (Williams et al., 1989) for review.

Axotomy of the septalhippocampal projection results in the rapid (i.e., within 2 weeks) down regulation of ChAT, p75, and trkA, expression in basal forebrain cholinergic neurons, which become atrophic and unrecognizable as neurons (Gage et al., 1986; Hagg et al., 1989; Hefti, 1986; Springer et al., 1987; Sofroniew et al., 1993). Although the loss of histological recognition was earlier interpreted to indicate death of the axotomized neurons (Daitz and Powell, 1954; Gage et al., 1986; Tuszynski et al., 1990), careful experiments using vital dyes have indicated that many of the axotomized neurons in fact do not die but exist in an atrophied zombie or hibernatory state (Hagg et al., 1988; Sofroniew et al., 1993; Peterson et al., 1992; Naumann et al., 1994), a state in which they may exist in a basal forebrain affected by Alzheimer's disease (Pearson et al., 1983). Using the fimbria/fornix axotomy model, it was shown that the axotomy-induced neuronal atrophy could be prevented and the cholinergic phenotype sustained or even augmented by treating the brains with intracerebroventricular doses of NGF, BDNF, or NT-4/5 (Hagg et al., 1989; Hefti, 1986; Knüsel et al., 1992a; Koliatsos et al., 1994; Kromer et al., 1987; Morse et al., 1993; Venero et al., 1994; Widmer et al., 1993b; Williams et al., 1986; Williams et al., 1989; Alderson et al., 1995). Most recently, GDNF has been reported to sustain the cholinergic phenotype of these neurons following axotomy (Williams et al., 1996). Please see Figures 1 and 2.

Cuello et al. (1989) developed a modified axotomy model for the basal forebrain projection to the cerebral cortex. Following terminal disruption by cortical devascularization, cholinergic neurons in the nucleus basalis also down-regulate their cholinergic phenotype. They have reported that treatment with NGF (Garofalo and Cuello, 1994, 1995; Burgos et al., 1995) but not BDNF or NT-3 (Skup et al., 1994) sustains the phenotype and stimulates sprouting in this model.

EFFECTS OF NEUROTROPHIC FACTORS ON NEUROCHEMICAL ACTIVITY IN LESION MODELS AND IN INTACT ANIMALS

NGF administration has profound effects on cholinergic neurochemistry in rodents. NGF treatment ($1-2$ μg/day for 2 weeks) stimulates ChAT activity (Dekker & Thal, 1992; Hefti et al., 1984; Williams and Oostveen, 1992; Williams, 1991b; Williams et al., 1989), high-affinity choline uptake (Williams and Rylett, 1990), and acetylcholine synthesis and release (Rylett and Williams, 1994; Rylett et al., 1993; Lapchak et al., 1993b; Lapchak, 1993; Garofalo and Cuello, 1995) in both intact ani-

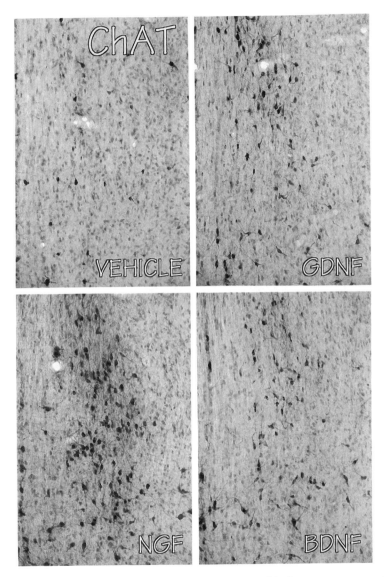

FIGURE 1. Effect of fimbrai/fornix axotomy and neurotrophic factor treatment on ChAT-positive neurons. The micrographs illustrate the ChAT-positive neurons in the medial septum ipsilateral to the axotomy and are representative of the results from animals treated with the maximally effective doses of neurotrophic proteins tested in these experiments. In vehicle-treated animals, there is an obvious loss of immunoreactive ChAT-positive neurons. Treatment with GDNF 1 μg/day. NGF 1 μg/day, and BDNF 10 μg/day significantly reduces the loss of ChAT-positive neurons, sustaining the cholinergic phenotype in the axotomized cells.

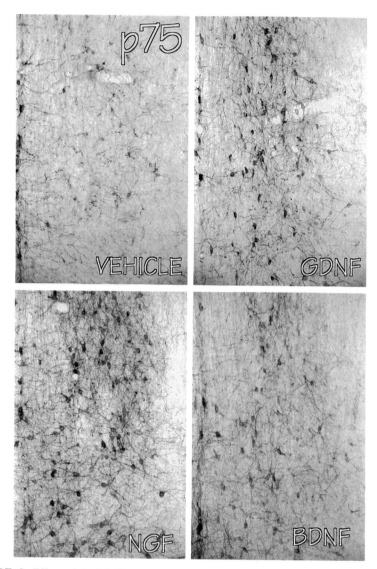

FIGURE 2. Effect of fimbria/fornix axotomy and neurotrophic factor treatment on p75-positive neurons. The micrographs illustrate the p75-positive neurons in the medial septum ipsilateral to the axotomy and are representative of the results from animals treated with the maximally effective doses of neurotrophic proteins tested in these experiments. In vehicle-treated animals, there is an obvious loss of immunoreactive p75-positive neurons. Treatment with GDNF 10 μg/day, NGF 1 μg/day, and BDNF 10 μg/day significantly reduces the loss of p75-positive neurons, sustaining the cholinergic phenotype in the axotomized cells.

mals and those with injury to hippocampal or cortical cholinergic projections. These effects of NGF on cholinergic activity can be relatively long lasting, particularly in the case of animals with injury or neurodegenerative changes in the basal forebrain. Septal ChAT activity was elevated in rats with fimbria/fornix lesions 10 weeks after the cessation of a 4-week period of intracerebroventricular (icv) NGF treatment (10 μg twice weekly) (Will and Hefti, 1985). Similarly, a recent study showed that hippocampal high affinity choline uptake (HACU) was augmented 7 weeks after cessation of a 4-week treatment regimen with intrahippocampally infused NFG (6 μg/day) in aged Long–Evans rats (Pelleymounter et al., 1995) (see Figure 3).

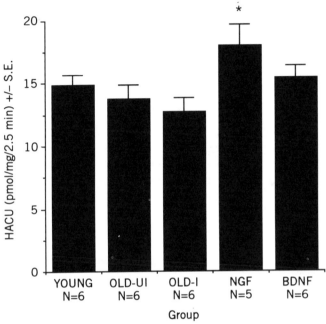

FIGURE 3. Effects of NGF and BDNF on hippocampal sodium-dependent, high-affinity choline uptake (SDHACU) in aged rats. Aged rats were separated into impaired and unimpaired subpopulations in the following manner: all rats were given 12 initial trials in the Morris maze task, with the twelfth trial acting as a "probe" trial for spatial bias, where the escape platform was removed, and the animal's swim path was observed. Based on the frequency of platform crossings, the proportion of time spent in the training quadrant, and the two latencies immediately preceding the probe trial, animals were identified as impaired or unimpaired. Impaired rats were counterbalanced across treatment groups for degree of impairment, and infused with either BDNF or NGF (6 μg/day) into the dorsal hippocampus. Unimpaired and young rats were infused with PBS. During the last 3 weeks of infusion, rats were allowed to continue training in the Morris task until they reached a learning criterion that was based on spatial bias during the probe trials. Rats were dropped from training when they met these criteria and were tested for retention of the escape platform location 7 weeks later. One week after the retention test, animals were sacrificed and hippocampal tissue was dissected and prepared for SDHACU analysis. OUI = old, unimpaired; OI = old, impaired. *ps < .0047, .02 compared to OI and OUI groups.

The neurochemical changes induced by NGF appear to reflect functional change in synaptic activity, since NGF also augments electrophysiologic transmission in the amygdala (Moises et al., 1995).

It is interesting to note that NGF can also restore noncholinergic neurochemical activity after injury to either the striatum or cortex. NGF normalized striatal dopamine and homovanillic acid levels in MPTP-treated mice (Garcia et al., 1992) and partially normalized cortical dopamine levels after a devascularizing cortical lesion (Maysinger et al., 1992). Unlike the effects of NGF on the cholinergic system, the effects of NGF on dopaminergic activity appeared to be dependent upon injury, since neither striatal or cortical dopamine (DA) were changed in normal rats treated with NGF.

Unlike NGF, BDNF has little or no effect on cholinergic neurochemistry (Lapchak and Hefti, 1992; Williams et al., 1996). BDNF, however, appears to stimulate noradrenergic, dopaminergic, and serotonergic activity. Nigral infusion of BDNF (12 μg/day for 2 weeks) has been shown to increased striatal DA (serotonin (5-HT) turnover in intact animals (Altar et al., 1994a, 1992; Martin-Iversen et al., 1992) and in animals with partial striatal DA depletions (Altar et al., 1994b). Intraventricular administration of BDNF (6 or 12 μg/day for 2 weeks) also increases striatal 5-hydroxyindoleacetic acid (5HIAA), nigral 5HIAA/5HT, cortical 5HIAA/5HT, 3,4 dihydroxyphenylacetic acid (DOPAC), and NE, hippocampal 5HIAA/5HT and DOAPC/DA (Siuciak et al., 1995), and hypothalamic 5HIAA/5HT (Pelleymounter et al., 1995; Siuciak et al., 1996). These BDNF-induced changes in monoamergic activity appear indicative of enhanced synaptic activity, since intranigral application of BDNF (11 μg/day) increased the average firing rate of pars compacta neurons by 32% (Shen et al., 1994). BDNF has also been shown to regulate central neuropeptides. Intraventricular infusion of BDNF for 2 weeks (12 μg/day) elevated striatal CCK, NPY, substance P (SP) and dynorphin, hippocampal, and cortical NPY and cholecystokinin (CCK), and reduced hippocampal dynorphin in adult rats (Croll et al., 1994). In contrast, NGF did not alter peptide levels in the above areas.

Similar to NGF, a 4-week intraventricular infusion of NT-3 (6 μg/day) has been shown to increase the size of AChE-staining neurons in the septum, striatum, and nMB of aged rats (Fischer et al., 1994). NT-3 also has limited effects on monoaminergic activity, affecting striatal 5-HIAA during intranigral infusion (Altar et al., 1994b). NT4/5 was without effect on AChE-staining neurons in the Fischer study, and its effects on other neurotransmitters have not been reported to date.

Intraventricular infusion of GDNF (6 mg/day) has been reported to stimulate septal ChAT activity in animals with fimbra/fornix lesions but not in intact animals (Williams et al., 1996). Further, a single bolus intraventricular or intranigral injection of GDNF (100 mg) augments nigral dopaminergic and serotonergic activity in intact animals and normalizes DA in animals with 6-OHDA lesions (Martin et al., 1996; Hoffer et al., 1994). Whether or not it has effects on other neurotransmitter systems remains to be seen.

NEUROTROPHINS AND COGNITION

Most of the evidence suggesting that neurotrophic factors improve learning and memory centers around the effects of NGF on spatial learning and memory in animals with injury- or age-induced neurodegeneration. One of the earliest reports describing the effects of NGF in a model of septohippocampal degeneration suggested that NGF could reduce lesion-induced cognitive deficits during, but not beyond, the treatment period. Radial arm maze acquisition rate was improved in rats with fimbria/fornix lesions that were injected (icv) twice a week, beginning at the time of the lesion. This improvement was not lasting, however; when the same rats were retested 6 weeks after NGF withdrawal. NGF-treated rats were as impaired as vehicle-treated counterparts (Will and Hefti, 1985).

The effects of NGF on learning in rats with septal lesions are somewhat equivocal and may depend upon (1) NGF injection site, (2) time of testing relative to injection, and (3) whether or not animals were pretrained prior to lesion and injection. A single intra*septal* injection of NGF (5 μg) at the time of lesion improved radial arm maze performance by facilitating the use of a different choice strategy for a period of 30 days after the injection (Janis et al., 1995), whereas a single intra*hippocampal* NGF injection (8 μg) at the time of septal lesions did not improve spatial alternation or radial arm maze acquisition 1, 5, or 9 months after injection; the deficits in radial arm acquisition actually appeared to be exacerbated by previous NGF administration (Pallage et al., 1986). Aside from the difference in injection sites, several major procedural differences in the two studies could explain the difference in results; animals had been extensively pretrained prior to the lesion in the Janis et al. (1995) study, and began testing 3 days after surgery and injection, whereas animals were novices to the task at the time of lesion and injection in the Pallage et al. (1986) study and did not begin testing until one month after surgery and injections. Thus, injection site, time of testing relative to injection, and stage of information processing were different in the two studies. It is not clear whether or not cholinergic stimulation was involved in the cognitive improvements observed in the Janis et al. (1995) study, since hippocampal HACU was not altered in NGF-treated rats 15 days after NGF injection. In contrast to the positive/equivocal nature of its effects in animals with fimbria/fornix or septal lesions, NGF was not shown to be at all efficacious in rats with hippocampal lesions (Kimble et al., 1979).

NGF has also shown efficacy in models involving degeneration of cortical fibers that originate in the nucleus basalis. Chronic, intraventricular administration of NGF (5 μg/day) delivered 3 weeks after the lesion via a subcutaneously implanted osmotic mini-pump (Alzet 2002) improved acquisition of the Morris maze task in rats with ibotenic acid-induced lesions of the nBM (Winkler and Thal, 1995). Water maze training/testing was conducted during the fourth week of NGF infusion. Interestingly, the cognition-enhancing effects of NGF in this study were dependent on the type of excitatory amino acid toxin that was used to injure nBM cells. NGF did not improve acquisition in rats where lesions were induced by either quisqualic acid or AMPA (Winkler and Thal, 1995). Cortical ChAT activity was partially normalized in these animals, which were sacrificed at the end of the NGF infusion period; the degree of ChAT normalization, however, did not correlate with degree of improvement in spatial learning.

NGF also improved cognition in animals with unilateral cortical lesions. Passive avoidance retention and spatial learning in the Morris water maze were improved in rats that were given continuous NGF infusions (6 µg/day) into the lateral ventricle at the time of lesion (Garofalo and Cuello, 1994). In this study, all animals had been pretrained in both tasks prior to lesion and were retested 2 weeks after NGF withdrawal. nBM ChAT activity was completely normalized and cortical ChAT and HACU were actually increased above control levels in NGF-treated rats, despite the fact that these animals were sacrificed 5 weeks after the end of drug infusions. Cortical or nBM GAD activity was not affected by NGF or the lesion.

Much of the literature describing the effects of NGF on learning center around its effects in aged rats, which show deficits in a variety of learning and memory paradigms that can be correlated with neurobiological impairments (Issa et al., 1990; Abdulla et al., 1995; Gallagher et al., 1990; Gallagher and Burwell, 1989; Ingram et al., 1981; Barnes, 1979). Aged rats can be separated into "impaired" and "unimpaired" subpopulations based on their acquisition rate in the Morris water maze (Gage et al., 1984; Rapp et al., 1987). It has been shown that chronic intraventricular infusion of NGF (1 µg/day) improved water maze performance in spatial learning-impaired 23–25-month-old Sprague–Dawley female rats during the fourth week of infusion but not during the second week. In addition, NGF increased nBM and striatal AChE-positive cell body size, suggesting a cholinergic mechanism of action (Fischer et al., 1987). It has been subsequently shown that these effects generalize to younger (18 month) and older (30 month) Fisher 344 female rats (Fischer et al., 1991). NGF also improved the performance of 23-month-old Fisher 344 males in a delayed alternation task and in the Morris maze task (Markowska et al., 1994). These rats had been pretrained in both tasks prior to the onset of NGF infusion (1.4 and 5.7 µg/day). Retest for both tasks occurred during the fourth week of infusion. Although both doses improved performance in the older rats, the low dose actually appeared to impair the performance of young rats in the delayed alternation task. Sensorimotor function was unaffected by NGF in young and old rats. In another study, however, a measure of motor function was affected by NGF infusion. In this study using an electrified Y-maze brightness discrimination paradigm, NGF did not improve brightness discrimination in aged rats, but did increase the number of avoidance attempts, suggesting an effect on motor, but not cognitive, function (Williams et al., 1991). Finally, NGF also improved object recognition in aged rats, along with increasing acetyalcoholic levels in cortex and hippocampus (Scali et al., 1994).

The effectiveness of NGF in learning-impaired aged rats led to the hypothesis that aged rats show evidence of neurodegeneration because they have reduced levels of NGF or do not respond to NGF as young animals do. Most reports, however, show no age-related change (or a slight increase) in hippocampal NGF levels (Crutcher and Weingartner, 1991; Hellweg et al., 1990). Considering the spatial learning heterogeneity in aged rats, it might be expected that if learning impaired and unimpaired rats were separated, one might observe differences in NGF levels that would correlate with spatial learning impairment. Indeed, there is a report that hippocampal NGF levels correlate (Henriksson et al., 1992) with spatial learning deficits. Another group finds no correlation, however (Hellweg et al., 1990). One group finds that NGF levels differed as a function of age in females but not in males (Nishizuka et al., 1991). Several other groups have found that spatial learning impairments in aged animals are accompanied by a loss in the low-affinity p75 NGF receptor (Koh et al., 1989; Markram and Segal, 1990), suggesting that aged animals cannot respond to NGF as well as young animals.

Very little information exists regarding the effects of other neurotrophins on cognition. One group has shown that intraventricular infusion of NT3 and NT4/5 (6 μg/day) improved acquisition/retention in aged, spatial learning-impaired female Sprague–Dawley rats (Fischer et al., 1994), whereas BDNF was not efficacious. One reason that BDNF might not have seemed efficacious is that BDNF does not diffuse well from the ventricles into the surrounding parenchyma, as measured by antibody staining or retrograde transport of iodinated material (Morse et al., 1993; Yan et al., 1994). In order to avoid this, one group delivered BDNF into the dorsal hippocampus, but still failed to observe a significant improvement in learning in aged, spatial learning-impaired male Long–Evans rats (Pelleymounter et al., 1996) (see Figure 4).

These negative results with BDNF and cognition are somewhat disappointing in view of earlier work showing that mRNA for BDNF was significantly reduced in the hippocampal formation of Alzheimer's patients (Phillips et al., 1991)). Further, mRNA for BDNF was reduced by manipulations that impair spatial memory, such as chronic atropine treatment or fimbria/fornix transections (Lapchak et al., 1993a), and increased in animals that had been exposed to enriched environments, which have been shown to improve spatial learning (Falkenberg et al., 1992). Finally, density of hypothalamic trkB mRNA has been shown to correlate with spatial learning impairments in aged Long–Evans rats (Williams et al., 1994). There are, of course, many reasons that BDNF might not improve cognition despite all of the correlative evidence presented above. It is also possible that the very limited diffusion properties of BDNF (even when infused into parenchyma) remain the basis for its lack of efficacy in aged rats. If limited diffusion is the reason for lack of efficacy, however, the potential for BDNF as a therapeutic in humans would remain low, since diffusion would be an even greater issue in organisms with a larger brain volume.

The only other neurotrophic factor that has been shown to affect cognition is basic FGF, (bFGF) (5–10 ng/side), administered at the time of lesion, ameliorated an acquisition deficit in an inhibitory avoidance paradigm that was induced by basal forebrain lesions in mice without reversing the lesion-induced cortical ChAT loss (Ishihara et al., 1992). To date, there is no published data describing the effects of GDNF on cognition. Table 1 summarizes the effects of the neurotrophic factors discussed here on cognition.

Although the above evidence suggest that neurotrophic factors can alleviate learning and memory deficits, it is important to recognize the limitations of the animal models and learning paradigms used to infer potential efficacy in humans. It is

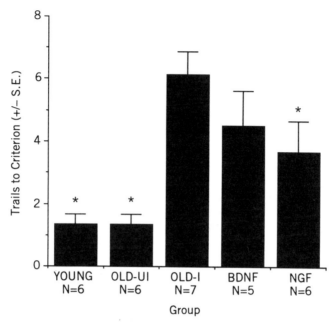

FIGURE 4. Effects of intrahippocampal BDNF and NGF infusion on trials to a spatial learning criterion in young, old impaired and old unimpaired rats. Aged rats were separated into subpopulations of impaired and unimpaired and then treated with either PBS, BDNF (6 mg/day), or NGF (6 mg/day) infused into the dorsal hippocampus, as described in Figure 3. They were then allowed to continue training on the Morris maze task during the last 3 weeks of a 4-week infusion period until they met a spatial bias criterion. Assessment of criterion performance was made on every sixth trial (probe trial). During the 40-sec probe trials, the escape platform was removed and swim path was evaluated, using quadrant time and number of platform crossings as measures of spatial bias. In order to meet criterion, rats were required to make at least two platform crossings and spend at least 30% of the trial in the training quadrant. OUI = old, unimpaired; OI = old, impaired. *$ps < .03, .001$ compared to OI rats.

commonly acknowledged that there are no animal models that closely mimic Alzheimer's disease, since neither lesions or aging have been shown to reliably produce the morphological changes (neuritic plaques and tangles) that provide definitive diagnosis of Alzheimer's disease (AD).

Further, most of the learning paradigms used to demonstrate efficacy of neurotrophic factors involve spatial learning and memory, where there is anecdotal evidence of deficits in Alzheimer's patients, primarily in familiar environments. The spatial learning paradigms used to test rodents, however, test the ability to reliably learn the location of a new place in a novel environment. While Alzheimer's patients would no doubt have difficulty with such a task, there is data suggesting that early-stage AD patients are no more impaired in spatial rotation tasks than are normal age-matched controls (Flicker et al., 1988). On the other hand, there is evi-

TABLE 1. Neurotrophic Factors: Distribution and Cognitive Effects

Neurotrophic Factor	Primary Distribution	Cell Population Rescued	Neurochemical Effects (intact animals)	Cognitive Effects
NGF	Cortex, hippocampus *trkA and p75 in:* Septum, nucleus basalis, thalamus, cerebellum, vestibular, and cochlear nuclei, SCG	Medial septum, nBM	Increase ChAT, AChE, HACU, ACh release	Reverse deficits in: radial arm maze (f/f, MS lesions), water maze (nBM, cortical lesions, aged rats), passive avoidance (nBM, cortical lesions), spatial alternation (aged rats)
BDNF	Hippocampus, cortex, locus coeruleus, mesencephalon, medial geniculate, vestibular n, cerebellum and brainstem *trkB in:* Olfactory bulb and cortex, neocortex, striatum, hippocampus, amygdala, ventromedial hypothalamus S. Nigra, VTA, cerebellum	S. nigra, medial septum	Increase DA, 5HT, NE release, increase TH activity	None
NT3	Hippocampus *trkC in:* Olfactory bulb and cortex, neocortex, basal forebrain, hippocampus, basal amygdala, ant. thalamus, hypothalamus S. nigra	Medial septum	Increase 5HIAA	Reverse deficits in water maze (aged rats)
NT4/5	Distribution unknown, evidence that NT4/5 uses trkB receptor			
GDNF	Striatum, septum, thalamus, spinal cord, medulla	Medial septum, S. nigra	Increase DA, 5HT release	Reverse deficits in water maze (aged rats) Not tested
bFGF	Hippocampus	Medial septum	None	Reversed deficits in passive avoidance (nBM lesions in mice)

dence that some AD patients do have profound visuo-spatial deficits that include difficulty with object recognition (Corkin, 1982) and spatial contrast sensitivity (Nissen et al., 1985). Therefore, it is difficult to say whether or not AD patients actually have a spatial memory deficit, as it is defined by the Morris maze task.

A hallmark of the memory loss in AD is rapid forgetting and a susceptibility to distractors (Irle et al., 1987; Reisberg et al., (1988). Therefore, while the Morris maze task may be a valid test for deficits observed in some AD patients, it might be more straightforward to use a task that taps into a deficit that is always observed in AD, such as rapid forgetting. Delayed match to sample or nonmatch to sample tasks can assess forgetting as a function of time, number of items to remember, and the addition of distractors without being confounded with learning, since all animals must be trained to a criterion prior to testing. An additional positive feature of the DMTS or DNMTS tasks is that they have been validated in AD patients, and correlate well with deficits in cognitive tasks commonly used to diagnose and follow AD patients (Irle et al., 1987). Further, animals with nBM lesions show deficits in these tasks, as do aged rats and primates (Irle et al., 1987), particularly as the number of items to be remembered is increased (Aggleton et al., 1989), similar to the early AD patient.

Thus, although aged animals with spatial learning impairments would certainly provide information about the ability of a therapeutic agent to improve learning, this model might not completely address the cognitive deficits that are observed in AD patients. Paradigms where animals are pretrained to a criterion and then tested for recognition or recall after a delay could address these more global cognitive deficits observed in AD patients.

With the above caveats in mind, the data discussed above suggest that neurotrophic factors may have some unique benefits in diseases that involve neurodegeneration with cognitive dysfunction, such as Alzheimer's disease.

DELIVERY OF NEUROTROPHIC FACTORS TO THE BRAIN

Bioactive protein neurotrophic factors have molecular weights greater than 20 kd and as such do not cross the blood–brain barrier. All of the efficacy studies on basal forebrain neurons in experimental animals have administered neurotrophic factors directly into the brain via an indwelling catheter or cannula. Efficacious use of neurotrophic factors in the clinic today would require similar direct administration of protein. Several groups are examining alternative methods of drug delivery. Friden et al. (1993) reported that a molecular complex of NGF conjugated to an antibody to endothelial cell transferrin receptor was able to cross the blood–brain barrier after systemic administration and affect a central target. Administration of such conjugates has been reported to affect basal forebrain neurons (Kordower et al., 1994; Granholm et al., 1994; Friden et al., 1995) and improve deficits in animal behavior (Backman et al., 1995). Other groups speculate that transplantation of cells transfected with a gene encoding a neurotrophic factor will enable therapeutic availability of protein. *Cytotherapeutics* has taken the approach of transplanting encapsulated transfected cells (Hammang et al., 1995; Emerich et al., 1994a,b; Winn et al., 1994), while *somatics* has transplanted transfected autologous primary fibroblasts or stem cells (Chen and Gage, 1995; Gage et al., 1995; Lucidi Phillip et al., 1995; Ray et al., 1995; Kawaja et al., 1992). Although the transfected cell strategy is technologically fantastic, there are very real pragmatic issues of dose control and mutagenic transformation that need to be resolved before such technology can be used in the clinic. Thus, direct administration to the brain via bolus injection or continuous infusion is the only viable method of drug administration currently available (Harbaugh, 1989a,b; Penn et al., 1988).

TREATMENT OF SDAT WITH NEUROTROPHIC FACTORS

Based on the positive efficacy of NGF in animal models of SDAT, several proposals have been put forth to test efficacy of NGF in humans (Phelps et al., 1989; Hefti, 1994; Olson, 1994). In fact, small-scale clinical trials testing for such efficacy are ongoing and beginning to be reported (cf Olson et al., (1992) and Petty et al. (1994)]. In these initial human clinical trials of NGF after systemic administration for peripheral neuropathy and central administration for Alzheimer's disease, untenable side effects have become evident. Peripheral administration of NGF at low doses causes severe muscle pain (Petty et al., 1994). Alzheimer's patients treated with intracerebroventricular infusions of NGF at the relatively low dose of 66 μg/day (Olson et al., 1992) [a dose comparable, based on brain weight, to a rat dose of 0.08 μg/day (Williams, 1991a)], show improvements in measures of cerebral blood flow and nicotinic binding. Unfortunately, these patients also experience peripheral rostral muscle pain similar to that reported after peripheral NGF administration, along with significant weight loss (L. Olson, personal communication).

NGF certainly activates the basal forebrain cholinergic system better than any other neurotrophic factor currently known (Williams et al., 1996), to the point of enhancing neurochemical and electrophysiological measures to supranormal levels. The reported alterations of cholinergic neuronal structure, abnormal sprouting, and abnormal neurotransmission induced by NGF in rodents may actually underlie some of the above undesirable clinical side effects (Butcher and Woolf, 1989; Williams et al., 1996).

BDNF has more modest effects on dystrophic cholinergic neurons than does NGF and, to date, has not been shown to reliably improve learning and memory in cognitively impaired animals (Fischer et al., 1994; Pelleymounter et al., in press). In addition, it induces the most severe weight loss of any neurotrophic factor discussed in this chapter (Pelleymounter et al., 1995). GDNF, however, is an order of magnitude more potent than BDNF on dystrophic cholinergic neurons and has minimal or no effect on uninjured normal cholinergic neurons (Williams et al., 1996). GDNF also has a wider spectrum of activity than does NGF, affecting normal catecholaminergic as well as serotonergic neuronal activity in vivo (Miller et al., 1994; Martin et al., 1996; Yan and Matheson, 1995). A very recent report showed that GDNF could also protect dorsal bundle noradrenergic neurons from 6-OHDA-induced degeneration (Arenas et al., 1995). As of this time, it is not known whether or not GDNF can improve learning in animals with cognitive deficits. Thus, GDNF has the potential to affect dystrophic cholinergic neurons, without inducing abnormal cholinergic activity, along with affecting the activity of normal and dystrophic monoaminergic neurons. Since Alzheimer's disease can involve degeneration of monoaminergic systems, along with the hallmark cholinergic degeneration, these attributes of GDNF suggest that it may provide an attractive alternative to NGF as a neurotrophic therapeutic for Alzheimer's disease.

In summary, NGF, BDNF, NT3, NT4/5, GNDE, and bFGF all have the capability of protecting neurons from injury-induced degeneration. These neurotrophic factors can also regulate the activity of cholinergic, serotonergic, and catecholaminergic neurons in intact animals. Finally, most of these neurotrophic factors also prevent or partially reverse the cognitive deficits that accompany degeneration of the above systems. In light of the fact that all of the systems affected by these neurotrophic factors undergo degenerative changes in AD, these proteins have the potential to (1) alleviate both the cognitive and affective symptoms of AD and (2) to slow the progression of the disease.

Unfortunately, these proteins may have untenable side effects, (as has been the case with the limited trials of NGF) and do not cross the blood–brain barrier, presenting a significant delivery issue. Therefore, it remains to be seen if the efficacy of these neurotrophic factors can outweigh the potential for side effects, along with the risk, cost, and inconvenience of intraventricular or intraparenchymal delivery. Providing evidence of such efficacy using models that realistically mimic the progression of both the biological and cognitive degeneration observed in AD is the challenge for the development of neurotrophic factors as realistic therapeutic agents.

REFERENCES

Abdulla F, Abu-Bakra M, Calaminici M, Stephenson J, Sinden J (1995): Importance of forebrain cholinergic and GABAergic systems to the age-related deficits in water maze performance of rats. Neurobiol Aging 16:41–52.

Alderson RF, Wiegand SJ, Anderson KD, Cai N, Cho J-Y, Lindsay RM, Altar CA (1995): Neurotrophin-4/5 maintains the cholinergic phenotype of axotomized septal neurons. Eur J Neurosci in press.

Aggleton J, Blindt H, Candy J (1989): Working memory in aged rats. Behav Neurosci 103:975–983.

Altar CA, Boyland CV, Fritsche M, Jackson C, Hyman C, Lindsay RM (1994a): The neurotrophins NT-4/5 and BDNF augment serotonin, dopamine, and GABAergic systems during behaviorally effective infusions to the substantia nigra. Exp Neurol 130:31–40.

Altar C, Boylan C, Fritsche M, Jones B, Jackson C, Wiegand S, Lindsay R, Hyman C (1994b): Efficacy of brain-derived neurotrophic factor and neurotrophin-3 on neurochemical and behavioral deficits associated with partial nigrostriatal dopamine lesions. J Neurochem 63:1021–1032.

Altar CA, Siuciak JA, Wright P, Ip NY, Lindsay RM, Wiegand SJ (1994c): *In situ* hybridization of *trk*B and *trk*C receptor mRNA in rat forebrain and association with high-affinity binding of [^{125}I]BDNF, [^{125}I]NT-4/5 and [^{125}I]NT-3. Eur J Neurosci 6:1389–1405.

Altar C, Boylan C, Jackson C, Hershenson S, Miller J, Wiegand S, Lindsay R, Hyman C (1992): Brain-derived neurotrophic factor augments rotational behavior and nigrostriatal dopamine turnover in vivo. Proc Natl Acad Sci U S A 89:11347–1351.

Ames BN, Shigenaga MK, Hagen TM (1993): Oxidants, antioxidants, and the degenerative diseases of aging. Proc Natl Acad Sci U S A 90:7915–7922.

Appel SH (1981): A unifying hypothesis for the cause of amyotrophic lateral sclerosis, Parkinsonism and Alzheimer disease. Ann Neurol 10:499–505.

Arenas E, Trupp M, Akerud P, Ibanez C (1995): GDNF prevents degeneration and promotes the phenotype of brain noradrenergic neurons in vivo. Neuron 15:1465–1473.

Backman C, Granholm A-C, Bartus R, Henry M, Hoffer B, Rose G (1995): Antitransferrin receptor antibody-NGF conjugate improves spatial memory and ameliorates cholingeric neuron atrophy in aged rats. Soc Neurosci Abst 21:546.

Barde YA (1990): The nerve growth factor family. Prog Growth Factor Res 2:237–248.

Barker PA, Murphy RA (1992): The nerve growth factor receptor: A multicomponent system that mediates the actions of the neurotrophin family of proteins. Mol Cell Biochem 110:1–15.

Barnes CA (1979): Memory deficits associated with senescence: A neurophysiological and behavioral study in the rat. J Comp Physiol Psych 93:74–104.

Bartus RT, Dean RL III, Beer B, Lippa AS (1982): The cholinergic hypothesis of geriatric memory dysfunction. Science 217:408–414.

Batchelor PE, Armstrong DM, Blaker SN, Gage FH (1989): Nerve growth factor receptor and choline acetyltransferase colocalization in neurons within the rat forebrain: Response to fimbria-fornix transection. J Comp Neurol 284:187–204.\

Batistatou A, Volonte C, Greene LA (1992): Nerve growth factor employs multiple pathways to induce primary response genes in PC12 cells. Mol Biol Cell Mar 3:363–371.

Beck KD, Valverde J, Alexi T, Poulsen K, Moffat B, Vandlen RA, Rosenthal A, Hefti F (1995): Mesencephalic dopaminergic neurons protected by GDNF from axotomy-induced degeneration in the adult brain. Nature 373:339–341.

Beal M, Mazurek M, Svendsen C, Bird E, Martin J (1986): Widespread reduction of somatostatin-like immunoreactivity in the cerebral cortex in Alzheimer's Disease. Ann Neurol 20:489–495.

Blottner D, Baumgarten HG (1992): Basic fibroblast growth factor prevents neuronal death and atrophy of retrogradely labeled preganglionic neurons *in vivo*. Exp Neurol 118:35–46.

Blum M, Weickert C (1995): GDNF mRNA expression in normal postnatal development, aging and in weaver mutant mice. Neurobiol. Aging 16:925–929.

Bothwell M (1995): Functional interactions of neurotrophins and neurotrophin receptors. Ann Rev Neurosci 18:223–253.

Bouras C, St. Hilaire-Kafi S, Constantinidis J (1986): Neuropeptides in Alzheimer's Disease: A review and morphological results. Prog Neuro-Psychopharmacol Biol Psychiatry 10:271–286.

Burgos I, Cuello AC, Liberini P, Pioro E, Masliah E (1995): NGF-mediated synaptic sprouting in the cerebral cortex of lesioned primate brain. Brain Res 692:154–160.

Butcher LI, Woolf NJ (1989): Neurotrophic agents exacerbate the pathologic cascade of Alzheimer's disease. Neurobiol Aging 10:557–570.

Buttke TM, Sandstrom PA (1994): Oxidative stress as a mediator of apoptosis. Immunol Today 15:7–10.

Carnahan J, Nawa H (1995): Regulation of neuropeptide expression in the brain by neurotrophins: Potential role in vivo. Mol Neurobiol 10:135–149.

Cecatelli S, Ernfors P, Villar M, Persson H, Hokfelt T (1991): Expanded distribution of mRNA for nerve growth factor, brain-derived neurotrophic factor and neurotrophin-3 in the rat brain after colchicine treatment. Proc Natl Acad Sci U S A 88:10352–10356.

Chao MV, Hempstead BL (1995): p75 and Trk: A two-receptor system. TINS 18:321–326.

Chen KS, Gage FH (1995): Somatic gene transfer of NGF to the aged brain: Behavioral and morphological amelioration. J Neurosci 15:2819–2825.

Cheng B, Mattson MP (1994): NT-3 and BDNF protect CNS neurons against metabolic/excitotoxic insults. Brain Res 640:56–67.

Cheng B, Goodman Y, Begley JG, Mattson MP (1994): Neurotrophin-4/5 protects hippocampal and cortical neurons against energy deprivation- and excitatory amino acid-induced injury. Brain Res 650:331–335.

Coleman PD, Flood DG (1987): Neuron number and dendritic extent in normal aging and Alzheimer's disease. Neurobiol Aging 8:521–545.

Corkin S (1982): Some relationships between global amnesia and the memory impairments in Alzheimer's Disease. In Corkin S, Davis K, Growden J, (eds): "Alzheimer's Disease: A Report of Progress in Research." New York: Raven, pp 149–164.

Cortes R, Probst A, Palacios J (1988): Decreased densities of dopamine D1 receptors in theputamen and hippocampus in senile dementia of the Alzheimer type. Brain Res 475:164–167.

Cotman CW, Whittemore ER, Watt JA, Anderson AJ, Loo DT (1994): Possible role of apoptosis in Alzheimer's disease. Ann N Y Acad Sci 747:36–49.

Coyle JT, Puttfarcken P (1993): Oxidative stress, glutamate, and neurodegenerative disorders. Science 262:689–695.

Croll S, Wiegand S, Anderson K, Lindsay R, Nawa H (1994): Regulation of neuropeptides in adult rat forebrain by the neurotrophins BDNF and NGF. Eur J Neurosci 6:1343–1353.

Crutcher K, Weingartner J (1991): Hippocampal NGF levels are not reduced in the aged Fischer 344 rat. Neurobiol Aging 12:449–454.

Daitz HM, Powell TPS (1954): Studies of the connexions of the fornix system. J Neurol Neurosurg Psychiatry 17:75–82.

Deckwerth TL, Johnson EM, Jr. (1993a): Neurotrophic factor deprivation-induced death. Ann N Y Acad Sci 679:121–131.

Deckwerth TL, Johnson EM, Jr. (1993b): Temporal analysis of events associated with programmed cell death (apoptosis) of sympathetic neurons deprived of nerve growth factor. J Cell Biol 123:1207–1222.

Dekker A, Thal L (1992): Effects of delayed treatment with nerve growth factor on choline acetyltransferase activity in the cortex of rats with lesions of the nucleus basalis magnocellularis: Dose requirements. Brain Res 584:55–63.

Dewar D, Chalmers D, Graham D, McCulloch J (1991): Glutamate metabotropic and AMPA binding sites are reduced in Alzheimer's disease: An autoradiographic study of the hippocampus. Brain Res 553:58–64.

Dragunow M, Faull RLM, Lawlor P, Beilharz EJ, Singleton K, Walker EB, Mee E (1995): *In situ* evidence for DNA fragmentation in Huntington's disease striatum and Alzheimer's disease temporal lobes. Neuroreport 6:1053–1057.

Eisen A, Calne DB (1992): Amyotrophic lateral sclerosis, Parkinson's disease and Alzheimer's disease: Phylogenetic disorders of the human neocortex sharing many characteristics. Can J Neurol Sci 19:117–120.

Emerich DF, McDermott PE, Krueger PM, Winn SR (1994a): Intrastriatal implants of polymer-encapsulated PC12 cells: Effects on motor function in aged rats. Prog Neuropsychopharmacol Biol Psychiatry 18:935–946.

Emerich DF, Winn SR, Harper J, Hammang JP, Baetge EE, Kordower JH (1994b): Implants of polymer-encapsulated human NGF-secreting cells in the nonhuman primate: Rescue and sprouting of degenerating cholinergic basal forebrain neurons. J Comp Neurol 349:148–164.

Escandón E, Burton LE, Szönyi É, Nikolics K (1993): Characterization of neurotrophin receptors by affinity crosslinking. J Neurosci Res 34:601–613.

Falkenberg T, Mohammed A, Henriksson B, Persson H, Winblad B, and Lindefors N (1992): Increased expression of brain-derived neurotrophic factor mRNA in rat hippocampus is associated with improved spatial memory and enriched environment. Neurosci Lett 138: 153–156.

Ferguson IA, Johnson EM, Jr. (1991): Fibroblast growth factor receptor-bearing neurons in the CNS: Identification by receptor-mediated retrograde transport. J Comp Neurol 313:693–706.

Fischer W, Sirevaag A, Wiegand SJ, Lindsay RM, Björklund A (1994): Reversal of spatial memory impairments in aged rats by nerve growth factor and neurotrophins 3 and 4/5 but not by brain-derived neurotrophic factor. Proc Natl Acad Sci U S A 91:8607–8611.

Fischer W, Björklund A, Chen K, Gage F (1991): NGF improves spatial memory in aged rodents as a function of age. J Neurosci 11:1889–1906.

Fischer W, Wictorin K, Björklund A, Williams LR, Varon S, Gage FH (1987): Amelioration of cholinergic neuron atrophy and spacial memory impairment in aged rats by nerve growth factor. Nature 329:65–68.

Flicker C, Ferris S, Crook T, Reisberg B, Bartus R (1988): Equivalent spatial-rotation deficits in normal aging and Alzheimer's disease. J Clin Exp Neuropsychol 10:387–399.

Friden PM, Walus LR, Watson P, Doctrow SR, Kozarich JW, Baeckman C, Bergman H, Hoffer B, Bloom F, Granholm AC, Biddle PT, Ebendal T, Gerhardt GA, Henry MA, Mackerlova L, Soederstroem S, Stroemberg I, Walus L (1995): Blood-brain barrier penetration and in vivo activity of an NGF conjugate: Effects of transferrin receptor antibody-NGF conjugate on young and aged septal transplants in oculo. Science Mar. 132:1–15.

Friden PM, Walus LR, Watson P, Doctrow SR, Kozarich HW, Bäckman C, Bergman H, Hoffer B, Bloom F, Granholm A-C (1993): Blood-brain barrier penetration and in vivo activity of an NGF conjugate. Science 259:373–377.

Frim DM, Uhler TA, Short MP, Ezzedine ZD, Klagsbrun M, Breakefield XO, Isacson O (1993): Effects of biologically delivered NGF, BDNF and bFGF on striatal excitotoxic lesions. Neuroreport 4:367–370.

Gage FH, Ray J, Fischer LJ (1995): Isolation, characterization, and use of stem cells from the CNS. Ann Rev Neurosci 18:159–192.

Gage FH, Wictorin K, Fischer W, Williams LR, Varon S, Björklund A (1986): Retrograde cell changes in medial septum and diagonal band following fimbriafornix transection: Quantitative temporal analysis. Neuroscience 19:241–255.

Gage G, Björklund A, Stenevi U, Dunnett S, Kelly P (1984): Intrahippocampal septal grafts ameliorate learning impairments in aged rats. Science 225:533–535.

Gallagher M, Burwell R (1989): Relationship of age-related decline across several behavioral domains. Neurobiol Aging 10:691–708.

Gallagher M, Burwell R, Kodsi M, McKinney M, Southerland S, Vella-Rountree I, Lewis M (1990): Markers for biogenic amines in the aged rat brain: Relationship to decline in spatial learning ability. Neurobiol Aging 11:507–514.

Garcia E, Rios C, Sotelo J (1992): Ventricular injection of nerve growth factor increases dopamine content in the striata of MPTP-treated mice. Neurochemical Res 17:979–982.

Garofalo L, Cuello AC (1995): Pharmacological characterization of nerve growth factor and/or monosialoganglioside GM1 effects on cholinergic markers in the adult lesioned brain. J Pharmacol Exp Ther 272:527–545.

Garofalo L Cuello AC (1994): Nerve growth factor and the monosialoganglioside GM1: Analogus and different in vivo effects on biochemical, morphological, and behavioral parameters of adult cortically lesioned rats. Exp Neurol 125:195–217.

Gash DM, Zhang Z, Cass WA, Ovadia A, Martin D, Russell D, Collins F, Hoffer BJ, Gerhardt GA (1995): Morphological and functional effects of intranigrally administered GDNF in normal rhesus monkeys. J Comp Neurol

Gash D, Zhang Z, Ovadia A, Cass W, Simmerman L, Russell D, Martin D, Lapchak P, Collins F, Hoffer B, and Gerhardt G (1996): Functional recovery in Parkinsonian monkeys treated with GDNF. Nature 380:252–255.

Goedert M, Fine A, Dawbarn D, Wilcock G, Chao M (1989): Nerve growth factor receptor mRNA distribution in human brain: Normal levels in basal forebrain in Alzheimer's disease. Brain Res Mol Brain Res 5:1–7.

Granholm AC, Baeckman C, Bloom F, Ebendal T, Gerhardt GA, Hoffer B, Mackerlova L, Olson L, Soederstroem S, Walus LR (1994): NGF and anti-transferrin receptor antibody conjugate: Short and long-term effects on survival of cholinergic neurons in intraocular septal transplants. J Pharmacol Exp Ther 268:448–459.

Hagg T, Fass-Holmes B, Vahlsing HL, Manthorpe M, Conner JM, Varon S (1989): Nerve growth factor (NGF) reverses axotomy-induced decreases in choline acetyltransferase. NGF receptor and size of medial septum cholinergic neurons. Brain Res 505:29–38.

Hagg T, Manthorpe M, Vahlsing HL, Varon S (1988): Delayed treatment with nerve growth factor reverses the apparent loss of cholinergic neurons after acute brain damage. Exp Neurol 101:303–312.

Hammang JP, Emerich DF, Winn SR, Lee A, Lindner MD, Gentile FT, Doherty EJ, Kordower JH, Baetge EE (1995): Delivery of neurotrophic factors to the CNS using encapsulated cells: developing treatments for neurodegenerative diseases. Cell Transplant 4(Suppl l):S27–28.

Harbaugh RE (1989a): Nerve growth factor as a potential treatment in Alzheimer's disease. Biomed Pharmacother 43:483–485.

Harbaugh RE (1989b): Novel CNS-directed drug delivery systems in Alzheimer's disease and other neurological disorders. Neurobiol Aging 10:623–629.

Hardy J, Adolfsson R, Alafuzoff I, Bucht G, Marcusson J, Nyberg P, Perdahl E, Wester P, Winblad B (1985): Transmitter deficits in Alzheimer's disease. Neurochem Intl 7: 545–563.

Hefti F (1994): Neurotrophic factor therapy for nervous system degenerative diseases. J Neurobiol 25:1418–1435.

Hefti F (1986): Nerve growth factor promotes survival of septal cholinergic neurons after fimbrial transections. J Neurosci 6:2155–2162.

Hefti F, Weiner WJ (1986): Nerve growth factor and Alzheimer's disease. Ann Neurol 20:275–281.

Hefti F, Hartikka J, Knusel B (1989): Function of neurotrophic factors in the adult and aging brain and their possible use in the treatment of neurodegenerative diseases. Neurobiol Aging 10:515–533.

Hefti F, Dravid A, Hartikka J (1984): Chronic intraventricular injections of nerve growth factor elevate hippocampal choline acetyltransferase activity in adult rats with partial septohippocampal lesions. Brain Res 293:305–311.

Hellweg R, Fischer W, Hock C, Gage F, Björklund A, Thoenen H (1990): Nerve growth factor levels and choline acetyltransferase activity in the brain of aged rats. Brain Res 537:123–130.

Henderson CE, Phillips HS, Pollock RA, Davies AM, Lemeulle C, Armanini M, Simpson LC, Moffet B, Vandlen RA, Koliatsos VE, Rosenthal A (1994): GDNF: A potent survival factor for motoneurons present in peripheral nerve and muscle. Science 266:1062–1064.

Henrikson B, Soderstrom S, Gower A, Ebendal T, Winblad B, Mohammed A (1992): Hippocampal nerve growth factor levels are related to spatial learning ability in aged rats. Behav Brain Res 48:15–20.

Higgins G, Mufson E (1989): NGF receptor expression is decreased in the nucleus basalis in Alzheimer's disease. Exp Neurol 106:222–236.

Hoffer BJ, Hoffman A, Bowenkamp K, Huettl P, Hudson J, Martin D, Lin L-FH, Gerhardt GA (1994): Glial cell line-derived neurotrophic factor reverses toxin-induced injury to midbrain dopaminergic neurons in vivo. Neurosci Lett 182:107–111.

Holtzman DM, Li Y, Parada LF, Kinsman S, Chen C-K, Valletta JS, Zhou J, Long JB, Mobley WC (1992): p140^{trk} mRNA marks NGF-responsive forebrain neurons: Evidence that *trk* gene expression is induced by NGF. Neuron 9:465–478.

Hudson J, Granholm A-C, Gerhardt GA, Henry MA, Hoffman A, Biddle P, Leela NS, Mackerlova L, Lile JD, Collins F, Hoffer BJ (1995): Glial cell line-derived neurotrophic factor augments midbrain dopaminergic circuits in vivo. Brain Res Bull 36:425–432.

Ingram D, London E, Goodrick C (1981): Age and neurochemical correlates of radial arm maze performance in rats. Neurobiol Aging 2:41–47.

Irle E, Kessler J, Markowitsch H (1987): Primate learning tasks reveal strong impairments in patients with presenile or senile dementia of the Alzheimer type. Brain Cogn 6:429–449.

Ishihara A, Saito H, Nishiyama N (1992): Basic fibroblast growth factor ameliorates learning deficits in basal forebrain-lesioned mice. Jpn J Pharmacol 59:7–13.

Issa A, Rowe W, Gauthier S, Meaney M (1990): Hypothalamic-pituitary-adrenal activity in aged, cognitively impaired and cognitively unimpaired rats. J Neurosci 10:3247–3254.

Jackson GR, Apffel L, Werrbach-Perez K, Perez-Polo JR (1990): Role of nerve growth factor in oxidant-antioxidant balance and neuronal injury. I. Stimulation of hydrogen peroxide resistance. J Neurosci Res 25:360–368.

Janis L, Glasier M, Martin G, Stackman R, Walsh T, Stein D (1995): A single intraseptal injection of nerve growth factor facilitates radial maze performance following damage to the medial septum in rats. Brain Res 679:99–109.

Jette N, Cole M, Fahnestock M (1994): NGF mRNA is not decreased in frontal cortex from Alzheimer's patients. Brain Res Mol Brain Res 25:242–250.

Johnson EM, Jr, Greenlund LJS, Akins PT, Hsu CY (1995): Neuronal apoptosis: Current understanding of molecular mechanisms and potential role in ischemic brain injury. J Neurotrauma 12:843–852.

Kaplan DR, Perkins A, Morrison DK (1992): Signal transduction by receptor tyrosine kinases. Cancer Treat Res 63P265-79:265–279.

Katzman R (1986): Alzheimer's disease. N Engl J Med 314:964–973.

Kawaja MD, Rosenberg MB, Yoshida K, Gage FH (1992): Somatic gene transfer of nerve growth factor promotes the survival of axotomized septal neurons and the regeneration of their axons in adult rats. J Neurosci 12:2849–2864.

Kimble D, Bremiller R, Perez-Polo J (1979): Nerve growth factor applications fail to alter behavior of hippocampal lesioned rats. Physiol Behav 23:653–657.

Kiss J, McGovern J, Patel AJ (1988): Immunohistochemical localization of cells containing nerve growth factor receptors in the different regions of the adult rat forebrain. Neuroscience 27:731–748.

Klein R, Conway D, Parada LF, Barbacid M (1990): The *trk*B tyrosine protein kinase gene codes for a second neurogenic receptor that lacks the catalytic kinase domain. Cell 61:647–656.

Knüsel B, Beck KD, Winslow JW, Rosenthal A, Burton LE, Widmer HR, Nikolics K, Hefti F (1992a): Brain-derived neurotrophic factor administration protects basal forebrain cholinergic but not nigral dopaminergic neurons from degenerative changes after axotomy in the adult rat brain. J Neurosci 12:4391–4402.

Knüsel B, Rabin S, Widmer HR, Hefti F, Kaplan DR, Hempstead BL, Rabin SJ, Kaplan L, Reid S, Parada LF (1992b): Neurotrophin-induced trk receptor phosphorylation and cholinergic neuron response in primary cultures of embryonic rat brain neurons. Overexpression of the trk tyrosine kinase rapidly accelerates nerve growth factor-induced differentiation. Neuroreport 3:885–888.

Koh S, Chang P, Collier T, Loy R (1989): Loss of NGF receptor immunoreactivity in basal forebrain neurons of aged rats: Correlation with spatial memory impairment. Brain Res 498:397–404.

Kokaia Z, Metsis M, Kokaia M, Elmér E, Lindvall O (1995): Co-expression of TrkB and TrkC receptors in CNS neurones suggests regulation by multiple neurotrophins. Neuroreport 6:769–772.

Koliatsos VE, Price DL, Gouras GK, Cayouette MH, Burton LE, Winslow JW (1994): Highly selective effects of nerve growth factor, brain-derived neurotrophic factor, and neurotrophins-3 on intact and injured basal forebrain magnocellular neurons. J Comp Neurol 343:247–262.

Kordower JH, Charles V, Bayer R, Bartus RT, Putney S, Walus LR, Friden PM (1994): Intravenous administration of a transferrin receptor antibody-nerve growth factor conjugate prevents the degeneration of cholinergic striatal neurons in a model of Huntington disease. Proc Natl Acad Sci U S A 91:9077–9080.

Kordower JH, Bartus RT, Bothwell M, Schatteman G, Gash DM (1988): Nerve growth factor receptor immunoreactivity in the nonhuman primate (Cebus apella): Distribution, morphology, and colocalization with cholinergic enzymes. J Comp Neurol 277:465–486.

Korsching S (1993: The neurotrophic factor concept: A reexamination. J Neurol 13: 2739–2748.

Korsching S, Auburger G, Heuman R, Scott J, Thoenen H (1985): Levels of nerve growth factor and its mRNA in the central nervous system of the rat correlate with cholinergic innervation. EMBO J 4:1389–1393.

Krieglstein K, Suter-Crazzolara C, Fischer WH, Unsicker K (1995): TGF-superfamily members promote survival of midbrain dopaminergic neurons and protect them against MPP^+ toxicity. EMBO J 14:736–742.

Kromer L (1987): Nerve growth factor treatment after brain injury prevents neuronal death. Science 235:214–235.

Lamballe F, Klein R, Barbacid M (1991): The trk family of oncogenes and neurotrophin receptors. Princess Takamatsu Symposia. 22:153–170.

Lamballe F, Smeyne RJ, Barbacid M (1994): Development expression of *trk*C, the neurotrophin-3 receptor, in the mammalian nervous system. J Neurosci 14:14–28.

Lapchak PA (1993): Nerve growth factor pharmacology: Application to the treatment of cholinergic neurodegeneration in Alzheimer's disease. Exp Neurol 124:16–20.

Lapchak PA, Hefti F (1992): BDNF and NGF treatment in lesioned rats: Effects on cholinergic function and weight gain. Neuroreport 3:405–408.

Lapchak PA, Araujo DM, Hefti F (1993a): Neurotrophins in the central nervous system. Rev Neurosci 3:1–10.

Lapchak PA, Araujo DM, Hefti F (1993b): Regulation of hippocampal muscarinic receptor function by chronic nerve growth factor treatment in adult rats with fimbrial transections. Neuroscience 53:379–394.

Levi-Montalcini R (1982): Developmental neurobiology and the natural history of nerve growth factor. Ann Rev Neurosci 5:341–362.

Levi-Montalcini R, Dal Toso R, Della Valle F, Skaper SD, Leon A (1995): Update of the NGF saga. J Neurol Sci 130:119–127.

Li Y, Holtzman DM, Kromer LF, Kaplan DR, Chu-Couzens J, Clary DO, Knüsel B, Mobley WC (1995): Regulation of TrkA and ChAT expression in developing rat basal forebrain: Evidence that both exogenous and endogenous NGF regulate differentiation of cholinergic neurons. J Neurosci 15:2888–2905.

Lin L-FH, Doherty DH, Lile JD, Bektesh S, Collins F (1993): GDNF: A glial cell line-derived neurotrophic factor for midbrain dopaminergic neurons. Science 260:1130–1132.

Lindholm D, Hartikka J, Da Penha Berzaghi M, Castrén E, Tzimagiorgis G, Hughes RA, Thoenen H (1994): Fibroblast growth factor-5 promotes differentiation of cultured rat septal cholinergic and raphe serotonergic neurons: Comparison with the effects of neurotrophins. Eur J Neurosci 6:244–252.

Loeb DM, Tsao H, Cobb MH, Green LA (1992): NGF and other growth factors induce an association between ERK1 and the NGF receptor, gp140prototrk. Neuron 9:1053–1065.

Louis J-C, Magal E, Gerdes W, Seifert W (1993): Survival-promoting and protein kinase C-regulating roles of basic FGF for hippocampal neurons exposed to phorbol ester, glutamate and ischaemia-like conditions. Eur J Neurosci 5:1610–1621.

Lucidi Phillipi CA, Gage GH, Shults CW, Jones KR, Reichardt LF, Kang UJ (1995): Brain-derived neurotrophic factor-transduced fibroblasts: Production of BDNF and effects of grafting to the adult rat brain. J Comp Neurol 354:361–376.

Maness LM, Kastin AJ, Weber JT, Banks WA, Beckman BS, Zadina JE (1994): The neurotrophins and their receptors: Structure, function, and neuropathology. Neurosci Biobehav Rev 18:143–159.

Markowska AL, Koliatsos VE, Breckler SJ, Price DL, Olton DS (1994): Human nerve growth factor improves spatial memory in aged but not in young rats. J Neurosci 14:4815–4824.

Markram H, Segal M (1990): Regional changes in NGF receptor immunohistochemical labeling in the septum of the aged rat. Neurobiol Aging 11:481–484.

Marsh HN, Scholz WK, Lamballe F, Klein R, Nanduri V, Barbacid M, Palfrey HC (1993): Signal transduction events mediated by the BDNF receptor gp145^{trkB} in primary hippocampal pyramidal cell culture. J Neurosci 13:4281–4292.

Martin-Iverson MT, Todd KG, Altar CA (1994): Brain-derived neurotrophic factor and neurotrophin-3 activate striatal dopamine and serotonin metabolism and related behaviors: Interactions with amphetamine. J Neurosci 14:1262–1270.

Martin D, Miller G, Fischer N, Dix D, Cullen T, Russell D (1996): Glial cell line-derived neurotrophic factor: The lateral cerebral ventricle is an effective site of administration for stimulation of the nigrostriatal system. European J Neurosci 8:1249–1255.

Mash D, Flynn D, Potter L (1985): Loss of M2 muscarinic receptors in the cerebral cortex in Alzheimer's disease and experimental cholinergic denervation. Science 228:1115–1117.

Mattson MP, Lovell MA, Furukawa K, Markesbery WR (1995): Neurotrophic factors attenuate glutamate-induced accumulation of peroxides, elevation of intracellular Ca^{2+} concentration, and neurotoxicity and increase antioxidant enzyme activities in hippocampal neurons. J Neurochem 65:1740–1751.

Maysinger D, Herrera-Marschitz M, Goiny M, Ungerstedt U, Cuello C (1992): Effects of nerve growth factor on cortical and striatal acetylcholine and dopamine release in rats with cortical devascularizing lesions. Brain Res 577:300–305.

Merlio J, Ernfors P, Jaber M, Persson H (1992): Molecular cloning of rat trkC and distribution of cells expressing messenger RNAs for members of the trk family in the rat central nervous system. Neuroscience 51:513–532.

Middlemas DS, Lindberg RA, Hunter T (1991): TrkB, a neural receptor protein-tyrosine kinase: Evidence for a full length and two truncated receptors. Mol Cell Biol 11:143–153.

Miller G, Martin D, Cullen T (1994): Central administration of rhGDNF causes augmentation of dopaminergic activity in vivo. Soc Neurosci Abstr 20:1300.

Moises HC, Womble MD, Washburn MS, Williams LR (1995): Nerve growth factor facilitates cholinergic neurotransmission between nucleus basalis and the amygdala in rat: An electrophysiological analysis. J Neurosci 15:8131–8142.

Morse JK, Wiegand SJ, Anderson K, You Y, Cai N, Carnahan J, Miller J, DiStefano PS, Altar CA, Lindsay RM, Alderson RF (1993): Brain-derived neurotrophic factor (BDNF) prevents the degeneration of medial septal cholinergic neurons following fimbria transection. J Neurosci 13:4146–4156.

Mountjoy CQ (1986): Correlations between neuropathological and neurochemical findings. Br Med J 42:81–85.

Naumann T, Kermer P, Frotscher M (1994): Fine structure of rat septohippocampal neurons. III. Recovery of choline acetyltransferase immunoreactivity after fimbria-fornix transection. J Comp Neurol 350:161–170.

Nawa H, Carnahan J, Gall C (1995): BDNF protein measured by a novel enzyme immunoassay in normal brain and after seizure: Partial disagreement with mRNA levels. Eur J Neurosci 7:1527–1535.

Nishizuka M, Katoh-Semba R, Eto K, Arai Y, Iizuka R, Kato K (1991): Age- and sex-related differences in the nerve growth factor distribution in the rat brain. Brain Res Bull 27:685–688.

Nissen M, Corkin S, Buonanno F, Growdon J, Wray S, Bauer J (1985): Spatial vision in Alzheimer's disease: General findings and a case report. Arch Neurol 42:667–671.

Nisticò G, Ciriolo MR, Fiskin K, Iannone M, deMartino A, Rotilio G (1992): NGF restores decrease in catalase activity and increases superoxide dismutase and glutathione peroxidase activity in the brain of aged rats. Free Radic Biol Med 12:177–181.

Nisticò G, Ciriolo MR, Fiskin K, Iannone M, De Martino A, Rotilio G (1991): NGF restores decrease in catalase and increases glutathione peroxidase activity in the brain of aged rats. Neurosci Lett 130:117–119.

Nordberg A, Winblad B (1986): Reduced number of ^{3}[H]nicotine and ^{3}[H]acetylcholine binding sites in the frontal cortex of Alzheimer brains. Neurosci Lett 72:115–119.

Ohsawa F, Widmer HR, Knüsel B, Denton TL, Heft F (1993): Response of embryonic rat hippocampal neurons in culture to neurotrophin-3, brain-derived neurotrophic factor and basic fibroblast growth factor. Neuroscience 57:67–77.

Olanow CW (1993); A radical hypothesis for neurodegeneration. TINS 16:439–444.

Olson L (1994): Neurotrophins in neurodegenerative disease: Theoretical issues and clinical trials. Neurochemistry 25:1–3.

Olson L, Nordberg A, von Holst H, Backman L, Ebendal T, Alafuzoff I, Amberla K, Hartvig P, Herlitz A, Lilja A, Lundqvist H, Langstrom B, Meyerson B, Perrson A, Viitanen M, Winblad B, Seiger A (1992): Nerve growth factor affects ^{11}C-nicotine binding, blood flow, EEG, and verbal episodic memory in an Alzheimer patient. J Neural Transm 4:79–95.

Oppenheim RW, Houenou LJ, Johnson JE, Lin L-FH, Li L, Lo AC, Newsome AL, Prevette DM, Wang S (1995): Developing motor neurons rescued from programmed and axotomy-induced cell death by GDNF. Nature 373:344–346.

Oppenheim RW, Qin-Wei Y, Prevette D, Yan Q (1992a): Brain-derived neurotrophic factor rescues developing avian motoneurons from cell death. Nature 360:755–757.

Oppenheim RW, Schwartz LM, Shatz CJ (1992b): Neuronal death, a tradition of dying. J Neurobiol 23:1111–1115.

Pacifici RF, Davies KJA (1991): Protein, lipid and DNA repair systems in oxidative stress: The free-radical theory of aging revisited. Gerontology 37:166–180.

Pallage V, Toniolo G, Will B, Hefti F (1986): Long-term effects of nerve growth factor and neural transplants on behavior of rats with medial septal lesions. Brain Res 386:197–208.

Pan Z, Perez-Polo JR (1993): Role of nerve growth factor in oxidant homeostasis: Glutathione metabolism. J Neurochem 61:1713–1721.

Parada LF, Tsoulfas P, Tessarollo L, Blair J, Reid SW, Soppet D (1992): The Trk family of tyrosine kinases: Receptors for NGF-related neurotrophins. Cold Spring Harb Symp Quant Biol 57:43–51.

Pearson RCA, Sofroniew MV, Cuello AC, Powell TPS, Eckenstein F, Esiri MM, Wilcock GK (1983): Persistence of cholinergic neurons in the basal nucleus in a brain with senile dementia of the Alzheimer's type demonstrated by immunohistochemical staining for choline acetyltransferase. Brain Res 289:375–379.

Pelleymounter MA, Cullen MJ (in press): The effects of intrahippocampal BDNF and NGF on spatial learning in aged Long-Evans rats. Mol Chem Neuropath.

Pelleymounter M, Cullen M, Wellmann C (1995): Characteristics of BDNF-induced weight loss. Exper Neurol 131:229–238.

Penn RD, Martin EM, Wilson RS, Fox JH, Savoy SM (1988): Intraventricular bethanechol infusion for Alzheimer's disease: Results of double-blind and escalating-dose trials. Neurology 38:219–222.

Perry EK, Johnson M, Kerwin JM, Piggott MA, Court JA, Shaw PJ, Ince PG, Brown A, Perry RH (1992): Convergent cholinergic activities in aging and Alzheimer's disease. Neurobiol Aging 13:393–400.

Peterson GM, Naumann T, Frotscher M (1992): Identified septohippocampal neurons survive axotomy: A fine-structural analysis in the rat. Neurosci Lett 138:81–85.

Petty BG, Cornblath DR, Adornato BT, Chaudhry V, Flexner C, Wachsman M, Sinicropi D, Burton LE, Peroutka SJ (1994): The effect of systemically administered recombinant human nerve growth factor in healthy human subjects. Ann Neurology 36:244–246.

Phelps CH, Gage FH, Growdon JH, Hefti F, Harbaugh R, Johnston MV, Khachaturian ZS, Mobley WC, Price DL, Raskind M, Simpkins J, Thal LJ, Woodcock J (1989): Potential use of nerve growth factor to treat Alzheimer's disease. Neurobiol Aging 10:205–207.

Phillips H, Hains J, Armanin M, Laramee G, Johnson S, Winslow J (1991): BDNF mRNA is decreased in the hippocampus of individuals with Alzheimer's disease. Neuron 7: 695–702.

Poulsen KT, Armanini MP, Klein RD, Hynes MA, Phillips HS, Rosenthal A (1994): TGF beta 2 and TGF beta 3 are potent survival factors for midbrain dopaminergic neurons. Neuron 13:1245–1252.

Rapp P, Roseberg R, Gallagher M (1987): An evaluation of spatial information processing in aged rats. Behav Neurosci 101:3–12.

Ratan RR, Baraban JM (1995): Apoptotic death in an *in vitro* model of neuronal oxidative stress. Clin Exp Pharmacol Physiol 22:309–310.

Ray J, Hogg J, Beutler AS, Takayama H, Baird A, Gage FH (1995): Expression of biologically active basic fibroblast growth factor by genetically modified rat primary skin fibroblasts. J Neurochem 64:503–513.

Reinikainen KJ, Riekkinen PJ, Paljarvi L, Soinen H, Helkala E-L, Jolkkonen J, Laakso M (1988): Cholinergic deficit in Alzheimer's disease: A study based on CSF and autopsy data. Neurochem Res 13:135–146.

Reisberg B, Ferris S, deLeon M, Sinaiko E, Franssen E, Kluger A, Mir P, Borenstein J, George A, Shulman E, Steinberg G, Cohen J (1988): Stage-specific behavioral, cognitive, and in vivo changes in community residing subjects with age-associated memory impairment and primary degenerative dementia of the Alzheimer type. Drug Devel Res 15:101–114.

Roberts-Lewis JM, Marcy VR, Zhao Y, Vaught JL, Siman R, Lewis ME (1993): Aurintricarboxylic acid protects hippocampal neurons from NMDA- and ischemia-induced toxicity in vivo. J Neurochem 61:378–381.

Rossor M, Iversen L, Reynolds G, Mountjoy C, Roth M (1984): Neurochemical characteristics of early and late onset types of Alzheimer's disease. Br Med J 288:961–964.

Rylett RJ, Williams LR (1994): Role of neurotrophins in cholinergic-neurone function in the adult and aged CNS. Trends Neurosci 17:486–490.

Rylett RJ, Goddard S, Schmidt BM, Williams LR (1993): Acetylcholine synthesis and release following continuous intracerebral administration of NGF in adult and aged Fischer-344 rats. J Neurosci 13:3956–3963.

Rylett RJ, Ball MJ, Colhoun EH (1983): Evidence for high affinity choline transport in synaptosomes prepared from hippocampus and neocortex of patients with Alzheimer's disease. Brain Res 289:169–175.

Sampath D, Jackson GR, Werrbach Perez K, Perez-Polo JR (1994): Effects of nerve growth factor on glutathione peroxidase and catalase in PC12 cells. J Neurochem 62:2476–2479.

Samples SD, Dubinsky JM (1993): Aurintricarboxylic acid protects hippocampal neurons from glutamate excitotoxicity in vitro. J Neurochem 61:382–385.

Scali C, Casamenti F, Pazzagli M, Bartolini L, Pepeu G (1994): Nerve growth factor increases extracellular acetylcholine levels in the parietal cortex and hippocampus of aged rats and restores object recognition. Neurosci Lett 170:117–120.

Sendtner M, Holtman B, Kolbeck R, Thoenen H, Barde Y-A (1992): Brain-derived neurotrophic factor prevents the death of motoneurons in newborn rat after nerve section. Nature 360:757–759.

Shen R, Altar C, Chiodo L (1994): Brain-derived neurotrophic factor increases the electrical activity of pars compacta dopamine neurons in vivo. Proc Natl Acad Sci U S A 91:8920–8924.

Siuciak J, Boylan C, Fritsche M, Altar C, Lindsay R (1996): BDNF increases monoaminergic activity in rat brain following intracerebroventricular or intraparenchymal administration. Brain Res 710:11–20.

Sofroniew MV, Cooper JD, Svendsen CN, Crossman P, Ip NY, Lindsay RM, Zafra F, Lindholm D (1993): Atrophy but not death of adult septal cholinergic neurons after ablation of target capacity to produce mRNAs for NGF, BDNF, and NT3. J Neurosci 13:5263–5276.

Spina MB, Squinto SP, Miller JA, Lindsay RM, Hyman C (1993): Brain-derived neurotrophic factor protects dopamine neurons against 6-hydroxydopamine and N-methyl-4-phenylpyridinium ion toxicity: Involvement of the glutathione system. J Neurochem 59:99–106.

Springer JE, Koh S, Tayrien MW, Loy R (1987): Basal forebrain magnocellular neurons stain for nerve growth factor receptor: Correlation with cholinergic cell bodies and effects of axotomy. J Neurosci Res 17:111–118.

Steininger TL, Wainer BH, Klein R, Barbacid M, Palfrey HC (1993): High-affinity nerve growth factor receptor (Trk) immunoreactivity is localized in cholinergic neurons of the basal forebrain and striatum in the adult rat brain. Brain Res 612:330–335.

Stephens RM, Loeb DM, Copeland TD, Pawson T, Greene LA, Kaplan DR (1994): Trk receptors use redundant signal transduction pathways involving SHC and PLC-gamma1 to mediate NGF responses. Neuron 12:691–705.

Su JH, Anderson AJ, Cummings BJ, Cotman CW (1994): Immunohistochemical evidence for apoptosis in Alzheimer's disease. Neuroreport 5:2529–2533.

Svendsen CN, Kew JNC, Staley K, Sofroniew MV (1994): Death of developing septal cholinergic neurons following NGF withdrawal *in vitro*: Protection by protein synthesis inhibition. J Neurosci 14:75–87.

Thoenen H (1991): The changing scene of neurotrophic factors. Trends Neurosci 14:165–170.

Tomac A, Lindqvist E, Lin L-FH, Ögren SO, Young D, Hoffer BJ, Olson L (1995): Protection and repair of the nigrostriatal dopaminergic system by GDNF *in vivo*. Nature 373:335–339.

Tuszynski MH, Armstrong DM, Gage FH (1990): Basal forebrain cell loss following fimbria/fornix transection. Brain Res 508:241–248.

Urschel B, Hulsebosch C (1992): Distribution and relative density of p75 nerve growth factor receptors in the rat brain as a function of age and treatment with antibodies to nerve growth factor. Brain Res 591:223–238.

Varon S, Manthorpe M, Williams LR (1984): Neuronotrophic and neurite promoting factors and their clinical potentials. Dev Neurosci 6:73–100.

Venero JL, Hefti F (1993): *Trk*A NGF receptor expression by non-cholinergic thalamic neurons. Neuroreport 4:959–962.

Venero JL, Knüsel B, Beck KD, Hefti F (1994): Expression of neurotrophin and *trk* receptor genes in adult rats with fimbria transections: Effect of intraventricular nerve growth factor and brain-derived neurotrophic factor administration. Neuroscience 59:797–815.

Volonte C, Angelastro JM, Greene LA (1993): Association of protein kinases ERK1 and ERK2 with p75 nerve growth factor receptors. J Biol Chem 268:21410–21415.

Whitehouse P, Vale W, Zweig R, Singer H, Mayeux R, Kuhar M, Price D, DeSouza E (1987): Reductions in corticotropin releasing factor-like immunoreactivity in cerebral cortex in Alzheimer's disease, Parkinson's disease and progressive supranuclear palsy. Neurology 37:905–909.

Whitehouse P, Martino A, Wagster M, Price D, Mayeux R, Atack J, Kellar K (1988): Reductions in [^{3}H]nicotinic acetylcholine binding in Alzheimer's disease and Parkinson's disease: An autoradiographic study. Neurology 38:720–723.

Whitehouse PJ, Price DL, Struble RG, Clark AW, Coyle JT, DeLong MR (1982): Alzheimer's disease and senile dementia: Loss of neurons in the basal forebrain. Science 215:1237–1239.

Whittemore SR, Seiger A (1987): The expression, localization and functional significance of B-nerve growth factor in the central nervous system. Brain Res Rev 12:439–464.

Whittemore ER, Loo DT, Cotman CW (1994): Exposure to hydrogen peroxide induces cell death via apoptosis in cultured rat cortical neurons. Neuroreport 5:1485–1488.

Widmer HR, Knüsel B, Hefti F (1992): Stimulation of phosphatidylinositol hydrolysis by brain-derived neurotrophic factor and neurotrophin-3 in rat cerebral cortical neurons developing in culture. J Neurochem 59:2113–2124.

Widmer HR, Kaplan DR, Rabin SJ, Beck KD, Hefti F, Knüsel B (1993a): Rapid phosphorylation of phospholipase Cgamma1 by brain-derived neurotrophic factor and neurotrophin-3 in cultures of embryonic rat cortical neurons. J Neurochem 60:2111–2123.

Widmer HR, Knüsel B, Hefti F (1993b): BDNF protection of basal forebrain cholinergic neurons after axotomy: Complete protection of p75NGFR-positive cells. Neuroreport 4:363–366.

Wilcock GK, Esiri MM, Bowen DM, Smith CCT (1982): Correlation of cortical choline acetyltransferase activity with the severity of dementia and histological abnormalities. J Neurol Sci 57:407–417.

Will B, Hefti F (1985): Behavioral and neurochemical effects of chronic intraventricular injections of nerve growth factor in adult rats with fimbria lesions. Behav Brain Res 17:17–24.

Williams LR (1995): Oxidative stress, age-related neurodegeneration, and the potential for neurotrophic treatment. Cerebrovasc Brain Metab Rev 7:55–73.

Williams LR (1991a): Hypophagia is induced by introcerebroventricular administration of nerve growth factor. Exp Neurol 113:31–37.

Williams LR (1991b): Exogenous nerve growth factor stimulates choline acetyl-transferase activity in aging Fischer 344 male rats. Neurobiol Aging 12:39–46.

Williams LR, Oostveen JA (1992): Sensitivity of Fischer 344 X Brown Norway hybrid rats to exogenous NGF: Weight loss correlates with stimulation of striatal choline acetyltransferase. Neurosci Lett 147:136–138.

Williams LR, Rylett RJ (1990): Exogenous nerve growth factor increases the activity of high affinity choline uptake and choline acetyltransferase in the brain of Fisher 344 male rats. J Neurochem 55:1042–1049.

Williams LR, Inouye G, Cummins V, Pelleymounter MA (1996): Glial cell line-derived neurotrophic factor sustains axotomized basal forebrain cholinergic neurons in vivo: Dose-response comparison to nerve growth factor and brain-derived neurotrophic factor. J Pharmacol Exp Ther 277:1140–1151.

Williams L, Rylett R, Moises H, Tang A (1991): Exogenous NGF affects cholinergic transmitter function and Y-maze behavior in aged Fischer 344 male rats. Can J Neurol Sci 18:403–407.

Williams LR, Jodelis KS, Donald MR (1989): Axotomy-dependent stimulation of choline acetyltransferase by exogenous mouse nerve growth factor in rat basal forebrain. Brain Res 498:243–256.

Williams LR, Varon S, Peterson GM, Wictorin K, Fischer W, Björklund A, Gage FH (1986): Continuous infusion of nerve growth factor prevents basal forebrain neuronal death after fimbriafornix transection. Proc Natl Acad Sci U S A 83:9231–9235.

Winkler J, Thal L (1995): Effects of nerve growth factor treatment on rats with lesions of the nucleus basalis magnocellularis produced by ibotenic acid, quisqualic acid and AMPA. Exper Neurol 136:234–250.

Woolf NJ, Gould E, Butcher LL (1989): Nerve growth factor receptor is associated with cholinergic neurons of the basal forebrain but not the pontomesencephalon. Neuroscience 30:143–152.

Yan Q, Matheson C, Sun J, Radeke M, Feinstein S, Miller J (1994): Distribution of intracerebral ventricularly administered neurotrophins in rat brain and its correlation with trk receptor expression. Exper Neurol 127:23–36.

Yan Q, Matheson CR (1995): Retrograde transport study of glial cell line-derived neurotrophic factor (GDNF) in adult rat nervous system. Soc Neurosci Abstr 15.

Yan Q, Matheson C, Lopez OT (1995): *In vivo* neurotrophic effects of GDNF on neonatal and adult facial motor neurons. Nature 373:341–344.

Yancopoulos GD, Maisonpierre PC, Ip NY, Aldrich TH, Belluscio L, Boulton TG, Cobb MH, Squinto SP, Furth ME (1990): Neurotrophic factors, their receptors, and the signal transduction pathways they activate. Cold Spring Harb Symp Quant Biol 55:371–379.

Zhang Y, Tatsuno T, Carney JM, Mattson MP (1993): Basic FGF, NFG, and IGFs protect hippocampal and cortical neurons against iron-induced degeneration. J Cereb Blood Flow Metab 13:378–388.

Zhou X-F, Parada LF, Soppet D, Rush RA (1993): Distribution of *trkB* tyrosine kinase immunoreactivity in the rat central nervous system. Brain Res 622:63–70.

Zubenko G, Moossy J (1988): Major depression in primary dementia: Clinical and neuropathologic correlates. Arch Neurol 45:1182–1186.

Zurn AD, Baetge EE, Hammang JP, Tan SA, Aebischer P (1994): Glial cell line-derived neurotrophic factor (GDNF), a new neurotrophic factor for motoneurones. Neuroreport 6:113–118.

Zweig R, Ross C, Hedreen J, Steele C, Cardillo J, Whitehouse P, Folstein M, Price D (1988): The neuropathology of aminergic nuclei in Alzheimer's Disease. Ann Neurol 24:233–242.

CHAPTER 21

Conceptual Issues In Research on Inflammation and Alzheimer's Disease

JOSEPH ROGERS

Sun Health Research Institute, 10515 West Santa Fe Drive, Sun City, Arizona 85372

INTRODUCTION

The possibility that inflammation might be involved in the pathology of Alzheimer's disease (AD) was first raised some 20 years ago with the seminal studies of Ishii and Haga (1976), who identified components of immunoglobulins in senile plaques of AD patients. Subsequent research, most notably by Eikelenboom's group (1982) and then by my own laboratory (Rogers et al., 1986, 1988a,b) and that of my colleague, Patrick McGeer (McGeer et al., 1987), added to this foundation and more sharply focused it toward inflammatory rather than autoimmune processes.

Today, a virtual textbook of inflammatory mechanisms has been observed in AD limbic and frontal cortex, with significant reductions or even absence of these processes in similar samples from the nondemented (ND) elderly (McGeer and Rogers, 1992; McGeer et al., 1994; Rogers et al., 1995). These advances have not come easily, however. At each step, worn out dogmas have had to be overcome and new arguments addressed. This chapter reviews some of the major issues that have confronted and continue to confront studies of inflammation and AD in an effort to establish a common ground of understanding from which subsequent research can progress.

IS THE BRAIN IMMUNOLOGICALLY PRIVILEGED?

As late as a decade ago, the concept of the immunologically privileged brain continued to influence many investigators [reviewed in Lampson (1987) and Fuchs and Bullard (1988)]. Thus, the identification of immunoreactivity to various inflamma-

Pharmacological Treatment of Alzheimer's Disease: Molecular and Neurobiological Foundations,
Edited by Brioni and Decker
ISBN 0-471-16758-4 © 1997 Wiley-Liss, Inc.

tory mediators in the AD brain was often viewed as a likely artifact—the product, for example, of nonspecific crossreactivity of the antibodies employed. Refutation of the dogma of brain immunologic privilege has come from numerous sources, with research on AD inflammation playing an important role in revising this notion.

In general, the idea of the immunologically privileged brain stemmed from research showing low rejection rates for central nervous system (CNS) grafts, absence of traditional lymphatic drainage, absence of intrinsic antigen-presenting cells [i.e., absence of endogenous major histocompatibility complex (MHC) expression], and a paucity or absence of certain key immune cells (Lampson, 1987; Fuchs and Bullard, 1988; Widner and Brunden, 1988; Lindvall, 1991; Sloan et al., 1991). For brain, many of these arguments were interrelated. Without lymphatic drainage, for example, adaptive immune responses would be difficult to mount since they depend on the cloning of lymphocytes in peripheral immune organs. A route of entry for peripheral leukocytes to the brain would also be necessary, and it was generally held that the blood–brain barrier prevented such invasion. Now, however, it is recognized that all these processes do occur in the context of the CNS, albeit in sometimes brain-idiosyncratic ways. The cerebrospinal fluid, for example, may serve as a substitute for peripheral lymphatics. Its great volume would be expected to result in considerable dilution of antigens, leading to much weakened adaptive immune responses in general and a diminished ability to reject grafts in particular. Nonetheless, studies over the last decade have shown that antigens introduced or specific to brain can make their way to peripheral immune organs (Wekerle et al., 1986). The blood–brain barrier notwithstanding, T-lymphocytes also routinely survey the brain (Wekerle et al., 1986) and brain microglia can profusely express MHC cell surface glycoproteins (Rogers et al, 1986, 1988a,b); McGeer et al., 1987). These latter phenomena suggest antigen-presenting and antigen-accepting capabilities that are resident in brain and could be functionally significant even if no form of lymphatic drainage were extant there. Finally, pathogenic adaptive immune responses can now be demonstrated in brain through such models as experimental autoimmune encephalitis (cf. Lassmann et al., 1993).

In summary, the dogma of brain-immunologic privilege has become outmoded. The brain may be immunologically dampened, but even this characterization could be considered inadequate because it may place undue emphasis on adaptive versus innate immune mechanisms.

ARE ADAPTIVE IMMUNE RESPONSES NECESSARY FOR THE EXPRESSION OF CNS IMMUNE-RELATED PATHOLOGY?

Because of early advances in multiple sclerosis research, including such models as experimental autoimmune encephalitis (cf Lassmann et al., 1993), neuroimmunology has long had a justified focus on adaptive immune mechanisms. To date, however, lymphocyte-mediated autoimmune mechanisms have been difficult to document in AD. Although brain-specific autoantibodies have been reported, necessary controls have proven elusive, the autoantibodies do not appear to have consistent targets (if they are defined at all), and not all patients appear to have them (reviewed in Rogers and Rovigatti, 1988). For example, a collaborative study (Mueller-Hill and Rogers, unpublished) found that approximately half of AD patients and half of nondemented controls (including the present author) had serum antibodies to amyloid β peptide (Aβ). Such findings did little to engender early enthusiasm for immune-related approaches to AD.

The adaptive immune response, however, is by no means all of the story. In fact, nature has endowed another major defense mechanism, the innate immune system (Stites and Terr, 1991; Constantinides, 1994). Here, the response is more dependent on direct attack of targets by phagocytes, is less specific with respect to particular antigens, and is typically more immediate than adaptive responses. Local tissue injury is one of the primary events that invokes the innate immune response, and inflammation, as in all immune responses, is a key player in the assault.

The innate pathway has substantial destructive potential even in the absence of adaptive immune responses, to include pathogenic reactions wherein the consequences of an innate system attack far outweigh any danger posed by the initiating event. Toxic shock syndrome and non-immune-mediated asthmatic responses provide obvious examples. In brain, innate immune responses to bacteria and to local tissue injury are always of grave concern. Survival of bacterial meningitis, for example, is about 50% with aggressive antibiotic therapy, but may improve to as much as 90% if steroidal or nonsteroidal anti-inflammatory drug therapy is concurrent to counter innate immune responses to the bacteria (Tuomanen, 1993).

In contrast to adaptive immune responses, there is now overwhelming evidence for a wide range of innate response mechanisms in AD (McGeer and Rogers, 1992; McGeer et al., 1994; Rogers et al., 1995). These include increased reactivity of microglia (Rogers et al, 1986; McGeer et al., 1987; Rogers et al., 1988a,b; Dickson et al., 1991, 1993), the brain's resident tissue phagocyte (Lassman et al., 1993), and increased expression of cytokines, cytokine receptors, complement, complement receptors, complement defense proteins, and acute-phase reactants [reviewed in McGeer and Rogers (1992), McGeer et al., (1994), and Rogers et al. (1995)].

In summary, although adaptive immune responses to brain-specific antigens have been the object of intense scrutiny in the context of multiple sclerosis research (cf Lassmann et al., 1993), and although there is little evidence so far of an autoimmune component to AD, there are still manifold opportunities for immune-mediated pathogenesis in AD through the innate immune response system.

IS INFLAMMATION A PRIMARY CAUSE OF AD, A SECONDARY RESPONSE, OR AN EPIPHENOMENON?

It is the author's long held view (Rogers, 1986) that for the last decade or so AD research has been characterized by an unproductive controversy over which pathologic events in AD are primary and which are secondary, with the implication being that only the former are important. Inflammation is almost certainly not a primary cause of AD. As in the periphery, it is most likely to arise as an innate immune response to local tissue injury—in this case, AD neurodegeneration. For this reason, AD inflammation has tended to be dismissed as a pathogenic source and to be regarded as some sort of interesting epiphenomenon. What is forgotten here is that, as in the periphery, once inflammatory mechanisms have been invoked by a primary pathogen, they can often become more pathogenic than the primary pathogen that gave rise to them. Thus, for example, the edema of head injury is often as likely to kill a patient as the head injury itself.

The most common expression of inflammation as a secondary, and therefore relatively trivial response in AD, is found in the idea that inflammation exists merely to clear the detritus of already existent AD pathology. This was initially a useful concept for those of us in the field because it provided an easily understood rationale through which others could accept the plethora of inflammatory mediators that were being demonstrated [reviewed in Rogers et al. (1988b), McGeer and Rogers (1992), McGeer et al. (1994); and Rogers et al. (1995)]. It has since, however, become a singular handicap.

Once released, many inflammatory mediators are toxic to cells regardless of the reason they were expressed. One of many examples of this is the phenomenon of bystander lysis, in which apparently healthy cells near the site of an inflammatory attack are damaged or destroyed (Kuby, 1994). Thus, we might expect at least some further damage to the AD brain even if the role of inflammation were limited to the removal of already existing tissue injury.

In addition, AD inflammation appears to be sustained beyond a detritus clearing role through both conventional and brain-idiosyncratic mechanisms. In particular, Aβ binds and activates complement in an antibody-independent fashion (Rogers et al., 1992; Jiang et al., 1994) and can therefore give rise to complement opsonins, anaphylotoxins, the membrane attack complex (Eikelenboom et al., 1989, 1991, 1994; Eikelenboom and Stam, 1984; Ishii and Haga, 1984; Ishii et al., 1988; Itagaki et al., 1994; McGeer et al., 1989a,b; Rogers et al., 1992; Webster et al., 1992), cytokines (Bauer et al., 1991; Buxbaum et al., 1992; Cacabelos et al., 1994; Fillit et al., 1991; Griffin et al., 1989; Shalit et al., 1994; Strauss et al., 1992), and acute-phase reactants (Abraham et al., 1990; Bauer et al., 1991; Coria et al., 1988; Duong et al., 1989; Gollin, 1992; Iwamoto et al., 1994; Kalaria and Kroom, 1992; Kisilevsky, 1994; Rozemuller et al., 1990; Strauss et al., 1992; Tennent et al., 1995; Van Gool et al., 1993; Wood et al., 1993), all of which have been detected in the AD brain and are reduced or absent in the ND brain. The fact that Aβ is present from preclinical to terminal stages of AD therefore provides an intrinsic means for producing all these inflammatory mediators throughout the course of AD even if more primary neurodegenerative events never occurred.

Exceptions to the above statement tend to prove the rule. For example, little inflammation occurs in the AD cerebellum despite sometimes profuse Aβ deposition. However, these deposits are typically diffuse (i.e., not in the cross β pleated Aβ configuration) and may predominately contain Aβ17–42 (Gowing et al., 1994). Aβ fragments not containing Aβ1–16 do not activate complement (Rogers et al., 1992), and complement activation by Aβ is directly correlated with its aggregation state (Webster et al., in preparation). Similarly, most Aβ deposits in ND patients are reported to be diffuse and are typically not associated with full inflammatory reactions (Lue et al., 1996).

Finally, there is now in vitro and in situ evidence that inflammation attacks living cells (i.e., not detritus) in the AD brain. Living cells, for example, attempt to ward off complement attack by secreting complement defense proteins. These are upregulated in AD (Akiyama et al., 1991; Choi-Miura et al., 1992; Eikelenboom et al., 1989; Kalaria and Kroon, 1992; May 1990; McGeer et al., 1991, 1992a; Tuohy, 1993; Walker et al., 1995). Such cells also attempt to shed complement on their membranes by blebbing and endocytosis, both of which can be observed with complement immunoelectron microscopy of AD cortical samples (Webster et al., 1992). A dead cell, detritus, does not bleb or endocytose; a living cell under active complement assault does. Culture studies also demonstrate *in vitro* that Aβ-mediated complement activation kills neurons with about 100 times the potency of Aβ alone (Schultz et al., 1994).

In summary, although AD inflammation is likely to arise initially as a detritus clearing mechanism, there are ample opportunities for sustaining inflammation so that it progressively assumes a pathogenic role in AD—a role it is fully capable of playing.

HOW POTENT IS AD INFLAMMATION?

One is often asked some form of this question as if it were necessary that the inflammatory response in AD brain be equivalent to that observed in toxic shock syndrome or some other acute inflammatory disorder. In fact, AD inflammation is probably relatively weak and, at least initially, highly localized. This is precisely what one should expect for an important pathogenic process in AD. Thus, the inflammation of toxic shock syndrome, which is acute, powerful, and systemic, can kill in a matter of hours. AD is a chronic, progressive disorder taking, on average, about 8–10 years to run its course.

Consider the phenomenon of Aβ-mediated complement activation (Rogers et al., 1992). Given the profuse deposition of Aβ in AD, an ability to activate complement equal to that of Ig itself would probably have lethal consequences for most patients in very short order. As it is, we were surprised to find (Webster et al., unpublished) that complement activation by Aβ and aggregated Ig could even be measured on the same scale, with Aβ being only about 2–3 times less potent. Similar findings should be obtained for many of the other inflammatory events, such as cytokine production, that occur in the AD brain. They are wholly consistent with the chronic, progressive nature of AD.

HOW SIGNIFICANT IS AD INFLAMMATION?

The extent to which inflammation contributes to the neurodegeneration that underlies AD remains an open question. However, given that there are now some 14 clinical studies that suggest anti-inflammatory drugs may slow or even delay the onset of AD (Andersen et al., 1995; Breitner et al., 1994, 1995; Broe et al., 1990; Graves et al., 1990; Jenkinson et al., 1989; Li et al., 1992; Lucca et al., 1994; McGeer et al., 1990, 1992b; Myllykangas-Luosujarvi and Isomaki, 1994; Rich et al., 1995; Rogers et al., 1993), it seems likely that the contribution is substantial. This is a therapeutically important point because it means we have decades of research and a pharmacopeia of existing drugs to draw on immediately, whereas it will likely be many years before we understand how to control or even understand the other potential pathogenic factors in AD.

CONCLUSIONS

It is both unproductive and foolish to assume that the particular pathogenic mechanism one happens to be working on is the only important process operative in AD. Extracellular ("tombstone") tangles give visible evidence of the toxicity of paired helical filaments. Culture studies, genetic mutations, and the dystrophic neurites coursing through cross β pleated amyloid deposits make clear the detrimental role Aβ plays in AD. Inflammation is inherently destructive, and treating the inflammation of AD is beneficial to patients. Whether or not these and other mechanisms are ultimately found to be primary in AD pathogenesis, there should be little doubt that they are pathogenic and worth addressing in any comprehensive program of AD research.

REFERENCES

Abraham CR, Shirahama T, Potter H (1990): α_1-Antichymotrypsin is associated solely with amyloid deposits containing the β-protein. Neurobiol Aging 11:123–129.

Akiyama H, Kawamata T, Dedhar S, McGeer PL (1991): Immunohistochemical localization of vitronectin, its receptor and beta-3 integrin in Alzheimer brain tissue. J Neuroimmunol 32:19–28.

Andersen K, Launer LJ, Ott A, Hoes AW, Breteler MMB, Hoffman A (1995): Do nonsteroidal antiinflammatory drugs decrease the risk for Alzheimer's disease? Neurology 45:1441–1445.

Bauer J, Strauss S, Schreiter-Gasser U, Ganter U, Schlegel P, Witt I, Volk B, Berger M (1991): Interleukin-6 and α_2-macroglobulin indicate an acute-phase state in Alzheimer's disease cortices. FEBS Lett 285:111–114.

Breitner JCS, Welsh KA, Helms MJ, Gaskell PC, Gau BA, Roses AD, Pericak-Vance (1995): Delayed onset of Alzheimer's disease with nonsteroidal anti-inflammatory and histamine H2 blocking drugs. Neurobiol Aging 16:523–520.

Breitner JCS, Gau BA, Welsh KA, Plassman BL, McDonald WM, Helmas MJ, Anthony JC (1994): Inverse association of anti-inflammatory treatments and Alzheimer's disease. Neurology 44:227–232.

Broe GA, Henderson AS, Creasey H, McCusker E, Korten HE, Jorm AF, (1990): A case-control study of Alzheimer's disease in Australia. Neurology 40:1698–1707.

Buxbaum JD, Oishi M, Chen HI, Pinkas-Kramarski R, Jaffe EA, Gandy SE, Greengard P (1992): Cholinergic agonists and interleukin-1 regulate processing and secretion of the Alzheimer β/A4 amyloid protein precursor. Proc Natl Acad Sci U S A 89:10075–10078.

Cacabelos R, Alvarez XA, Fernandez-Novoa L, Franco A, Mangues R, Pellicer A, Nishimura T (1994): Brain interleukin-1 beta in Alzheimer's disease and vascular dementia. Meth Find Exp Clin Pharmacol 16:141–145.

Choi-Miura NH, Ihara Y, Fukuchi K, Takeda M, Nakano Y, Tobe T, Tomita M (1992): SP-40,40 is a constituent of Alzheimer's amyloid. Acta Neuropathol 83:260–264.

Constantinides P (1994): "General Pathobiology." Norfolk, CT: Appleton & Lange.

Cooper NR (1985): The classical complement pathway: Activation and regulation of the first complement component. Adv Immunol 37:151–171.

Coria F, Castano E, Prelli F, Larrondo-Lillo M, Van Duinen S, Shelanski ML, Frangione B (1988): Isolation and characterization of amyloid P component from Alzheimer's disease and other types of cerebral amyloidosis. Lab Invest 58:454–458.

Dickson DW, Lee SC, Mattiace LA, Yen SC, Brosnan C (1993): Microglia and cytokines in neurological disease, with special reference to AIDS and Alzheimer's disease. Glia 7:75–83.

Dickson DW, Mattiace LA, Kure K, Hutchins K, Lyman WD, Brosnan C (1991): Microglia in human disease, with an emphasis on acquired immune deficiency syndrome. Lab Invest 64:135–156.

Duong T, Pommier EC, Schiebel AB (1989): Immunodetection of the amyloid P component in Alzheimer's disease. Acta Neuropathol 78:429–437.

Eikelenboom P, Stam FC (1984): An immunohistochemical study on cerebral vascular and senile plaque amyloid in Alzheimer's dementia. Virch Arch B (Cell Pathol) 47:17–25.

Eikelenboom P, et al (1994): Inflammatory mechanisms in Alzheimer's disease. Trends Pharmacol Sci 15:447–450.

Eikelenboom P, Rosemuller JM, Kraal G, Stam FC, McBride PA, Bruce ME, Fraser H (1991): Cerebral amyloid plaques in Alzheimer's disease but not in scrapie-affected mice are closely associated with a local inflammatory process. Virch Archiv B Cell Pathol 60:329–336.

Eikelenboom P, Hack CE, Rozemuller JM, Stam FC (1989): Complement activation in amyloid plaques in Alzheimer's dementia. Virch Arch B Cell Pathol 56:259–262.

Eikelenboom P, Stam FC (1982): Immunoglobulins and complement factors in senile plaques. An immunoperoxidase study. Acta Neuropath 57:239–242.

Fillit H, Ding W, Buee L, Kalman J, Alstiel L, Lawlor B, Wolf-Klein G (1991): Elevated circulating tumor necrosis factor levels in Alzheimer's disease. Neurosci Lett 129:318–320.

Fuchs HE, Bullard DE (1988): Immunology of transplantation in the central nervous system. Appl Neurophysiol 51:278–296.

Gollin PA, (1992): α_1-Antitrypsin and α_1-antichymotrypsin are in the lesions of Alzheimer's disease. Neuroreport 3:201–203.

Gowing E, Roher AE, Woods AS, Cotter RJ, Channey M, Little SP, Ball MJ (1994): Chemical characterization of Aβ17–42 peptide, a component of diffuse amyloid deposits of Alzheimer disease. J Biol Chem 269:10987–10990.

Graves AB, White E, Koepsell TD, Reifler BV, Van Belle G, Larson EB, Raskind M (1990): A case-control study of Alzheimer's disease. Ann Neurol 28:766–774.

Griffin WST, Sheng JG,, Roberts GW, Mrak RE (1989): Brain interleukin-1 and S-100 immunoreactivity are elevated in Down syndrome and Alzheimer's disease. Proc Natl Acad Sci U S A 86:7611–7615.

Ishii T, Haga S (1984): Immuno-electron-microscopic localization of complements in amyloid fibrils of senile plaques. Acta Neuropathol (Berl) 63:296–300.

Ishii T, Haga S (1976): Immuno-electron microscopic localization of immunoglobulins in amyloid fibrils of senile plaques. Acta Neuropathol (Berl) 336:243–249.

Ishii T, Haga S, Kametani F (1988): Presence of immunoglobulins and complements in the amyloid plaques in the brain of patients with Alzheimer's disease. In Pouplard-Barthelaix A, Emile J, Christen Y (eds): "Immunology and Alzheimer's Disease." Berlin: Springer-Verlag, pp 17–29.

Itagaki S, Ariyama H, Saito H, McGeer PL (1994): Ultrastructural localization of complement membrane attack complex (MAC)-like immunoreactivity in brains of patients with Alzheimer's disease. Brain Res 645:78–84.

Iwamoto N, Nishiyama E, Ohwada J, Arai H (1994): Demonstration of CRP immunoreactivity in brains of Alzheimer's disease: Immunohistochemical study using formic acid pretreatment of tissue sections. Neurosci Lett 177:23–26.

Jenkinson MI, Bliss MR, Brain AT, Scott DL (1989): Rheumatoid arthritis and senile dementia of the Alzheimer's type. Br J Rheumatol 28:86–87.

Jiang H, Burdick D, Glabe CG, Cotman CW, Tenner AJ (1994): β-Amyloid activates complement by binding to a specific region of the collagen-like domain of the C1q A chain. J Immunol 152:5050–5059.

Kalaria RN, Kroon SN (1992): Complement inhibitor C4-binding protein in amyloid deposits containing serum amyloid P in Alzheimer's disease. Biochem Biophys Res Commun 186:461–466.

Kisilevsky R (1994): Inflammation-associated amyloidogenesis: Lessons for Alzheimer's amyloidogenesis. Mol Neurobiol 8:65–66.

Kuby J (1994): "Immunology," 2nd ed. New York: WH Freeman, p 402.

Lampson LA (1987): Molecular basis of the immune response to neural antigens. Trends Neurosci 10:211–216.

Lassman H, Schmied M, Vass K, Hickey WF (1993): Bone marrow derived elements and resident microglia in brain inflammation. Glia 7:19–24.

Li G, Shen YC, Chen CH, Zhau YW (1992): A case-control study of Alzheimer's disease in China. Neurology 42:1481–1482.

Lindvall O (1991): Prospects of transplantation in human neurodegenerative disease. Trends Neurosci 14:376–384.

Lucca U, Tettamanti M, Forloni G, Spagnoli A (1994): Nonsteroidal antiinflammatory drug use in Alzheimer's disease. Biol Psychiatry 36:854–856.

Lue L, Brachova L, Walker DG, Rogers J (1996): Characterization of glial cultures from rapid autopsies of Alzheimer's and control patients. Neurobiol Aging 17:421–429.

May PC (1990): Dynamics of gene expression for a hippocampal glycoprotein elevated in Alzheimer's disease and in response to experimental lesions in rat. Neuron 5:831–839.

McGeer PL, Rogers J (1992): Anti-inflammatory agents as a therapeutic approach to Alzheimer's disease. Neurology 42:447–449.

McGeer PL, Rogers J, McGeer EG (1994): Neuroimmune mechanisms in Alzheimer disease pathogenesis. Alzheimer Dis Assoc Disord 8:149–165.

McGeer PL, Kawamata T, Walker DG (1992a): Distribution of clusterin in Alzheimer brain tissue. Brain Res 579:337–341.

McGeer PL, Harada N, Kimura H, McGeer EG, Schulzer M (1992b): Prevalence of dementia amongst elderly Japanese with leprosy: Apparent effect of chronic drug therapy. Dementia 3:146–149.

McGeer PL, Walker DG, Akiyama H, Kawamata T, Guan AL, Parker CJ, Okada N, McGeer EC (1991): Detection of the membrane inhibitor of reactive lysis (CD59) in diseased neurons of Alzheimer brain. Brain Res 544:315–319.

McGeer PL, McGeer EG, Rogers J, Sibley J (1990): Anti-inflammatory drugs and Alzheimer's disease. Lancet 335:1037.

McGeer PL, Akiyama H, Itagaki S, McGeer EG (1989a): Activation of the classical complement pathway in brain tissue of Alzheimer patients. Neurosci Lett 107:341–346.

McGeer PL, (1989b): Immune system response in Alzheimer's disease. Can J Neurol Sci 16: 516–527.

McGeer PL, Itagaki S, Tago H, McGeer EG (1987): Reactive microglia in patients with senile dementia of the Alzheimer type are positive for histocompatibility glycoprotein HLA-DR. Neurosci Lett 79:195–200.

Myllykangas-Luosujarvi R, Isomaki H (1994): Alzheimer's disease and rheumatoid arthritis. Br J Rheumatol 33:501–502.

Rich JB, Rasmusson DX, Folstein MF, Carson KA, Kawas C, Brandt J (1995): Nonsteroidal anti-inflammatory drugs in Alzheimer's disease. Neurology 45:51–55.

Rogers J (1986): Key concepts in a modern view of Alzheimer's pathogenesis. Neurobiol Aging 7:518–520.

Rogers J, Rovigatti U (1988): Immunologic and tissue culture approaches to the neurobiology of aging. Neurobiol Aging 9:759–762.

Rogers J, Lue LF, Brachova L, Webster SD, Schultz J (1995): Inflammation as a response and a cause of Alzheimer's pathophysiology. Dementia 9:133–138.

Rogers J, Kirby LC, Hempelman SR, Berry DL, McGeer PL, Kaszniak AW, Zalinski J, Cofield M, Mansukhani L, Willson P, Kogan F, (1993): Clinical trial of indomethacin in Alzheimer's disease. Neurology 43:1609–1611.

Rogers J, Cooper NR, Webster SD, Schultz J, McGeer PL, Styren SD, Civin WH, Brachova L, Bradt B, Ward P, Lieberburg I (1992): Complement activation by β-amyloid in Alzheimer disease. Proc Natl Acad Sci U S A 89:10016–10020.

Rogers J, Luber-Narod J, Styren SD, Civin WH (1988a): Expression of immune system-associated antigen by cells of the human central nervous system. Relationship to the pathology of Alzheimer disease. Neurobiol Aging 9:339–349.

Rogers J, Luber-Narod J, Muffson EJ, Styren SD, Civin WH (1988b): Presence of immune system markers in human brain and their potential role as a primary pathogenetic mechanism in Alzheimer's disease. In Finch CE and Davies P (eds): "Molecular Biology of Alzheimer's Disease" (Banbury Report 21). Cold Spring Harbor, NY: Cold Spring Harbor Laboratories, pp 51–56.

Rogers J, Singer RH, Luber-Narod J, Bassell GL (1986): Neurovirologic and neuroimmunologic considerations in Alzheimer's disease. Neurosci Abstr 12:944.

Rozemuller JM, Stam FC, Eikelenboom P (1990): Acute phase proteins are present in amorphous plaques in the cerebral but not in the cerebellar cortex of patients with Alzheimer's disease. Neurosci Lett 119:75–78.

Schultz J, Schaller J, McKinley MP, Bradt B, Cooper N, May P, Rogers J (1994): Enhanced cytotoxicity of amyloid β-peptide by a complement dependent mechanism. Neurosci Lett 175:99–102.

Shalit F, Sredni B, Stern L, Kott E, Huberman M. (1994): Elevated interleukin-6 secretion levels by mononuclear cells of Alzheimer's patients. Neurosci Lett 174:130–132.

Sloan DJ, Wood MJ, Charlton HM (1991): The Immune response in intracerebral neural grafts. Trends Neurosci 14:341–346.

Sites DP, Terr AI (1991): "Basic and Clinical Immunology," 7th ed. Norfolk, CT: Appleton & Lange.

Strauss S, Bauer J, Ganter U, Jonas U, Berger M, Volk B. (1992): Detection of interleukin-6 and α_2-macroglobulin immunoreactivity in cortex and hippocampus of Alzheimer's disease patients. Lab Invest 66:223–230.

Tennent GA, Loval LB, Pepys MB (1995): Serum amyloid P component prevents proteolysis of the amyloid fibrils of Alzheimer disease and systemic amyloidosis. Proc Natl Acad Sci U S A 92:4299–4303.

Tuohy JM (1993): Evidence of increased levels of C4 binding protein in Alzheimer's disease. Soc Neurosci Abst 19:834.

Tuomanen E (1993): Breaching the blood-brain barrier. Sci Am 268:80–84.

Van Gool D, De Strooper B, Van Leuven F, Triau E, Dom R (1993): α_2-macroglobulin expression in neuritic-type plaques in patients with Alzheimer's disease. Neurobiol Aging 14:233–237.

Walker DG, Yasuhara D, Patston PA, McGeer EG, McGeer PL (1995): Complement C1 inhibitor is produced by brain tissue and is cleaved in Alzheimer disease. Brain Res 675:75–82.

Wekerle H, Linnington C, Lassman H, Meyerman R (1986): Cellular immune reactivity within the CNS. Trends Neurosci 9:171–277.

Webster SD, Lue LF, McKinley MP, Rogers J (1992): Ultrastructural localization of complement proteins to neuronal membranes and β-amyloid peptide containing Alzheimer's disease pathology. Neurosci Abstr 18:765.

Winder H, Brundin P (1988): Immunological aspects of grafting in the mammalian central nervous system. A review and speculative synthesis. Brain Res Rev 13:287–324.

Wood JA, Wood PL, Ryan R, Graff-Radford NR, Pilapil C, Robitaille Y, Quirion R (1993): Cytokine indices in Alzheimer's temporal cortex: No changes in mature IL-1β or IL-1RA but increases in the associated acute phase proteins IL-6, α_2-macroglobulin and C-reactive protein. Brain Res 629:245–252.

CHAPTER 22

Fundamental Role for Estrogens in Cognition and Neuroprotection

JAMES W. SIMPKINS, PATTIE S. GREEN, and KELLY E. GRIDLEY

Department of Pharmacodynamics and the Center for the Neurobiology of Aging, University of Florida, Gainesville, Florida 32610

ROLE OF ESTROGENS IN COGNITION, MEMORY, AND NEURODEGENERATION

Women, Estrogen, and the Risk of Alzheimer's Disease

The average age at menopause is 54 years and the current life expectancy for a woman is 78 years. Therefore, most women will spend about 30% of their life in an estrogen-deprived state, with this percentage increasing with life expectancy. Recent evidence supports a role for ovarian steroids in normal maintenance of brain function and suggests that the loss of these steroids at menopause may play a role in cognitive decline and neurodegeneration found in Alzheimer's disease (AD).

Age-matched epidemiological studies reveal that women are twice as likely as men to develop AD. This observation is irrespective of geographical location as studies in the United States (Aronson et al., 1990), Europe (Rocca et al., 1991), Japan (Rocca et al., 1986), and China (Zhang et al., 1990) find an increased prevalence of AD among women. Further, Aronson et al. (1990) found a significant interaction between sex and history of myocardial infarction in the risk of AD. Women with a history of myocardial infarction were five times more prone to AD than other women while a myocardial infarction history had no effect on the risk of men.

Other epidemiological studies have examined the role of estrogen in the risk of AD in women. Henderson et al. (1994) found that AD patients were less likely to use estrogen replacement therapy than controls, although the groups did not differ in age or the total number of prescribed medications. Furthermore, the AD patients who were estrogen users showed a significantly better cognitive performance as

Pharmacological Treatment of Alzheimer's Disease: Molecular and Neurobiological Foundations,
Edited by Brioni and Decker
ISBN 0-471-16758-4   © 1997 Wiley-Liss, Inc.

measured by the Mini-Mental State Examination while there was no significant difference in the age, education, or symptom duration between estrogen users and nonusers. A retrospective study by Paganini-Hill and Henderson (1994) found not only that estrogen use reduced the risk of AD and related senile dementia diagnoses but that this effect was both dose and duration dependent. One study found no significant correlation between current and former estrogen use and the incidence of AD (Brenner et al., 1994). However, the odds ratio of current estrogen use in the risk of AD in this study (0.6 with a 95% confidence interval of 0.3 to 1.2) was similar to that found by Paganini-Hill and Henderson (0.67 with a 95% confidence interval of 0.38 to 1.17). Further, Tang et al. (1996) found in a prospective study not only that ERT reduces the risk of AD but its effects were consistent among Caucasian, Hispanic, and African-American populations.

Estrogen and Alzheimer's Disease: Clinical Trials

Several small clinical trials have examined the effects of estrogen therapy on cognition and memory in AD patients. Fillit et al. (1986) treated seven women with Alzheimer's-type dementia with estradiol for a 6-week period. Scores on a variety of psychometric tests were evaluated prior to estrogen treatment and at 3 and 6 weeks of treatment. Three of the women responded to the estrogen therapy with improved scores on three of the psychometric tests. The scores returned to baseline as serum estradiol levels declined in the posttreatment period. The scores of the other women were not different from baseline at either time point. The estrogen-responsive group differed from the nonresponsive group with an older age at dementia onset and less severe dementia. A higher rate of osteoporosis and lower posttreatment serum estradiol levels were also found in the responder group, suggesting that an estrogen-deficiency may contribute to dementia in some women.

Similarly, Honjo et al. (1989) found that 6 weeks of estrogen therapy improved cognition of women with AD. This improvement was not due to practice effects as the scores of untreated women with AD did not change. Furthermore, the pretreatment serum estrogen levels of women with AD were lower than for age-matched, nondemented controls suggesting that low serum estrogen levels could contribute to Alzheimer's-type dementia. Low-dose, long-term estrogen therapy has also been shown to be effective in preventing the cognitive decline of AD patients (Honjo et al., 1994). Over the study period, the cognitive performance of untreated AD patients declined while those of patients receiving low-dose estrogen treatment improved or remained constant. The mean scores between groups were not significantly different prior to treatment on either the Mini-Mental State Examination or the Hasegawa Dementia Scale. At 5 months, the scores on both tests were significantly higher in the estrogen group.

Together these studies suggest that postmenopausal estrogen deficiency may contribute to and that estrogen replacement therapy may prevent cognitive dysfunction later in life. It also suggests that estrogen treatment can benefit at least a subset of women with senile dementia. Further clinical trials are merited in continuing to elucidate these beneficial effects of estrogens.

Estrogen and Cognition: Nondemented Subjects

The effect of estrogen on cognition is not limited to forms of dementia. Estrogen has also been shown to improve performance of nondemented postmenopausal women on some tests of memory. A controlled study of surgically menopausal women showed that postoperative estrogen treatment improved the performance on paragraph recall tests when compared to placebo treatment (Sherwin, 1988). The scores of the estrogen-treated group were comparable to presurgical baseline scores and the scores of an ovary intact control group. In a separate study that compared pre- and postsurgical menopause performance of women treated with estrogen or a placebo, estrogen replacement therapy prevented the delcine in both immediate and delayed recall of paired associates (Phillips and Sherwin, 1992). Furthermore, estrogen increased the scores on immediate paragraph recall above the pretreatment baseline. Postmenopausal women on estrogen replacement therapy have significantly better proper name recall than age- and education-matched control subjects (Robinson et al., 1994). There was also a trend toward improved word recall in subjects taking estrogen. Collectively, these results indicate that estrogen has cognitive effects and is important in normal brain function.

Estrogen and Learning/Memory Behaviors in Rats

Estrogen's role in learning and memory-related behaviors in rodent models has been studied; however, the results are conflicting. Some researchers have found that ovariectomy (OVX) reduces the performance of rats in learning/memory tasks (Cannizzaro et al., 1970; Davis et al., 1976; Singh et al., 1994) while others have seen no effect (Joseph et al., 1978; van Oyen et al., 1981; van Hest et al., 1988). One group has even seen an increase in performance on memory tasks (Diaz-Veliz et al., 1989, 1991). These studies are difficult to interpret as verification that intact control animals were cycling normally or that the serum estrogen levels of these control animals were higher than that of the ovariectomized animals was not consistently performed. These factors are important since Diaz-Veliz et al. (1989) has shown that performance in rats differs over the estrous cycle using an active avoidance task. In the active avoidance paradigm, rats are given some visual or auditory signal followed by a short electric shock; an avoidance is scored if the rat leaves the area when signaled, thus avoiding the shock. The rats had a significantly higher number of avoidances in the proestrus and diestrus phases, when estrogen levels are high, versus the estrus and menstrus phases when estrogen levels are lower.

Data on the effects of estrogen therapy on learning/memory behaviors is likewise discrepant. Cannizzaro et al. (1970) found that OVX inhibited avoidance learning in young and adult female rats and that treatment with estrogen or estrogen–progestin normalized the behavior. Singh et al. (1994) demonstrated a decrease in avoidance learning in rats ovariectomized for either 5 or 28 weeks that was reversed with either 3 or 25 weeks of estrogen replacement (Figure 1).

Estrogen treatment has also been reported to increase or decrease performance on avoidance tasks in a dose-dependent manner (Diaz-Veliz et al. 1991). They

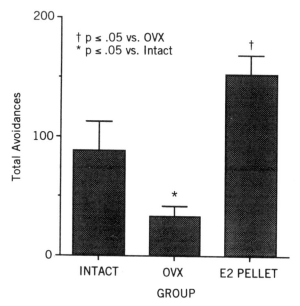

FIGURE 1. Active avoidance performance following 28 weeks of ovariectomy in intact, ovariectomized, and E2 replaced animals. Total number of avoidances made over the 14-day testing period were recorded for each animal group. Sample size was 6 in intact and ovariectomized groups and 3 in the E2 pelleted group. Overall group difference was assessed using the Kurskal–Wallis one-way ANOVA followed by Mann Whitney U test for individual group comparisons. (*$p \leq 0.05$ vs. intact; †$p \leq 0.05$ vs. OVX). [Figure from Singh et al. (1994) with permission.]

demonstrated an increase in the number of correct avoidances in response to OVX. A single 20-μg/rat dose of estradiol (E2) improved performance over that of untreated OVX rats; however, a 2-μg/rat dose decreased the number of correct avoidances and a 0.2-μg/rat dose had no discernable effect. Luine and Rodriguez (1994) found no effect of E2 on the performance of young OVX female rats in the radial arm maze, a test of spatial learning/memory.

There are two significant differences between the studies demonstrating estrogen enhancement of performance and the studies that found no effect. The first difference is the hormonal environment during the training sessions. Both Cannizzaro et al. (1970) and Singh et al. (1994) began estrogen treatment before initiating training sessions for the task. In the studies of Diaz-Veliz et al. (1991) and Luine and Rodriguez (1994), the animals were trained before estrogen treatment began, and the rats were tested for their retention of that training after receiving estrogen. Furthermore, the Diaz-Veliz et al. (1991) and Luine and Rodriguez (1994) studies looked at the effect of OVX and estrogen on memory as they tested the rat's ability to remember their pretreatment training. In contrast, both Cannizzaro et al. (1970) and Singh et al. (1994) looked at the ability of estrogen to improve the learning of

TABLE 1. Effect of Short-Term and Long-Term Ovariectomy and Steroid Replacement on Learning and Retention

	5 wk	28 wk
Treatment Group	Days to Reach Criteria	
Intact	14 ± 1.0	9 ± 2.8
Ovariectomized	15 ± 0.0	15 ± 0.0
E2 pellet	9.5 ± 2.1^a	1.3 ± 0.3^a

[a]$p \leq 0.05$ vs. ovariectomized animals using the Mann–Whitney U nonparametric statistic. Values represent means $\pm$ SEM for the days needed for animals to exhibit 11 correct avoidances in 15 attempts.

Animals were tested for 14 consecutive days beginning at 5 weeks and were retested at 28 weeks.

Table from Singh et al. (1994) with permission.

the task where, in addition, Singh et al. (1994) found an effect of E2 treatment on long-term memory of the task as well (Table 1).

Overall, these studies indicate that estrogen does function in learning/memory behaviors in female rats. However, these effects are complex and affected by many variables, including dose and duration of treatment and the age and strain of the animal tested. Positive effects of estrogen treatment on spatial memory has also been demonstrated in both young and old male rats (Luine and Rodriguez 1994).

In particular reference to AD, estrogen has also been shown to reverse the negative effects of scopolamine on T-maze alteration (Dohanich et al., 1994). Scopolamine blocks cholinergic muscarinic receptors with high affinity and treatment with scopolamine results in confusion and memory loss in human subjects that resembles early AD symptoms (Katzman, 1986).

ESTROGEN AND THE CHOLINERGIC SYSTEM

Cholinergic System

It is widely accepted that the basal forebrain plays a pivotal role in cognitive performance, and deficits in the basal forebrain cholinergic system are among the most consistently found pathologies in AD. An estrogen effect on basal forebrain cholinergic neurons may explain the aforementioned cognitive enhancing actions of estrogens.

A short review of the brain-cholinergic system anatomy is in order. The major nuclei of the cholinergic system in the rat brain are comprised of six regions and are referred to as Ch1–Ch6. These correspond to the medial septum (MS), nucleus of the vertical limb of the diagonal band of Broca (VDB), nucleus of the horizontal limb of the diagonal band of Broca (HDB), nucleus basalis magnocellularis

(NBM), pedunculopontine nucleus, and the lateral dorsal tegmental nucleus, respectively. Acetylcholine (ACH) neurons, situated primarily in the basal forebrain, send projections to the cortical, hippocampal, and amygdala regions. In rats, NBM provides the major innervation to cortical regions.

ACH is synthesized at the nerve ending in a one-step enzymatic reaction from choline and acetyl coA by choline acetyltransferase (ChAT). Following release of ACH into the synapse, acetylcholinesterase (ACE) hydrolyzes ACH into choline and acetate. Approximately 35–50% of the choline that is liberated is recycled back into the synapse. Two mechanisms exist for choline uptake into the cell— high-affinity choline uptake (HACU) and low-affinity choline uptake (LACU). HACU is specific for cholinergic terminals and is a saturable carrier-mediated process dependent on temperature and sodium concentration. Choline supply, via HACU, is thought to be rate limiting in ACH synthesis. LACU is found in cell bodies and in some nonneuronal tissue, participating in the synthesis of choline-containing phospholipids.

Cholinergic impairment, demonstrated by a reduction in ChAT activity, was correlated with the extent of intellectual impairment as assessed by a memory information test in patients with senile dementia (Perry et al., 1978). In animals models, discrete lesions of forebrain nuclei lead to deficits in learning/memory (Decker et al., 1992). Scopalamine significantly lowers T maze performance in OVX female rats, while administration of estrogen steroid replacement counteracts these effects (Dohanich et al., 1994). This evidence, linked with previously described behavioral effects, suggests that estrogens may exert their influence through modulation of basal forebrain cholinergic function.

Estrogen and the Cholinergic System

The effects of estrogen status on cholinergic function can be studied by measuring HACU, ChAT activity and expression, and regulation of nerve growth factor receptors. HACU is regarded as reflecting the moment to moment activity of the cholinergic population being investigated, while ChAT activity and mRNA production reflect the degree of target tissue innervation or, alternatively, the relative number of viable cholinergic neurons.

In response to estrogen deprivation, frontal cortex HACU shows decreases of 24–50% when compared to intact animals (Singh et al., 1994; O'Malley et al., 1987; Figure 2) Similarly, ovariectomy causes HACU decreases of 34% in the hippocampus (Singh et al., 1994). Interestingly, estrogen treatment in both studies resulted in normalization of HACU even though treatments varied from 5 days to 2 weeks in animals that were OVX for 3 weeks before treatment.

In addition to effects on HACU, estrogens have been shown to increase ChAT activity and production of ChAT protein. Previous studies by Luine (1985) show increases in ChAT activity in the HDB, VDB, MS, CA1 region of the hippocampus, and frontal cortex of 88, 8, 19, 21, and 43%, respectively, after 10 days of estrogen treatment. When specifically studying the preoptic area, increases in ChAT activity of 24% were noted after 24 hours of treatment with estrogens and 32% when mea-

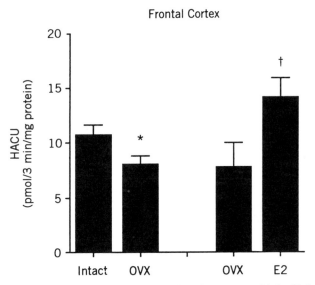

FIGURE 2. Effect of 5-week ovariectomy and E2 replacement on high-affinity choline up-take in the frontal cortex of behaviorally naive rats. The results are a compilation of two sep-arate experiments comparing intact and ovariectomized animals in one and ovariectomized and E2 pelleted animals in the other. Sample sizes were 5 for the intact group and 6 for both ovariectomized and E2 pelleted groups. Differences between groups were assessed using an unpaired, two-tailed *t* test, inasmuch as INTACT vs. OVX and OVX vs. E2-pelleted were separate studies. [Figure from Singh et al. (1994) with permission.]

sured after 3 days (Luine, 1980). In this latter study, ChAT enzyme production in the preoptic area (POA) was also elevated. We extended this work to include chronic estrogen treatment, with ChAT activity measured at 2 and 25 weeks of es-trogen replacement (Singh et al., 1994). When compared to OVX animals, mea-surements in the frontal cortex remained unchanged after 2 weeks of treatment but showed increases of 105% at the 25-week time point. It is important to point out that intact controls and OVX animals had equal ChAT activity at this 25-week time point, suggesting that unopposed estrogen treatment slowed the rate of decline of ChAT activity (Table 2). In hippocampus, increases in ChAT activity of 23–29% were seen at 2 and 25 weeks of estrogen treatment (Table 3). Since ChAT may be present in excess in cholinergic neurons, it is possible that increases in activity in projection areas may occur as a result of axonal transport, for example, cell bodies in the MS send projections to the hippocampus. Early work by Luine et al. (1975) further suggests that the effects of estrogens are dose dependent and present in hy-pophysectomized rats; other studies support a biphasic time course, dependent on dose of estrogen and length of treatment (Gibbs, 1994). We believe that the length of time from OVX to treatment is an additional variable to be considered as Luine et al. generally begins estrogen treatment 4–7 days following OVX (Luine, 1985; Luine et al., 1975) while Singh et al. (1994) begins 21 days later.

TABLE 2. Effect of Short-Term and Long-Term Ovariectomy and Estradiol Replacement on Choline Acetyltransferase Activity in the Frontal Cortex[a]

Treatment Group	5 wk	28 wk
	ChAT Activity (nmol/30 min/mg protein)	
Intact	10.2 ± 0.5	4.0 ± 0.1
Ovariectomized	9.2 ± 0.6	4.0 ± 0.2
E2 pellet	9.8 ± 0.6	8.2 ± 0.8[b]

[a] $n = 6$ for ovariectomized and E2 pellet groups and $n = 5$ for intact group for the 5-week time period. For the 28-week time period, $n = 6$ for all treatment groups.
[b] $p \leq 0.05$ vs. intact and OVX.

Table from Singh et al. (1994) with permission.

In summary, while distinct differences in technique were utilized (e.g. strain of rat, length of estrogen treatment, length of time from OVX to treatment), estrogen consistently upregulates HACU and ChAT activity within specific regions of the basal forebrain and their projections.

NEUROTROPHINS AS MEDIATORS OF THE NEUROPROTECTIVE EFFECTS OF ESTROGENS

Neurotrophins and Basal Forebrain Cholinergic Neurons

The past 10 years have witnessed an explosion in our knowledge of the trophic factors that are responsible for the development of cholinergic neurons, their maintenance in adulthood, and their decline in vitality during aging. These studies have

TABLE 3. Effect of Short-Term and Long-Term Ovariectomy and Estradiol Replacement on Choline Acetyltransferase Activity in the Hippocampus[a]

Treatment Group	5 wk	28 wk
	ChAT Activity (nmol/30 min/mg protein)	
Intact	13.2 ± 0.8	5.7 ± 0.3
Ovariectomized	10.3 ± 0.3[b]	6.2 ± 1.1
E2 pellet	12.7 ± 0.5	8.0 ± 1.1

[a] $n = 6$ for ovariectomized and E2 pellet groups and $n = 5$ for intact group for the 5-week time period. For the 28-week time period, $n = 6$ for all treatment groups.
[b] $p \leq 0.05$ vs. intact and E2 pellet.

Table from Singh et al. (1994) with permission.

also indicated the potential role of trophic factors in the response of neurons to injury. From this knowledge, we are now in a position to assess the physiology of the cholinergic system from the perspective of their life-long survival and dysfunctional events that lead to their atrophy and death following injury, during aging, and with neurodegenerative disease.

The prototypic neurotrophic factor, nerve growth factor (NGF) was identified more than 30 years ago (Levi-Montalcini, 1952) and has subsequently been recognized as one of a family of such neurotrophins that include brain-derived neurotrophic factor (BDNF) and neurotrophin 3 (NT 3), NT 4/NT 5 (Maisonpierre et al., 1990a; Friedman et al., 1991; Ebemdal, 1992). NGF injections have been shown to support cholinergic growth and connectivity during development (Gnahn et al., 1983; Hsiang et al., 1989; Maisonpierre et al., 1990b; Phillips et al., 1990; Knusel et al., 1991), to protect cholinergic neurons from the effects of axotomy of pathways projecting from the nucleus basalis and the septum (Hefti et al., 1984; Hefti, 1986; Martinez et al., 1987; Hagg et al., 1989; Higgins et al., 1989; Junard et al., 1990; Kromer, 1987; Lapchak and Hefti, 1991), and to improve basal forebrain cholinergic neuronal function and memory during aging (Fischer et al., 1991; Williams et al., 1991). This neuroprotective effect of NGF, which is well described in rodent models, is now apparent in subhuman primates (Tuszynski et al., 1990; Koliatsos et al. 1990, 1991). Further, the protective effects of NGF appears to be independent of the mode of administration, as implantation of NGF secreting cells (Rosenberg et al., 1988; Piccardo et al., 1992) or of biopolymers containing NGF secreting cells (Emerich et al., 1994) into the brain produces the same protection of cholinergic neurons.

Similar to NGF, BDNF appears to be involved in the maintenance and connectivity of adult neurons (Phillips et al., 1990; Knusel et al., 1991), and BDNF have been shown to protect medial septal cholinergic neurons after axotomy (Alderson et al., 1990). BDNF neurons are distributed in close association with cholingeric neurons and has trophic influences on noncholinergic neurons as well, suggesting a more widespread neurotrophic role in the central nervous system.

Neurotrophins exert their effects on neurons by binding to specific membrane-spanning proteins. The pan-neurotrophin receptor, p75, is a 75-Kd transmembrane protein that binds all neurotrophins with low affinity (Rodriguez-Tebar et al., 1990; Hempstead et al., 1991) and is broadly distributed in the adult forebrain, midbrain, hindbrain, and cerebellum (Gibbs et al., 1989; Koh et al., 1989). Relevant to cholinergic neuronal function, p75 receptors are localized in about 90% of cholinergic neurons in the nucleus basalis, medial septum and diagonal band of Broca (Dawbarn et al., 1988; Woolf et al., 1989).

The trk family of transmembrane receptors—which now includes trk A, trk b, trk C, and trk D—are tyrosine kinases that bind different neurotrophins. Coincident with the localization of the p75 receptor in the adult forebrain is the NGF prefering, trk A receptor (Gibbs and Pfaff, 1994; Raivich and Kreutzberg, 1987; Richardson et al., 1986). Again, about 90% of basal forebrain cholinergic neurons express the trk A receptor (Gibbs and Pfaff, 1994). Trk B receptors preferentially bind BDNF (Squinto et al., 1991) and, consistent with the broader effects of this neurotrophin in the brain, is more widely distributed than trk A receptors. However, trk B receptors have been localized in basal forebrain cholinergic neurons and appear to mediate the effects of BDNF on this important set of neurons (Alderson et al., 1990; Phillips et al., 1990; Knusel et al., 1991).

Effects of Estrogens on Neurotrophins

Estrogens have been shown to exert trophic influences in a variety of brain regions but in particular the hypothalamus. Toran-Allerand (1980) first demonstrated a striking growth of hypothalamic/preoptic area explants in vitro when cultures were exposed to 17 β-E2. This growth response was shown to be due to the induction of dendrites arising from the cell body of neurons in the explant (Toran-Allerand et al. 1982). This effect was shown to be antagonized by tamoxifen (Chowen et al., 1992) suggesting a classical estrogen-receptor involvement in the response. Inasmuch as the sprouting and cytoprotective effects of estrogens were similar to those reported for the neurotrophins, a neurotrophic mediation of the estrogen effect on hypothalamic neurons was proposed.

NGF and estrogen have been shown to be closely related in the regulation of brain-cholingeric neurons. Estrogen-receptors are colocalized in a subset of basal forebrain neurons with the p75 receptor and the high-affinity trkA and trkB receptors (Toran-Allerand et al., 1992; Miranda et al., 1993). Similarly, colocalization of E2-receptor, neurotrophin and neurotrophin receptors mRNAs were observed in various areas of the cerebral cortex and the hippocampal formation (Miranda et al.,

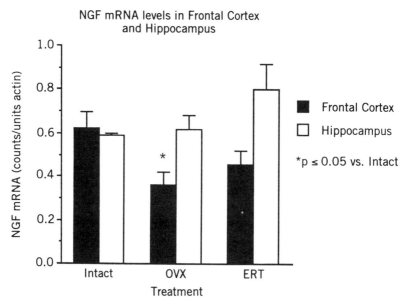

FIGURE 3. Effects of 3 months of ovariectomy (OVX) and replacement with 17 β-estradiol (ERT) on concentrations of NGF mRNA in the frontal cortex and hippocampus.

1993). Additionally, physiological estradiol concentrations differentially regulate both the p75 receptor (Sohrabji et al., 1994a) and upregulate trkA receptors in the dorsal root ganglion (Sohrabji et al., 1994a). NGF similarly upregulates estrogen receptors in PC12 cells (Sohrabji et al., 1994b) and in hypothalamic explants (Toran-Allerand, personal communication). Finally, we have reported that estrogen treatment increases the expression of mRNAs for both NGF and BDNF in the cortex and hippocampus of OVX rats (Singh et al., 1993, 1995). Gibbs (1994) has suggested that estrogens down-regulate the expression of NGF and its receptors, as he observed that exposure to estradiol at concentrations that increase ChAT expression, reduced p75 and trk A receptors and NGF mRNA expression. Gibbs proposed that the estrogen-induced increase in acetylcholine release causes a decrease in NGF neuronal function.

This reciprocal regulation of estrogen and NGF receptors and neurotrophins strongly suggests a role of estrogens in the normal maintenance of cholinergic neurons. We used long-term ovariectomy and estradiol-replacement (ERT) to assess the effects of steroid environment on the expression of mRNAs for the neurotrophins, NGF, and BDNF in the target regions of basal forebrain cholinergic neurons, the cerebral cortex, and the hippocampus. The study paradigm was intended to determine if the expected length of steroid deprivation and ERT in postmenopausal women (10–20% of their life) influenced the expression of these important neurotrophins in brain regions known to be essential for normal maintenance of cholinergic neurons.

We evaluated the effects of ovariectomy and E2-replacement on NGF mRNA levels in the brains of adult female Sprague–Dawley rats. At 14 weeks of steroid modification (a time roughly equivalent to 10% of the rats' mean life span of 130 weeks), RNA was isolated from the frontal cortex and the hippocampus. It then was subjected to dot blot analysis following a demonstration by northern analysis of a single species of RNA, which hybridized with the cDNA probe used to detect the NGF mRNA. OVX reduced by 45% and ERT resulted in a partial recovery of NGF mRNA in the frontal cortex (Figure 3, Singh et al., 1993). In the hippocampus, no effect of OVX was observed, but the steroid caused a mean increase in NGF mRNA levels (Singh et al., 1993).

Subsequently, we conducted a detailed analysis of the effects of 29 weeks of OVX and ERT (a time equivalent to 22% of the rats mean life span) on BDNF mRNA in various brain regions of adult rats (Singh et al., 1995). Long-term OVX reduced BDNF mRNA in all hippocampal subregions evaluated, with significant reductions seen in CA 2, CA 3, CA 4 and the dentate gyrus (Table 4). Estrogen treatment at physiological doses restored BDNF mRNA in each region evaluated. In the cortical regions evaluated, OVX reduced BDNF mRNA significantly in the frontal and temporal cortex. Long-term estrogen replacement was ineffective in restoring BDNF mRNA in any cortical region. A subsequent analysis (unpublished observation) revealed that shorter term treatment was effective in restoring BDNF mRNA in the cortex. Collectively, these studies demonstrate that estrogens regulate the expression of BDNF mRNA and thereby could exert dramatic effects on brain-cholinergic neurons and memory-related behaviors.

TABLE 4. The Effect of 28 weeks of Ovariectomy and Estradiol Replacement on BDNF mRNA in the Hippocampus

Treatment	BDNF mRNA (dpm/mm2)[a]				
	CA 1	CA 2	CA 3	CA 4	Dentate Gyrus
INTACT	4.1 ± 0.3	5.5 ± 0.2	10.5 ± 0.3	8.7 ± 0.2	8.6 ± 0.2
(n = 5)	(n = 41)	(n = 41)	(n = 52)	(n = 42)	(n = 47)
OVX	3.3 ± 0.3[b]	3.8 ± 0.2[b]	6.4 ± 0.2[b]	5.6 ± 0.2[b]	5.9 ± 0.3[b]
(n = 5)	(n = 32)	(n = 32)	(n = 40)	(n = 32)	(n = 32)
E2 PELLET	3.8 ± 0.2	4.8 ± 0.2[c]	8.8 ± 0.3[b,c]	7.5 ± 0.3[b,c]	9.5 ± 0.4[a]
(n = 5)	(n = 39)	(n = 39)	(n = 47)	(n = 40)	(n = 40)

[a]Numbers in parenthesis represent the total number of slices analyzed from five brains per treatment group.
[b]$p \leq 0.05$ vs. INTACT
[c]$p \leq 0.05$ vs. OVX

Table modified from Singh et al. (1995) with permission.

Taken together with the observations that E2 receptors are colocalized with both the high-affinity and the low-affinity neurotrophin receptors (Sohrabji et al., 1994a), the present results indicate that estrogens could serve to maintain basal forebrain cholinergic neurons during adulthood, and the loss of estrogens at the menopause might result in the removal of important trophic support of cholinergic neurons. Long-term loss of neurotrophin input to these cells could contribute to their selective vulnerability and the resulting decline in cognitive function during aging and with neurodegenerative disease, such as Alzheimer's disease.

NEUROPROTECTIVE EFFECTS OF ESTROGENS IN VITRO

An alternative mechanism through which estrogens could slow the progression of age-related cognitive loss and that associated with Alzheimer's disease is by directly affecting neurons to enhance their viability. To address this possibility, we developed in vitro models for neuronal viability that allowed control of the level and nature of the insult applied to the cells and concentration and type of neuroprotectant agents applied to the media. These in vitro models have the additional advantage of the homogeneity of the cell type used. By selecting human-derived neurons devoid of glia and endothelial cells, we could assess the direct effects of estrogens on neurons.

We first developed an in vitro model for neuroprotection based on the survival of human SK-N-SH neuroblastoma cells under conditions of serum deprivation. These cells were chosen for a number of features: they are human in origin, exhibit a neuronal phenotype upon differentiation, and are sensitive to environmental insults such as serum deprivation, β-amyloid toxicity, and hypoglycemia. Additionally, this nervous-system-derived cell line is responsive to and has receptors for nerve growth factor and estrogens (Ratka et al., 1995). The observed neuroprotective effects of β-E2 in SK-N-SH cells are also seen in rat primary cortical neurons in culture, at similar doses of the estrogens (Singer et al., 1995; Green et al., 1995).

Initial studies were conducted using the SK-N-SH cell line to determine the effects of estrogen treatment on the survival of cultured cells when subjected to serum-deprivation (Bishop and Simpkins 1994; Simpkins et al., 1994). When cells are challenged in this fashion, we observe a 50% reduction in live cell number by 24 hours and an 80–90% reduction by 48 hours. This consistent and robust kill provides the opportunity to assess continuous estradiol treatment on cell survivability. Treatment with 2 nM β-E2 is effective in preventing the cell loss associated with 24 and 48 hr of serum deprivation. This neuroprotective effect of β-E2 is due to the preservation of live cells, which increases the fraction of total cells in the culture. A mitotic effect of the estrogen on this cell line has been discounted since treatment with β-E2 for 24 and 48 hr did not increase the incorporation of tritiated thymidine into SK-N-SH cells (Bishop and Simpkins, 1994). These results support that continuous exposure to physiological concentrations of native estrogen, β-E2, can protect this cell line from the neurodegenerative effects of serum deprivation.

We compared the effects of the potent estrogen, 17 β-E2, and the weak estrogen, 17 α-E2, on serum deprivation induced toxicity in SK-N-SH cells to assess the relationship between the estrogenic potency and the neuroprotectivity of estrogens (Green et al., 1996; Simpkins et al., 1995). Both isomers of estradiol caused a dose-dependent protection of SK-N-SH cells at both low (0.25 × 10^6 cells/well) and high (1.0 × 10^6 cells/well) initial plating density. Both estradiol isomers show equal potency in protecting SK-N-SH cells from the serum deprivation insult. In cultures plated at low density with 48 hr of serum deprivation and estrogen treatment (0.2 and 2 nM doses), SK-N-SH cells were protected by 86–106% and 172–189%, respectively (Simpkins et al., 1995; Figure 4).

We used tamoxifen, the mixed estrogen agonist–antagonist, to determine the extent to which antagonism of the estrogen receptor was blocking the effects of the estradiol isomers. We coadministered tamoxifen (20 nM) with 17 β-E2 or 17 α-E2 (2 nM), and cultures were evaluated 48 hr later. This dose of tamoxifen had no effect on SK-N-SH cell number when administered alone and blocked only 32–39% of the neuroprotective effect of either isomer. These data dictate that two-thirds of estradiol's neuroprotective activity in our model is mediated through a mechanism that is not blocked by this estrogen antagonist.

A variety of other steroids including cholesterol, progesterone, testosterone, dihydrotestosterone, and corticosterone (2 nM concentrations) were evaluated for their neuroprotectivity to determine the specificity of estrogen's effect (Simpkins et al., 1995: data not shown). At 48 hr in culture, when peak effects of both α-E2 and β-E2 were seen, none of these steroids demonstrated neuroprotection. Progesterone and corticosterone were also tested at concentrations ranging from 0.1 to 200 nM, and neither steroid protected SK-N-SH cells at any of the tested concentrations.

Exploring the potential role of a genomic mechanism in the neuroprotective effects of estrogens, we assessed the interaction of progestins in the cytoprotective ef-

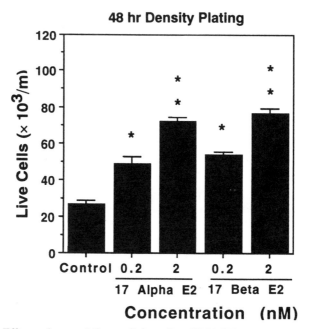

FIGURE 4. Effects of α- and β-estradiol on live SK-N-SH cell number following low-density plating. Cells were plated at 0.25×10^6 cells per well and cell number was determined 48 hr later. All wells were deprived of serum for the entire incubation period. Wells were either treated with no steroid (control) or with α-estradiol or β-estradiol at the concentrations indicated. *Indicates $p < 0.05$ vs. control. **Indicates $p < 0.05$ vs. control and both isomers at the 0.2 nM concentration.

fects of estrogen. SK-N-SH cells were administered 17 β- or 17 α-E2 and progesterone (all at 2 nM) at the time of serum deprivation. As reported above, both estradiol isomers caused a dose-dependent protection and progesterone alone did not protect SK-N-SH cells. Addition of progesterone at the time of the initial estradiol exposure had no effect on the neuroprotective effects of either 17β- or 17 α-E2 (data not shown). We conclude that progesterone neither suppresses nor potentiates the neuroprotective effects of estradiol, suggesting that an interaction between estrogen and progestin receptors is not involved in the neuroprotective effects of estrogens.

ESTROGENS AND β-AMYLOID PEPTIDE

To further assess the neuroprotective role of estrogens, we tested the effectiveness of estrogens against β-amyloid (Aβ) toxicity in vitro. Aβ toxicity is of interest as this peptide is a core component of senile plaques, the hallmark of postmortem diagnosis of AD (Blessed et al., 1968). The Aβ25–35 fragment has been shown to be the toxic portion of the 1–40 peptide (Behl et al., 1994; Mattson et al., 1994;

Hensley et al., 1994) causing cell death in primary neuronal cultures with a dose–response and time course similar to Aβ1–40. Furthermore, the Aβ25–35 fragment does not require preaggregation as does the 1–40 peptide.

SK-N-SH cells were exposed to Aβ25–35 at doses ranging from 0 to 80 μ*M* for 4 days. Aβ25–35 caused a dose-dependent reduction in live SK-N-SH cell number ranging from 36% at the 10 μ*M* concentration to 83% at the 80 μ*M* concentration. This extent of cell loss is similar to that reported for Aβ25–35 in primary neuronal cultures (Goodman and Mattson, 1994) and PC-12 cells (Behl et al., 1994). The addition of 2 n*M* β-E2 concurrently with the Aβ25–35 (20 μ*M*) reduced the fragment toxicity by 83 and 51% in two separate studies (Figure 5). This indicates that estrogen treatment can reduce the neurotoxicity of Aβ to cultured human cells and suggests that estrogens may have efficacy in preventing neuronal death associated with the accumulation of amyloid plaques during the progression of AD.

Estrogens may also play a role in the processing of amyloid precursor protein (APP). Jaffe et al. (1994) demonstrated that treatment with 1.8×10^{-9} M 17 β-estradiol directs processing of APP toward a nonamyloidogenic fragment. Such an affect could further reduce cell damage and loss of neurons as an individual ages. Taken together, these data indicate that estrogen exposure could reduce β-amyloid production and its toxicity, resulting in the lower incidence of Alzheimer's disease observed in postmenopausal subjects on estrogen replacement therapy.

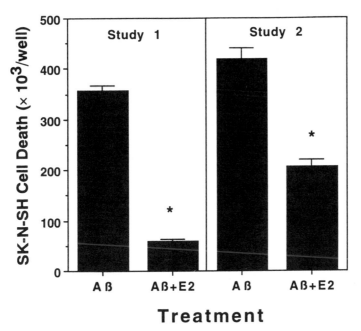

FIGURE 5. Effects of 17 β-estradiol (2 n*M*) on the toxicity induced by Aβ 25–35 (20 μ*M*). Cells were plated at 10^6 cells/mL and were exposed to 17 β-estradiol and Aβ 25–35. Four days later, the number of trypan blue-excluding cells were determined. Depicted are mean ± SEM for 4–5 wells/group. *= $p < 0.05$ vs. Aβ group.

ACKNOWLEDGEMENT

The research described was supported by NIH grants AG P01 10485 and T32 NS 07333 and a grant from Apollo Genetics, Inc., Cambridge, MA

REFERENCES

Alderson RF, Alterman AL, Barde YA, Lindsay RM (1990): Brain-derived neurotrophic factor increases survival and differentiated functions of rat septal cholinergic neurons in culture. Neuron 5:297–306.

Aronson MK, Ooi WL, Morgenstern H, Hafner A, Masur D, Crystal H, Frishman WH, Fisher D, Katzman R (1990): Women, myocardial infarction, and dementia in the very old. Behav Neural Biol 40:1102–1106.

Behl C, Davis JB, Klier FG, Schubert D (1994): Amyloid β peptide induces necrosis rather than apoptosis. Brain Res 645:253–264.

Bishop J, Simpkins JS (1994): Estradiol treatment increases viability of glioma and neuroblastoma cells in vitro. Mol Cell Neurosci 5:303–308.

Blessed G, Tomlinson BE, Roth M (1968): The association between quantitative measures of dementia and of senile changes in the cerebral gray matter of elderly subjects. Br J Psychol 114:797–811.

Brenner DE, Kukull WA, Stergachis A, van Belle G, Bowen JD, McCormick WC, Teri L, Larson EB (1994): Postmenopausal estrogen replacement therapy and the risk of Alzheimer's disease: A population-based case-control study. Am J Epidemiol 140: 262–267.

Cannizzaro G, Provenzano PM, Nigito S (1970): The effects of castration and of progestin-oestrogen combinations upon avoidance conditioning in female rats. Pharmacol Res Commun 2:267–276.

Chowen JA, Torres-Aleman I, Garcia-Segura LM (1992): Trophic effects of estradiol on fetal rat hypothalamic neurons. Neuroendocrinology 56:895–901.

Davis H, Porter JW, Burton J-A, Levine S (1976): Sex and strain differences in leverpress shock escape behavior. Physiol Psych 4:351–356.

Dawbarn D, Allen SJ, Semenenko FM (1988): Coexistence of choline acetyltransferase and nerve growth factor receptors in the rat forebrain. Neurosci Lett 94:138–144.

Decker MW, Marjchrzak MJ, Anderson DJ (1992): Effects of nicotine on spatial memory deficits in rats with septal lesions. Brain Res 572:281–285.

Diaz-Veliz G, Fabio U, Dussaubat N, Mora S (1991): Effects of estradiol replacement in ovariectomized rats on conditioned avoidance responses and other behaviors. Physiol Behav 50:61–65.

Diaz-Veliz G, Soto V, Dussaubat N, Mora S (1989): Influence of the estrous cycle, ovariectomy and estradiol replacement upon the acquisition of conditioned avoidance responses in rats. Physiol Behav 46:397–401.

Dohanich GP, Fader AJ, Javorsky DJ (1994): Estrogen and estrogen-progesterone treatments counteract the effect of scopolamine on reinforced T-maze alteration in female rats. Behav Neurosci 108:988–992.

Ebemdal T (1992): Function and evolution in the NGF family and its receptors. J Neurosci Res 32:461–470.

Emerich DF, Winn SR, Harper J, Hammang JP, Baetge EE, Kordower JH (1994): Implants of polymer-encapsulated human NGF-secreting cells in the nonhuman primate: rescue and sprouting of degenerating cholinergic basal forebrain neurons. J Comp Neurol 349: 148–164.

Fillit H, Weinreb H, Cholst I, McEwen B, Amador R, Zabriskie J (1986): Observations in a preliminary open trial of estradiol therapy for senile dementia—Alzheimer's type. Psychoneuroendocrinology 11:337–345.

Fischer W, Bjorkland A, Chen K, Gage FH (1991): NGF improves spatial memory in aged rodents as a function of age. J Neurosci 11:1889–1906.

Friedman WJ, Ernfors P, Persson H (1991): Transient and persistent expression of NT-3/HDNF mRNA in the rat brain during postnatal development. J Neurosci 11: 1577–1584.

Gibbs RB (1994): Estrogen and nerve growth factor-related systems in brain: Effects on basal forebrain cholinergic neurons and implications for learning and memory processes and aging. Ann N Y Acad Sci 743:165–196.

Gibbs RB, Pfaff DW (1994): In situ hybridization detection of trkA mRNA in brain: Distribution, co-localization with p75NGFR and up-regulation by nerve growth factor. J Comp Neurol 341:324–339.

Gibbs RB, McMabe JT, Buck CR, Chao MV, Pfaff DW (1989): Expression of NGF receptor in the rat forebrain detected with in situ hybridization and immunohistochemistry. Mol Brain Res 6:275–287.

Gnahn H, Hefti F, Heumann R, Schwab M, Thoenen H (1983): NGF-mediated increase in choline-acetyltransferase (ChAT) in the neonatal forebrain: Evidence for a physiological role of NGF in the brain. Dev Brain Res 9:45–52.

Goodman Y, Mattson MP (1994): Secreted forms of β-amyloid precursor protein protect hippocampal neurons against amyloid β-peptide-induced oxidative injury. Exp Neurol 123:1–12.

Green PS, Bishop J, Simpkins JW (1996): 17α-estradiol exerts neuroprotective effects on SK-N-SH cells. J Neurosci (in press).

Hagg T, Fass-Holmes B, Vahlsing HL, Manthrope M, Conner JM, Varon S (1989): Nerve growth factor (NGF) reverses axotomy-induced decreases in choline-acetyltransferase, NGF-receptor and size of medial septum cholinergic neurons. Brain Res 505:29–38.

Hefti F (1986): Nerve growth factor promotes survival of septal cholinergic neurons after fimbrial transections. J Neurosci 6:2155–2162.

Hefti F, Dravid A, Hartikka J (1984): Chronic intraventricular injections of nerve growth factor elevates choline acetyltransferase activity in adult rats with partial septo-hippocampal lesion. Brain Res 293:305–311.

Hempstead BL, Martin-Zanca D, Kaplan DR, Chao MV (1991): High affinity NGF binding requires co-expression of the trk proto-oncogene and the low affinity NGF receptor. Nature 350:678–683.

Henderson VW, Paganini-Hill A, Emanuel CK, Dunn ME, Buckwalter JG (1994): Estrogen replacement therapy in older women: Comparisons between Alzheimer's disease cases and nondemented control subjects. Arch Neurol 51:896–900.

Hensley K, Carney JM, Mattson MP, Aksenova M, Harris M, Wu JF, Floyd RA, Butterfield DA (1994): A model for β-amyloid aggregation and neurotoxicity based on free radical generation by the peptide: relevance to Alzheimer's disease. Proc Natl Acad Sci U S A 91:3270–3274.

Higgins GA, Koh S, Chen KS, Gage FH (1989): NGF induction of NGF receptor genes expression and cholinergic neuronal hypertrophy within the basal forebrain of the adult rat. Neuron 3:247–256.

Honjo H, Tanaka K, Kashigawa T, Urabe M, Hayashi M, Hayashi K (1994): Senile dementia-Alzheimer's type and estrogen. Horm Metabol Res 27:204–207.

Honjo H, Ogino Y, Naitoh K, Urabe M, Yasuda J (1989): In vivo Effects by estrone sulfate on the central nervous system-senile dementia (Alzheimer's type). J Steroid Biochem 34:521–525.

Hsiang J, Heller A, Hoffmann PC, Mobley WC, Wainer BH (1989): The effects of nerve growth factor on the development of septal cholinergic neurons in reaggregate cell cultures. Neuroscience 29:209–223.

Jaffe AB, Toran-Allerand D, Greengard P, Gandy SE (1994): Estrogen regulated metabolism of Alzheimer amyloid β precursor protein. J Biol Chem 269:13065–13068.

Joseph R, Hess S, Birecree E (1978): Effects of hormone manipulations and exploration on sex differences in maze learning. Behav Biol 26:364–377.

Junard EO, Montero CNM, Hefti F (1990): Long-term administration of mouse nerve growth factor to adult rats with partial lesions of the cholinergic septohippocampal pathway. Exp Neurol 110:25–38.

Katzman R (1986): Alzheimer's disease. N Engl J Med 314:964–973.

Knusel B, Winslow JW, Rosenthal A, Burton LE, Seid DP, Nikolics K, Hefti F (1991): Promotion of central cholinergic and dopaminergic neuron differentiation by brain derived neurotrophic factor but not neurotrophin 3. Proc Natl Acad Sci U S A 88:961–965.

Koh S, Oyler GA, Higgins GA (1989): Localization of nerve growth factor receptor messenger RNA and protein in the adult rat brain. Exp Neurol 106:209–221.

Koliatsos VE, Clatterbuck RE, Nauta HJW, Knusel B, Burton LE, Hefti F, Mobley WC, Price DL (1991): Human nerve growth factor prevents degeneration of basal forebrain cholinergic neurons in primates. Ann Neurol 30:831–840.

Koliatsos VE, Nauta HJW, Clatterbuck RE, Holtzman DM, Mobley WC, Price DL (1990): Mouse nerve factor prevents degeneration of axotomized basal forebrain cholinergic neurons in the monkey. J Neurosci 10:3801–3813.

Kromer LF (1987): Nerve growth factor treatment after brain injury prevents neuronal death. Science 235:214–216.

Lapchak P, Hefti (1991): Effects of recombinant human nerve growth factor on presynaptic cholinergic function in rat hippocampal slices following partial septohippocampal lesions: Measures of Ach synthesis and release. Neuroscience 42:639–649.

Levi-Montalcini R (1952): Effects of mouse tumor transplantation on the nervous system. Ann N Y Acad Sci 55:330–343.

Luine VN (1985): Estradiol increases choline acetyltransferase activity in specific basal forebrain nuclei and projection areas of female rats. Exp Neurol 89:484–490.

Luine VN (1980): Immunochemical demonstration of increased choline acetyltransferase concentration on rat preoptic area after estradiol administration. Brain Research 191: 273–277.

Luine V, Rodriguez M (1994): Effects of estradiol on radial arm maze performance of young and aged rats. Behav Neural Biol 62:230–236.

Luine VN, Khylchevskaya RI, McEwen BS (1975): Effects of gonadal steroids on activities of monoamine oxidase and choline acetyltransferase in rat brain. Brain Res 86:293–306.

Maisonpierre PC, Belluscio L, Squinto S, Ip NY, Furth ME, Lindsay RM, Yancopoulos GD (1990a): Neurotrophin-3: A neurotrophic factor related to NGF and BDNF. Science 247:1446–1451.

Maisonpierre PC, Belluscio L, Friedman B, Alderson RF, Wiegand SJ, Furth ME, Lindsay RM, Yancopoulos (1990b): NT-3, BDNF and NGF in the developing rat nervous system: Parallel as well as reciprocal patterns of expression. Neuron 5:501–509.

Martinez HJ, Dreyfus CF, Jonakit CM, Black IB (1987): Nerve growth factor selectively increases cholinergic markers but not neuropeptides in rat forebrain in culture. Brain Res 412:295–301.

Mattson MP, Tomaselli KJ, Rydel RE (1994): Calcium-destablizing and neurodegenerative effects of aggregated beta-amyloid peptide are attenuated by basic FGF. Brain Res 621:35–39.

Miranda RC, Sohrabji F, Toran-Allerand CD (1993): Presumptive estrogen target neurons express mRNAs for both the neurotrophins and neurotrophin receptors: A basis for potential development interactions of estrogen with the neurotrophins. Mol Cell Neurosci 4:510–525.

O'Malley CA, Hautamaki RD, Kelley M, Meyer EM (1987): Effects of ovariectomy and estradiol benzoate on high affinity choline uptake, Ach synthesis, and release from rat cerebral cortical synaptosomes. Brain Res 403:389–392.

Paganini-Hill A, Henderson VW (1994): Estrogen deficiency and risk of Alzheimer's disease in women. Am J Epidemiol 140:256–261.

Perry EK, Tomlinson BE, Blessed G, Bergmann K, Gibson PH, Perry RH (1978): Correlation of cholinergic abnormalities with senile plaques and mental test scores in senile dementia. Br Med J 2:1457–1459.

Phillips HJ, Hains M, Laramee GR, Rosenthal A, Winslow JW (1990): Widespread expression of BDNF but not NT-3 by target areas of basal forebrain cholinergic neurons. Science 250:290–294.

Phillips SM, Sherwin BB (1992): Effects of estrogen on memory function in surgically menopausal women. Psychoneuroendocrinology 17:485–495.

Piccardo P, Maysinger D, Cuello AC (1992): Recovery of nucleus basalis cholinergic neurons by grafting NGF secreting fibroblasts. Neuroreport 3:353–356.

Raivich G, Kreutzberg GW (1987): The localization and distribution of high affinity β-nerve growth factor binding sites in the central nervous system of the adult rat. A light microscopic autoradiographic study using [^{125}I]-nerve growth factor. Neuroscience 20:23–36.

Ratka A, Mambourg SE, Singh M (1995): Effects of estradiol on luteinzing hormone-releasing hormone in SK-N-SH neuroblastoma cells. Neurosci Abst 21:1394.

Richardson PM, Issa MKV, Riopelle RJ (1986): Distribution of neuronal receptors for nerve growth factor in the rat. J Neurosci 6:2312–2321.

Robinson D, Friedman L, Marcus R, Tinklenberg J, Yeasavage J (1994): Estrogen replacement therapy and memory in older women. J Am Geriatr Soc 42:919–922.

Rocca WA, Hofman A, Brayne C, Breteler MM, Clarke M, Copeland JR, Dartigues J, Engedal K, Hagnell O, Heeren TJ, Jonker C, Lindesay J, Lobo A, Mann AH, Molsa PK, Morgan K, O'Connor DW, Droux A, Sulkava R, Kay DW, Amaducci L (1991): Frequency and distribution of Alzheimer's disease in Europe: A collaborative study of 1980–1990 prevalence findings. Ann Neurol 30:381–390.

Rocca WA, Amaducci LA, Schoenberg BS (1986): Epidemiology of clinically diagnosed Alzheimer's disease. Ann Neurol 19:415–424.

Rodriguez-Tebar A, Dechant G, Barde Y-A, (1990): Binding of brain-derived neurotrophic factor to the nerve growth factor receptor. Neuron 4:487–492.

Rosenberg MB, Friedman T, Robertson RC, Tuszynski M, Wolff JA, Breakfield, XO, Gage FH (1988): Grafting genetically modified cells to the damaged brain: Restorative effects of NGF expression. Science 242:1575–1578.

Sherwin BB (1988): Estrogen and/or androgen replacement therapy and cognitive functioning in surgically menopausal women. Psychoneuroendocrinology 13:345–357.

Simpkins JW, Green PS, Bishop J (1995): 17 α-estradiol exerts neuroprotective effects on SK-N-SH cells. Soc Neurosci Abstracts 21:1979.

Simpkins JW, Singh M, Bishop J (1994): The potential role for estrogen replacement therapy in the treatment of the cognitive decline and neurodegeneration associated with Alzheimer's disease. Neurobiol Aging 15:s1–s3.

Singer CA, Strickland TM, Rogers KL, Dorsa DM (1995): Estrogen protects primary cortical neurons from glutamate neurotoxicity. Neurosci Abst 21:882.

Singh M, Meyer EM, Simpkins JW (1995): The effect of ovariectomy and estradiol replacement on brain-derived neurotrophic factor messenger ribonucleic acid expression in cortical and hippocampal brain regions of female Sprague-Dawley rats. Endocrinology 136:2320–2324.

Singh M, Meyer EM, Millard WJ, Simpkins JW (1994): Ovarian steroid deprivation results in a reversible learning impairment and compromised cholinergic function in female Sprague-Dawley rats. Brain Res 644:305–312.

Singh M, Meyer EM, Huang FS, Millard WJ, Simpkins JW (1993): Ovariectomy reduces ChAT activity and NGF mRNA levels in the frontal cortex of female Sprague-Dawley Rats. Soc. Neurosci Abst 19:254.

Sohrabji F, Miranda RC, Toran-Allerand CD (1994a): Estrogen differentially regulates estrogen and nerve growth factor receptor mRNAs in adult sensory neurons. J Neurosci 14:459–471.

Sohrabji F, Green LA, Miranda RC, Toran-Allerand CD (1994b): Reciprocal regulation of estrogen and NGF receptors by their ligands in PC12 cells. J Neurobiol 25:974–988.

Squinto SP, Stitt TN, Aldrich TH, Davis S, Bianco SM, Radziewjewski C, Glass DJ, Masiakowski P, Furth ME, Valenzuela DM, DiStefano PS, Yancopoulos GD (1991): trkB encodes a functional receptor for brain-derived neurotrophic factor and neurotrophin 3 but not nerve growth factor. Cell 65:885–893.

Tang MX, Jacobs D, Stern Y, Marder K, Schofield P, Gurland B, Andrews H, Mayeux R (1996): Effect of oestrogen during menopause on risk and age at onset of Alzheimer's disease. Lancet 348:429–432.

Toran-Allerand CD (1980): Sex steroids and the development of the newborn mouse hypothalamus and preoptic area in vitro. II. Morphological correlates and hormonal specificity. Brain Res 189:413–427.

Toran-Allerand CD (1995): personal communication.

Toran-Allerand CD, Miranda RC, Bentham WD, Sohrabji F, Brown TJ, Hochberg RB, MacLusky NJ (1992): Estrogen receptors colocalize with low-affinity nerve growth factor receptors in cholinergic neurons of the basal forebrain. Proc Natl Acad Sci 89:4668–4672.

Toran-Allerand CD, Hashimoto K, Greenough WT, Saltarelli M (1982): Sex steroids and the development of the newborn mouse hypothalamus and preoptic area in vitro. III. Effects of estrogen on dendritic differentiation. Dev Brain Res 7:97–101.

Tuszynski MH, U HS, Amaral K, Gage FH (1990): Nerve growth factor infusion in the primate brain reduces lesion-induced cholinergic neuronal degeneration. J Neurosci 10: 3604–3614.

van Hest A, van Kempen M, van Haaren F, van de Poll NE (1988): Memory in male and female Wistar rats: effects of gonadectomy, and stimulus presentations during the delay interval. Behav Brain Res 29:103–110.

van Oyen H, Walg H, van de Poll NE (1981): Discriminated lever press avoidance conditioning in male and female rats. Physiol Behav 26:313–317.

Williams LR, Rylett RJ, Moises HC, Tang AH (1991): Exogenous NGF affects cholinergic transmitter function and Y-mase behavior in aged Fischer 344 male rats. Can J Neurol Sci 18:403–407.

Woolf NJ, Gould E, Butcher LL (1989): Nerve growth factor receptor is associated with cholinergic neurons of the basal forebrain but not the pontomesencephalon. Neuroscience 30:143–152.

Zhang M, Katzman R, Salmone D, Jin H, Cai G, Wang Z, Qu G, Grant I, Yu E, Levy P, Klauber MR, Liu WT (1990): The prevalence of dementia and Alzheimer's disease in Shanghai, China: Impact of age, gender, and education. Ann Neurol 27:428–437.

CHAPTER 23

Alzheimer's Disease: Prospects for Treatment in the Next Decade

MICHAEL WILLIAMS AND STEPHEN P. ARNERIC

Neuroscience Discovery, Pharmaceutical Products Division, Abbott Laboratories, Abbott Park, Illinois 60064-3500

INTRODUCTION

In the last decade of the twentieth century, the sophisticated tools of molecular biology, pharmacology, biochemistry, and genomics have generated enormous amounts of information related to various aspects of the Alzheimer's disease (AD) process (Schenk et al., 1995; Siman and Greenberg, 1996; Williams and Davis, 1996).

This heterogeneous, progressive disease of the central nervous system still is of unknown etiology with the exception of the rare familial cases of autosomal-dominant inheritance of gene defects (Schellenberg, 1995). It is characterized by a progressive impairment of cognitive function with associated attentional deficits, anxiety, agitation, and depression and a significant burden on society, especially the immediate caregiver. AD affects upward of 4 million people in the United States and is the fourth leading cause of death behind heart disease, cancer, and stroke.

A key biochemical hallmark of AD is a selective loss of basal forebrain cholinergic function (Coyle et al., 1983) manifested by a loss of cholinergic neurons and the enzyme choline acetyltransferase (ChAT), which is responsible for acetylcholine (ACh) synthesis. Associated with these neurochemical changes are the classical amyloid plaques and associated tangles that remain the definitive, albeit postmortem, diagnostic markers for the disease. These observed pathologies have accordingly focused potential therapies for AD into four main areas: palliative cholinergic replacement or augmentation, restorative trophic factor treatment, modulation of brain amyloid processing, and modulation of tau phosphorylation. Since the dis-

Pharmacological Treatment of Alzheimer's Disease: Molecular and Neurobiological Foundations,
Edited by Brioni and Decker
ISBN 0-471-16758-4   © 1997 Wiley-Liss, Inc.

ease etiology is unknown, the drug discovery process for AD is, at the present time, one of hypothesis testing. When potent and selective modulators of a given molecular target are available for evaluation and are shown to be effective in disease treatment, this may be anticipated to enhance the understanding of the disease process.

Complimenting these drug discovery efforts are ongoing activities to develop reliable and predictive tests that diagnose the disease at an early enough stage that the neuronal loss can be arrested or reversed and the development of animal models that are predictive of the human disease state. Both diagnostics and animal models are critical to advancing drug discovery efforts.

PALLIATIVE CHOLINERGIC REPLACEMENT THERAPIES

Compounds that have the potential to restore the cholinergic tone that is lost in AD include: acetylcholinesterase (AChEase) inhibitors that prevent ACh breakdown, directly acting muscarinic and nicotinic receptor agonists that replace ACh, and ACh releasing agents that promote release of the remaining endogenous ACh stores. Conceptually, the effects of AChEase inhibitors and ACh releasers are limited by the availability of endogenous ACh. As AD is a progressive disorder, these approaches are comparable to the use of L-Dopa in the treatment of Parkinson's disease.

A number of compounds that had activity in animal models predictive in one or more of these various categories reached clinical trials in the past decade only to fail because of lack of efficacy or limiting, class-related side effect liabilities. While the former reflects the inherent difficulty of clinical trials in this area (Cutler et al., 1994), the latter frequently reflects wishful thinking on the part of the company sponsoring the trials, hoping that the well-established side effects of a particular compound class will not extrapolate from animals to humans. This is especially true of muscarinic agonists where the side effect liabilities with the M_1 agonist, xanomeline, have led Lilly to develop a patch formulation to reduce peak dosing.

Until the approval of Aricept (Pfizer/Eisai) this year, the only compound specifically approved for the treatment of AD was the acetylcholinesterase inhibitor, tacrine (Parke-Davis/CoCencys). Tacrine has to be given four times a day and has limited efficacy with significant side effect liability, particularly nausea and hepatotoxicity. Despite its U.S. approval in 1993 (Williams, 1993), the compound has not been approved in countries like England. Sales of tacrine never achieved the estimates that led to its clinical development and have decreased to approximately $40 million per year in 1995. Parke-Davis gave marketing rights for tacrine to CoCencys in late 1995 as part of a collaborative research agreement. However, a 2-year follow-up study of the original 30-week, randomized, placebo-controlled studies, examined the relationship between short-term symptomatic relief and long-term outcome measures such as nursing home placement and mortality (Gracon et al., 1996). Patients receiving >80 mg/day of tacrine were significantly less likely to have entered a nursing home than those receiving <80 mg/day, and those receiving >120 mg/day were significantly less likely to have died than those receiving <80 mg/day. These redeeming qualities of tacrine may give renewed hope to caregivers for improved effective future therapies.

Acetylcholinesterase Inhibitors

A number of second-generation AChEase inhibitors that show improved efficacy with reduced effect liability are currently in late-stage clinical trials or have been recently approved. These have been divided into three types: reversible, including Aricept (donepezil, E2020 which was approved by the FDA in September, 1996; Pfizer/Eisai; Figure 1); the pseudoirreversible that include physostigmine (Forrest; Figure 1), Evalon (SDZ ENA-713; Novartis; Figure 1), NXX 066 (Astra Arcus), eptastigmine (MF-201; Mediolanum), which is presently in extended Phase III trials and the backup, MF 268; and irreversible, represented by the dichlorvos prodrug, metrifonate (Bayer; Figure 1), which is also in Phase III trials. Galanthamine (Waldheim/Janssen/Shire/Synaptec; Figure 1), S-9977 (Servier), and Cl 1002 (Parke-Davis, Figure 1) are other AChEase inhibitors in clinical trials. P 11467 (HMR) is an AChEase inhibitor with $\alpha 2$ adrenoceptor antagonist activity that is structurally related to bespiridine.

Cholinergic Agonists

A number of directly acting cholinergic agents, both muscarinic and nicotinic, are also currently in clinical trials. The muscarinics are primarily M_1/m_1 selective with the cardiovascular and gastrointestinal side effects typically associated with this compound class. Of these, xanomeline (Lilly/Novo Nordisk; Figure 1) is the most advanced. It is a potent, full M_1/m_1 agonist, with low intrinsic activity at the other receptor subtypes. The compound has shown efficacy as measured by a two-point decrease in the Alzheimer's Disease Assessment Scale—cognitive (ADAS-COG) scale at 75 mg three times per day (tid) in a 6-month, double-blinded, Phase II trial in 373 patients. However, significant dropouts occurred in the first month of the trials due to mAChR-related peripheral side effects that included a greater than 20% incidence of syncope. The clinical trials for xanomeline are currently on hold as the compound is being developed as a transdermal formulation to overcome poor bioavailability and to avoid the peak loading that may contribute to its observed side effect profile. LY 287041 is a follow-on compound.

Mirilamine (Parke Davis/HMR; Figure 1) is a muscarinic agonist that is in Phase III clinical trials. It apparently exhibited typical mAChR-related peripheral side effects in Phase I. Tasaclidine (WAL 2014-FU; Boehringer Ingelheim/Pharmacia & Upjohn) is an orally active M_1 receptor agonist that is presently in Phase II trials. SDZ ENA 163 (thiopilopcarpine; Novartis; Figure 1) has a similar biochemical profile to mirilamine and can also enhance ACh release. It is currently in Phase I trials. FKS 508 (Teva/Snow Brand) is yet another acronym for the perennial M_1 receptor agonist, AF 102B, that is active in animal models of cognitive impairment. The compound has been extensively profiled for its effects on cellular responses thought to be beneficial in ameliorating the AD process. Thus FKS 508/AF 102B can: (i) prevent the formation of amyloid and promoting the normal processing of APP; (ii) enhance neurotrophin production; (iii) prevent paired helical filament (PHF) formation by decreasing tau phosphorylation; (iv) inhibit apoptosis; and (v) improve mnemonic processes in various animal models of cognition trials as well as replace

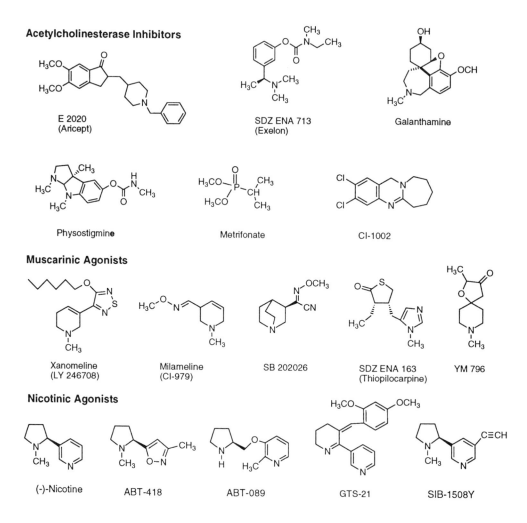

Acetylcholinesterase Inhibitors

E 2020
(Aricept)

SDZ ENA 713
(Exelon)

Galanthamine

Physostigmine

Metrifonate

CI-1002

Muscarinic Agonists

Xanomeline
(LY 246708)

Milameline
(CI-979)

SB 202026

SDZ ENA 163
(Thiopilocarpine)

YM 796

Nicotinic Agonists

(-)-Nicotine

ABT-418

ABT-089

GTS-21

SIB-1508Y

Miscellaneous Approaches

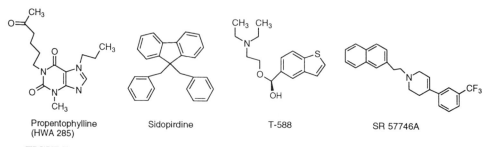

Propentophylline
(HWA 285)

Sidopirdine

T-588

SR 57746A

FIGURE 1. Structures of selected AChEase inhibitors, muscarinic agonists, nicotinic agonists, and other miscellaneous agents in clinical trials.

the ACh lost as a result of the disease process. In the light of such promising data at the molecular level and reports that the compound has shown a 5–10% improvement in the ADAS-Cog score in 50% of patients examined in Phase II clinical trials, it is somewhat surprising that FKS 508 has been in clinical trials since the late 1980s. AF 150(S) is a follow-up compound. YM 796 (Yamanouchi; Figure 1), PD 151832 (Parke-Davis), and Lu 25-109 (Lundbeck) are other M_1 receptor agonists also in, or entering, clinical trials. SB 202026 (SmithKline Beecham) has an interesting preclinical profile (Loudon et al., 1996) and apparently had entered Phase II trials in 1995.

The nicotinic agonist approach to AD therapy is relatively recent compared to the 20 or so years that have been dedicated to exploiting the somewhat unsuccessful campaign to develop a muscarinic agonist. Based on the reported effects of nicotine in improving cognitive performance in AD patients (Newhouse et al., 1988; Sahakian and Coull, 1994), a number of companies including Abbott, Bayer, Pfizer, Taiho, Japan Tobacco, R.J. Reynolds, SIBIA, Novo Nordisk, Astra, and CytoMed have been examining the potential for nAChR ligands in the treatment of AD and other disorders. Four compounds of this class of compound, termed cholinergic channel modulators (ChCMs) to avoid the negative connotations associated with nicotine as the addictive component of cigarette smoking and to embrace the ability to have agonist/antagonist activities for different subtypes of nAChRs in the same molecule (Arneric et al., 1996b), have entered or are being readied for clinical trials. ABT-418 (Abbott; Figure 1) is presently in Phase II trials for AD and is an isoxazole bioisostere of nicotine with a markedly reduced cardiovascular side effect profile (Arneric et al., 1995b). Reports from a limited Phase II trial, showed that ABT-418 demonstrated a dose-dependent enhancement of attention in AD patients (Newhouse et al., 1996). ABT-089 (Abbott; Figure 1) is an orally active ChCM that is a potential follow-up on ABT-418 (Arneric et al. 1996a). GTS-21 (Taiho/University of Florida; Figure 1) is a ChCM with activity at α4 and α7, but not α3, containing nAChRs (Meyer et al., 1994) that is active in animal models of cognition and has neuroprotective properties in vitro. It is rumored to be in Phase I trials in Europe. The bioavailability of this compound, however, is poor. SIB-1508Y (SIBIA; Figure 1), the active isomer of SIB 1765F (Lloyd et al., 1995), is the third ChCM reported by SIBIA. Like ABT-418, it is relatively selective for the human α4β2 nAChR. It is inactive in a monkey delayed matching-to-sample task of cognition, but reversed behavioral despair in a learned helplessness model suggesting some potential antidepressant activity. Neurochemically, it releases ACh and dopamine in animal microdialysis models. It is currently rumored to be entering Phase II trials for the treatment of Parkinson's disease. RJR 2403 (R.J. Reynolds) is another α4β2 selective ChCM under active evaluation (Lippiello et al., 1996).

Acetylcholine Releasers

While several ACh-releasing agents have entered clinical trials, all have been dropped due to efficacy issues. Aviva (linopirdine), the palindromic compound from Dupont-Merck, was dropped in early Phase III in 1992. Sidopiridine is a follow-on compound that is rumored to have entered clinical trials. Bespirdine (HP 749; HMR; Figure 1) reached Phase III before being dropped due to lack of efficacy in late 1995. JTP 2942 (Japan Tobacco) is a long-acting analog of thyrotropin-releasing hormone (TRH) that can release ACh and is active in animal models of cognition. It is in Phase I trials in Japan. Other TRH analogs that have reached clinical trials like MK 771 have had limiting cardiovascular side effects. Ondansetron (Glaxo-Wellcome) is a $5HT_3$ receptor antagonist currently marketed for the treatment of migraine. The compound promotes the release of ACh and has cognition enhancing activity in animal models. It has been in Phase III trials for age-associated dementia; its present development status is unclear. However T-588 (Toyama; Figure 1) is a benzamide that enhances the release of ACh and norepinephrine and is active in animal models of cognition. It has also been reported to enhance the actions of NGF in vitro. A number of angiotensin-converting enzyme inhibitors and angiotensin-II antagonists which have been shown to release ACh in animal models, have also been claimed in patents as potential treatments for AD.

NEURORESTORATIVE APPROACHES

Longer-term research efforts are presently focused on identifying compounds that have the potential to interfere with the AD-associated degenerative process by delaying, halting, or potentially reversing neuronal death. The major approaches of this type involve: (i) modulation of aberrant amyloid deposition. This can theoretically be achieved by preventing amyloid fibril formation; inhibiting amyloid precursor protein (APP) processing and, as a consequence, amyloid β peptide (Aβ) production; facilitating Aβ removal; promoting degradation of Aβ; blocking of Aβ toxicity; (ii) modulation of tau protein phosphorylation; and (iii) trophic factor modulation of cell viability.

Modulation of Aberrant Amyloid Deposition

The pathophysiology of AD is inextricably linked to high densities of amyloid-containing neurofibrillary plaques that are found in postmortem brain samples. Brain amyloid is comprised of two major forms of the neurotoxic amyloid β-peptide, Aβ1-40 and Aβ1-42 (Schenk et al., 1995) and is formed from the glycoprotein, APP via proteolysis by cathepsin-like proteases termed β- and γ-secretase. While a number of candidate enzymes for this protease role have been identified, including cathepsins D and G and chymotrypsin, none has unequivocally been identified as the key enzyme responsible for Aβ formation.

APP appears to be a normal product of human neurons and is associated with synaptogenesis. APP is increased threefold in rats raised in an enriched behavioral environment (e.g., with litter mates as opposed to living alone). These animals learned new tasks more readily than impoverished litter mates who display a delay in learning performance. Anti-βAPP antibody given intracerebroventricular (i.c.v.) can impair passive avoidance behavior. Thus APP may play an important role normally as a synaptic facilitatory molecule (Huber et al., 1996).

APP appears to be overproduced in individuals genetically predisposed to AD and in vitro, various forms of Aβ have been shown to be neurotoxic and proinflammatory, although such studies are confounded by considerable variability in the physical form of Aβ (Ma et al., 1994; Williams et al., 1995), most notably its aggregation form, which affects protein–protein interactions and the subsequent biological properties of Aβ. This has significantly confounded research activities in the area of drug discovery. Furthermore, despite considerable research efforts, it is still unclear as to whether Aβ is a cause of the neuronal loss associated with AD or a result of the disease process (Selkoe, 1993). Nonetheless, compounds that reduce brain Aβ deposition or its production from APP may be potential neurorestorative approaches and, given the paucity of knowledge related to AD etiology, will probably require evaluation in clinical trials to gain unequivocal proof of principle for this approach.

A series of candidate inhibitors of Aβ formation include MDL 28170 (HMR), brefeldin A, monesin, bafilomycin A, leupeptin, and E-64 that can inhibit the cleavage of Aβ from APP in cell culture. Companies such as Athena/Elan (in collaboration with Lilly), Cephalon (in collaboration with Schering-Plough), SIBIA Neurosciences (in collaboration with BMS), and Scios-Nova (in collaboration with HMR) are no doubt using high throughput screening to identify more potent and bioavailable compounds.

Another approach to blocking amyloid deposition is the identification of compounds that can complex Aβ and prevent its aggregation into plaques. Such agents include the polyanionic dye, Congo Red, and the nonsulfated analog, Chrysamine G, the antibiotic, rifampicin, a series of anthracyclinones from Pharmacia, and the clearance chaperones (Potter et al., 1995), α-chymotrypsin and apolipoprotein E (apoE) (Strittmatter and Roses, 1996).

Alternatively, activation of M_1 muscarinic receptors can modulate APP processing and result in a shift away from aberrant Aβ formation. However, it has been shown that this M_1 response rapidly diminishes with repeated exposure to full agonists. It remains to be determined whether partial agonists of m_1 receptors may overcome the apparent limitation to this approach.

In light of the reported neurotoxicity of Aβ and the varied biological activity depending on its physical form, there has been considerable speculation that there might be an "Aβ receptor" or partner protein. Several groups have reported on binding assays for Aβ (Roch and Puttfarken, 1996), but none have been sufficiently robust to unequivocally support the concept of a neurotoxic amyloid receptor linked to intracellular events modulating neuronal survival and death. If an Aβ receptor did exist, it would provide another drug target, albeit downstream from APP cleavage, for AD treatment.

Tau Phosphorylation

Tau phosphoprotein is a major hallmark of the neurofibrillary tangles that is also associated with AD pathology. The phosphorylation state of tau is altered in AD and also in ApoE-deficient mice. It has been suggested that M_1 agonists may also modulate the rate of tau phosphorylation. The pharmacology of this approach is just emerging.

Trophic Factors

Trophic factors or neurotrophins are endogenous peptides that promote the growth and/or survival of neurons in the nervous system by acting to prevent the constitutive effects of cell death receptors such as p75 or TGF-R1. They include nerve growth factor (NGF), brain-derived neurotrophic factor (BDNF), the neurotrophins NT-3, NT-4 and NT-5, and glial-derived neurotrophic factor (GDNF). Withdrawal of NGF from primary cultures of human neurons leads to their death, suggesting that NGF and other neurotrophins have a permissive role in maintaining neuronal survival.

These natural peptides have been advanced to clinical trials either as nonimmunogenic cell transplants (CytoTherapeutics; CereCRIB) or as intrathecal infusions for various neurodegenerative diseases, including AD, Parkinson's disease (PD), and amyotrophic lateral sclerosis (ALS). Such studies have given mixed results to date as side effects, for example, diffuse pain and reactivation of viral infection, appear to limit their utility. However, the use of GDNF in methyl-4-phenyl-1,2,3,6-tetrahydropyridine (MPTP)-lesioned primate model of PD has shown favorable results lasting for 4–5 months (Gash et al., 1996).

An alternative approach to the direct administration of peptides is to identify compounds that are able to stimulate the production of trophic factors via receptor-mediated activation of early gene responses. Both muscarinic and nicotinic agonists are neuroprotective (Arneric et al., 1996b) and may have this inherent property, suggesting that palliative approaches, if begun at the early stages of the disease, may promote early gene induction and trophic factor expression. The phosphodiesterase inhibitor/adenosine uptake blocker, propentofylline (HMR; Figure 1), which has demonstrated efficacy in the treatment of stroke and AD (Rudolphi, 1996), can also induce NGF production (Shinoda et al., 1990). Other agents with effects on NGF production include NS-506 (NeuroSearch), a series of protein kinase inhibitors including CEP-427 (Cephalon), the 5HT ligand, SR-57746A (Sanofi; Figure 1), and the hypoxanthine analog, AIT-082.

The nootropics, a class of compounds related to piracetam (UCB, launched in 1972) with a controversial mechanism of action related to glutamate receptor modulation, can enhance ACh release. While approved for use for the treatment of age-associated dementias in Europe and Japan, they have not been approved in the United States due to concerns related to efficacy. Chemically related agents, the so-called Ampakines (Cortex), have reemerged as enhancers of excitatory amino acid neurotransmission and are being examined in the clinic for potential cognitive activity.

Miscellaneous Approaches

A variety of pharmacological agents and/or molecular targets have been implicated in the pathophysiology of AD and in broad patent claims. These include compounds that modulate apotosis or programmed cell death (Thompson, 1995; Davies, 1995), especially apopain inhibitors (Nicholson et al., 1995), cerebrovasodilators, calcium channel blockers, angiotensin converting enzyme (ACE) inhibitors and angiotensin-II antagonists (EXP-655, DuPont-Merck), protein kinase C inhibitors

(K252a, Kyowa Hakko/Cephalon; nicergoline, Pharmacia & Upjohn), inhibitors of oxidative stress and spin trap reagents [monoamine oxidase (MAO) inhibitors, e.g., deprenyl], galanin antagonists, adenosine receptor antagonists (Apafylline; Boehringer Ingelheim/Pharmacia & Upjohn; MDL 102503; HMR), modulators of mitochondrial energy function (Davis, in press), anti-inflammatory agents (Parker et al., 1990), cytokine antagonists (Eikelenboom et al., 1994), histamine H_3 receptor antagonists (GT-2016, Gliatech; GlaxoWellcome), RS 56812 (Roche) (Baudy, 1996), and corticotrophin releasing factor (CRF) binding protein inhibitors (Neurocrine/Lilly; Behan et al., 1995).

It should be noted that the molecular processes related to the neuronal cell death and microglia activation associated with the ischemia following stroke are often viewed as being similar to those involved in AD and other neurodegenerative disorders. As such, compounds active in stroke models may also be of use in AD. Thus data from transgenic mice deficient in the serine protease, tissue plasminogen activator (tPA), suggest that tPA may mediate glutamate-induced neurotoxicity, a key event in stroke-mediated cell death (Tsirka et al., 1995). Nicergoline, and propentophylline are representative compounds having this type of potential dual utility through common pathophysiologic events.

GENETIC ASPECTS OF AD

Several genes have been linked to various forms of AD (Schellenberg, 1995). Trisomy 21 patients who demonstrate early-onset AD have an extra copy of both the APP gene on chromosome 21 and Cu-SOD gene. Transfection of missense mutations of the APP770 protein that occur in familial AD (FAD) of the Swedish type, either a single (V7171) or a double mutation (K670N, M671L), can alter the amount of Aβ produced from APP or the proportion of the more toxic Aβ 1-42 (Schenk et al., 1995) providing additional evidence for a role for Aβ in AD etiology. An FAD locus on chromosome 14 (Schellenberg, 1995) produces mutated forms of S182 (also known as STM1), a seven-region spanning protein that may be involved in either intracellular protein transport (Schellenberg, 1995) or in the intracellular signal processes involving the *Notch* family (Levitan and Greenwald, 1995). STM2 is a related gene on chromosome 1, a mutation in the protein product of which has been associated with FAD of the Volga German type (Artavnis-Tsakonas et al., 1995).

Other potential molecular approaches to AD have been documented in the excellent overviews of Baudy (Baudy, 1993, 1994, 1995a,b,c; 1996).

Thus while genetic studies have resulted in the identification of two proteins, S182 and STM2 that are the product of genes linked to AD, the functional role of these proteins has yet to be elucidated (Dewji and Singer, 1996). As the molecular basis of AD is not well understood and validated models are not available, the proof of principle for the involvement of many of these molecular approaches in AD will require potent, selective, and bioavailable compounds for examination in the clinical setting.

TRANSGENIC ANIMAL MODELS OF AD TO DEVELOP AND TEST NEW DRUGS

A number of groups have reported on the development of transgenic models of Alzheimer's disease over the last 5 years (Greenberg et al., 1996). The reports to date have focused on the histopathological changes in these animals and have been notable by the lack of behavioral data reported. Representative advances on the development of transgenic animal models of AD are summarized below.

Athena/Elan (Games et al., 1995) continues to provide evidence for the neuropathological hallmarks associated with a transgenic mouse overexpressing a mutant form of the β-amyloid precursor protein (βAPP 717V-F). At present there are several hundred homozygous and several thousand heterozygous transgenic mice. Region and age-dependent (3 vs. 12 months) changes in the development of amyloid plaques in the neocortex and hippocampus, vascular amyloidosis, astrocytosis, and microgliosis have been documented. Other features of Aβ plaques including apoE, cathepsin D, and proteoglycan immunoreactivity are particularly associated with the plaques in older mice (12 months). Additionally, altered phosphorylation of cytoskeletal elements (i.e., tau and neurofilaments) are evident as are signs of apoptosis present in the aged mice. Although the mice have been said to be "behaviorally disturbed," no data are currently available for review (Hsiao et al., 1996). It is rumored that Athena has 50 nM compounds that block Aβ toxicity in vitro that serve as lead compounds to evaluate in vivo efficacy in this transgenic model.

Behavioral data are available for a second transgenic mouse overexpressing the 751 amino acid isoform of human β-APP (Moran et al., 1995, 1996), a model available to HMR/Scios. Behavioral data comparing "young" (5–6 months) and "old" (9–12 months) transgenic mice to similarly aged wild-type mice indicate no group differences in the string test or rotorod tests of muscle strength or motor coordination. In the water maze paradigm of spatial learning, hidden and visible platforms have been used to show significant deficits in acquisition of learning in both the young and old transgenic mice. In contrast, when the platform was visible, no significant deficits are observed. In a probe trial, significant deficits between the wild-type and 12-month transgenic mice are observed. Deficits in the 12-month group are also observed in an avoidance learning paradigm (Y maze task). Apart from a slight hypoactivity that was seen in both young and old transgenic mice over a 24-hour period, there are no group differences seen in tests of behavioral despair or anxiety. At present the correlation between the cognitive deficits and histopathology remains unclear.

Hsiao et al. (1996) have recently described a transgenic mouse model overexpressing APP$_{695}$ (βAPP 670K-N, 671M-L) that showed behavioral impairment at 9–10 months of age which was associated with 5–14 fold increases in Aβ production and Aβ plaque formation.

To date, the utility of these scientifically interesting genetic models of aberrant APP processing/expression for drug discovery efforts remains unproven. Preclinical proof of principle awaits the testing of compounds known to inhibit the aberrant processing of APP. Only after moving forward an effective compound into clinical evaluation will the hypothesis that Aβ plays an important link in the etiology and progression of the disease come to some level of resolution.

DIAGNOSTICS

Clinical diagnosis of AD is a critical issue in addressing the disease. It is still, to a major extent, exclusionary in nature, sometimes inaccurate, and often not useful until the disease process is considerably advanced (Cutler et al., 1994) when drug intervention may have limited, if any efficacy. Postmortem examination of brain tissue remains the most reliable diagnostic by definition where high densities of amyloid-containing neurofibrillary plaques and tau-protein-associated senile tangles represent a characteristic hallmark of AD (Siman and Greenberg, 1996; Schenk et al., 1995). Changes in the cerebrospinal fluid content of Aβ (Schenk et al., 1995), α-secretase amyloid precursor protein (α-sAPP; 30), tau (Arai et al., 1995; Lannfelt et al., 1995) and tau protein phosphorylation (Vigo-Pelfrey et al., 1995), AD associated protein (ADAP, Alz50), artificial neuron network positron tomography (Defiguieredo et al., 1995), brain amyloid deposits (Saito et al., 1995), and mitochondrial gene defects (Davis, in press) have all been reported as potential tools for AD diagnosis. There is, however, currently no accepted test for the disease (Kolata, 1996). Allelic variation of the housekeeping gene, apoE, affects the mean age of onset of AD but is not diagnostic for the disease (Tsirka et al., 1995; Strittmatter and Roses, 1996). The apoE4 allele is associated with an earlier onset for sporadic and late-onset FAD forms of AD. ApoE3 and apoE2 may have a potential protective role in delaying AD onset. Interestingly, apoE4-negative AD patients are more responsive to cholinergic palliative therapy than apoE4 carriers (Porier et al., 1995) and may support the suggestion that tacrine is only effective in a subpopulation of dementia patients (Davis, in press). The apoE approach to AD therapeutics developed by Roses and co-workers (Stittmaltz and Roses, 1996) has been licensed to GlaxoWellcome.

FUTURE TRENDS IN CLINICAL TRIALS

One facet of the approval of safer AChEase inhibitors will be the conduct of placebo-controlled clinical trials. Should such entities be widely established, the current patient population which is essentially drug naive in the context of palliative AD therapy, will soon be on an AChEase inhibitor that may require appropriately novel approaches to clinical trial design.

The utility of "the bridging study" as a means of overcoming the variability between normal elderly and AD populations in maximum tolerated doses (MTDs) and ultimately decreasing the time required to achieve the optimal dose for evaluating Phase II/III efficacy is becoming increasingly recognized (Cutler and Sramek, 1996). For example, the recent Phase II trials for xanomeline

(Lilly) indicated that the highest dose tested (75 mg tid) was the only dose show-ing superiority over placebo—a dose that would not have been investigated since healthy elderlies had a MTD of 50 mg tid, whereas AD patients had a MTD of 100 tid.

There are ongoing efforts to develop more sensitive instruments to evaluate clinically meaningful changes in cognitive function. In particular, data has been collected as part of the Alzheimer's Disease Cooperative Study (ADCS) and the Mt. Sinai AD Research Center indicating the limitations of the ADAS as a sensitive measure of every aspect of cognitive function affected by AD (Mohs et al., 1996). This is especially pronounced for mild and severe patients. Measures that showed high reliability and/or sensitivity are a letter cancellation test of vi-sual attention and a delayed recall memory test. Tests with poor reliability in-clude a test of facial recognition, praxis items from the Boston Diagnostic Apha-sia Exam, a maze completion test, and additional word list learning trials. The data support the addition of one or more attention/concentration items to the ADAS, a measure of delayed recall for studies of mild or at-risk subjects, and reinforced the view that AD treatment should focus primarily on cognitive symptoms.

Future AD trials will need to focus on evaluating the impact of primary preven-tion because of the substantial cost required for caring for AD patients (Thal, 1996). As a strategy to overcome the prohibitive costs of time (>5 years) and money of such trials, it has been suggested that an alternative strategy that targets individuals at risk for AD having mild cognitive impairment (MCI) be used. These individuals would be expected to convert at a rate of 15% per annum. Using this approach a 3-year study involving 500 subjects would allow sufficient individuals to develop di-agnosable AD for the detection of a 30% decrease in risk. Candidate compounds for such a trial include vitamin E, vitamin C, coenzyme Q, and the MAO-B-inhibitor, selegeline.

The globalization of effective AD therapies will require that consistent crite-ria be established to evaluate compounds that may slow down the progression of symptoms or modify the disease process (Gauthier et al., 1996). Although there is near global consensus of the value of Diagnostic and Statistical Manual of Mental Disorders, 4th edition (DSM-IV) and National Institute of Neurological and Communicative Diseases and Stroke—Alzheimer's Disease and Related Disorders Association (NINCDS—ADRDA) criteria for early-stage diagnosis, there is more divergence in establishing a trial design that can differentiate be-tween placebo and active treatment over 12–18 months. It has been suggested that the Clinical Dementia Rating (CDR) scale, and at least one domain-specific measure related to cognition, activities of daily living, or behavior be a minimal requirement. Alternatively, trials could be conducted starting at a given disease stage and a longer follow-up would continue until critical end points were reached, such as loss of skills in instrumental tasks, in self-care activities, or need for institutionalization. As a means to establish whether a treatment causes an irreversible stabilization effect, trials containing a blind 6-month washout would be required. Finally, with the probable advent of multiple drugs having the same mechanism of action, it may be necessary to also evaluate the pharmacoeconomic impact of the treatment.

SUMMARY AND HORIZONS

Research into the causative factors of AD and related neurodegenerative diseases continues at an ever-increasing rate with considerable focus on the genetics (Schellenberg, 1995) and genomics of the disease, the latter benefiting from the considerable body of data existing for gene function in *Caenorhabditis elegans* (Schellenberg, 1995; Levitan and Greenwald, 1995).

The etiology of AD remains unknown, although there is considerable evidence linking various genetic mutations associated with chromosomes 1, 14, 19, and 21 (Schellenberg, 1995). Cognitive decline due to nerve cell death appears to be an inevitable part of the aging process, with the age of onset and degree of severity of the disease and associated neuronal loss being affected by genetic predisposition and environmental insult. Thus, AD may be a disease reflecting on acceleration of the aging process. Environmental insults may be a factorial reflection of the accumulated results of the assorted brain traumas associated with physical, chemical, and/or viral insults (Levy-Lahad et al., 1995). Accordingly, the increased life expectancy in the technologically advanced nations due to improved health care may be anticipated to increase the occurrence of AD, related dementias, and neurological disorders.

Research in the area of AD therapy has been focused in large pharmaceutical companies on cholinergic replacement therapy with little success in the past 15–20 years. It has been noted (Williams, 1993) that the approval of tacrine was due more to persistence than the efficacy of the compound. Preclinical research has been hampered by the inadequacy of the available animal models, the cost and unpredictability of clinical trials, and the lack of any useful diagnostic procedure. The recent reports (Greenberg et al., 1996) of transgenic animals overexpressing Aβ that show the histological and some of the behavioral hallmarks of AD may be a promising advance, although the proprietary nature of these models limits their widespread use. A caveat of these models is that there is an *a priori* assumption that Aβ is THE cause of AD. While there is suggestive evidence to this effect, no conclusive data exists. Overproduction of Aβ may simply follow cellular dysfunction. Thus compounds showing efficacy in any of the various transgenic models will need clinical testing to provide proof of principle that Aβ is the causative factor in the human situation. The various hurdles to preclinical and clinical research in the area of AD therapeutics hae been addressed in the thoughtful review of Greenberg and Murphy (1994).

As the shape and focus of the major pharmaceutical companies has changed as the result of health care reform and competitive issues (Williams and Reed, 1997), it is likely that the several biotech companies focused on CNS disease opportunities will continue to be a major force in driving research in this area. Athena Neurosciences (with Lilly), Scios (with HMR), Cephalon (with Schering-Plough), SIBIA

Neurosciences (with BMS), NeuroSearch, Cortex, Darwin, Mitokor, Sequana, Neurocrine (with Lilly), and Gliatech (with Janssen) are companies specifically focusing on AD therapeutics or diagnosis while companies like Idun (with Novartis) are focusing on basic mechanisms of apoptosis that may also be anticipated to advance the area beyond palliative, symptomatic approaches.

Ultimately, clinical designs over the next decade that address scientific, medical, and regulatory aims will be paramount in demonstrating a product has some beneficial effect on the signs and symptoms or course of dementia, and enable the drafting of reliable and useful instructions to guide clinicians in the safe use of drugs for the treatment of Alzheimer's disease (Leber, 1996).

A report from the most recent meeting on Alzheimer's disease in Osaka (Kolata, 1996) has put a realistic spin on the escalating hyperbole related to Alzheimer's disease research, noting that scientists in the area "confess that much of what may seem to the public to be breakthroughs is instead science in progress . . ." With this in mind, it is important that the hypotheses related to Alzheimer's disease etiology be treated as such rather than as starting points for the invocation of ever more fanciful and intricate intracellular signal transduction pathways for Aβ when the initial events of amyloid neurotoxicity are so poorly characterized and understood. This will then provide a more realistic basis for developing the sorely needed diagnostic tests that are crucial to a successful clinical development program.

Note: E2020 (donepezil, Aricept) received approval from the FDA on 11/26/96 for the treatment of Alzheimer's disease. This is the second agent approved in the United States.

REFERENCES

Arai H, Terajimia M, Miura M, Higuchi S, Muramatsu T, Machida N, Seiki H, Takase S, Clark CM, Lee VM-Y, Trojanowski JQ, Saski H (1995): Tau in cerebrospinal fluid: A potential diagnostic marker in Alzheimer's disease. Ann Neurol 38:649–652.

Americ SP, Bannon AW, Briggs CA, Brioni JD, Buccafusco JJ, Decker MW, Gopalakrishnan M, Holladay MW, Kyncl J, Lin NH, Marsh KG, Qiu YU, Radek R, Donnelly-Roberts DL, Sullivan JP and Williams M (1996a): ABT-089: An orally active cholinergic channel modulator (ChCM) with cognition enhancing and neuroprotective activity. Fourth Int. Springfield Symp. on Adv. in Alzheimer's Disease, Nice France, April 10–14, p 69.

Americ SP, Holladay MW, Sullivan JP (1996b): Cholinergic channel modulators as a novel therapeutic strategy for Alzheimer's disease. Exp Opin Invest Drugs 5:79–100.

Americ SP, Sullivan JP, Williams M (1995a): Neuronal nicotinic acetylcholine receptors. Targets for new therapeutic agents. In "Psychopharmacology, the Fourth Generation of Progress." Bloom FE, Kupfer DJ (eds): New York: Raven pp 94–110.

Americ SP, Sullivan JP, Briggs CA, Donnelly-Roberts D, Decker MW, Brioni JD, Marsh KC, Rodrigues AD (1995b): Preclinical pharmacology of ABT-418: A prototypical cholinergic channel activator for the potential treatment of Alzheimer's disease. CNS Drug Rev 1:1–26.

Artavanis-Tsakonas S, Matsuno K, Fortini M (1995) Notch signaling. Science 268:225–268.

Baudy RB (1996): Agents for the treatment of neurodegenerative diseases. Part 6. Curr Opin Ther Patents 3:313–343.

Baudy RB (1995a): Agents for the treatment of neurodegenerative diseases. Part 5. Curr Opin Ther Patents 5:1027–1059.

Baudy RB (1995b): Agents for the treatment of neurodegenerative diseases. Part 4. Curr Opin Ther Patents 5:1173–1206.

Baudy RB (1995c): Agents for the treatment of neurodegenerative diseases. Part 3. Curr Opin Ther Patents 4:343–378.

Baudy RB (1994): Agents for the treatment of neurodegenerative diseases. Part 2. Curr Opin Ther Patents 4:343–378.

Baudy RB (1993): Agents for the treatment of neurodegenerative diseases. Part 1. Curr Opin Ther Patents 3:1763–1786.

Behan DP, Heinrichs SC, Troncoso JC, Liu X-J, Kawas CH, Ling N, De Souza EB (1995): Displacement of corticotrophin releasing factor from its binding protein as a possible treatment for Alzheimer's disease. Nature 378:284–287.

Coyle JT Price DI, Delong MR (1983): Alzheimer's disease: A disorder of cholinergic innervation. Science 219:1184–1190.

Cutler NR, Sramek JJ (1996): The bridging study: Optimizing the dose for phase II/III. Fourth Int. Springfield Symp. on Adv. in Alzheimer's Disease, Nice France, April 10–14, p 88.

Cutler NR, Sramke JJ, Veroff AE (1994): "Alzheimer's Disease. Optimizing Drug Development Strategies." Chichester, UK: Wiley, pp 38–39.

Davies AM (1995): The bcl-2 family of proteins, and the regulation of neuronal survival. Trends Neurosci 18:355–358.

Davis RE, Miller S, Herrnstadt C, Ghosh SS, Fahy E, Shinobu L, Galasko D, Thal LJ, Beal MF, Howell N, Parker Jr, WD (1996): Mutations in mitochondrial cytochrome C oxidase genes segregate with late-onset Alzheimer's disease. Proc Natl Acad Sci U S A 93, (in press).

Defiguieredo RJP, Shankle WR, Maccato A, Dick MB, Mundkur P, Mena I, Cotman CW (1995): Neural-network-based classification of cognitively normal, demented, Alzheimer disease and vascular dementia from single photon emission with computed tomography image data from brain. Proc Natl Acad Sci U S A 92:5530–5534.

Dewji NN, Singer SJ (1996): Genetic clues to Alzheimer's disease, Science 271:159–160.

Eikelenboom P, Zhan S-S, Van Gool WA, Allsop D. (1994): Inflammatory mechanisms in Alzheimer's disease. Trends Pharmacol Sci 15:447–450.

Games D, Adams D, Alessandrini R, Barbour R, Berthelette P, Blackwell C, Carr T, Celmens J, Donaldson T, Gillespie F, Guido T, Hagpian S, Johnson, Wood K, Khan K, Lee M, Liebowitz P, Lieberberg I, Little S, Masliah E, Mcconologue L, Montoya-Zavala M, Mucke L, Paganini L, Penniman E (1995): Alzheimer-type neuropathology in transgenic mice overexpressing v717f β-amyloid precursor protein. Nature, 373:523–527.

Gash DM, Zhang Z, Ovadia A, Cass WA, Yi A, Simmerman L, Russell D, Martin D, Lapcheck PA, Collins F, Hoffer BJ, Gerhardt GA (1996): Functional recovery in parkinsonian monkeys treated with GDNF. Nature 380:252–255.

Gauthier S, Gray J, Poirier J (1996): Effects on decline or deterioration. Fourth Int. Springfield Symp. on Adv. in Alzheimer's Disease, Nice France, April 10–14, p 87.

Gracon S, Knopman D, Schneider L, Davis K, Smith F (1996): Long term tacrine treatment: Nursing home placement and mortality. Fourth Int. Springfield Symp. on Adv. in Alzheimer's Disease, Nice France, April 10–14, p 53.

Greenberg BD, Murphy MF (1994): Toward an integrated discovery and development program in Alzheimer's disease: The amyloid hypothesis. Neurobiol Aging 15 (Supp 2):S105–S109.

Greenberg BD, Savage MJ, Howland DS, Ali SM, Siedlak SL, Perry G, Siman R, Scott RW (1996): APP trangenesis: Approaches toward the development of animal models for Alzheimer's disease neuropathology. Neurobiol Aging 17:153–172.

Hsiao K, Chapman P, Nilsen S, Eckman C, Harigaya Y, Younkin S, Yang F, Cole G (1996): Correlative memory deficits, Aβ elevation, and amyloid plaques in transgenic mice. Science 274:99–102.

Huber G, Martin JR, Bailly Y, Mariani J, Brugg B (1996): β-Amyloid precursor protein— role in cognitive brain function? Fourth Int. Springfield Symp. on Adv. in Alzheimer's Disease, Nice France, April 10–14, p 47.

Kolata G (1996): Hopes are rosy on Alzheimer's, but results slim. New York Times Midwest Edition, Science Times, July 30, 1996, B5/B6.

Lannfelt L, Basun H, Wahlund L-O, Rowe BA, Wagner S (1995): Decreased α-secretase cleaved amyoid precursor protein as diagnostic marker for Alzheimer's disease. Nature Med 1:829–832.

Leber P (1996): U.S. Regulatory approaches to the evaluation of anti-dementia drug products. Fourth Int. Springfield Symp. on Adv. in Alzheimer's Disease, Nice France, April 10–14, p 97.

Levitan D, Greenwald I (1995): Facilitation of lin-12-mediated signalling by sel-12, a Caenorhabditis elegans S182 Alzheimer's disease gene. Nature 377:351–354.

Levy-Lahad E, Wasco W, Poorkaj P, Romano DM, Oshima J, Pettingell WH, Yu C-E, Jondro PD, Schmidt SD, Wang K, Crowley AC, Fu Y-H, Guenette SY, Galas D, Nemens E, Wijsman EM, Bird TD, Schelleneberg GD, Tanzi RE (1995): Candidate gene for the chromosome 1 familial Alzheimer's disease locus. Science 269:973–977.

Lippiello PM, Bencherf M, Caldwell WS, Arrington S, Fowler K, Louvett ME, Reeves L (1996): RJR-2403: A CNS selective nicotinic agonist with therapeutic potential. Fourth Int. Springfield Symp. on Adv. in Alzheimer's Disease, Nice France, April 10–14, p 68.

Loudon J, Clark M, Brown F, Bromidge S, Harries M, Hawkins J, Hatcher J, Noy G, Riley G (1996): SB 202026: A muscarinic partial agonist with functional selectivity. Fourth Int. Springfield Symp. on Adv. in Alzheimer's Disase, Nice France, April 10–14, p 158.

Lloyd GK, Rao TS, Sacaan A, Reid RT, Correa LD, Whelan K, Risbrough V, Menzaghi FM (1995): SIB-1765F, a novel nicotinic agonist: profile in models of extrapyramidal motor function. Soc Neurosci Abtr 21:11.10.

Ma J, Yee A, Brewer Jr HB, Das S, Potter H (1994): Amyloid-associated proteins α1-antichymotrypsin and apolipoprotein e promote assembly of Alzheimer β-protein into filaments. Nature 372:92–94.

Meyer EM, De Fiebre CM, Hunter BE, Simplins CE, Frauworth N, De Fiebre NEC (1994): Effects of anabaseine-related analogs on rat brain nicotinic receptor binding and on avoidance behaviors. Drug Develop Res 31:127–134.

Mohs R, Marin D, Green C, Knopman D, Petersen R, Ferris S, Thal L, Davis K (1996): Revisions in the Alzheimer's disease assessment scale (ADAS). Fourth Int. Springfield Symp. on Adv. in Alzheimer's Disease, Nice France, April 10–14, p. 89.

Moran P, Higgins L, Cordell B, Moser P (1996): B-APP751 Transgenic mice: Deficits in learning and memory. Fourth Int. Springfield Symp. on Adv. in Alzheimer's Disease, Nice France, April 10–14, p 29.

Moran PM, Higgins LS, Cordell B, Moser PC (1995): Age-related learning deficits in transgenic mice expressing the 751-amino acid isoform of human β-amyloid precursor protein. Proc Natl Acad Sci U S A 92:5341–5345.

Newhouse PA, Sunderland T, Tariot P, Blumhardt CL, Weingartner H, Mellow A (1988): Intravenous nicotine in Alzheimer's disease: A pilot study. Psychopharmacology 95:171–175.

Newhouse PA, Potter A, Corwin J (1996): Acute administration of the cholinergic channel activator ABT-418 improves learning in Alzheimer's disease. Society for Research on Nicotine and Tobacco, March 16, Washington, D.C. Abstract A39.

Nicholson DW, Ali A, Thornberry NA, Vaillancourt JP, Ding CK, Gallant M, Gareau Y, Griffin PR, Labelle M, Lazebnik YA, Munday NA, Raju SM, Smulson ME, Yamin T-T, Lu VI, Miller DK (1995): Identification and inhibition of the ICE/ced-3 protease necessary for mammalian apoptosis. Nature 376:37–43.

Parker WD, Filley CF, Parks JK (1990): Cytochrome oxidase deficiency in Alzheimer's disease. Neurology 40:1302–1303.

Porier J, Delisle M-C, Quirion R, Aubert I, Farlow M, Lahari S, Hui S, Bertrand P, Nalbantoglu J, Gilfix BG, Gauthier S (1995): Apoprotein e4 allele as a predictor of cholinergic deficits and treatment of outcome in Alzheimer's disease. Proc Natl Acad Sci U S A 92:10227–10231.

Roch JM, Puttfarcken P (in press): Biological actions of the Aβ amyloid protein and precursor. Curr Drugs.

Rothwell NJ, Hopkins SJ (1995): Cytokines and the nervous system ii. Actions and mechanisms of action. Trends Neurosci 18:130–136.

Rudolphi K (1996): Propentophylline (HWA 285)—Preclinical data. Fourth Int. Springfield Symp. on Adv. in Alzheimer's Disease, Nice France, April 10–14, p 82.

Sahakian BJ, Coull JT (1994): Nicotine and tetrahydroaminoacridine: evidence for improved attention in patients with dementia of the Alzheimer type. Drug Dev Res 31:80–88.

Saito Y, Buciak J, Yang J, Pardridge WM (1995): Vector-mediated delivery of ^{125}I-labeled β-amyloid peptide $A\beta_{1-40}$ through the blood brain barrier and binding to Alzheimer disease amyloid of the $A\beta_{1-40}$/vector complex. Proc Natl Acad Sci U S A 92:10227–10231.

Schellenberg GD (1995): Genetic dissection of Alzheimer disease, a heterogenous disorder. Proc Natl Acad Sci U S A 92:8552–8559.

Schenk DB, Rydel RE, May P, Little S, Panetta J, Lieberberg I, Sinha S (1995): Therapeutic approaches related to amyloid-β peptide and alzheimer's disease. J Med Chem 38:4141–4154.

Selkoe DJ (1993): Physiological production of the β-amyloid protein and the mechanism of Alzheimer's disease. Trends Neurol Sci 16:403–409.

Sherrington R, Rogaev EL, Liang Y, Rogaeva EA, Levesque G, Ikeda M, Chi H, Lin C, Li G, Holman K, Tsuda T, Mar L, Foncin J-F, Bruni AC, Montesi MP, Sorbi S, Rainero I, Pinessi L, Nee L, Chumakov I, Pollen D, Brookes A, Sanseau P, Polinsky RJ, Wasco W, Da Silva Har, Haines JL, Pericak-Vance MA, Tanzi RE, Roses AD, Fraser PE, Rommens JM, St George-Hyslop PH (1995): Cloning of a gene bearing missense mutations in early-onset familial alzheimer's disease. Nature 375:754–760.

Shinoda I, Furukawa Y, Furukawa S (1990): Stimulation of nerve growth factor synthesis secretion by propentofylline in cultured mouse astroglial cells. Biochem Pharmacol 39:1813–1816.

Siman R, Greenberg BD (1996): Alzheimer's disease. In "Neurotherapeutics: Emerging Strategies" Pullan L, Patel J (eds): Totowa, NJ: Humana, pp 389–428.

Strittmatter WJ, Roses AD, (1996): Apolipoprotein E and Alzheimer's disease. Ann Rev Neurosci 19:53–77.

Thal LJ (1996): Trials to prevent Alzheimer's disease in a population at risk. Fourth Int. Springfield Symp. on Adv. in Alzheimer's Disease, Nice France, April 10–14, p 86.

Thompson CB (1995): Apoptosis in the pathogenesis and treatment of disease. Science, 267:1456–1462.

Tsirka SE, Gualandris A, Amaral DG, Strickland S (1995): Excitotoxin-induced neuronal degeneration and seizure are mediated by tissue plasma activator. Nature 377:340–344.

Vigo-Pelfrey C, Seubert P, Barbour R, Blomquist C, Lee M, Lee D, Coria F, Chang L, Miller B, Lieberberg I, Schenk D (1995): Elevation of microtubule-associated protein tau in the cerebrospinal fluid of patients with Alzheimer's disease, Neurol 45:788–793.

Williams M (1993): Tacrine—recommendation for approval. Curr Opin Invest New Drugs 2: 541–544.

Williams M, Shiosaki K, Puttfarcken P (1995): Amyloid β peptide in Alzheimer's disease pathology: towards a rational basis for drug discovery? Exp Opin Invest Drugs. 4: 263–270.

Williams M and Davis RE (1996): Alzheimer's disease and related dementias: Prospects for Treatment. Fitzgerald JD, Bowman WC, Taylor JB (eds): In "Emerging Drugs: The Prospects for Improved Medicines." London: Ashley, pp 137–166.

Williams M and Reed R (1997): The pharmaceutical industry in the 21st century. Williams M, McAfee DA (eds): In "Pharmaceutical Research and Development: Applied Biomedical Research in the Drug Discovery Process." New York: Wiley, in press.

Yamaguchi F, Richards SJ, Beyreuther K, Salbaum M, Carlson GA, Dunnett SA. (1991): Transgenic mice for the amyloid precursor protein 695 isoform have impaired spatial memory. Neuroreports 2:781–784.

DATE DUE